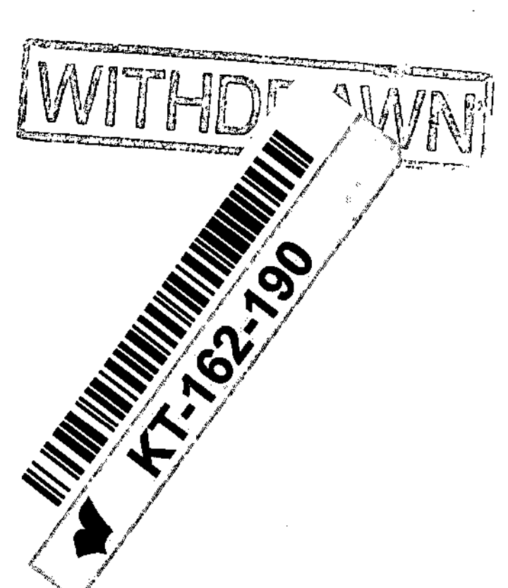
WITHDRAWN
KT-162-190

NAPIER UNIVERSITY LIS

PRIMARY CARE OF THE PREMATURE INFANT

PRIMARY CARE OF THE PREMATURE INFANT

Dara Brodsky, MD

Department of Neonatology
Beth Israel Deaconess Medical Center;
Department of Pediatrics
Harvard Medical School
Boston, MA

&

Mary Ann Ouellette, MS, APRN, IBCLC

Pediatric Nurse Practitioner
Beth Israel Deaconess Medical Center
Boston, MA;
Westwood-Mansfield Pediatric Associates
Westwood/Mansfield, MA

SAUNDERS

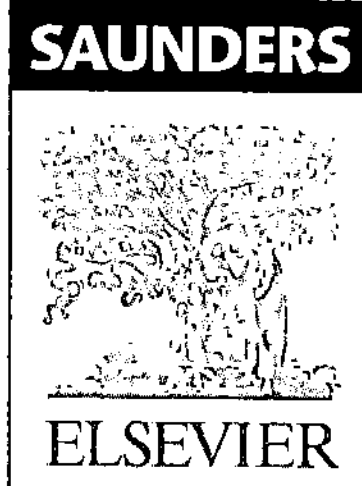

SAUNDERS
ELSEVIER

1600 John F. Kennedy Boulevard
Suite 1800
Philladelphia, PA 19103-2899

PRIMARY CARE OF THE PREMATURE INFANT
ISBN-13: 978-1-4160-0039-6

Notice

Knowledge and best practice in this field are constantly changing. As new research and experience broaden our knowledge, changes in practice, treatment and drug therapy may become necessary or appropriate. Readers are advised to check the most current information provided (i) on procedures featured or (ii) by the manufacturer of each product to be administered, to verify the recommended dose or formula, the method and duration of administration, and contraindications. It is the responsibility of the practitioner, relying on their own experience and knowledge of the patient, to make diagnoses, to determine dosages and the best treatment for each individual patient, and to take all appropriate safety precautions. To the fullest extent of the law, neither the Publisher nor the Editors assume any liability for any injury and/or damage to persons or property arising out of or related to any use of the material contained in this book.

The Publisher

Library of Congress Cataloging-in-Publication Data
Primary care of the premature infant / [edited by] Dara Brodsky, Mary Ann Ouellette. — 1st ed.
p.; cm.
Includes bibliographical references.
ISBN-13: 978-1-4160-0039-6
ISBN-10: 1-4160-0039-9
1. Premature infants—Medical care. 2. Primary care (Medicine) I. Brodsky, Dara. II. Ouellette, Mary Ann.
[DNLM: 1. Infant, Premature. 2. Infant Care. 3. Infant, Premature, Diseases. 4. Primary Health Care. WS 410 P952 2008]

RJ250.P75 2008
618.92'011—dc22
2006036045

Acquisitions Editor: Rebecca Gaertner
Editorial Assistants: Suzanne Flint, Liz Hart
Project Manager: Bryan Hayward
Design Direction: Ellen Zanolle

Printed in the United States of America

Last digit is the print number: 9 8 7 6 5 4 3 2 1

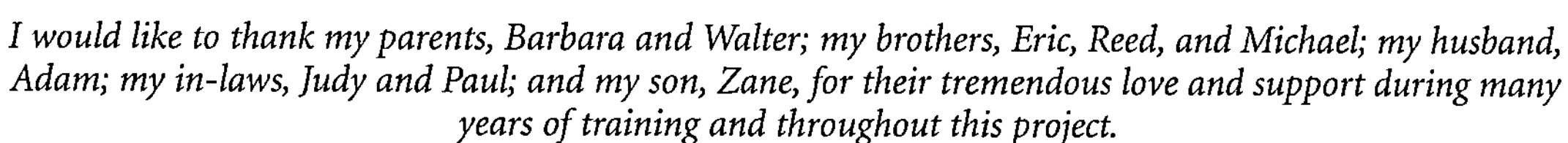

I would like to thank my parents, Barbara and Walter; my brothers, Eric, Reed, and Michael; my husband, Adam; my in-laws, Judy and Paul; and my son, Zane, for their tremendous love and support during many years of training and throughout this project.

Dara Brodsky, MD

I dedicate this book to my husband Mike and daughter Catherine for their unconditional love, patient understanding, and endless support that made this all possible. I would like to thank my parents Michael and Rita Fahey, my sister Ruth, and my four brothers for their boundless faith and trust in my abilities, as well as all the children, their families, friends, and colleagues, especially at Westwood-Mansfield Pediatrics, who encouraged me to undertake this project.

Mary Ann Ouellette, MS, APRN, IBCLC

Five percent of the authors' proceeds will be donated to the March of Dimes in support of their mission to improve the health of babies by preventing birth defects, premature birth, and infant mortality.

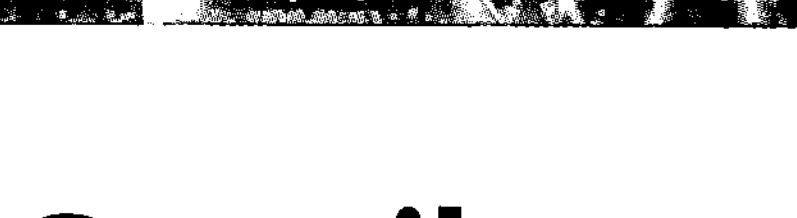

Contributors

We would like to acknowledge the following people for their invaluable contributions to this book.

Pankaj B. Agrawal, MD, MMSc
Division of Newborn Medicine
Children's Hospital, Boston, MA
Harvard Medical School

Yvette Blanchard, ScD, PT
University of Hartford, West Hartford, CT
Brazelton Institute, Children's Hospital,
Boston, MA

Mandy Brown Belfort, MD, MPH
Division of Newborn Medicine
Children's Hospital, Boston, MA
Harvard Medical School

Rosalind S. Brown, MD
Division of Endocrinology
Children's Hospital, Boston, MA
Harvard Medical School

Rosanne K. Buck, RNC, MS, NNP
Department of Neonatology
Beth Israel Deaconess Medical Center,
Boston, MA

Oguz Cataltepe, MD
Director of Pediatric Neurosurgery
Division of Neurosurgery
University of Massachusetts,
Worcester, MA

Sule Cataltepe, MD
Department of Newborn Medicine
Brigham & Women's Hospital, Boston, MA
Harvard Medical School

Marcy Chant, AuD
Department of Neonatology
Beth Israel Deaconess Medical Center,
Boston, MA

Emily Jean Davidson, MD, MPH
Department of Medicine, Division
of General Pediatrics
Children's Hospital, Boston, MA
Harvard Medical School

Michele DeGrazia, RNC, PhD, NNP
Division of Newborn Medicine
Children's Hospital, Boston, MA

Ruben Diaz, MD, PhD
Division of Endocrinology
Children's Hospital, Boston, MA
Harvard Medical School
Chief, Division of Endocrinology
Hospital Sant Joan de Deu, Barcelona,
Spain

Elizabeth Doherty, MD
Division of Newborn Medicine
Winchester Hospital,
Winchester, MA; Children's Hospital,
Boston, MA
Harvard Medical School

Eric C. Eichenwald, MD
Medical Director, Newborn Center
Texas Children's Hospital, Houston, TX
Baylor College of Medicine

Deirdre M. Ellard, MS, RD/LDN, CNSD
Department of Nutrition
Brigham & Women's Hospital, Boston, MA

Jill S. Fischer, MD
Westwood-Mansfield Pediatric Associates, Westwood/Mansfield, MA
Pediatric Physicians Organization of Children's Hospital, Boston, MA

Munish Gupta, MD
Department of Neonatology
Beth Israel Deaconess Medical Center, Boston, MA
Harvard Medical School

Mary H. Horn, RN, MS, RRT
Surgical Clinical Nurse Specialist
Surgical Program
Children's Hospital, Boston, MA

Jennifer Hyde, MD
Westwood-Mansfield Pediatric Associates, Westwood/Mansfield, MA
Pediatric Physicians Organization of Children's Hospital, Boston, MA

Julie Iglesias, RN, MS, CPNP
Nurse Coordinator
Liver, Intestine & Multivisceral Transplant Center and Short Bowel Program
Children's Hospital, Boston, MA

Deborah S. Kerr, MSW, LICSW
Social Work/Case Management Department
South Shore Hospital
South Weymouth, MA 02190

Kimberly G. Lee, MD, MSc, IBCLC, FABM
Department of Pediatrics
Medical University of South Carolina, Charleston, SC

Kristen E. Lindamood, RNC, MS, NNP
Division of Newborn Medicine
Children's Hospital, Boston, MA

J.S. Lloyd, MD
Director of the Neonatal Intensive Care Unit
Department of Pediatrics
South Shore Hospital, Weymouth, MA
Affiliated with Children's Hospital, Boston, MA

Camilia R. Martin, MD, MS
Associate Director, Neonatal Intensive Care Unit, Beth Israel Deaconess Medical Center
Department of Neonatology
Beth Israel Deaconess Medical Center, Boston, MA
Harvard Medical School

Jack Maypole, MD
Director of Pediatrics, South End Community Health Center
Division of Developmental and Behavioral Pediatrics
Boston Medical Center, Boston
Boston University School of Medicine

Catherine Noonan, RN, MS, CPNP
Pediatric Nurse Practitioner
Children's Hospital, Boston, MA

J. Kevin Nugent, PhD
Director of the Brazelton Institute
Children's Hospital, Boston, MA
Harvard Medical School
University of Massachusetts at Amherst

Steven Parker, MD
Division of Developmental and Behavioral Pediatrics
Boston Medical Center, Boston
Boston University School of Medicine

Xianhua Piao, MD, PhD
Division of Newborn Medicine
Children's Hospital, Boston, MA
Harvard Medical School

Sandy Quigley, MS, CWOCN, CPNP
Clinical Specialist in Wound, Ostomy & Continence Care
Children's Hospital, Boston, MA

Mary Quinn, NNP, IBCLC
Neonatal Nurse Practitioner Coordinator
Department of Neonatology
Beth Israel Deaconess Medical Center, Boston, MA

Lawrence Rhein, MD
Director, Center for Healthy Infant Lung Development
Division of Newborn Medicine, Division of Respiratory Diseases
Children's Hospital, Boston, MA
Harvard Medical School

Steven A. Ringer, MD, PhD
Chief, Division of Newborn Medicine
Brigham & Women's Hospital, Boston, MA
Harvard Medical School

Vincent C. Smith, MD, MPH
Associate Director, Neonatal Intensive Care Unit, Beth Israel Deaconess Medical Center
Department of Neonatology
Beth Israel Deaconess Medical Center, Boston, MA
Harvard Medical School

Jane E. Stewart, MD
Director, Infant Follow-Up Program, Children's Hospital
Department of Neonatology
Beth Israel Deaconess Medical Center, Boston, MA
Harvard Medical School

John A.F. Zupancic, MD, ScD
Director, Harvard Neonatal Fellowship Program
Department of Neonatology
Beth Israel Deaconess Medical Center, Boston, MA
Harvard Medical School

Contents

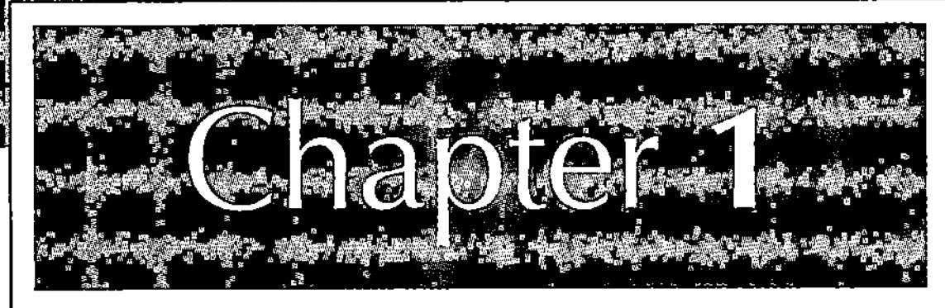

Introduction: Transition of the Premature Infant from Hospital to Home

Dara Brodsky, MD, and Mary Ann Ouellette, MS, APRN, IBCLC

In 1963, President John F. Kennedy's wife Jacqueline delivered an infant at 34 weeks' gestation. The President's child must have received the most advanced medical care but was unable to survive because of severe lung disease caused by surfactant deficiency. Today, medical technology has dramatically improved the survival rate of premature infants, and now almost 100% of infants born at 34 weeks' gestation survive.

At the same time that more premature infants are surviving, the rate of premature deliveries has increased to the point that almost 500,000 infants are born premature each year, accounting for ≈12% of all births in the United States.[1] A significant number of these premature infants are born between 34 and 37 weeks' gestation. This rise of premature births is partly attributable to a greater number of multiple pregnancies, which, in turn, is due to the increased number of older women who are interested in having children. Older women are more inclined to seek assisted reproductive methods that often result in multiple births, many of which are preterm. In fact, approximately half of twin pregnancies and nearly all pregnancies of triplets (or greater) lead to deliveries before 37 weeks' gestation. Other causes of prematurity include cervical incompetence, placental or uterine anomalies, trauma, advanced maternal illness, chorioamnionitis, and subclinical infection.[2,3] In spite of the increased understanding of the various factors leading to preterm deliveries, in most cases an etiology for the premature birth remains unknown.

Even though physicians cannot always identify the cause of premature delivery, medical advancements in obstetric and neonatal care have led to dramatically greater chances for survival of extremely premature infants. Infants born at 24 weeks' gestation currently have a survival rate of approximately 40% to 60%.[4] Unfortunately, the morbidities of these extremely premature infants have not decreased significantly. Indeed, gestational age at birth is inversely correlated with the chance that the infant will experience physical, developmental, and/or psychosocial sequelae.

Because of the increased number of premature deliveries and the greater number of extremely premature infants who are surviving, primary care providers are taking care of a growing population of former premature infants. Therefore it is critical that primary care providers understand the special difficulties facing these infants and their families. Depending on the infant's degree of prematurity and the number of complications the infant encounters in the neonatal intensive care unit (NICU), he or she is at risk for a wide variety of physical and developmental problems. Some of these medical problems may be identified in the NICU and require further monitoring for a significant period of time, whereas others may manifest clinically later in infancy or in childhood.[5] Thus the primary care provider should understand both how to follow problems that NICU clinicians have already identified and how to be attentive to new issues that may develop.

Discharge Planning

Before discharge from the NICU, the premature infant must demonstrate physiologic maturity by predefined criteria (Table 1-1). Whereas the premature

Table 1-1 Discharge of a Premature Infant from the Neonatal Intensive Care Unit

	Specific Topics	Comments
Discharge Criteria	Thermoregulation	Focus is on infant's ability to maintain a normal body temperature when infant is clothed in an open crib.
	No apnea or bradycardia of prematurity for a defined period	Number of hospital observational days that are spell free varies by unit.
	Exclusively taking oral feedings with adequate weight gain	There is no longer a specific weight requirement for discharge.
Discharge Teaching	Teach good handwashing and minimize exposure to crowded places	Instruct families to carry an antibacterial solution in case soap and water are not easily accessible.
	Infants must sleep on their backs	It is important to discuss with families of premature infants that although their infant might have been placed on their abdomen and/or side in the neonatal intensive care unit, infants were being monitored with a cardiorespiratory monitor at the time. After discharge, the American Academy of Pediatrics recommends that infants sleep on their backs to decrease the risk for sudden infant death syndrome.*
	When to call the primary care clinician	Instruct parents to contact their pediatric provider if the infant has any abdominal issues, breathing difficulties, feeding intolerance, fever, and/or decreased activity that could represent an illness.
	Medication administration	Parents should fill prescriptions before the infant leaves the hospital, and the family should be taught how to administer the medication(s).
	Caloric supplementation	Provide written instructions for formula/milk preparation.
Discharge Checklist	Car safety seat screening	This is usually assessed in all infants born <37 weeks' gestation (see Chapter 12B).
	Phone contact with primary care provider	In addition to phone contact, provide a written summary of the infant's medical course for the provider.
	Newborn hearing screening	Perform prior to discharge and, if needed, arrange for outpatient follow-up.
	Newborn state screening	Premature infants often have initial newborn screening results that are "out of range," requiring follow-up testing.
	Immunizations	In addition to routine immunizations, assess need for respiratory syncytial virus prophylaxis and determine whether caregivers should receive influenza vaccination.
	Cardiopulmonary resuscitation (CPR)	Ideally, all care providers should learn CPR.
Follow-up Appointments and/or Referrals	Primary care provider Referral to Early Intervention Program and/or Infant Follow-up Program If possible, visiting nurse Ophthalmologist Other consultant(s) as needed	Consider arranging postdischarge appointments at times that would decrease exposure to children with infections.
Discharge Paperwork to Families	Discharge summary (including infant's recent weight, length, and head circumference) Immunization record Growth curve List of medications and doses Appointments and contact numbers of consultants, including lactation consultant	If possible, supply the family with a copy of the infant's discharge summary in case the family needs to go to an emergency department.

*American Academy of Pediatrics Task Force on Sudden Infant Death Syndrome: *Pediatrics* 116(5):1245-1255, 2005; and Oyen N, Markestad T, Skaerven R, et al: *Pediatrics* 100(4):613-621, 1997.

infant usually meets these requirements at an approximate postmenstrual age (PMA) of 40 weeks, infants who are born closer to 24 weeks' gestation usually are discharged later, and infants born closer to 37 weeks' gestation often are discharged before 40 weeks' PMA. The premature infant is not required to attain a certain weight before being discharged to home; rather, the infant should demonstrate a sustained pattern of weight gain.

The infant's transition from the NICU to home should correspond with a shift in parental thinking from viewing their infant as receiving "illness care" to "primary care."[6] In addition to teaching families about this change, the NICU staff is responsible for discharge teaching, ensuring that specific tests are completed prior to discharge, developing a home care plan, and arranging for the appropriate follow-up appointments and/or referrals for surveillance and support services (Table 1-1). The NICU staff should provide families with a copy of the infant's discharge summary, immunization record, growth curve, medication list, and contact numbers.

Primary Care Provider Role

Primary care providers often are responsible for directly managing the "late preterm" infant, previously known as the "near-term" infant, in the newborn nursery. These infants are born between 34 and 36 6/7 weeks' gestation, which accounts for the majority of all singleton preterm births. This population of infants has a broad range of potential short-term morbidities, including respiratory distress, jaundice, feeding difficulties, hypoglycemia, temperature instability, and sepsis.[7] Although these infants may be admitted directly to the NICU, some may be admitted to the newborn nursery under the supervision of the primary care physician. Some infants in this latter group may develop complications and require subsequent transfer to the NICU for management of their medical issues. Those infants who are not transferred to the NICU and are discharged to home directly from the newborn nursery still have a higher rate of rehospitalization, within the first 2 weeks after discharge, than do full-term infants, mostly because of feeding difficulties and jaundice.[8] Table 1-2 provides guidelines for the primary care clinician in caring for these late preterm infants, both in the hospital and after discharge.

Because primary care providers are the principal clinicians for the premature infant and the infant's family, they are in a unique position to help families normalize their childbirth experience. Therefore it is important that clinicians provide continuity of care with an emphasis on a team approach. Indeed, the premature infant whose family uses a large pediatric practice might benefit from a core team of providers.

During the first office visit, the primary care provider should focus on the issues listed in Table 1-3.

Table 1-2 Guidelines for the Primary Care Provider Caring for the Late Preterm Infant

Newborn Nursery Care	Monitor for feeding difficulties, respiratory distress, jaundice (use different guidelines than full-term infant recommendations, as noted in Chapter 6B), temperature instability, hypoglycemia, and signs/symptoms of sepsis. Have lower threshold for supplementing breastfeeding and obtaining a lactation consultant who can continue to advise the mother after discharge (see Chapter 3B). Perform car safety seat screening. Determine whether infant meets current requirements for respiratory syncytial virus prophylaxis (see Chapter 2C). Routine newborn care: newborn state screening, hepatitis B vaccine, hearing screening. Educate family about differences between late preterm and full-term infants (see below).
Family Education*	• Feeding Late preterm infants usually eat less and may need to be fed more often. These infants have difficulty coordinating sucking, swallowing, and breathing during the feeding and thus may need to be observed closely while eating. Some late preterm infants may feed well initially while in the hospital and then become tired and feed poorly. Families should contact their primary care provider if the infant has decreased oral intake. Infants should have 5–6 wet diapers in every 24-hour period. • Sleeping Late preterm infants may be sleepier than full-term infants and sleep through feedings, in which case the family should awaken the infant to feed. All infants, including late preterm infants, should sleep on their backs.

*Guidelines modified from National Nurses' Association Announces Initiative to Improve Care of Near-Term Infants and Educate Parents, Nurses about Their Needs. Available at: *http://www.dentalplans.com/Dental-Health-Articles/What-the-Parents-of-Near-Term-Infants-Need-to-Know.asp.*

Continued

Table 1-2 Guidelines for the Primary Care Provider Caring for the Late Preterm Infant—cont'd

	• Temperature Regulation Late preterm infants have decreased subcutaneous fat and may have more difficulty regulating their body temperature than do full-term infants. If the environment is cool, late preterm infants should wear hats to decrease heat loss. Families should be aware of their primary care provider's protocol for assessing an infant's temperature. • Jaundice Late preterm infants are at greater risk for jaundice than are full-term infants, so families should be taught how to look for jaundice and about the need for close follow-up. • Infection Late preterm infants are at greater risk for developing infections than are full-term infants, so families should watch for signs of infection, such as fever, difficulty breathing, and/or lethargy. Families should minimize exposure of late preterm infants to crowded places. Families should practice good handwashing. • Car Safety Seat Minimize the amount of time late preterm infants are placed in car seats until the infants demonstrate they have achieved good head control.
Follow-up	Instruct family to schedule appointment within 1–2 days after discharge (infants who are breastfeeding exclusively should be evaluated, if possible, the day after discharge by a visiting nurse and/or primary care provider). At the first office visit, the primary care provider should: • Assess for dehydration with weight check and physical examination. • Evaluate for jaundice. • Arrange for continued close follow-up in the exclusively breastfeeding infant (see Chapter 3B). • See Table 1-3 for other aspects of care that might be applicable. Re-emphasize educational points noted above. Record the results of the newborn screening test.

Table 1-3 Initial Visit with Primary Care Provider

History	Review prenatal information (pregnancy history, maternal medications during pregnancy). Review postnatal information (gestational age, birth weight, head circumference and length at birth, delivery course, hospital course). Document discharge weight, head circumference, and length.
Feeding Issues	Note amount of milk per feeding and per day. Discuss length of time of feedings. Document caloric content of milk and type of milk.
Medications	Note name(s) of medications (trade and generic). Emphasize dosage, method of administration, and frequency. Discuss indications for PRN medications. Discuss protocol if dose is omitted or if dose is repeated. Discuss potential side effects. Discuss storage. Confirm that the family is comfortable administering medications.
Other Questions for the Family	Discuss infant's sleeping patterns. Address any other parental concerns.
Physical Examination	Chart weight, head circumference, and length (refer to growth curves in Chapter 3A); chart by chronological and corrected gestational age.
Documentation (see Table 1-4)	Review and assemble the following documents: Discharge summary Immunization record Growth curve in the hospital Newborn screening test results Hearing screen results Recent laboratory data (including hematocrit and reticulocyte count, recent electrolyte levels if infant is receiving diuretics, recent alkaline phosphatase level) Cranial ultrasound results Ophthalmologic examination results Echocardiogram results, if applicable List of home equipment, if applicable Confirm that cardiopulmonary resuscitation (CPR) was taught to all care providers. Document names, appointment dates, and contact numbers of other consultants.

Table 1-3 Initial Visit with Primary Care Provider—cont'd

Assessment	If infant meets state criteria for Early Intervention, a referral should be made. Determine if an Infant Follow-Up Program is needed (if so, make a referral if not already done). Assess need for other community services (e.g., visiting nurse, physical therapy). In addition to routine immunizations, assess need and timing of respiratory syncytial virus prophylaxis and determine whether caregivers should receive influenza vaccination. Determine when the family needs to schedule next ophthalmologic examination. Determine if the family requires written documentation for insurance support (e.g., specialized prescribed formulas, nonformulary medications). Assess psychosocial and support needs. Assess financial support needs (see Chapter 13, "Resources for Clinicians and Families").
Education	Discuss with family that although their infant might have been placed on the abdomen and/or side in the neonatal intensive care unit, infants were being monitored with a cardiorespiratory monitor at the time. After discharge, the American Academy of Pediatrics recommends that infants sleep on their backs to decrease the risk for sudden infant death syndrome.* Review good handwashing technique. Review when to call the primary care clinician. Recommend that families schedule future visits at times that would decrease exposure to children with infections. Discuss with families their need to maintain a low threshold for calling the primary care provider. Suggest to families with an infant who had a prolonged NICU course that they carry a copy of the discharge summary with them and that they provide a copy to any day care provider. Suggest to families with infants who are being discharged home on oxygen that they should contact the local fire and police departments to alert those services that their infant is receiving oxygen. Suggest to families with infants who have special needs that they should contact the local utility companies of the need for uninterrupted electrical and phone service.

*American Academy of Pediatrics Task Force on Sudden Infant Death Syndrome. *Pediatrics* 116(5):1245-1255, 2005; and Oyen N, Markestad T, Skaerven R, et al: *Pediatrics* 100(4):613-621, 1997.
NICU, Neonatal intensive care unit.

Primary care providers should summarize the infant's hospital course, similar to the sample provided in Table 1-4, to be able to quickly access this information at future visits. The provider should encourage families to schedule appointments at times that would decrease the chance of exposure to sick children and similarly should advise families to minimize the infant's exposure to people with respiratory illnesses. The primary care provider might recommend that an infant have more than one slotted appointment time if that infant has multiple complicated medical issues. Because premature infants are at increased risk for rehospitalization during the first few years of life, primary care providers should encourage families to take atypical behavior seriously and contact the office immediately if they are concerned. The primary care provider should continue to schedule frequent follow-up visits to assess for adequate weight gain, particularly in the smallest infants, during the weeks immediately after discharge.[9]

Throughout the rest of the infant's clinical care, primary care providers should prioritize the following responsibilities (outlined in Table 1-5)[10]:

1. Manage complications of prematurity;
2. Monitor for potential new problems;
3. Support the family;
4. Coordinate various medical and social services needed;
5. Educate the family by providing anticipatory guidance and list of resources.

A Resource for Pediatric Primary Care Providers

We have designed this book to be a resource for primary care providers who are caring for premature infants. Throughout this book we have used standard terminology (Table 1-6) to describe premature infants. The chapters in this book discuss the most common medical complications facing premature

Table 1-4 Sample Documentation of the Hospital Course of a Premature Infant

Infant Name ______________ **Infant's Last Name in Hospital, if Different** ______________
Gestational Age ______________ **EDC** ________ **Date of Birth** ______________

Birth Information:
Birth hospital __________ Delivery mode ______ Vacuum/Forceps (circle if applicable)
Apgar score ____(1 min) _____ (5 min) ____ (10 min) Chest compressions and/or epi required: Yes No
Birth measurements and percentiles: Weight ________ Length ________ HC ________
Relevant maternal information (e.g., maternal medications): ______________

Hospital Course: NICU hospital __________ Date of discharge ________
Respiratory: *Intubated:* Yes No *RDS/Surfactant:* Yes No *Date extubated:* ______
Date off CPAP: _____ *BPD:* Yes No *Date off oxygen:* _____ *Baseline blood gas:* ______
Postnatal steroids: Yes No *Apnea:* Yes No *Caffeine:* Yes No *Date discontinued caffeine:* ______
Nutrition: *Calories & amount/type of oral intake at discharge:* ______________ *Copy of growth curve:* Yes No
Recent growth (dates & centiles): Weight ____ *Length* _____ *HC* ______
Gastro: *Reflux:* Yes No *Oral aversion:* Yes No *Constipation:* Yes No
NEC: Yes No *Surgery:* Yes No *Ostomy:* Yes No
Current need for enteral tube: Yes No *Cholestasis:* Yes No
Neurology: *HUS results:* __________ *Gestational age of most recent HUS:* ______________
Hematology: *Anemia:* Yes No *Lowest Hct:* _____ *Phototherapy:* Yes No *Date of last blood transfusion:* ____
Cardiology: *Echo results:* ______ *Indocin:* Yes No *Murmur:* Yes No *Surgical ligation of PDA:* Yes No
Endocrine: *Osteopenia of prematurity:* Yes No *Hypothyroidism:* Yes No
Ophthal: *ROP:* Yes No *Surgery:* Yes No *Retina mature:* Yes No
Surgical: *Cryptorchidism:* Yes No *Inguinal hernia:* Yes No
Infections: ______________ **Other Issues:** ______________
Recent Labs, Date: Hgb/Hct _____ Retic ____ Lytes _____ AlkP______ Ca/P _____ I/D bilirubin _____ Other____

Discharge Information: Received discharge summary: Yes No
Medications: ______________
Home equipment: ______________
Car safety seat results: __________
Hearing screen results: ________ Referral made? Yes No If yes, date of appointment ______________
Newborn state screen results: __________ (Attach official report from state lab) Follow-up needed: Yes No
Immunizations received and dates: ______________
Candidate for RSV immunoprophylaxis: Yes No If candidate, did infant receive first dose? Yes No Date of next dose: _____
Family taught CPR: Yes No If not taught, recommend CPR ______________
EI candidate: Yes No If candidate, referral made: Yes No If Yes, name of EI program: ______________
IFUP available and candidate: Yes No If Yes, date of appointment: ______________
Names & phone numbers of all consultants with next recommended appointment:
Pulmonary: ______________ Ophthalmologist: ______________
Surgery: ______________ Lactation consultant: ______________
Visiting Nurse: __________ Nutritionist: __________ Other: ______________

Other Follow-up Needed (circle all that apply): Further imaging (HUS and/or MRI and other________)
Hearing screen (all infants born ≤32 weeks' gestation should be retested at ≈12 months' chronological age)
Ophthalmologic examination (all infants born <32 weeks' gestation should be retested at 6–9 months' chronological age)
Dental examination (by age 12 months)
Laboratory monitoring: Hgb/Hct/Retic Lytes AlkP Ca/P bilirubin Other: ______________

AlkP, alkaline phosphatase; *BPD,* bronchopulmonary dysplasia; *cal,* calories; *Ca/P,* calcium/phosphate; *CPAP,* continuous positive airway pressure; *CPR,* cardiopulmonary resuscitation; *echo,* echocardiogram; *EDC,* estimated date of confinement; *EI,* Early Intervention; *Gastro,* gastroenterology; *HC,* head circumference; *Hct,* hematocrit; *Hgb,* hemoglobin; *HUS,* head ultrasound; *I/D,* indirect/direct; *IFUP,* Infant Follow-Up Program; *Labs,* laboratory results; *lytes,* electrolytes; *MRI,* magnetic resonance imaging; *NEC,* necrotizing enterocolitis; *NICU,* neonatal intensive care unit; *Ophthal,* ophthalmology; *PDA,* patent ductus arteriosus; *RDS,* respiratory distress syndrome; *retic,* reticulocyte count; *ROP,* retinopathy of prematurity; *RSV,* respiratory syncytial virus.
Note: This is a guideline that does not represent a professional standard of care.

Table 1-5 Guidelines for the Primary Care Provider Caring for the Premature Infant

- Manage complications of prematurity
- Monitor for potential new problems
  - Poor growth
  - Reflux
  - Pulmonary problems
  - Nutritional deficiencies
  - Bone mineralization abnormalities
  - Developmental delays
  - Hearing and vision deficits
  - Child abuse or neglect
  - Behavior disturbances
  - Learning disabilities
- Support the family
- Coordinate various medical and social services needed
  - Refer infant to an Early Intervention Program (in most states, neonatal intensive care unit graduates are eligible for this program)
  - Determine whether an Infant Follow-Up Program is needed (if so, make a referral if not already done)
- Educate the family by providing anticipatory guidance and a list of resources

infants, with particular emphasis on specific systems, including respiratory, growth and nutrition, gastrointestinal, neurologic, hematologic, endocrine, neurosensory, and surgical issues (Table 1-7). Each chapter discusses the pathophysiology of the specific disease, current NICU management, and potential complications. The chapters emphasize how the primary care provider should manage these complications and monitor for potential new problems during the first few years of the premature infant's life. Because primary care providers need to use community resources to educate themselves and to provide ongoing support for families and their infants, we include a list of resources in most chapters and summarize them in Chapter 13, "Resources for Clinicians and Families."

Currently, few up-to-date resources are available to help the primary care provider manage a premature infant in the office setting. Yet, as the rate of premature delivery and the number of premature infants who survive are increasing, primary care clinicians are caring for a greater number of premature infants. We hope that this book will serve as a useful guide for primary care providers caring for this growing population.

Table 1-6 Terms Commonly Used to Describe Premature Infants

Term	Definition
Premature Infant	**Infant born before 37 weeks' estimated gestational age**
Late Preterm	**Previously known as "near-term" infant** Infant born between 34 (some use 35) and 36 6/7 weeks' gestation
Low Birth Weight (LBW)	**Birth weight <2500 g (5 lb 8 oz)**
Very Low Birth Weight (VLBW)	**Birth weight <1500 g (3 lb 5 oz)**
Extremely Low Birth Weight (ELBW)	**Birth weight <1000 g (2 lb 3 oz)**
Gestational Age	**Age based on time elapsed between the first day of the last menstrual period and the day of delivery** Reliable by ±1 week if based on first-trimester ultrasound
Chronological Age	**Age based on time elapsed after birth** = postnatal age
Postmenstrual Age*	**Age based on time elapsed between the first day of the last menstrual period and birth plus time elapsed after birth** = gestational age + chronological age For example, a 26-week-gestational-age infant who is 10 weeks' chronological age would have a postmenstrual age of 36 weeks
Corrected Age*	**Age of the infant based on the expected delivery date** Calculated by subtracting the number of weeks born before 40 weeks' gestation from the chronological age Used to describe children up to age 3 years who were born preterm For example, a 12-month-old, former 28-week-gestational-age infant has a corrected age of 9 months

*Engle WA, Committee on Fetus and Newborn: *Pediatrics* 114(5):1362-1364, 2004.

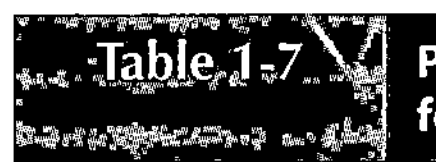

Potential Medical Problems for Premature Infants

Respiratory
- Bronchopulmonary dysplasia
- Ventilator-dependent with need for tracheostomy tube
- Apnea of prematurity

Growth and Nutrition
- Inadequate nutrition and/or growth
- Difficulty with breastfeeding
- Nutritional deficiencies
- Complications intrauterinegrowth restriction

Gastrointestinal
- Gastroesophageal reflux
- Colic
- Oral aversion
- Constipation
- Need for enteral tubes
- Necrotizing enterocolitis and/or short bowel syndrome
- Direct hyperbilirubinemia

Neurologic
- Intraventricular hemorrhage and posthemorrhagic hydrocephalus
- Hydrocephalus
- White matter injury
- Cerebral palsy
- Delayed neurodevelopment

Hematologic
- Anemia of prematurity
- Indirect hyperbilirubinemia

Endocrine
- Hypothyroidism
- Osteopenia of prematurity

Neurosensory
- Retinopathy of prematurity
- Other ophthalmologic issues
- Hearing loss

Surgical
- Cryptorchidism
- Inguinal or umbilical hernia

REFERENCES

1. Martin JA, Kochanek KD, Strobino DM, et al: Annual summary of vital statistics. *Pediatrics* 115(3):619-634, 2005.
2. Romera R, Espinoza J, Chaiworapongsa T, et al: Infection and prematurity and the role of preventive strategies. *Semin Neonatol* 7(4):259-274, 2002.
3. Locksmith G, Duff P: Infection, antibiotics, and preterm delivery. *Semin Perinatol* 25(5):295-309, 2001.
4. Data from Vermont Oxford Network 2004, and Lemons JA, Bauer CR, Oh W, et al: Very low birth weight outcomes of the National Institute of Child Health and Human Development Neonatal Research Network, January 1995 through December 1996. NICHD Neonatal Research Network. *Pediatrics* 107(1):e1, 2001.
5. Trachtenbarg DE, Golemon TB: Office care of the premature infant: part II. Common medical and surgical problems. *Am Fam Physician* 57(10):2383-2390, 1998.
6. Tufts G: Primary care of the premature infant. *Am J Nurse Practitioners* 8(10):25-42, 2004.
7. Wang ML, Dorer DJ, Fleming MP, et al: Clinical outcomes of near-term infants. *Pediatrics* 114(2):372-376, 2004.
8. Escobar GJ, Joffe S, Gardner MN, et al: Rehospitalization in the first two weeks after discharge from the neonatal intensive care unit. *Pediatrics* 104(1):e2 1999
9. American Academy of Pediatrics. Committee on Fetus and Newborn: hospital discharge of the high-risk neonate—proposed guidelines. *Pediatrics* 102(2):411-417, 1998.
10. Engle WA, American Academy of Pediatrics Committee on Practice and Ambulatory Medicine and Committee on Fetus and Newborn: The role of the primary care pediatrician in the management of high-risk newborn infants. *Pediatrics* 98(4):786-788, 1996.

GENERAL REFERENCES

Berger SP, Holt-Turner I, Cupoli JM, et al: Caring for the graduate from the neonatal intensive care unit: at home, in the office, and in the community. *Pediatr Clin North Am* 45(3):701-712, 1998.

Bernstein S, Heimler R, Sasidharan P: Approaching the management of the neonatal intensive care unit graduate through history and physical assessment. *Pediatr Clin North Am* 45(1):79-105, 1998.

Goldenberg RL, Iams JD, Mercer BM, et al: What we have learned about the predictors of preterm birth. *Semin Perinatol* 27(3):185, 2003.

Sherman MP, Steinfeld MP, Philipps AF, et al: Follow-up of the NICU patient. *Emedicine,* 2004. Available at: http://www.emedicine.com/ped/topic2600.htm

Verma RP, Sridhar S, Spitzer AR: Continuing care of NICU graduates. *Clin Pediatr* 42(4):299-315, 2003.

Chapter 2A

Pulmonary Issues in the Premature Infant

Lawrence Rhein, MD, and Sule Cataltepe, MD

Respiratory issues are among the most common long-term complications in children born prematurely. This chapter reviews the current understanding of the pathophysiology of chronic lung disease in premature infants and discusses the current interventions used to manage the disease.

The term *bronchopulmonary dysplasia* (BPD) is commonly used interchangeably with *chronic lung disease of prematurity*. The term BPD was first used by Northway et al.[1] in 1967 to describe clinical, radiologic, and pathologic findings in premature infants who were exposed to high concentrations of oxygen and prolonged mechanical ventilation. Advances in neonatal care, such as use of antenatal steroids, surfactant replacement therapy, gentler ventilation techniques, and optimal nutritional support, have resulted in both an increased survival of extremely premature infants and an increased incidence of BPD.[2,3] However, the clinical presentation of the "new BPD" is milder than that described originally by Northway et al. Many infants with this new form have mild to moderate initial respiratory distress and receive ventilation with low pressures and oxygen concentration. Subsequently, some of these infants develop progressive deterioration in lung function and ultimately develop BPD.

The original definition of BPD described by Northway et al. has changed over time in parallel with the changes in the epidemiology and clinical presentation of the disease. Bancalari et al.[4] modified the definition of BPD to include respiratory failure early in the neonatal period requiring assisted ventilation for a minimum of 3 days, radiographic abnormalities, and continuing respiratory symptoms and oxygen dependence at 28 days' postnatal age. With improvements in survival rates of infants at even lower gestational ages, many infants who met these criteria were clinically asymptomatic by the time of discharge from the hospital. Therefore Sheehan et al.[5] proposed a change in definition from oxygen dependence at 28 days' postnatal age to oxygen dependence at 36 weeks' postmenstrual age. A severity-based definition now has been proposed.[6]

For the purposes of this review, BPD is defined as follows:

1. Supplemental oxygen requirement at 36 weeks' postmenstrual age,
2. Persistent abnormalities on chest radiograph, and
3. Clinical signs of respiratory compromise persisting after age 28 days.

Epidemiology

The incidence of BPD varies significantly among neonatal intensive care units (NICUs)[7] and based on the definition used. Most cases occur in infants with birth weights <1500 g or who are born at gestational age ≤28 weeks. Approximately 30% to 40% of infants born weighing <1000 g develop BPD.[8]

Pathophysiology

The pathogenesis of BPD is multifactorial but can be attributed to a combination of three major factors:

1. Lung immaturity, leading to abnormal development of the lung,
2. Injury from inflammatory mediators caused by a variety of inciting factors, and
3. Inadequate repair response due to abnormal development of repair mechanisms.

Lung development is a highly structured and sequential process. Alveoli undergo septation, which allows the alveoli to bud out or branch from existing alveoli. Interruption of this process leads to arrested alveolarization. In infants with BPD, airways have the same total volume but fewer total alveoli, resulting in larger airspaces. Multiple mediators can disrupt alveolarization, including glucocorticoids, mechanical ventilation, extreme hypoxia or hyperoxia, poor nutrition, and high levels of various cytokines.[9]

Numerous factors induce an inflammatory response in the airways and pulmonary interstitium of preterm infants with BPD.[10] This inflammatory response is characterized by the accumulation of neutrophils, macrophages, and proinflammatory mediators. Oxygen toxicity and barotrauma/volutrauma from mechanical ventilation are associated with inflammation. In addition, volutrauma and atelectrauma cause abnormal stretch of the alveolar capillaries, leading to leakage of intravascular blood and protein. Leakage of these proteins causes mechanical obstruction, attracts other inflammatory cells, and inactivates surfactant, leading to further lung injury.

Regardless of the initial insult, the final common pathway is release of inflammatory cytokines and chemokines that results in more inflammatory cell recruitment and fibrosis. The antioxidant and antiprotease enzymes in premature infants are immature and cannot easily reverse any damage that has incurred. Other factors that contribute to the development of BPD include the presence of a patent ductus arteriosus, antenatal and postnatal infections, and relative surfactant deficiency. Figure 2A-1 outlines the factors that influence antenatal and postnatal lung development in premature infants.

Other Pulmonary Complications Associated with BPD (Table 2A-1)

Subglottic stenosis is a common complication in infants who require intubation, particularly if they have undergone prolonged or multiple intubations. Use of inappropriately large endotracheal tubes also contributes to the prevalence of subglottic stenosis. Common symptoms are stridor, hoarseness, cyanosis, and apnea.

Tracheal or bronchial granulomas may occur and may be related to aggressive suctioning techniques and/or extended endotracheal intubation.

Acquired tracheobronchomalacia, or central airway collapse, is an extremely common complication in infants with BPD. It is due to barotrauma

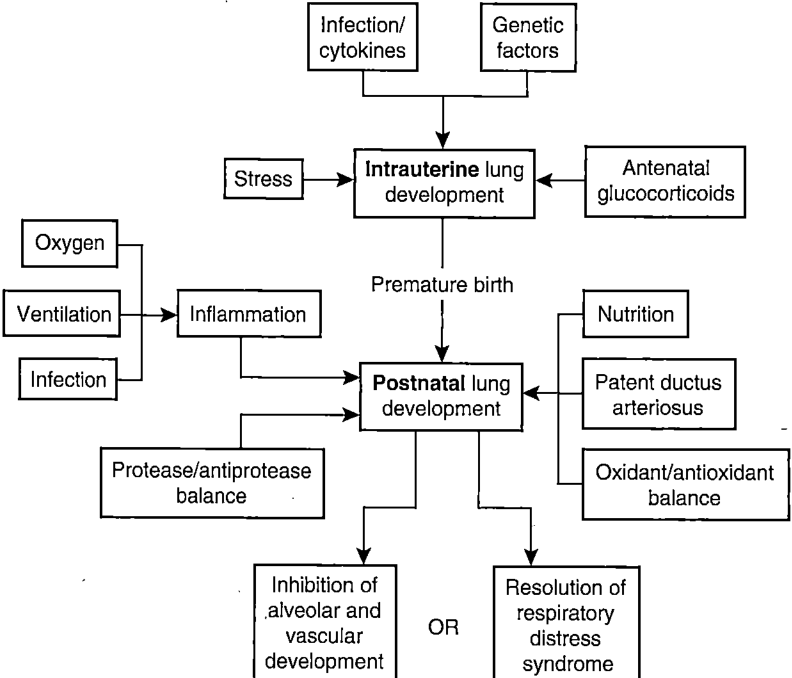

FIGURE 2A-1 This schematic shows the multiple potential factors that can influence antenatal and postnatal lung development in premature infants. Depending on the timing, combination, and severity of these insults, the premature infant can have alveolar and pulmonary maldevelopment or minimal lung disease.

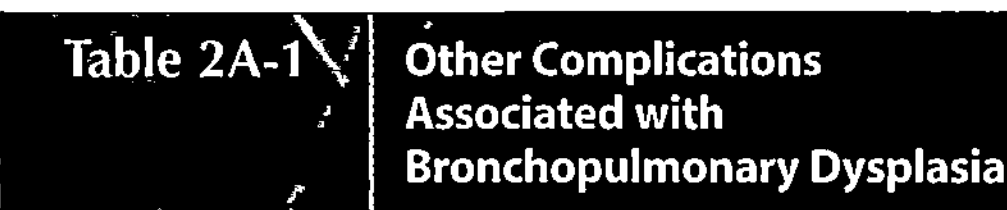

Table 2A-1 Other Complications Associated with Bronchopulmonary Dysplasia

Pulmonary	Nonpulmonary
Subglottic stenosis	Poor growth
Tracheal or bronchial granulomas	Altered renal function (directly or indirectly)
Acquired tracheobronchomalacia	Developmental delay
Cor pulmonale and pulmonary hypertension	

and airway deformation caused by positive pressure ventilation. Symptoms include homophonous wheezing and cyanosis.

Sleep disturbances with prolonged episodes of hypoxemia are common.

Cor pulmonale and *pulmonary hypertension* are serious complications that most commonly develop in infants with BPD who were born at less than 25 weeks' gestation or have a birth weight <1000 g. As described previously, children with BPD have fewer alveoli and abnormalities of the pulmonary vasculature.[11] Disordered pulmonary vascular growth along with acute vasoconstriction by hypoxia, hypercarbia, and/or acidosis lead to vascular structural changes that contribute to the development of pulmonary hypertension.

Nonpulmonary Problems Associated with BPD (Table 2A-1)

In addition to the lung and airway problems associated with BPD, infants often have issues with other organs. As a result, these infants have poor growth for various reasons, including renal insufficiency, decreased intake because of fluid restriction or tiring with feedings, swallowing dysfunction or dysphagia, recurrent hypoxemic episodes, and/or increased energy requirements. Renal dysfunction can occur, particularly if nephrocalcinosis develops as a complication of prolonged use of loop diuretics. Infants with BPD are at increased risk for developing long-term neurodevelopmental difficulties.[12]

Transitioning the Child with BPD from Hospital to Home

Children with BPD can be successfully transitioned to home when the care team has determined that the family, with appropriate resources, can adequately and safely meet the therapeutic needs of the infant. Some of the factors to consider are infant-related issues, family-related issues, and community-related issues.

Infant issues

1. Infants must have a stable respiratory status and be able to maintain acceptable oxygen saturations. If oxygen is still required, the oxygen flow rate to maintain saturations >93% should not have changed significantly within the week prior to discharge. Any apnea must be medically controlled or resolved prior to discharge.
2. Infants should demonstrate appropriate weight gain on enteral feedings. For children with difficulty growing on full oral feeding, placement of a gastrostomy tube is preferable to prolonged use of a nasogastric tube because of the risks of trauma from repeated placement of the tube and an altered ability to swallow. Aspiration can occur in infants with delayed development of oromotor coordination and can result in further lung injury.
3. Medication regimens should not have any recent changes that would cause adverse effects.
4. Respiratory syncytial virus (RSV) and influenza prophylaxis should be administered during appropriate high-risk months.

Family factors

An extensive teaching protocol should be followed before the infant with BPD is discharged home (Table 2A-2). Parents must be instructed to appropriately identify signs and symptoms of respiratory distress. Families must be able to count the respiratory rate as well as identify retractions, nasal flaring, and grunting. The family's ability to appropriately administer medications, including oxygen, must be established. All family caregivers must be certified in infant cardiopulmonary resuscitation (CPR) and have the ability to provide emergency management. Finally, the family must have the ability to transport the child for follow-up appointments.

Community factors

The neonatologist must contact the primary care provider before an infant with BPD is discharged and discuss the home care plan. If infants will require home nursing care or oxygen equipment, these services must be arranged and discussed with the pediatrician.

Consideration of alternatives to home discharge should be given to some infants with severe BPD requiring continuous ventilation and frequent care. These alternatives include rehabilitation centers, chronic care facilities, and hospice programs.

Table 2A-2 Discharge Teaching to Families of Infants with Bronchopulmonary Dysplasia

Discharge Focus	Teaching Points
Overall discussion of bronchopulmonary dysplasia	Describe the disease process, management, and potential sequelae Discuss importance of weight gain
Assessment of infant	Assess respiratory status Evaluate for cyanosis Monitor neurologic status Be attentive to changes in appetite and/or behavior Monitor for signs of dehydration
Medications	Denote name(s) of medications (trade and generic) Emphasize dosage, method of administration, and frequency Discuss indications for PRN medications Discuss protocol if dose is omitted or repeated Discuss potential side effects Discuss storage
Oxygen (if needed)	Describe purpose Explain flow rate, method of administration, and how to read the flow meter Teach how to maintain and clean equipment Discuss oximetry technique and interpretation Address safety considerations Discuss handicapped placard Discuss weaning protocol
Emergency management	All caregivers should be taught cardiopulmonary resuscitation Post emergency contact numbers near phone For infants who are being discharged home on oxygen therapy, suggest to the family that they contact the local fire, police, and utility departments to alert these services that their infant is receiving oxygen
Infection control	Practice frequent handwashing Minimize exposure to people Care providers should receive influenza vaccine Infants should receive respiratory syncytial virus and influenza prophylaxis during appropriate months
Other specific issues, if needed	Discuss tracheostomy care, mechanical ventilation, and cardiorespiratory monitoring

Modified from: Allen J, Zwerdling R, Ehrenkranz R, et al: *Am J Respir Crit Care Med* 168(3):373, 2003.

Specific Common Therapies Continued After Discharge

Oxygen therapy

Goals of oxygen therapy are multifold and aim to limit pulmonary artery hypertension and right ventricular workload; to provide adequate exercise tolerance; and to promote appropriate growth and repair of the developing lungs. Maintaining oxygen saturations >95% may have beneficial effects, such as promoting growth,[13] reducing the frequency of central apnea,[14] and reducing the transient elevations in pulmonary artery pressures associated with intermittent hypoxemia.[11] Oxygen is most often delivered by nasal cannula. We recommend using humidified 100% oxygen at titrated low-flow levels to maintain saturation >95% rather than using higher flow rates of blended oxygen. Methods for weaning an outpatient from supplemental oxygen are described later in this chapter.

Currently, the potential toxic effects of oxygen are of tremendous concern. However, oxygen toxicity in the first few weeks of life is much more of a concern than is the potential toxicity to premature infants approaching readiness for discharge from an NICU, near 36 weeks' postmenstrual gestational age. Oxygen flow through a nasal cannula combines with room air (21%) inhaled through the mouth, resulting in lower net oxygen concentration reaching the lungs. Minute ventilation for infants averages 200 to 250 ml/kg, or approximately 400 to 600 ml for the average premature infant approaching readiness for discharge. For the infant with flow rates ≤200 ml, the contribution of oxygen concentration of the cannula flow is low, and the amount of room air breathed through the mouth is high. In this case, the amount of supplemental oxygen is low, so oxygen toxicity should be minimal.[15] Although the Benefits of Oxygen Saturation Targeting (BOOST) trial demonstrated an increased number of pulmonary exacerbations in infants with higher oxygen saturation targets,[16] it is important to remember that for infants who are out of the nursery and are older than the infants described in the trial, their risk for sequelae from high oxygen saturations likely is minimal.

Bronchodilators

In theory, beta-sympathomimetics improve pulmonary function by reducing bronchospasm. In ventilated infants, these drugs have been shown to increase dynamic compliance, decrease airway resistance, and improve lung function.[17] However, the bronchodilator response is not universal. No studies have demonstrated consistent efficacy or improvement in outcome in nonventilated infants. Studies are limited by variations in effective drug delivery to the lungs. Variability in effects also may reflect variable genetic response. Infants with recurrent episodes of wheezing, cough, or respiratory distress may benefit from a trial of bronchodilators. Providers should determine clear assessment of efficacy (reduction in work of breathing or coughing episodes) when prescribing bronchodilators because these agents have side effects such as tachycardia. Furthermore, infants with BPD may have associated tracheobronchomalacia, and beta-agonist therapies may exacerbate obstructive episodes by relaxing the upper smooth muscle in airways that already are floppy. In addition, beta-agonists can cause pulmonary vasodilation and potentially worsen ventilation/perfusion mismatch. Therefore, use of ipratroprium, a competitive muscarinic acetylcholine receptor antagonist, may be a better bronchodilator choice for infants with BPD.

Review of the appropriate delivery technique for inhaled bronchodilators is critical. In our clinic, we prefer to use a meter-dosed inhaler (MDI) and spacer instead of nebulizer treatments. The MDI with a spacer is more convenient, requires less delivery time, and achieves comparable deposition.

Diuretic therapy

Although diuretics are widely used in NICUs, little is known about their effect on survival or duration of oxygen support. Similar to bronchodilators, the response to diuretics is not universal. Side effects of all diuretics include hypokalemia and metabolic alkalosis, which can exacerbate carbon dioxide retention. Potential side effects with prolonged use of furosemide are hypocalcemia, rickets, hearing loss, and renal calcinosis.

For infants who appear to benefit from diuretic treatment, we recommend monitoring electrolyte levels monthly, assuming that the infants remain on a constant dose of diuretic. Electrolyte supplementation (i.e., potassium chloride) often is required for infants receiving diuretic therapy, and the dose should be adjusted to maintain potassium levels between 4 and 5.5 mEq/L and chloride levels between 95 and 110 mEq/L. Because electrolyte preparations are available in several different concentrations, it is critical to be explicit about the volume and dose that has been ordered.

Because of the significant side effects associated with furosemide, we attempt to wean this medication first if it is being administered daily. Thiazides are not dose adjusted for weight. Rather, they are weaned by allowing the infant to outgrow the dose. When the infant has grown to a weight that corresponds to a dosage of 30 mg/kg/day, we decrease the dose by half for several days, then discontinue the thiazides completely. Decreases in thiazide dosing should be mirrored by weans in electrolyte supplementation. Close follow-up to monitor weight, oxygen saturation, and work of breathing is important during this weaning phase.

Corticosteroids

Systemic steroids can decrease the need for persistent bronchodilator therapy, but they are associated with several negative side effects, including hypertension, hyperglycemia, and cataracts. Furthermore, studies have found an association between early use of dexamethasone for treatment of BPD and neurologic problems in childhood.[18,19] Systemic steroids have been shown to decrease alveolarization.[9]

Because of the numerous potential side effects of systemic steroids, inhaled steroids have been used. Inhaled steroids may provide some benefit for obstructive pulmonary disease. However, the effects of inhaled steroids on alveolarization are not established. Given the other known side effects of inhaled steroids, including impaired growth, adrenal suppression, oral candidiasis, and cataracts, we do not recommend inhaled steroid use unless repeated episodes of respiratory distress clearly are uncontrollable with other therapies. Further long-term studies of inhaled steroid use are warranted.

Evaluation of the Infant with BPD after Discharge from the NICU

The exact schedule of follow-up visits depends on the severity of illness and the availability of home nursing services. A care provider (primary care provider or pulmonologist) should see most infants every 2 to 4 weeks. Certain information is critical to obtain during the visit, as outlined in Table 2A-3. Optimal growth is essential to improve BPD, and supplemental calories are often necessary.

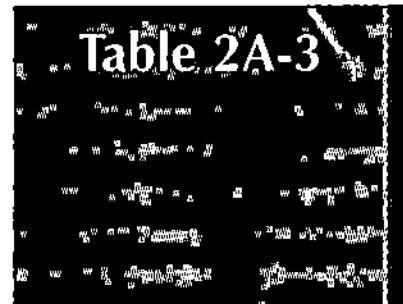

Table 2A-3 Evaluation of the Infant with Bronchopulmonary Dysplasia after Discharge by Primary Care Clinician and/or Pulmonologist

EVERY 2–4 WEEKS

- Weight, length, and head circumference, plotted on a growth chart
- Pulse oximetry on baseline oxygen regimen and on room air (*note:* this may not be possible in the primary care setting)
- List of medications, including dosages and calculated dose per weight
- Intercurrent illnesses, emergency room visits, and/or hospitalizations
- Feeding regimen, including fluid and caloric intake
- Vital signs, including respiratory rate and blood pressure
- Physical examination, with focus on presence of retractions, crackles, wheezing, or edema
- Review of immunization status (eligibility for respiratory syncytial virus prophylaxis and influenza vaccine)

EVERY 3 MONTHS

- Electrocardiography to monitor for right axis deviation, right atrial enlargement, or right ventricular hypertrophy, which is particularly important for infants born <25 weeks' gestation, birth weight <1500 g, history of prolonged mechanical ventilation, or requirement for continuous positive airway pressure
- Echocardiography may be needed for patients with poor growth

Infant Pulmonary Function Testing

Pulmonary function testing can help to assess severity of disease, response to therapies, and long-term course of lung function. Unfortunately, few centers perform these tests regularly to make them useful for follow-up patient care. Currently, pulmonary function tests are important in research protocols but are not yet clinically useful for most infants.

Weaning from Supplemental Oxygen (Figure 2A-2)

At every visit to the pulmonologist, oxygen saturations are measured when the infant is receiving his or her baseline oxygen regimen. If the primary care provider has access to a pulse oximeter, he or she should check the infant's oxygen saturation at each visit.

A. For infants with stable growth and baseline work of breathing who are receiving flows >100 ml/min, we also check saturations after infants are given 100 ml for 20 minutes. If the infants can maintain saturations in this test, then they are maintained on 100-ml flow for 4 weeks until the next visit (see B).

B. For infants receiving flow ≤100 ml, oxygen saturations are measured on the baseline oxygen regimen and again after 20 minutes on room air mist.

When the infant can maintain saturations >95% after 20 minutes on room air mist, we allow the family to attempt a trial with the infant off oxygen for 30 min/day for the next several days, keeping the infant on the oximeter and monitoring for increased work of breathing. If this trial is successful, we allow the family to extend the mist trials to 1 hr/day for 3 to 5 days. If the trials continue to be successful, we allow the family to extend the mist trial by 1 hour, to 2 hr/day for 3 to 5 days. We recommend limiting extensions to increments of 1 hr/day, with no more frequent than one extension every 3 days to monitor for tiring or poor growth. Final goals of the mist trial extensions at home are to discontinue the oxygen except with feedings and overnight. At any point, if the infant demonstrates desaturations, poor growth, or increased work of breathing, extensions are halted.

Once the infant is able to achieve the goal of discontinued oxygen except during feedings and overnight, we arrange a home oximetry test off oxygen to verify that overnight saturations are maintained at >92%. If an infant cannot be weaned from supplemental oxygen, further evaluation may be indicated (Table 2A-4).

Travel Advice

Infants with BPD can travel safely if appropriate precautions are taken. For the child undergoing oxygen therapy, several considerations are critical, including ensuring a sufficient amount of oxygen, securing the oxygen safely, and preparing appropriate monitoring. Airline travel carries the additional issue of decreased inspired oxygen concentration in the room-air component of inspired air, making the need for additional nasal cannula flow probable. This can be determined by using Equation 1:

$$F_{IO_2}\ \#1 \times (\text{Barometric Pressure} - 47) \text{ at Ground Level} = F_{IO_2}\ \#2 \times (\text{Barometric Pressure} - 47) \text{ at New Altitude.} \quad (1)$$

Direct flights are recommended, and prior arrangements with the airlines to explain oxygen needs may be helpful. For car travel, most states provide handicapped parking placards for families with children who require oxygen supplementation. The form is obtained through the state registry of motor vehicles.

OUTPATIENT WEANING OF AN INFANT WITH BPD FROM SUPPLEMENTAL OXYGEN*

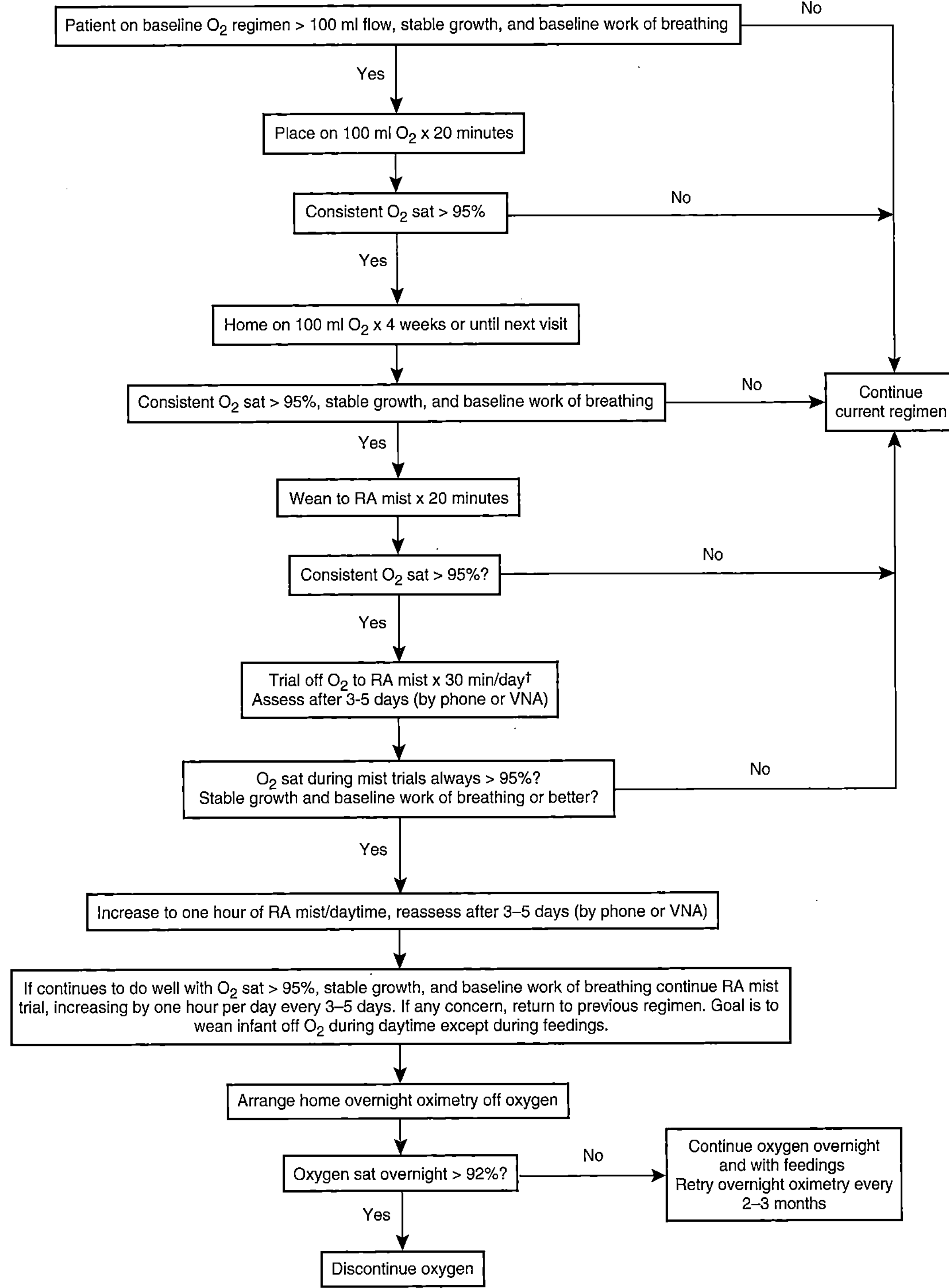

FIGURE 2A-2 *O_2,* oxygen; *RA,* room air; *sat,* saturation; *VNA,* Visiting Nurse Association
*This is an algorithm that is usually followed by the infant's pulmonologist. The goal of this algorithm is to wean the infant off oxygen during the day when not feeding, then to discontinue oxygen overnight, and finally to discontinue oxygen during feedings. An oxygen sat > 95% is recommended to maintain a low pulmonary vascular resistance and minimize right ventricular workload.
†Trial should occur when the infant is awake and not feeding. If infant has a respiratory infection, increased oxygen is often recommended and weaning should be put on hold.
Please note that this is a recommended algorithm that does not represent a professional standard of care; care should be revised to meet individual patient needs.

Table 2A-4 Differential Diagnosis of Patients with Bronchopulmonary Dysplasia

Diagnosis	Symptoms	Evaluation
Gastroesophageal reflux	Recurrent wheezing Recurrent lower respiratory infections	pH probe, barium swallow Assess response to empiric treatment Possible endoscopy If patient has a tracheostomy, consider adding coloring to milk and monitor color of secretions
Cardiovascular abnormalities	Poor growth Edema	Electrocardiography, echocardiography
Aspiration	Recurrent wheezing Recurrent lower respiratory infections	Barium swallow Endoscopy
Tracheomalacia	Wheezing	Flexible bronchoscopy
Upper airway obstruction	Stridor, apnea Weak cry	Radiographs Bronchoscopy
Immunodeficiencies	Recurrent and/or atypical infections	Immune evaluation
Cystic fibrosis	Recurrent lower respiratory infections Failure to thrive	Sweat test Genetic testing

Modified from: Allen J, Zwerdling R, Ehrenkranz R, et al: *Am J Respir Crit Care Med* 168(3):358, 2003.

Infection Prevention

For optimal social development and familial psychological comfort, it is important for the infant to be exposed to other people. However, anyone who contacts a premature infant should wash his or her hands before holding or touching the infant. Exposure to anyone with obvious viral respiratory symptoms should be avoided. Vaccination and RSV prophylaxis guidelines are discussed in detail in other sections of this book. Caretakers and children with BPD should be vaccinated for influenza.

Evaluation of the Infant with BPD and Recurrent Respiratory Issues

Whenever a child is doing poorly on the maintenance regimen that had stabilized him or her previously or is unable to wean from supplemental oxygen, several possible explanations must be considered:

1. Because many diagnoses mimic the symptoms of severe BPD, an evaluation for other causes may be necessary (Table 2A-4).
2. Perhaps the infant is not receiving the recommended regimen. This could be attributable to loss of oxygen supply, a blocked tube or valve, and/or disconnected cannula. Incomplete receipt of medications may be the result of noncompliance because of lack of understanding of the regimen, stressors on the family, or intolerable side effects not revealed by the parents. A thorough review of the caregivers' understanding of medications and the specific delivery techniques is critical.
3. The infant's disease may be more severe than previously thought. The infant may have severe BPD, and although the infant is receiving the appropriate medications, more aggressive therapy may be needed.

Long-Term Pulmonary Outcomes

With rapid changes in neonatal care and survival, lung disease in premature infants born less than 10 years ago may be different from the lung disease observed in premature infants today. Results from follow-up studies indicate that infants with BPD are more likely to be hospitalized in the first 2 years of life and are at higher risk for obstructive lung disease.[20] Prospective, long-term follow-up studies are needed to better predict outcomes for the new generations of premature infants with BPD.

The infants born at the earliest gestational ages (<28 weeks) or with a birth weight <1000 g require follow-up even if they do not require oxygen prior to discharge. In addition, any gestational-age infant who has weaned rapidly from therapies needs to be followed for the long term because decreased alveolarization may have long-term sequelae that are not evident in early infancy.

Summary

Pulmonary sequelae of prematurity are significant issues for many infants. Close follow-up in collaboration with a pulmonologist can limit the long-term sequelae and lead to improved long-term pulmonary outcomes for many children. Primary care providers should refer to the detailed official statement from the American Thoracic Society that addresses many of the issues discussed in this chapter.[21] More research about the pulmonary management of premature infants and therapeutic options for infants with BPD is needed to decrease the incidence and improve outcomes.

Resource for Families and Clinicians

www.nhlbi.nih.gov/health/dci/Diseases/Bpd/Bpd_WhatIs.html

The web site of the National Heart, Lung and Blood Institute provides information about bronchopulmonary dysplasia to families.

REFERENCES

1. Northway WJ, Rosan RC, Porter DY: Pulmonary disease following respirator therapy of hyaline-membrane disease. Bronchopulmonary dysplasia. *N Engl J Med* 276:357-368, 1967.
2. Bancalari E, Claure N, Sosenko IR: Bronchopulmonary dysplasia: changes in pathogenesis, epidemiology and definition. *Semin Neonatol* 8:63-71, 2003.
3. Bancalari E: Changes in the pathogenesis and prevention of chronic lung disease of prematurity. *Am J Perinatol* 18:1-9, 2001.
4. Bancalari E, Abdenour GE, Feller R, et al: Bronchopulmonary dysplasia: clinical presentation. *J Pediatr* 95:819-823, 1979.
5. Shennan AT, Dunn MS, Ohlsson A, et al: Abnormal pulmonary outcomes in premature infants: prediction from oxygen requirement in the neonatal period. *Pediatrics* 82:527-532, 1988.
6. Jobe AH, Bancalari E: Bronchopulmonary dysplasia. *Am J Respir Crit Care Med* 163:1723-1729, 2001.
7. Van Marter LJ, Pagano M, Allred EN, et al: Rate of bronchopulmonary dysplasia as a function of neonatal intensive care practices. *J Pediatr* 120:938-946, 1992.
8. Stevenson DK, Wright LL, Lemons JA, et al: Very low birth weight outcomes of the National Institute of Child Health and Human Development Neonatal Research Network, January 1993 through December 1994. *Am J Obstet Gynecol* 179:1632-1639, 1998.
9. Jobe AJ: The new BPD: an arrest of lung development. *Pediatr Res* 46:641-643, 1999.
10. Speer CP: Inflammation and bronchopulmonary dysplasia. *Semin Neonatol* 8:29-38, 2003.
11. Parker TA, Abman SH: The pulmonary circulation in bronchopulmonary dysplasia. *Semin Neonatol* 8:51-61, 2003.
12. Yeo CL, Choo S, Ho LY: Chronic lung disease in very low birthweight infants: a 5-year review. *J Paediatr Child Health* 33:102-106, 1997.
13. Groothuis JR, Rosenberg AA: Home oxygen promotes weight gain in infants with bronchopulmonary dysplasia. *Am J Dis Child* 141:992-995, 1987.
14. Sekar KC, Duke JC: Sleep apnea and hypoxemia in recently weaned premature infants with and without bronchopulmonary dysplasia. *Pediatr Pulmonol* 10:112-116, 1991.
15. Fan LL, Voyles JB: Determination of inspired oxygen delivered by nasal cannula in infants with chronic lung disease. *J Pediatr* 103:923-925, 1983.
16. Askie LM, Henderson-Smart DJ, Irwig L, et al: Oxygen-saturation targets and outcomes in extremely preterm infants. *N Engl J Med* 349:959-967, 2003.
17. Cabal LA, Larrazabal C, Ramanathan R, et al: Effects of metaproterenol on pulmonary mechanics, oxygenation, and ventilation in infants with chronic lung disease. *J Pediatr* 110:116-119, 1987.
18. O'Shea TM, Kothadia JM, Klinepeter KL, et al: Randomized placebo-controlled trial of a 42-day tapering course of dexamethasone to reduce the duration of ventilator dependency in very low birth weight infants: outcome of study participants at 1-year adjusted age. *Pediatrics* 104:15-21, 1999.
19. Yeh TF, Lin YJ, Lin HC, et al: Outcomes at school age after postnatal dexamethasone therapy for lung disease of prematurity. *N Engl J Med* 350:1304-1313, 2004.
20. Gross SJ, Iannuzzi DM, Kveselis DA, et al: Effect of preterm birth on pulmonary function at school age: a prospective controlled study. *J Pediatr* 133:188-192, 1998.
21. Allen J, Zwerdling R, Ehrenkranz R, et al: Statement on the care of the child with chronic lung disease of infancy and childhood. *Am J Respir Crit Care Med* 168:356-396, 2003.

Chapter 2B

Apnea of Prematurity

Eric C. Eichenwald, MD

Apnea of prematurity represents a striking disorder of respiratory control. With the increased survival of less mature infants over the past 20 years, it is one of the most frequently diagnosed problems in the special care nursery. Waiting for resolution of recurrent apnea, a typical discharge criterion, is a common reason for prolonged hospital stays in premature infants. The specific etiology of apnea in individual infants often is elusive and likely multifactorial; however, research on the development of respiratory control has increased our understanding of factors that contribute to this disorder and forms the basis for a rational approach to therapy. This chapter reviews the epidemiology, pathogenesis, evaluation, and management of apnea of prematurity.

Control of Breathing Rhythm

The central pattern generator is the part of the brainstem comprising inspiratory and expiratory neurons thought to control rhythmic breathing.[1] These respiratory neurons are located primarily in the ventral lateral region of the medulla. Separate populations of these neurons control inspiration and expiration. Central inspiratory activity results from release of inhibition and progressive excitation of inspiratory neurons, leading to contraction of the respiratory muscles and ultimately an increase in lung volume. Inspiration terminates when a critical threshold, or "off-switch," is reached. This critical threshold is determined in part by feedback from the pulmonary stretch receptors, which increase their discharge when lung volume increases. Input from chemoreceptors, which respond to changing Po_2 and PCo_2 levels, affects the rate of rise of central inspiratory activity and can change the critical threshold for the inspiratory off-switch.

Expiration results from central inhibition, which suppresses inspiratory activity. The power of central inhibition decays with time. Expiration is divided into two different phases. During quiet breathing, expiration is mainly passive, with airflow determined by the elastic recoil forces that have developed during active inspiration. During the first phase of expiration, however, the inspiratory muscles, primarily the diaphragm, are activated again. This postinspiratory inspiratory activity partially offsets the initial elastic recoil forces of the inflated lungs and serves to retard or brake the rate of expiratory airflow. Laryngeal muscles also are activated and help to regulate expiratory airflow by controlling upper airway resistance. The second phase of expiration, in contrast, is generally completely passive unless circumstances such as exercise demand active expiration.

The duration of expiration is determined when a second critical threshold is reached. This occurs because central inspiratory inhibition decreases in a time-dependent fashion and also is influenced by input from pulmonary stretch receptors, which respond to changes in lung volume. When the threshold is reached, central inhibition of inspiration is abruptly terminated, and inspiration ensues again. Disorders of respiratory control in premature infants may be secondary to central effects or result from the way in which afferent information from the periphery impacts on the central pattern generator.

Definition and Epidemiology of Apnea of Prematurity

An apneic spell usually is defined as the cessation of airflow for ≥20 seconds or interruption of breathing for a shorter duration accompanied by bradycardia (heart rate <100 beats/min) or cyanosis. Apnea can be classified as (1) central apnea, which is associated with no respiratory efforts; (2) obstructive apnea, which is associated with continued respiratory efforts without air flow; or (3) mixed apnea, in which a central respiratory pause is preceded or followed by upper airway obstruction. The majority of apneic spells in premature infants are mixed apnea, although in an individual infant one type may predominate.

It is important to differentiate true apneic spells from the periodic breathing normally observed during infancy. Periodic breathing commonly is defined as an episode of three or more respiratory pauses of ≥3 seconds with intervening periods of normal respiration of <20 seconds.[2] Periodic breathing occurs frequently in premature infants but also is seen in normal-term infants and diminishes with age.[2-4] The number and duration of periodic breathing episodes, however, are greater in premature infants compared with term infants.[2] The presence of periodic breathing does not appear to be related to the risk of prolonged apneic spells in premature infants.[2,3]

In premature infants with apnea, the time interval between the start of an apneic spell and onset of bradycardia and cyanosis is variable. In one study of closely monitored premature infants, the interval between the onset of apnea and the onset of bradycardia was brief (approximately 8 seconds) and was not related to preceding hypoxemia.[5] Heart rate usually reached its lowest value at approximately 30 seconds after the onset of apnea. PO_2 assessed by a transcutaneous monitor began to fall soon after the onset of apnea and continued to fall for an average of 26 seconds after reinitiation of regular breathing. These results suggest that bradycardia after an apneic spell is centrally mediated. However, more recent studies using pulse oximetry to assess for hypoxemia suggest that the bradycardia associated with recurrent apnea may be more closely related to the fall in oxygenation caused by the apnea spell than previously thought.[6]

The incidence of apnea of prematurity is inversely related to gestational age. Clinically significant recurrent apneic spells occur in virtually all infants born at 24 to 29 weeks' gestation, in approximately half of those born at 30 to 32 weeks' gestation, and in approximately 25% of infants born at 34 to 35 weeks' gestational age (Figure 2B-1).[7] In contrast, apnea occurs only rarely in term infants (37–41 weeks' gestation) and usually is associated with a serious contributing cause, such as birth asphyxia, intracranial disease, or respiratory depression caused by medications.

In premature infants who develop apnea, spells usually begin during the first 2 days of life. In general, if apneic spells do not begin in the first week of life, they are unlikely to occur later unless illness develops.[7] However, apnea may not be detected in infants with lung disease until after mechanical ventilation is no longer required. Although apneic spells can persist for variable periods postnatally, they generally cease by 37 weeks' postmenstrual age in infants delivered at ≥28 weeks.

Pathogenesis of Apnea of Prematurity

In the healthy premature infant the cause of apneic spells is likely multifactorial. Many factors influence breathing by impacting on the central pattern generator and thus ultimately affecting the respiratory muscles and rhythmic breathing. These factors include influences from higher centers, neuromodulators, central and peripheral chemoreceptors, and reflexes from the upper airway. In turn, many of these influences on breathing are affected by immaturity. Our knowledge of how these influences interact to result in disturbances in the control of breathing in the premature newborn is

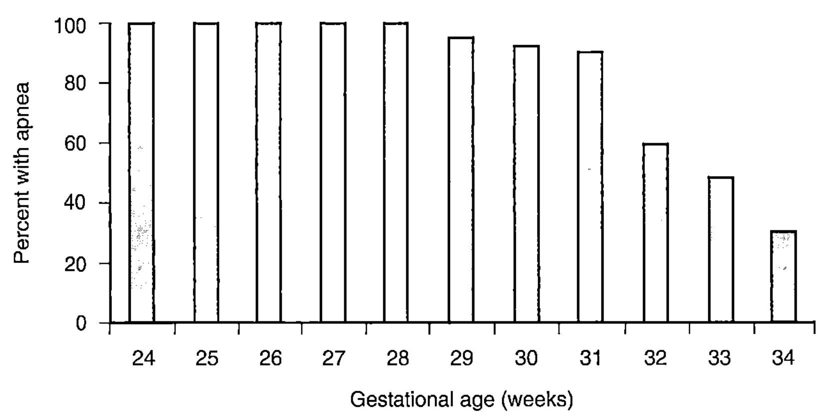

FIGURE 2B-1 The incidence of apnea decreases with advancing gestational age. Data from references 42 and 43.

derived from clinical observations and limited studies of the responses of human infants to respiratory stimuli.

Developmental immaturity

The important role of maturation is suggested by the high prevalence of apnea in infants born at low gestational ages. Histologically, the immature brain has fewer synaptic connections and dendritic arborizations and poor myelination compared with the brain of older infants. Physiologic evidence also indicates a relationship between clinical apnea and brainstem neuronal function. Premature infants with apnea have prolonged brainstem conduction of auditory evoked responses compared with infants of similar gestational age without apnea.[8] This finding suggests that overall brainstem immaturity may partly explain respiratory rhythm abnormalities in premature infants.

Neuromodulators

Several neurotransmitters and neuromodulators have been identified that may influence breathing control in the newborn.[9,10] These substances can be either inhibitory (e.g., endorphins, prostaglandins, adenosine) or excitatory (e.g., substance P) to breathing. An imbalance between excitatory and inhibitory neuromodulators has been hypothesized to promote instability of respiratory control in newborn infants.[10]

Sleep state

Cortical influences, such as changes with sleep state, also affect breathing control in premature infants.[11] Breathing during active (rapid eye movement [REM]) sleep, which represents 50% to 60% of sleep time in premature infants, tends to be highly irregular in both tidal volume and frequency. Breathing in quiet (non-REM) sleep, in contrast, tends to be more regular. Apneic spells are more common in active sleep than in either quiet sleep or wakefulness.[12] The increased frequency of apnea in active sleep likely is influenced by central neural mechanisms that impact on the central pattern generator. In addition, active sleep is characterized by decreased skeletal muscle tone, which accentuates the already highly compliant chest wall of newborn infants. This results in inspiratory chest wall distortion and the characteristic paradoxical breathing pattern observed in infants during active sleep. As a result, a substantial amount of diaphragmatic work is wasted on distortion of the chest wall instead of lung inflation.[13] At the extreme, this might result in diaphragmatic fatigue.[14] Distortion of the chest wall also may terminate inspiration early by activation of an intercostals-to-phrenic inhibitory reflex.[15]

Chemoreceptor responses

Premature infants with apnea are less sensitive to increased carbon dioxide levels than are gestational age-matched infants without apnea.[16] This decreased sensitivity to CO_2 may be indicative of greater central immaturity in infants with apnea, although decreased respiratory muscle function also may play a role. Maturation also affects the ventilatory response to hypoxia. Although adults respond to an hypoxic challenge with sustained hyperventilation, premature newborns respond with transient hyperventilation followed by hypoventilation and sometimes apnea.[17] It is possible that the failure of premature infants to sustain a hyperventilatory response to hypoxia promotes instability of breathing and contributes to the development of apneic spells.

Respiratory muscle coordination

Development affects the coordinated activity of the upper airway dilating and inspiratory pump muscles. The majority of apneic spells in premature infants have a component of airway obstruction, and most prolonged apneas tend to be of the mixed type.[18] The primary site of spontaneously occurring obstruction during apnea is the upper pharynx.[19] Apneic spells occur more frequently in premature infants when they assume a position of neck flexion, which presumably narrows the already vulnerable neonatal airway.[20] If upper airway muscle activity is decreased, as it appears to be in premature infants with apnea,[21] negative pressure in the pharynx generated during inspiration may result in pharyngeal collapse and obstruction to air flow.

Laryngeal reflexes

Some apneic spells may be part of an upper airway protective response to stimulation of laryngeal chemoreceptors by fluids such as milk or oral secretions. This reflex response is potent in newborns and consists of swallowing, airway obstruction, and central apnea. Apnea induced by instilling small amounts of water into the retropharynx of premature infants closely resembles spontaneously occurring spells.[22] This suggests that airway protective reflexes may play a role in some apneic spells and may explain the association of apnea with oral feeding.

Other factors

Neonatal apnea may be a frequent manifestation of specific pathophysiologic disorders in both term and premature infants. Conditions that have been clinically associated with apnea include (1) infection, both local and systemic; (2) intracranial pathology; (3) drug depression (both from maternal peripartum analgesics and from illicit drugs); (4) metabolic disorder; and (5) respiratory

Table 2B-1 Disorders Precipitating Apnea

Infection
- Sepsis
- Meningitis
- Necrotizing enterocolitis

Intracranial Pathology
- Asphyxia
- Seizures
- Intraventricular/parenchymal hemorrhage
- Central nervous system malformation
- Ventriculoperitoneal shunt malfunction

Drug Effect
- Anesthetics
- Maternal drug uses
- Hypermagnesemia

Metabolic Disorder
- Hypoxia
- Hyperthermia/hypothermia
- Hypoglycemia
- Electrolyte disorder

Respiratory Disorder
- Upper airway obstruction
- Parenchymal lung disease

disorder (Table 2B-1). The association of apnea with a variety of pathophysiologic states suggests that the respiratory centers responsible for generating regular breathing in newborns are more sensitive than those in older infants to a wide array of internal and external stimuli that may precipitate apnea.[23]

Clinicians frequently observe that recurrent apnea may occur in association with a gavage feeding, or that formula is visible in the mouth of infants after an apneic event. This has led some to conclude that gastroesophageal reflux, a common clinical condition in premature infants, contributes to the pathogenesis of apnea of prematurity. Although it is possible that activation of the laryngeal chemoreflex by reflux of gastric fluids could precipitate apnea, data suggest that this is, at best, a rare cause of recurrent apnea in premature infants. Although both occur frequently, several studies have shown no temporal relationship between reflux episodes and apnea in premature infants.[24] In one study, when apnea and reflux occurred closely together, more commonly the apnea event began before the reflux episode.[25] This finding suggests that the apnea itself may precipitate relaxation of the gastroesophageal junction, which could explain the frequency of finding milk in the pharynx of premature infants after an apneic spell.

Apneic spells typically worsen (or recur) after general anesthesia.[26] One common scenario for such an effect is inguinal hernia repair in a premature infant either before or after discharge from the hospital. This risk may persist up to 60 weeks' postmenstrual age, so it is advisable for older premature infants to be monitored for apnea after anesthesia administration. Apnea may be associated temporally with routine vaccinations given to hospitalized extremely premature infants at 2 months after birth.

Evaluation and Therapy

It generally is recommended that all infants born at <35 weeks' gestational age be monitored for apnea.[27] The duration of monitoring depends on the gestational age at birth. Heart rate should be monitored in addition to or instead of respiratory movements, because impedance monitors cannot reliably differentiate normal breathing from obstructed efforts.[28] The role of continuous pulse oximetry for all premature infants diagnosed with, or at risk for, apnea is unclear. In a study in which oximetry was used in addition to standard cardiorespiratory monitoring of seemingly well, convalescent, preterm infants, 10% of these infants experienced prolonged episodes of hypoxemia without associated bradycardia or prolonged apnea.[29] However, many units do not routinely use pulse oximeters as standard monitoring for infants without a supplemental oxygen requirement.

A thorough investigation for an underlying cause should be undertaken after a premature infant has severe or recurrent apneic episodes (Tables 2B-2 and 2B-3). The extent of the evaluation requires clinical judgment and depends on the clinical status of the infant and the timing and severity of the spells. Only after specific pathophysiologic disorders that can precipitate apnea have been excluded should the apneic episodes be considered idiopathic. In contrast, apnea in term infants is never normal, and a serious identifiable cause usually can be found.

A number of therapeutic options for apnea of prematurity are available to the clinician. If an underlying cause is identified, specific therapy should be instituted. Anticipatory care to avoid triggering reflexes known to precipitate apnea, such as extreme neck flexion or deep pharyngeal suctioning, is advisable. In many infants, intermittent tactile stimulation alone, such as rubbing the

Table 2B-2 Evaluation of Infant with Apnea

History	Physical Examination
Maternal	Lethargy or irritability
Labor and delivery	Cyanosis or pallor
Neonatal	Peripheral perfusion
	Abnormal movements/tone
	Respiratory distress
	Assessment of gestational age

Table 2B-3 Laboratory Evaluation of Apnea

Potential Cause	Evaluation
Infection	Complete blood cell count Cultures (blood, cerebrospinal fluid, urine)
Impaired oxygenation	Arterial blood gas, oximeter
Respiratory distress	Chest radiograph
Metabolic disorders	Glucose, calcium, electrolyte levels
Drugs	Toxic screen, magnesium level
Intracranial pathology	Cranial ultrasound, computed tomographic scan
Seizures	Electroencephalogram

back or feet, may be sufficient to interrupt occasional apneic spells. In infants who have frequent apneic spells or require vigorous stimulation or bag-and-mask ventilation for resuscitation, additional therapy usually is begun. Pharmacologic therapy with the methylxanthines (theophylline and caffeine) is effective in reducing the frequency of apneic spells in most premature infants.[30,31] The methylxanthines act by a central stimulatory effect, thought to be mediated by a rise in brainstem levels of cyclic adenosine monophosphate (cAMP). They also are antagonistic to the inhibitory effects on breathing of the neuromodulator adenosine[32] and may increase diaphragmatic contractility.[33] Pharmacologic therapy with the methylxanthines does not replace the need to continuously monitor the premature infant with apnea.

Aminophylline administered intravenously or theophylline given orally are the drugs most commonly used. They are given as an initial loading dose of 5 to 6 mg/kg, followed by 6 mg/kg/day divided every 6 or 8 hours. Adequate therapeutic plasma levels range from 5 to 12 μg/mL; few infants demonstrate an additional response at higher levels.[34] Frequent monitoring of plasma levels is essential with the methylxanthines because metabolism may be unpredictable in premature infants. Toxicity, which includes jitteriness, tachycardia, and gastrointestinal distress, is directly related to plasma levels. No long-term toxicity has been documented with methylxanthine use in premature infants, although this remains poorly studied and is the subject of an ongoing multicenter trial.

Caffeine may have less cardiovascular toxicity than theophylline in premature infants.[31] Caffeine citrate can be given as a loading dose of 20 mg/kg either intravenously or orally, followed by 5 to 7 mg/kg once daily starting 24 hours after the loading dose. Serum levels should be maintained between 10 to 15 μg/mL. Doxapram, a potent respiratory stimulant, is used in some units, although its use as a pharmacologic agent to help control apnea in infants who do not respond to the methylxanthines remains investigational.[35,36]

Although data suggest that little, if any, relationship exists between gastroesophageal reflux and apnea of prematurity, antireflux medications often are prescribed for infants with apnea. However, in one retrospective study, no improvement in apnea was seen after institution of cisapride or metoclopramide therapy.[37] It is doubtful that these medications have any role in the routine management of recurrent apnea.

Apnea in convalescent premature infants may be related to anemia of prematurity. However, results of studies attempting to correlate specific hematocrit levels to the frequency of apnea and bradycardias are inconclusive. Nevertheless, blood transfusions to correct anemia have been a conventional component of therapy for apnea. Data on the response of apnea of prematurity to packed red blood cell transfusions are sparse as well. Blood transfusions may lead to improvement in the frequency of apnea in small premature infants, but the effect appears to be short-lived.[38] Several studies have been unable to demonstrate a reduction in prolonged apneic spells after transfusions, although occurrences of periodic breathing and short apnea episodes (5–15 seconds) may be reduced.[38-40] The potential benefits and risks of blood transfusions should be weighed in individual infants.

In infants receiving methylxanthine therapy who continue to have apneic spells, a trial of nasal continuous positive airway pressure (CPAP) at 2 to 5 cm H_2O may be useful. In the laboratory, CPAP reduces the incidence of obstructive but not central apnea in premature infants.[41] The additional airway care required with CPAP and the frequent feeding difficulties encountered limit long-term CPAP use in some patients. Some infants with severe or very frequent apnea spells, particularly very-low-birth-weight infants, may fail to sustain effective breathing despite such therapy and require endotracheal intubation and mechanical ventilation.

Persistent Apnea and Home Monitoring

Most premature infants become free of apnea by 35 to 37 weeks' postmenstrual age and no longer require therapy or monitoring.[7] However, in extremely premature infants, apnea frequently persists beyond term gestation. A significant proportion of infants delivered between 24 and 28 weeks continue to have recurrent apneic spells beyond 40 weeks' postmenstrual age, especially those diagnosed with chronic lung disease.[42] Usually further evaluation of these infants is not necessary unless their apnea persists beyond 42 to 43 weeks' postmenstrual age.

In general, consideration should be given to discontinuation of methylxanthine therapy when infants reach 33 to 34 weeks' postmenstrual age and are not experiencing frequent or severe apneic episodes. Therapy for persistent idiopathic apnea in infants remains controversial. Because all premature infants eventually develop cardiorespiratory maturity, continued hospitalization for monitoring may be the best approach in most cases, especially if persistent episodes require caretaker intervention. Continued use of methylxanthines may control persistent apnea in infants whose spells recur when the drug is discontinued. For patients discharged on methylxanthine therapy, caffeine is preferred because of its longer half-life. With adjustments for weight gain while undergoing therapy, determinations of blood caffeine levels rarely are indicated (Figure 2B-2 shows a possible

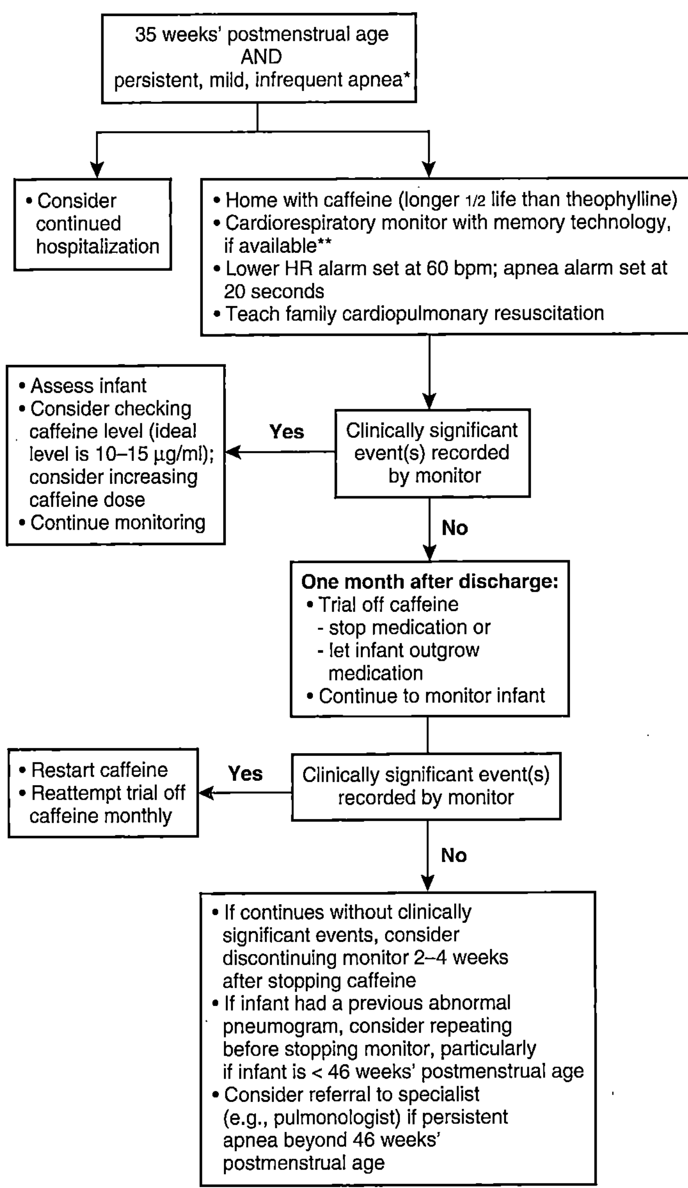

FIGURE 2B-2 *An apneic spell is defined as the cessation of airflow for >20 seconds or interruption of breathing for <20 seconds accompanied by HR < 100 beats/minute or cyanosis.
**Educate family that home monitoring does not prevent Sudden Infant Death Syndrome (SIDS) or Apparent Life Threatening Events (ALTEs).
Please note that this is a recommended algorithm that does not represent a professional standard of care; care should be revised to meet individual patient needs.

algorithm for discharging a premature infant with apnea). A trial off therapy should be performed monthly while the infant is monitored at home; if no clinically significant events occur in the 2 to 4 weeks after discontinuation of caffeine, then consideration should be given to stopping the home monitor.

Common sense dictates that some interval pass between the last documented apnea and discharge to home. Most neonatologists recommend an apnea-free period of 5 to 7 days, although this approach is based more on cumulative clinical experience than on systematic study.[42-44] Using this approach, the vast majority of premature infants can be sent home without pharmacologic therapy or a home monitor. Recordings of impedance pneumography and electrocardiograms ("pneumograms") can be used to document the occurrence of apnea during the recording period if the incidence cannot be determined using standard monitoring in the newborn intensive care unit. However, routine use of predischarge pneumograms in convalescent preterm infants should be discouraged. The significance of episodes of apnea or periodic breathing on pneumogram recordings that are not detected clinically remains uncertain, and they do not predict the risk of subsequent apnea.[45,46] Furthermore, apnea of prematurity is not an independent risk factor for sudden infant death syndrome (SIDS) or for apnea of infancy.[46,47]

Some centers routinely use home cardiorespiratory monitoring for infants with persistent apnea who are otherwise ready for discharge, as well as for those discharged home after discontinuation of methylxanthine therapy or with an abnormal pneumogram. At this time, few data are available on the effectiveness of home monitoring programs in these infants.[45,47] No evidence indicates that home apnea monitoring reduces the number of deaths from SIDS or the number of apparent life-threatening events (ALTEs) in any monitored population. Home monitor use at discharge in premature infants appears to be dependent more on physician preference than on medical indication and does not lead to earlier discharge.[48] In a large study of preterm infants monitored at home after discharge, although some infants had significant apneic events monitored at home, the occurrence of these events did not predict risk of ALTEs or SIDS. In this study, almost all infants ceased having significant apnea by 43 weeks' postmenstrual age.[49]

Because data supporting home monitor use are not available, the devices should not be routinely prescribed for healthy preterm infants with a history of apnea of prematurity. However, they may be useful in isolated circumstances, such as infants with persistent apnea being discharged home on methylxanthine therapy or infants with isolated, infrequent minor apnea/bradycardia events. If a home monitor is being used, both heart rate and respiratory rate should be recorded; in general, continuous monitoring of oxygen saturation in this population is impractical. Newer "memory" technology, which allows clinicians to download recorded events, always should be used if a home monitor is prescribed. Such recordings allow the clinician to determine if alarms reported by the parents are artifact or clinically relevant. In most circumstances, home monitors should be discontinued at approximately 43 to 46 weeks' postmenstrual age or in older infants after 1 month without clinically relevant events.

REFERENCES

1. von Euler C: On the central pattern generator for the basic breathing rhythmicity. *J Appl Physiol* 55:1647, 1983.
2. Glotzbach SF, Baldwin RB, Lederer NE et al: Periodic breathing in preterm infants: incidence and characteristics. *Pediatrics* 84:785, 1989.
3. Barrington KJ, Finer NN: Periodic breathing and apnea in preterm infants. *Pediatr Res* 27:118, 1990.
4. Barrington KJ, Finer NN, Wilkinson MH: Progressive shortening of the periodic breathing cycle duration in normal infants. *Pediatr Res* 21:247, 1987.
5. Hiatt IM, Hegyi T, Indyk L, et al: Continuous monitoring of PO_2 during apnea of prematurity. *J Pediatr* 98:288, 1988.
6. Poets CF, Stebbens VA, Samuels MP, et al: The relationship between bradycardia, apnea, and hypoxemia in preterm infants. *Pediatr Res* 34:144, 1993.
7. Henderson-Smart DJ: The effect of gestational age on the incidence and duration of recurrent apnoea in newborn babies. *Aust Paediatr J* 17:273, 1981.
8. Henderson-Smart DJ, Pettigrew AG, Campbell DJ: Clinical apnea and brainstem neural function in preterm infants. *N Engl J Med* 308:353, 1983.
9. Lagercrantz H: Neuromodulators and respiratory control in the infant. *Clin Perinatol* 14:683, 1987.
10. Moss IR, Inman JG: Neurochemicals and respiratory control during development. *J Appl Physiol* 67:1, 1989.
11. Eichenwald EC, Stark AR: Respiratory motor output: effect of state and maturation in early life. In Haddad GG, Farber JP, editors: *Developmental neurobiology of breathing*. New York, 1991, Marcel Dekker.
12. Gabriel M, Albani M, Schulte FJ: Apneic spells and sleep states in preterm infants. *Pediatrics* 57:142, 1976.
13. Heldt GP, McIlroy MB: Distortion of the chest wall and work of diaphragm in preterm infants. *J Appl Physiol* 62:164, 1987.
14. Muller N, Gulston G, Cade D, et al: Diaphragmatic muscle fatigue in the newborn. *J Appl Physiol* 46:688, 1979.
15. Hagan R, Bryan AC, Bryan MH, et al: Neonatal chest wall afferents and regulation of respiration. *J Appl Physiol* 42:362, 1977.
16. Gerhardt T, Bancalari E: Apnea of prematurity. I. Lung function and regulation of breathing. *Pediatrics* 74:58, 1984.
17. Sankaran K, Wiebe H, Seshia MM, et al: Immediate and late ventilatory response to high and low O_2 in preterm infants and adult subjects. *Pediatr Res* 13:875, 1979.
18. Butcher-Puech MC, Henderston-Smart DJ, Holley D, et al: Relation between apnea duration and type and neurological status of preterm infants. *Arch Dis Child* 66:953, 1985.
19. Mathew OP, Roberts JL, Thach BT: Pharyngeal airway obstruction in preterm infants during mixed and obstructive apnea. *J Pediatr* 100:964, 1982.
20. Thach BT, Stark AP: Spontaneous neck flexion and airway obstruction during apneic spells in preterm infants. *J Pediatr* 94:275, 1979.

21. Gauda EB, Miller MJ, Carlo WA, et al: Genioglossus response to airway occlusion in apneic versus nonapneic infants. *Pediatr Res* 22:683, 1987.
22. Pickens DL, Schefft G, Thach BT: Prolonged apnea associated with upper airway protective reflexes in apnea of prematurity. *Am Rev Respir Dis* 137:113, 1988.
23. Martin RJ, Miller MJ, Carlo WA: Pathogenesis of apnea in preterm infants. *J Pediatr* 109:733, 1986.
24. Barrington KJ, Tan K, Rich W: Apnea at discharge and gastroesophageal reflux in the preterm infant. *J Perinatal* 22:8, 2002.
25. Arad-Cohen N, Cohen A, Tirosh E: The relationship between gastroesophageal reflux and apnea in infants. *J Pediatr* 137:321, 2000.
26. Krane EJ, Haberkern CM, Jacobson LE: Postoperative apnea, bradycardia, and oxygen desaturation in formerly premature infants: prospective comparison of spinal and general anesthesia. *Anesth Analg* 80:7, 1995.
27. Stark AR: Apnea. In Cloherty JP, Eichenwald EC, Stark AR, editors: *Manual of neonatal care*, ed 5. Philadelphia, 2004, Lippincott-Williams.
28. Warbuton D, Stark AR, Taeusch HW: Apnea monitor failure in infants with upper airway obstruction. *Pediatrics* 60:742, 1977.
29. Poets CF, Stebbens VA, Richard D, et al: Prolonged episodes of hypoxemia in preterm infants undetectable by cardiorespiratory monitoring. *Pediatrics* 95:860, 1995.
30. Shannon DC, Gotay F, Stein IM, et al: Prevention of apnea and bradycardia in low-birth weight infants. *Pediatrics* 55:589, 1975.
31. Aranda JV, Gorman W, Bergsteinsson, et al: Efficacy of caffeine in treatment of apnea in the low-birth-weight infant. *J Pediatr* 90:467, 1977.
32. Lagercrantz H, Yamamoto Y, Fredholm, et al: Adenosine analogues depress ventilation in rabbit neonates. Theophylline stimulation of respiration via adenosine receptors? *Pediatr Res* 18:387, 1984.
33. Murciano D, Aubier M, Lecocguic Y, et al: Effects of theophylline on diaphragmatic strength and fatigue in patients with chronic obstructive pulmonary disease. *N Engl J Med* 311:349, 1984.
34. Muttitt SC, Tierney AJ, Finer NN: The dose response of theophylline in the treatment of apnea of prematurity. *J Pediatr* 112:115, 1988.
35. Barrington KJ, Finer NN, Peters KL, et al: Physiologic effects of doxapram in idiopathic apnea of prematurity. *J Pediatr* 108:125, 1986.
36. Barrington KJ, Finer NN, Torok-Both G, et al: Dose-response relationship of doxapram in the therapy of refractory idiopathic apnea of prematurity. *Pediatrics* 80:22, 1987.
37. Kimball AL, Carlton DP: Gastroesophageal reflux medications in the treatment of apnea of prematurity. *J Pediatr* 138:355, 2001.
38. Joshi A, Gerhardt T, Shandloff P, et al: Blood transfusion effect on respiratory pattern of preterm infants. *Pediatrics* 80:79, 1987.
39. DeMaio JG, Harris MC, Deuber C, et al: Effect of blood transfusion on apnea frequency in growing premature infants. *J Pediatr* 114:1039, 1989.
40. Keyes WG, Donohue PK, Spivak JL, et al: Assessing the need for transfusion of premature infants and role of hematocrit, clinical signs, and erythropoietin level. *Pediatrics* 84:412, 1989.
41. Miller MJ, Carlo WA, Martin RJ: Continuous positive pressure selectively reduces obstructive apnea in preterm infants. *J Pediatr* 106:91, 1985.
42. Eichenwald EC, Aina A, Stark AR: Apnea frequently persists beyond term gestation in infants delivered at 24 to 28 weeks. *Pediatrics* 100:354, 1997.
43. Eichenwald EC, Blackwell M, Lloyd JS, et al: Inter-neonatal intensive care unit variation in discharge timing: influence of apnea and feeding management. *Pediatrics* 108:928, 2001.
44. Darnall RA, Kattwinkel J, Nattie C, et al: Margin of safety for discharge after apnea in preterm infants. *Pediatrics* 100:795, 1997.
45. Rosen CL, Glaze DG, Frost JD: Home monitor follow-up of persistent apnea and bradycardia in preterm infants. *Am J Dis Child* 140:547, 1986.
46. Southall DP, Richards JM, Rhoden KJ, et al: Prolonged apnea and cardiac arrhythmias in infants discharged from neonatal intensive care units: failure to predict an increased risk for sudden infant death syndrome. *Pediatrics* 70:844, 1982.
47. Committee on Fetus and Newborn: Apnea, sudden infant death syndrome, and home monitoring. *Pediatrics* 111:914, 2003.
48. Perfect-Sychowski SP, Dodd E, Thomas P: Home apnea monitor use in preterm infants discharged from newborn intensive care units. *J Pediatr* 139:245, 2001.
49. Ramanathan R, Corwin, MJ, Hunt CE et al: Cardiorespiratory events recorded on home monitors: comparison of healthy infants with those at increased risk for SIDS. *JAMA* 285:2199, 2001.

Use of Immunoprophylaxis for Prevention of Severe Respiratory Syncytial Virus Bronchiolitis

J.S. Lloyd, MD

Respiratory syncytial virus (RSV) bronchiolitis is a common and potentially life-threatening infection in children younger than 2 years and nationally accounts for approximately 90,000 hospitalizations and 4500 deaths per year.[1-3] Nearly every child in the United States becomes infected with RSV in their first 2 years of life, and up to 2% of these children require hospitalization.[4]

Young children and infants whose medical histories have been complicated by prematurity, congenital heart disease (CHD), bronchopulmonary dysplasia (BPD), pulmonary hypertension, or immune deficiency are at greatest risk for severe or fatal RSV infection.[5-9] In this vulnerable pediatric population, the likelihood of being hospitalized with RSV bronchiolitis rises to nearly 20%,[10] with infants younger than 1 year at greatest risk for dying of RSV.[11]

Epidemiology

RSV infections follow a seasonal pattern, which typically lasts from November to March. The timing and severity of this 5-month "RSV season" varies from year to year and is characterized by a peak incidence of infection in January and February. RSV infections, clinically indistinguishable from those of influenza, adenovirus, or rhinovirus, often present as a "common cold." However, in the youngest infants RSV infections develop into a serious lower respiratory tract disease known as *bronchiolitis.*

Because of the antigenic variability of RSV, different strains of the virus may coexist within a given season and vary from one RSV season to another. Consequently, an infected individual may develop only partial immunity to the virus and remain susceptible to RSV in subsequent seasons. In general, the first infection is the most severe, with severity decreasing over time.[12]

Because RSV is found in oral and nasal secretions, it is easily transmitted from one individual to another. Close physical proximity plays a significant role in transmission. Several risk factors increase the risk for RSV infection: crowded living situations, day care centers, toddler siblings, and environmental pollutants (e.g., tobacco smoke).[12] In fact, it is not uncommon to find that 100% of the children in a busy day care center develop an RSV infection following exposure to an index case.[13]

The Viral Genome

RSV is a 120- to 300-nm enveloped single-strand RNA paramyxovirus made up of 11 proteins. Two of these proteins—glycoproteins G and F—are clinically significant. Glycoprotein G confers both genetic variability and infectivity to the virus by attaching to the airway epithelium. It is this portion of the virus that allows different strains to develop in a given RSV season. Glycoprotein F produces the characteristic syncytial formations in respiratory epithelium by causing infected respiratory cells to fuse with healthy cells in the respiratory tract.

This portion of the viral genome is well conserved, thus making the glycoprotein F an ideal target for antibody prophylaxis.[14]

Transmission and Prevention

RSV is transmitted by both direct and indirect means. *Direct transmission* occurs when noninfected individuals inhale RSV-laden respiratory droplets generated by the cough or sneeze of an infected person. *Indirect transmission* occurs when contaminated fomites, such as infected hands, utensils, or toys, come into contact with the mucosal surfaces (e.g., mouth, nose, eyes) of a noninfected person.

RSV is stable in the environment for only a few hours and is readily controlled with simple measures such as soap, water, and disinfectants. Prevention programs are based on fundamental principles of good handwashing, limiting exposure to infected persons, and educating children on the importance of covering their mouths and noses when coughing or sneezing. Unfortunately, excluding children with cold symptoms is not an effective infection control measure because the transmission of RSV often occurs in the asymptomatic phase of RSV infection.[4]

Strict adherence to universal contact precautions by healthcare workers remains the most effective means of controlling nosocomial infections.[15] If an RSV outbreak is documented in a high-risk unit, control measures should focus on cohorting and isolating the infected patient. Every effort should be made to prevent the admission of a noninfected high-risk infant to a hospital floor with known RSV-positive patients. No recommendations have been made by either the Centers for Disease Control and Prevention (CDC) or the American Academy of Pediatrics (AAP) regarding the use of immunoprophylaxis in preventing nosocomial RSV disease.[14]

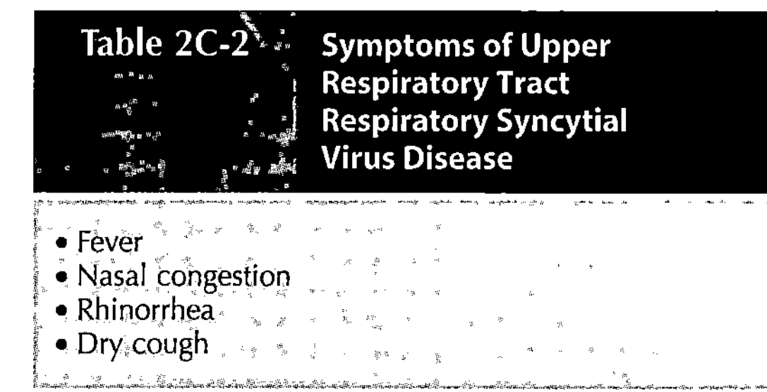

Table 2C-2 Symptoms of Upper Respiratory Tract Respiratory Syncytial Virus Disease

- Fever
- Nasal congestion
- Rhinorrhea
- Dry cough

Anticipatory guidance for parents plays an important role in limiting exposure and transmission of RSV to their high-risk infants. Many neonatal intensive care units (NICUs) offer classes and provide educational material regarding RSV infection prior to discharge from the NICU (Table 2C-1).

Infection with RSV

An incubation period of 2 to 8 days follows inoculation of the mucosal surfaces by the RSV virus. During this time, the virus replicates in the nasopharyngeal epithelium, causing common clinical symptoms of fever, rhinorrhea, cough, and nasal congestion (Table 2C-2).

RSV spreads either by direct extension or by migration of infected macrophages to the distal airways,[16] resulting in lower airway disease and symptoms of bronchiolitis: hypoxia, tachypnea, retractions, coughing, and wheezing (Table 2C-3). The chest radiograph of a child with bronchiolitis is typified by hyperinflation with perihilar infiltrates, peribronchial wall thickening, and patchy atelectasis. Lobar, segmental, and subsegmental pneumonia also may be found.

Apnea complicates RSV bronchiolitis in up to 20% of hospitalized infants younger than 2 months.[16] Apnea may be the only presenting symptom of RSV infection in the infant and is most common in the

Table 2C-1 Anticipatory Guidance for Parents of High-Risk Infants

- Review importance of thorough handwashing
- Educate parents on techniques for cleaning countertop surfaces and toys with soap, water, and disinfectants
- Review the importance of proper "respiratory etiquette" with parents: cover mouth/nose during sneeze or cough, then wash hands
- Encourage parents to teach handwashing and respiratory etiquette to their other children
- Encourage limiting exposure of infants to all crowds and to persons with respiratory infections
- Provide educational material on RSV prevention and transmission prior to and during the RSV season

RSV, Respiratory syncytial virus.

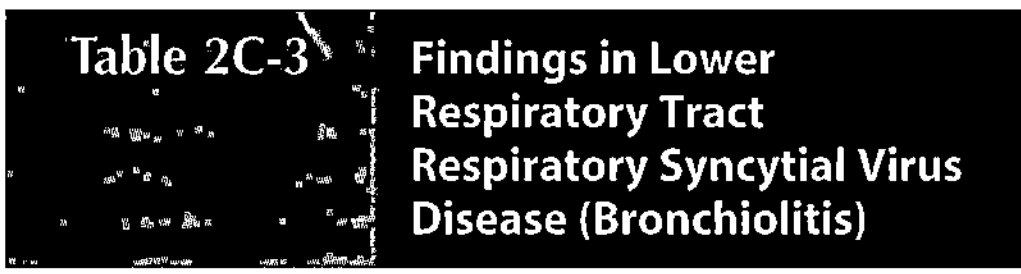

Table 2C-3 Findings in Lower Respiratory Tract Respiratory Syncytial Virus Disease (Bronchiolitis)

- Tachypnea
- Retractions (mild: intercostals; moderate to severe: subcostal, supraclavicular)
- Congested cough
- Wheezing (expiratory > inspiratory)
- Prolonged expiratory phase
- Apnea (most common in infants <2 months old)
- Hypoxia
- Chest radiograph: hyperinflation with perihilar infiltrates, peribronchial wall thickening, patchy atelectasis

Table 2C-4 Patients at Increased Risk for Apnea

- History of prematurity
- Prior history of apnea of prematurity
- Respiratory syncytial virus infection at ≤2 months' corrected gestational age

former premature infant with a history of apnea of prematurity (Table 2C-4).

An RSV infection in the bronchiole tree causes necrosis, mucosal inflammation, sloughing of the epithelium, microvascular leak, edema, and increased mucus production. These pathologic changes result in small airway obstruction producing the prolonged expiratory phase and wheezing characteristic, especially in small infants, of RSV bronchiolitis. In autopsies of fatal cases of bronchiolitis, pathologists have noted a pattern of predominantly peribronchial lymphocytic infiltrations.[16,17]

The likelihood of an infant's RSV infection progressing from an upper respiratory infection to that of bronchiolitis is based on the severity of the presenting clinical signs and the infant's medical history. The degree of hypoxia and respiratory distress in conjunction with a history of prematurity and a postnatal age ≤6 months increases the infant's risk of developing bronchiolitis (Table 2C-5).[16] The single best predictor of severe disease is an initial pulse oximetry reading <95% in room air.[16]

Although viral pneumonia is the best recognized complication of RSV infection, uncommon manifestations such as meningitis, ataxia, myelitis, myocarditis, and third-degree heart block have been documented (Table 2C-6).[16] Acute otitis media is a common finding in infants diagnosed with RSV and other viral infections.[18,19]

Infants at increased risk for respiratory failure from an RSV infection often have a premorbid diagnosis of extreme prematurity (≤28 weeks' gestation), extremely low birth weight ≤750 g, BPD, immunodeficiency, neuromuscular compromise, or hemodynamically significant CHD (Table 2C-7).[5-9]

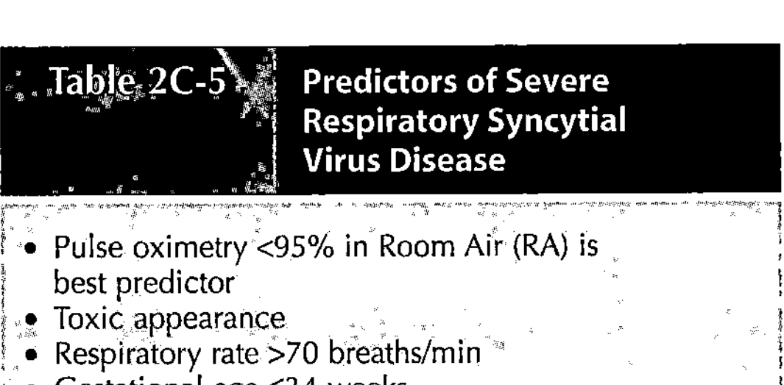
Table 2C-5 Predictors of Severe Respiratory Syncytial Virus Disease

- Pulse oximetry <95% in Room Air (RA) is best predictor
- Toxic appearance
- Respiratory rate >70 breaths/min
- Gestational age ≤34 weeks
- Postnatal age ≤6 months

Table 2C-6 Unusual Manifestations of Respiratory Syncytial Virus Infection

- Meningitis
- Ataxia
- Myocarditis
- Myelitis
- Third-degree heart block

Diagnosis of RSV Infection

An understanding of the epidemiology and symptomotology of RSV infection allows for a presumptive diagnosis in the outpatient setting. However, a definitive diagnosis is generally preferred for the inpatient setting, as the presence of RSV-positive patients will impact on the care of other hospitalized patients.

Large quantities of RSV are found in the respiratory droplets of infected individuals, thus making nasal secretions an ideal specimen for diagnostic testing. Although culture of the nasal washings for the virion provides a definitive diagnosis, direct immunofluorescence or enzyme-linked immunoabsorbent assays have become the preferred techniques because they provide results within a few hours. These latter techniques are reliable and accurate and offer 80% to 95% specificity and sensitivity for the presence of RSV.[20]

Development of Immune Prophylaxis

In light of the significant morbidity and mortality of RSV in the high-risk infant population, immunologic prophylaxis became a clinical priority in the 1980s.[21] Attention was placed on developing a vaccine for RSV, and in 1996 the Food and Drug Administration (FDA) approved the intravenous polyclonal antibody RSV immune globulin (RSV-IGIV; RespiGam).

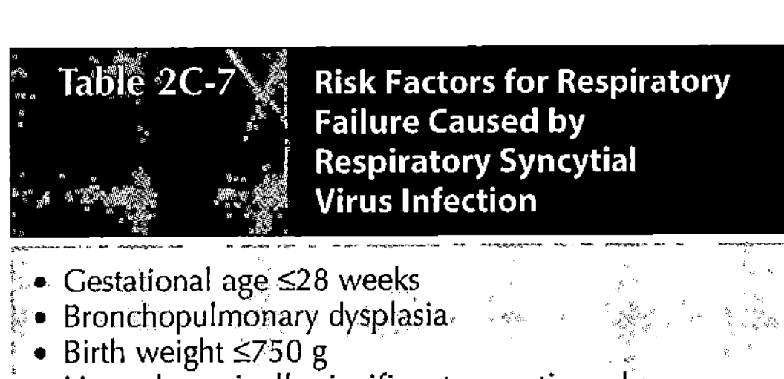
Table 2C-7 Risk Factors for Respiratory Failure Caused by Respiratory Syncytial Virus Infection

- Gestational age ≤28 weeks
- Bronchopulmonary dysplasia
- Birth weight ≤750 g
- Hemodynamically significant cyanotic and acyanotic heart disease
- Immune deficiency
- Neuromuscular disease
- Cystic fibrosis

Clinical Trials Involving RSV-IGIV

A number of large randomized clinical trials have looked at the safety and efficacy of RSV-IGIV as immunoprophylaxis for RSV infection. In 1993, Groothius et al.[22] reported the results of a multicenter, randomized controlled trial in which children younger than 4 years with underlying BPD, CHD, or a history of prematurity (≤35 weeks' gestation) were randomized to receive five monthly low-dose RSV-IGIV infusions (150 mg/kg), high-dose RSV-IGIV infusions (750 mg/kg), or no RSV-IGIV. Results showed that infants who received five monthly 750 mg/kg low doses of RSV-IGIV had significantly fewer hospital admissions, less severe lower respiratory tract disease, and fewer intensive care days (Table 2C-8). Patients with a history of prematurity and BPD were found to benefit most. Adverse reactions were considered mild and included decreased oxygen saturation, evidence of fluid overload, and fever.

A second multicenter, randomized placebo-controlled clinical trial was undertaken by the PREVENT study group.[23] In this study, 510 infants younger than 24 months with BPD and/or a history of prematurity were randomized to receive either 750 mg/kg RSV-IGIV or placebo (1% albumin) once per month during the RSV season in 1994 to 1995. Outcome measures included the number of (1) RSV hospitalizations, (2) RSV-related hospital days, and (3) days receiving supplemental oxygen. The incidence of all outcome measures was decreased in the group that received RSV-IGIV (Table 2C-9).[23]

The PREVENT study also suggested that infants and children with BPD derived a greater benefit from RSV-IGIV than did infants with a history of prematurity alone.[21] Additional clinical findings included a decreased rate of hospitalizations for respiratory illness from any cause and fewer concomitant episodes of acute otitis media.[24]

Table 2C-8 Clinical Trial Results Comparing RSV-IGIV with Placebo

Outcome Measure	Decrease (%)	p Value
Hospitalizations	63	.02
Respiratory disease score	32	.01
Total intensive care unit days per 100 children	97	.05

Modified from: Groothius JR, Simoes EA, Levin MJ, et al: *N Engl J Med* 329:1524-1530, 1993. *RSV-IGIV*, Respiratory syncytial virus immune globulin intravenous.

Table 2C-9 The PREVENT Study: Clinical Trial Results Comparing RSV-IGIV with Placebo (1% Albumin)

Outcome Measure	Decrease (%)	p Value
RSV hospitalizations	41	.047
RSV hospital days per 100 patients	53	.045
RSV hospital days receiving oxygen per 100 patients	60	.007

Modified from: The PREVENT Study Group: *Pediatrics* 99:93-97, 1997.
RSV, Respiratory syncytial virus; *RSV-IGIV*, respiratory syncytial virus immune globulin intravenous.

Clinical Trials Involving Palivizumab

In 1998 the FDA approved palivizumab (Synagis), the first monoclonal antibody developed into a vaccine, for use as immunoprophylaxis for children ≤2 years at risk for severe RSV infection.

One large multicenter clinical trial, conducted at 139 centers in the United States, Canada, and the United Kingdom during the 1996 to 1997 RSV season, demonstrated the efficacy and safety of palivizumab in premature, high-risk infants and children.[25]

In this Impact-RSV study, 1502 children younger than 2 years with a diagnosis of BPD (requiring continuing medical therapy) or former preterm infants (≤35 weeks' gestation) younger than 6 months were randomized to receive five monthly intramuscular (IM) injections of either palivizumab (15 mg/kg) or placebo at the onset of the RSV season. The results demonstrated that immunoprophylaxis with palivizumab decreased RSV hospitalizations by 55% compared with the placebo-controlled group. Not surprisingly, premature children without BPD showed the largest decrease in rates of hospitalizations compared with infants having BPD (78% vs 39%). Additional study endpoints included: number of hospital days (proxy for severity of illness), number of days requiring supplemental oxygen, and number of intensive care unit (ICU) admissions (Table 2C-10).[25]

Immunoprophylaxis of Infants and Children with CHD

From 1998 to 2002, investigators enrolled 1287 infants with hemodynamically significant CHD

Table 2C-10 Clinical Trial Results Comparing Palivizumab with Placebo

Outcome Measure	Decrease (%)	*p* Value
RSV hospitalizations	55	<.001
With BPD	39	.038
Premature without BPD	78	<.001
RSV hospital days receiving oxygen per 100 children	40	<.001
RSV intensive care unit admissions	57	.026

From: The Impact-RSV Study Group: *Pediatrics* 102:531-537, 1998.
BPD, Bronchopulmonary dysplasia; *RSV*, respiratory syncytial virus.

Table 2C-11 RSV Prophylaxis of Infants and Children with Congestive Heart Disease Comparing Palivizumab with Placebo

Outcome Measure	Decrease (%)	*p* Value
RSV-related hospitalization	45	.003
Total days of RSV-associated hospitalization per 100 children	56	.003
Total RSV-associated hospital days with supplemental oxygen per 100 children	73	.014

From: Feltes TM, Cabala AK, Meisner HC, et al: *J Pediatr* 143:532-540, 2003.
RSV, Respiratory syncytial virus.

into a double-blind, placebo-controlled clinical trial and randomized them to receive either palivizumab or placebo.[26] The subjects were stratified at study entry to cyanotic or acyanotic heart disease. The results demonstrated that infants who received palivizumab had a 45% decrease in RSV-related hospitalizations and a 73% decrease in the total number of RSV-related hospital days requiring supplemental oxygen per 100 children compared with the placebo group (Table 2C-11). There was no statistical difference in the number of adverse events between the two groups. This study concluded that palivizumab was a safe and effective means for providing RSV immunoprophylaxis for infants and children with hemodynamically significant CHD.[26]

The results of these various clinical trials helped to prove that immunoprophylaxis is safe and effective in decreasing the incidence of hospitalization attributable to RSV infections in high-risk infants and children. No studies have been undertaken to compare the relative efficacy of the two immunoprophylactic agents.

It is important to note that none of these clinical studies showed a decrease in the incidence of RSV infection.

Comparison of RSV-IGIV and Palivizumab

Although both RSV-IGIV and palivizumab have proved effective in the immunoprophylaxis of infants and children at risk for RSV bronchiolitis, RSV-IGIV has a number of clinical shortcomings: (1) it is administered intravenously, (2) the required 4-hour infusion is time consuming for both healthcare workers and parents, (3) it is a blood product, (4) it is contraindicated for infants with CHD, and (5) it represents a fluid challenge for infants with BPD.

Palivizumab, as an IM injection, has largely supplanted RSV-IGIV because it is easy to administer. Palivizumab, like RSV-IGIV, is administered monthly during the typical 5-month RSV season from November to March. Additional differences between palivizumab and RSV-IGIV are summarized in Table 2C-12.

Table 2C-12 Comparison of RSV-IGIV with Palivizumab

Characteristics	RSV-IGIV (RespiGam)	Palivizumab (Synagis)
Type of immunoglobulin	Polyclonal	Monoclonal
Method of administration	Intravenous	Intramuscular
May be administered to infants with hemodynamically significant congestive heart disease	No	Yes
Protects against other viral infections	Yes	No
Associated with decreased incidence of acute otitis media	Yes	No
Risk of fluid overload in infants with bronchopulmonary dysplasia	Yes	No
Blood product	Yes	No
Interferes with routine childhood immunization schedule	Yes	No
Dosage	750 mg/kg/dose	15 mg/kg/dose
Dosing interval	Monthly	Monthly
No. doses per "RSV season"	5	5

RSV, Respiratory syncytial virus; *RSV-IGIV*, respiratory syncytial virus immune globulin intravenous.

Table 2C-13 Risk Factors for Rehospitalization of a Preterm Infant

- Gestational age ≤32 weeks
- Discharge from NICU <3 months before start of "RSV season"
- Need for ≥28 days of supplemental oxygen during stay in neonatal intensive care unit

RSV, Respiratory syncytial virus.

Controversies in RSV Immunoprophylaxis

The primary benefit of RSV immunoprophylaxis is a decreased rate of RSV-related hospitalizations. To date, none of the randomized clinical trials have demonstrated a significant decrease in the rate of mortality attributable to RSV infection in infants who received prophylaxis.

Clinical investigators have noted that although the risk of developing RSV infection in the first year of an infant's life remains high at 40% to 60%, the risk of being hospitalized for RSV is low at 0.5% to 2%.[4] Within the high-risk premature infant group, the overall risk of hospitalization for RSV bronchiolitis increases to 3.2%.[27] The risk of developing severe bronchiolitis requiring hospitalization increases to 25% if that infant has specific risk factors: (1) gestational age ≤32 weeks, (2) discharge from the NICU <3 months before start of "RSV season," and (3) past need for supplemental oxygen ≥28 days during NICU stay (Table 2C-13).[10,27]

Most infants diagnosed with RSV bronchiolitis, however, are appropriate for gestational age, term infants.[11,28] Multiple economic analyses of RSV immunoprophylaxis have not shown offering immunoprophylaxis to all infants at risk for RSV infection to be cost effective.[27,29-31] Joffe et al.[27] studied the at-risk, preterm population and concluded that, for even the most premature infants, the cost of RSV prophylaxis was high relative to the benefits obtained.

For these reasons RSV immunoprophylaxis is recommended for a specific group of high-risk infants and children.

Recommendations for Immunoprophylaxis for RSV Disease

Based on an analysis of the risks and benefits of immunoprophylaxis, the CDC and the AAP have concluded that immunoprophylaxis is most appropriate for a select subgroup of infants. Their 1998 recommendations for RSV immunoprophylaxis were revised in 2003 to reflect the addition of palivizumab (Synagis) to the therapeutic options[13] (Table 2C-14). Additional updates can be found at the following websites: *http://www.cdc.gov/* and *http://www.aap.org/*.

Table 2C-14 Summary of 2003 Recommendations by the American Academy of Pediatrics (AAP) for Use of Immunoprophylaxis in RSV Infection*

Without BPD†	With BPD†
FORMER PREMATURE INFANTS	**IRRESPECTIVE OF PREMATURITY**
Gestational age ≤28 weeks, who are ≤12 months old at the start of the RSV season Gestational age >28 to ≤32 weeks, who are ≤6 months old at the start of the RSV season Gestational age >32 to ≤35 weeks, who are ≤6 months old at the start of the RSV season AND have two or more of the following risk factors: a. Child care attendance b. School-aged siblings c. Exposure to environmental air pollutants (e.g., tobacco smoke) d. Congenital abnormalities of the airways e. Severe neuromuscular disease	≤12 months old at the start of the 1st RSV season ≤24 months old with persistent signs of BPD* at the start of the second RSV season

*Refer to the AAP web site for updated recommendations.
†Bronchopulmonary dysplasia (BPD) is defined as use of supplemental oxygen, bronchodilators, diuretics, or corticosteroids within 6 months of the start of the RSV season.
RSV, Respiratory syncytial virus.

Table 2C-14 Summary of 2003 Recommendations by the American Academy of Pediatrics (AAP) for Use of Immunoprophylaxis in RSV Infection—cont'd

INFANTS AND CHILDREN WITH CONGENITAL HEART DISEASE (PALIVIZUMAB ONLY):

At the start of RSV season:
≤12 months old and receiving medications to control congestive heart failure
≤12 months old with either uncorrected or partially corrected cyanotic heart disease who remain cyanotic
≤24 months old with hemodynamically significant cyanotic and acyanotic heart disease
Note: Consider a postoperative dose of palivizumab (15 mg/kg) when patient is medically stable[13]

INFANTS AND CHILDREN WITH PULMONARY HYPERTENSION:

At the start of RSV season:
≤12 months old with moderate pulmonary hypertension
≤24 months old with severe pulmonary hypertension

INFANTS AND CHILDREN NOT CONSIDERED AT RISK FOR SEVERE RSV (IMMUNOPROPHYLAXIS NOT INDICATED):

Infants with nonhemodynamically significant heart disease

1. Atrial septal defect
2. Small ventricular septal defect
3. Pulmonic stenosis
4. Patent ductus arteriosus

Infants with corrected cardiac lesions without cyanosis or congestive heart failure
Infants with mild cardiomyopathy who are not receiving medical therapy

Appendix

ADDITIONAL AAP REMARKS:

- Once a child qualifies for immunoprophylaxis, administration should continue for the remainder of the RSV season, even if the child no longer meets the clinical criteria or age requirement prior to completion of the RSV season.
- Even if a child develops RSV during immunoprophylaxis, he or she should complete the drug course.
- Neither RSV-IGIV nor palivizumab is indicated or licensed for the *treatment* of RSV infection.
- RSV prophylaxis should begin before the onset of the RSV season (November) and terminate at the end of the RSV season (March), allowing for 6 months of protection.
  i. Physicians should consult their local health department for the epidemiology of their local RSV strain.
- All high-risk infants and their contacts should be immunized against influenza beginning at age 6 months.
- There is insufficient information regarding the immunoprophylaxis of infants with cystic fibrosis (CF), severe combined immunodeficiency (SCID), or acquired immunodeficiency syndrome (AIDS). However, these patients may benefit from prophylaxis.
- RSV-IGIV is contraindicated in children with CHD.
- There are no recommendations regarding the administration of palivizumab as a means of preventing nosocomial RSV infection.

INTERFERENCE OF IMMUNOPROPHYLAXIS ON THE ROUTINE CHILDHOOD IMMUNIZATION SCHEDULE:

- RSV-IGIV does interfere with childhood immunization schedules.
  i. The MMR (measles-mumps-rubella (MMR) vaccine should be deferred for 9 month after the last dose of RSV-IGIV.
  ii. The varicella vaccine should be deferred for 9 months after the last dose of RSV-IGIV.
- Palivizumab does not interfere with the routine childhood immunization schedule.

REGARDING RISK FACTORS FOR INFECTION:

- High-risk infants should NEVER be exposed to environmental pollutants (e.g., tobacco smoke).
- High-risk infants should be kept away from crowds and situations where exposure to infected individuals cannot be controlled.
- Participation of high-risk infants in child care should be restricted during the RSV season, whenever feasible.

Conclusion

Targeted immunoprophylaxis of the most vulnerable infants, application of basic infection control measures, and parent education should greatly reduce the incidence of severe RSV disease. Although premature infants with specific risk factors remain at highest risk for hospitalization and death as a result of RSV infection, most infants who develop RSV bronchiolitis are not premature or small for gestational age.

RSV bronchiolitis is an important healthcare issue worldwide, affecting virtually all infants by their second birthday. The development of safe, affordable, and effective vaccines for respiratory viral infections in all infants younger than 2 years would substantially reduce the incidence of childhood disease.[32]

Resources for Families and Clinicians

For recent updates about RSV:

http://www.cdc.gov/
http://www.aap.org/

REFERENCES

1. Hall CB: Respiratory syncytial virus. What we know now. *Contemp Pediatr* November:2-11, 1993.
2. Glezen WP, Taber LH, Frank AL, et al: Risk of primary infection and reinfection with respiratory syncytial virus. *Am J Dis Child* 140:543-546, 1986.
3. Institute of Medicine Committee on Issues and Priorities for New Vaccine Development: Prospects for immunizing against respiratory syncytial virus. In *New vaccine development, establishing priorities.* Washington DC, 1988, 1: 397-409, National Academy of Sciences Press.
4. Respiratory syncytial virus. Available at: *www.cdc./gov/ ncidod/dvrd/revb/respiratory/rsvfeat.htm.*
5. Groothius JR, Guiterrez KM, Lauer BA: Respiratory syncytial virus infection in children with bronchopulmonary dysplasia. *Pediatrics* 82:199-203, 1988.
6. Cunningham CK, McMillan JA, Gross SJ: Rehospitalization for respiratory illness in infants less than 32 weeks gestation. *Pediatrics* 88:527-532, 1991.
7. Ogra PL, Patel JP: Respiratory syncytial virus infection and the immunocompromised host. *Pediatr Infect Dis J* 7: 246-249, 1988
8. MacDonald NE, Hall CB, Suffin SC, et al: Respiratory syncytial virus infection in infants with congenital heart disease. *N Engl J Med* 307:397-400, 1982.
9. Simoes EAF, Sondheimer HM, Top FH Jr, et al: Respiratory syncytial virus immune globulin for prophylaxis against respiratory syncytial virus disease in infants and children with congenital heart disease. The Cardiac Study Group. *J Pediatr* 133:492-499, 1998.
10. Joffe S, Escobar G, Black SB, et al: Rehospitalization for respiratory syncytial virus among premature infants. *Pediatrics* 104:894-899, 1999.
11. Holman RC, Shay DK, Curns AT, et al: Risk factors for bronchiolitis-associated deaths among infants in the United States. *Pediatr Infect Dis J* 22:483-489, 2003.
12. American Academy of Pediatrics Committee on Environment Health: Environmental tobacco smoke: a hazard to children. *Pediatrics* 99:639-642, 1997.
13. Anderson LJ, Parker RA, Strikas RA et al: Day care attendance and hospitalization for lower respiratory tract illness *Pediatrics* 82:300-308, 1988.
14. American Academy of Pediatrics. Committee on Infectious Disease and Committee on Fetus and Newborn: Policy statement. Revised indication for the use of palivizumab and respiratory syncytial virus immune globulin intravenous for the prevention of respiratory syncytial virus infections. *Pediatrics* 112:1442-1446, 2003.
15. CDC MMRW recommendations and reports. Guidelines for prevention of nosocomial pneumonia. 1997;46:1-79. Available at: *www.cdc.gov/epo/mmwr/preview/mmwrhtml/ 00045365.htm.*
16. Hall C: Respiratory syncytial virus. In Feigen RD, Cherry JC, editors: *Textbook of pediatric infectious disease,* ed 4. Philadelphia, 1998, WB Saunders.
17. Mbawuike IN, Wells J, Byrd R, et al: HLA-restricted CD8+ cytotoxic T lymphocyte, interferon-g, and interleukin-4 responses to respiratory syncytial virus infection in infants and children. *J Infect Dis* 183:687-696, 2001.
18. Heikkinen T, Thint M, Chonmaitree T: Prevalence of various respiratory viruses in the middle ear during acute otitis media. *N Engl J Med* 340:260-264, 1999.
19. Pass RF: Respiratory virus infection and otitis media. *Pediatrics* 102:400-401, 1998.
20. American Academy of Pediatrics: *Red book. 2003 report of the Committee on Infectious Diseases,* ed 26. Elk Grove Village, Illinois, 2003, American Academy of Pediatrics.
21. Boyce TG, Mellen BG, Mitchell EF, et al: Rates of hospitalization for respiratory syncytial virus. In *New vaccine development: establishing priorities. Biol I.* Washington, DC, 1986, National Academy Press.
22. Groothius JR, Simoes EA, Levin MJ, et al: Prophylactic administration of respiratory syncytial virus immune globulin to high-risk infants and young children. The Respiratory Syncytial Virus Immune Globulin Study Group. *N Engl J Med* 329:1524-1530, 1993.
23. The PREVENT Study Group: Reduction of respiratory syncytial virus hospitalization among premature infants and infants with bronchopulmonary dysplasia using respiratory syncytial virus immune globulin prophylaxis. *Pediatrics* 99:93-97, 1997.
24. Simoes EA, Groothius JR, Tristam DA, et al: Respiratory syncytial virus-enriched globulin for the prevention of acute otitis media in high-risk children. *J Pediatr* 129: 214-219, 1996.
25. The Impact-RSV Study Group: Palivizumab, a humanized respiratory syncytial virus monoclonal antibody, reduces hospitalization from respiratory syncytial virus infection in high-risk infants. *Pediatrics* 102:531-537, 1998.
26. Feltes TM, Cabala AK, Meisner HC, et al: Palivizumab prophylaxis reduces hospitalization due to respiratory syncytial virus in young children with hemodynamically significant congenital heart disease. *J Pediatr* 143:532-540, 2003.
27. Joffe S, Ray GT, Escobar GJ, et al: Cost-effectiveness of respiratory syncytial virus prophylaxis among preterm infants. *Pediatrics* 104:419-427, 1999.
28. Prais D, Schonfeld T, Amir J: Admission to the intensive care unit for respiratory syncytial virus bronchiolitis: a national survey before palivizumab use. *Pediatrics* 112:548-552, 2003.
29. Atkins JT, Karimi P, Morris BH, et al: Prophylaxis for RSV-IGIV among preterm infants of thirty-two weeks gestation or less: reduction in incidence, severity of illness and cost. *Pediatr Infect Dis J* 19:138-143, 2002.
30. Kamal-Bahl S, Doshi J, Campbell J: Economic analysis of respiratory syncytial virus immunoprophylaxis in high-risk infants. *Arch Pediatr Adolesc Med* 156:1034-1041, 2002.
31. Yount LE, Mahle WT: Economic analysis of palivizumab in infants with congenital heart disease. *Pediatrics* 114: 1606-1611, 2004.
32. Piedra PA: Future directions in vaccine prevention of respiratory syncytial virus. *Pediatr Infect Dis J* 21:482-487, 2002.

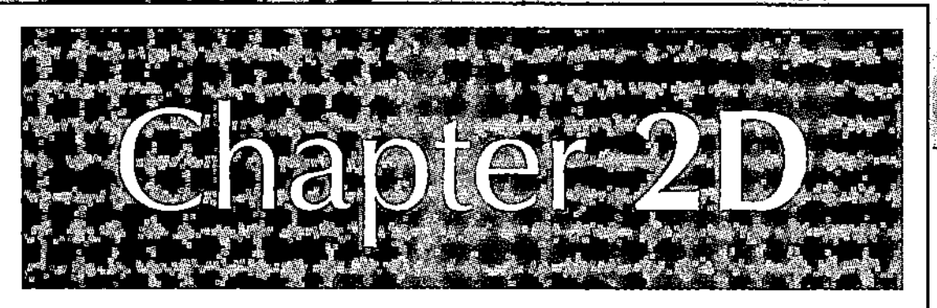

Chapter 2D

Tracheostomy Tubes in the Neonate

Mary H. Horn, RN, MS, RRT, and Catherine Noonan, RN, MS, CPNP

Because an increasing number of premature infants with severe pulmonary disease are surviving, chronic ventilatory support is becoming more common. As a result of this ventilator dependence, many of these infants require tracheostomies. Therefore it is increasingly important for primary care providers to have a good understanding of how to care for an infant with a tracheostomy tube. This chapter discusses indications for a tracheostomy tube, types of tubes, routine tracheostomy care, skin care, potential complications, discharge planning and teaching, and the decannulation process.

Indications for a Tracheostomy Tube

There are multiple indications for tracheostomy placements in neonates.[1-4] These indications include ventilator-dependent lung disease, anatomic concerns, risk for aspiration, central nervous system disorders, and neuromuscular disease (Table 2D-1). In rare cases, other surgical procedures may provide a better outcome than placement of a tracheostomy tube (Table 2D-2).[5,6] Many factors may contribute to ventilator dependence and should be evaluated before a tracheostomy or surgical procedure. These factors include transient pulmonary dysfunction, anemia, poor nutrition, inadequate pain management, and discomfort from the endotracheal tube.

Table 2D-1 Indications for Tracheostomy Tubes in Infants

- Ventilator dependence
  - Severe chronic lung disease of prematurity
  - Subglottic stenosis
  - Severe laryngotracheomalacia
- Chronic aspiration
- Trauma
- Muscle weakness
- Neurologic impairment
- Anomalies
  - Craniofacial anomalies
  - Pierre Robin sequence
  - Congenital anomalies
  - Vascular anomalies
- Tumors

Types of Tracheostomy Tubes

A tracheostomy is performed by an otolaryngologist or ear/nose/throat specialist while the child is sedated in the operating room. An otolaryngologist selects a tracheostomy tube mostly on the basis of anatomy. This decision is important because an appropriately sized tube will minimize complications.[7,8] Tracheostomy tubes (Figure 2D-1) are available in various types and sizes, with specific internal diameters (IDs), outer diameters (ODs), tube lengths, and flange types (Tables 2D-3 and 2D-4). The majority of

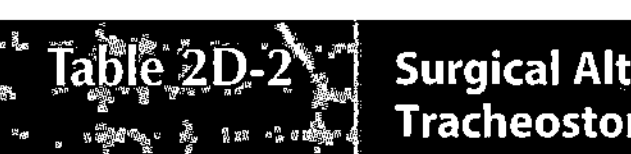

Table 2D-2 Surgical Alternatives to Tracheostomy Placement

- Endoscopic correction of anomaly
- Mandibular distraction
- Laryngotracheal reconstruction
- Ex utero intrapartum treatment (procedure at time of newborn delivery)

FIGURE 2D-1 Components of a Tracheostomy Tube. This image shows a tracheostomy tube delineating a 15-mm adaptor, flanges, and holes for ties. Adjacent to the image is a schematic showing the inner and outer diameter of the tube.

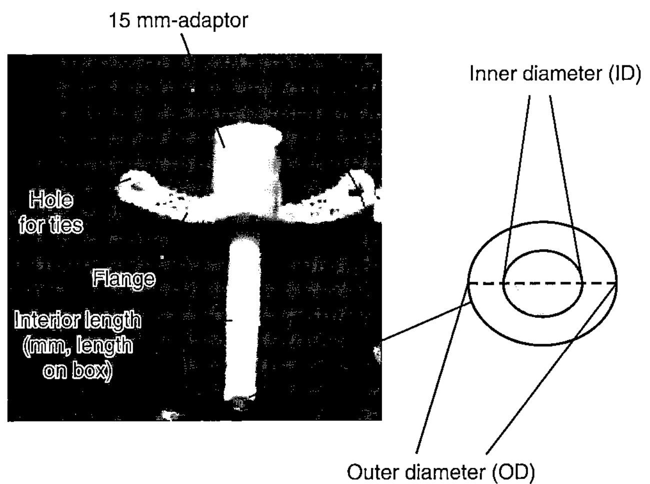

Table 2D-3 Types of Tracheostomy Tubes: Neonatal / Pediatric

Type	Sizes/Cuffs	Advantages	Disadvantages
Shiley	Neonatal Pediatric Cuffed Uncuffed	Comfortable flange, flat and beveled internally	Cuff is wider than trach tube, so less comfortable at removal
Sims Portex	Neonatal Pediatric Uncuffed	(15-mm) adaptor angle extends down, preventing obstruction	Cuff not available Flange slightly V-shaped
Bivona	Neonatal Pediatric Cuffed (TTS) Uncuffed	Can special order or adapt length, flange and/or extension Cuff same width as trach tube Flex tube available	Metal lined, so cannot be used in MRI. Must use other style of tracheotomy tube or airway V-shaped flange may cause discomfort, create ulcers due to pressure at stoma site, lead to difficulty when threading ties
Metal trach tubes	Neonatal Pediatric	Inner cannula available	Outer diameter (OD) is larger, so an inner cannula can be used

Table 2D-4 Neonatal and Pediatric Cuffless Tube Sizes

Specific Neonatal Cuffless Tube Sizes											
Shiley Size*	ID (mm)	OD (mm)	Shaft Length (mm)†	Bivona Size*	ID (mm)	OD (mm)	Shaft Length (mm)	Portex Size*	ID (mm)	OD (mm)	Shaft Length (mm)
				2.5	2.5	4.0	30	2.5	2.5	4.5	30
3.0	3.0	4.5	30	3.0	3.0	4.7	32	3.0	3.0	5.2	32
3.5	3.5	5.2	32	3.5	3.5	5.3	34	3.5	3.5	5.8	34
4.0	4.0	5.9	34	4.0	4.0	6.0	36				
4.5	4.5	6.5	36								
Specific Pediatric Cuffless Tube Sizes											
Shiley Size*	ID (mm)	OD (mm)	Shaft Length (mm)†	Bivona Size*	ID (mm)	OD (mm)	Shaft Length (mm)	Portex Size*	ID (mm)	OD (mm)	Shaft Length (mm)
				2.5	2.5	4.0	38	2.5	2.5	4.5	30
3.0	3.0	4.5	39	3.0	3.0	4.7	39	3.0	3.0	5.2	36
3.5	3.5	5.2	40	3.5	3.5	5.3	40	3.5	3.5	5.8	40
4.0	4.0	5.9	41	4.0	4.0	6.0	41	4.0	4.0	6.5	44
4.5	4.5	6.5	42	4.5	4.5	6.7	42	4.5	4.5	7.1	48
5.0	5.0	7.1	44	5.0	5.0	7.3	44	5.0	5.0	7.7	50
5.5	5.5	7.7	46	5.5	5.5	8.0	46	5.5	5.5	8.3	52

ID, Internal diameter; *OD*, outer diameter.
*Both neonatal and pediatric Shiley and Bivona tubes are available cuffed or uncuffed. Portex tubes are available only uncuffed.
†Shaft length is the internal length of the tracheostomy tube inside the stoma.

neonatal and pediatric tracheostomy tubes consist of a single cannula. Some tubes are reinforced with wire for stability and cannot be used during magnetic resonance imaging (MRI). The flange is the neck plate region that contains two openings to secure the tube with ties. Ideally, the flange should provide minimal pressure to the soft tissues of the neck. Flanges can be beveled, sitting comfortably on the neck without tension. Flanges also can be V-shaped and may push into the stoma as the ties are tightened, potentially causing skin or stoma erosion. Tracheostomy tubes may require adjustment as the infant grows because of corresponding airway changes.

Tracheostomy tubes can be uncuffed or cuffed. The cuff provides a seal so that only a small amount of air can escape around the tube. Because infants have a narrow cricoid ring that creates a seal, cuffed tubes usually are not needed. In addition, cuffed tubes usually are not placed in infants because of the potential for tracheal erosion. However, cuffed tubes may be indicated in infants on ventilators who cannot maintain appropriate inspiratory pressures with an uncuffed tracheostomy tube. A cuffed tube also may be necessary if the next uncuffed tube size is too large but too much air is escaping from the present uncuffed tube size to allow for adequate mechanical ventilation. Occasionally, a cuffed tube is needed temporarily in infants with severe chronic aspiration. The two types of cuffed neonatal tubes are air cuffed and tight to the shaft. When deflated, the air cuffed tube has more excess material than the tight to the shaft tube, potentially making it more difficult to remove. Solid metal and fenestrated tubes are available, but these variations are rarely used in infants.

Speaking valves can be used in conjunction with the tracheostomy tube to maximize speech development. Speech occurs when air passes around the tube, enabling air to escape past the vocal cords. The valves can be used as early as infancy and play an important role in facilitating communication. Two possible types of valves are the Shiley and the Passy-Muir (Table 2D-5). A speech pathologist or respiratory therapist should be consulted to determine the appropriate type of valve. When applying these speaking valves, inspiratory and expiratory effort must be assessed. The tube should always remain uncuffed, and movement of the valve with each breath should be monitored. No distention of the valve or blockage of airflow (either externally or internally) should occur because distention may create excessive positive end-expiratory pressure. Therefore oxygen (O_2) saturation levels and heart rate should be monitored while a speaking valve is being used. Both parameters should remain stable if the valve is functioning correctly. Because the valve does not provide moisture, its use should be limited to brief observed periods (up to 1 hour), and the

Table 2D-5 Types of Speaking Valves

Shiley valve (with or without O_2 adapter)	Passy-Muir valve (with or without O_2 adapter)
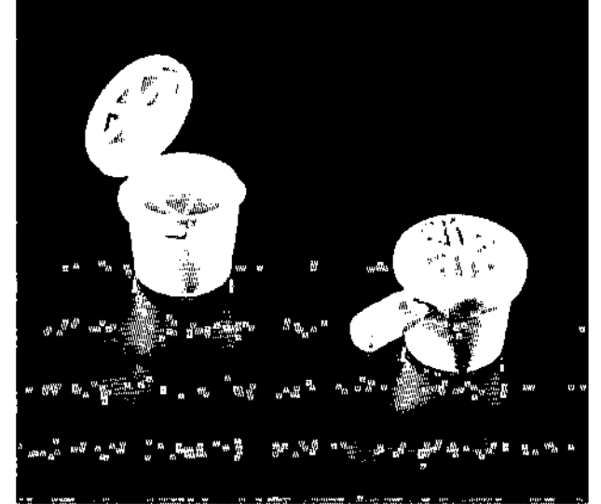	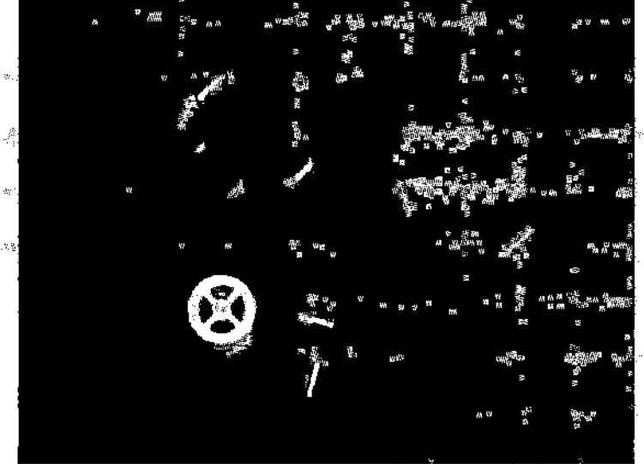
Shiley with O_2 adapter is on the **right**.	
www.Mallinckrodt.com	*www.passymuir.com*

need for this valve should be assessed regularly; indeed, some infants may not be able to tolerate a valve at all.

Tracheostomy Care

Humidity is essential to tracheotomy maintenance and care. Most infants benefit from a tracheostomy mask attached to a heated or cooled humidified air or oxygen system. Heat-moisture exchangers (HMEs) or "artificial noses" also can provide humidification when the infant is traveling. Heat moisture exchangers are composed of hydrophilic paper or foam material that collects heat and moisture. Neonatal-sized HMEs have less dead space, minimizing the amount of breathing effort needed by the infant. Because occlusion from secretions can occur, these devices must be used when the infant is being observed. Other humidity devices also are available (Table 2D-6). Appropriate humidification will prevent tube obstruction from dried or thick secretions. Inadequate humidification can lead to thick secretions, and excessive humidification can create loose secretions. Abnormal secretions also can result from other causes (Table 2D-7).

Suctioning is critical for optimal tracheostomy care and can help to ensure patency of the airway. Suctioning should be performed as clinically needed with a minimum frequency of every 4 hours in infants. The suction distance is determined by the length of the tracheostomy tube and the height of the outside adaptor and flange. An additional 3 to 5 mm should be added to allow the suction catheter to slightly clear the end of the tracheostomy tube. A sign defining the safe length to suction should be placed near the infant for viewing by care providers. Vigorous suctioning can cause trauma and should be avoided.[9,10] The use of saline instillation with suctioning is controversial, and recommendations vary.[11]

Recommendations for changing tracheostomy tubes can vary among providers. The frequency ranges from daily to monthly; however, most providers recommend weekly tracheostomy changes.[8] Frequent tube changes provide several advantages, including decreasing the risk for infection or granuloma formation, minimizing the risk of occlusion by blocked secretions, and maintaining the skills of the caregiver. However, tubes should be changed with great care because frequent tube changes may lead to stretching of the stoma and/or discomfort to the infant.[8]

Skin Care

Infants tend to have more skin complications associated with a tracheostomy tube than do adults. The flanges of the neonatal tube cover a proportionately larger skin area compared with adults, so the chances of surface breakdown are greater. Ventilator tubing, securing devices, adaptors, and inline monitors are proportionally heavier in neonates than in adults and therefore lead to greater skin problems. Unfortunately, the design of a tracheostomy tube does not often prioritize the neonate's needs. In addition, the more delicate skin of the neonate can lead to deeper tissue erosion from pressure.[12] Chin erosion is a distinct complication in infants.[13] Children with neuromuscular or developmental disorders are at greater risk for skin complications because of limited head and neck movement as well as decreased awareness of excessive pressure.[13]

Infants with tracheostomy tubes should have a routine skin assessment. The entire circumference of the neck, stoma site, chin, and skin folds should be inspected at least twice per day. The skin should be cleaned with a diluted ¼-strength hydrogen

Table 2D-6 Methods of Humidification

Method	Uses	Contraindications
Heat-moisture exchanger (HME) is a thermodiluter device, frequently called an "artificial nose;" it is a portable humidification filter Air enters or is exhaled through the filter, and moisture is retained in the device (see image below) 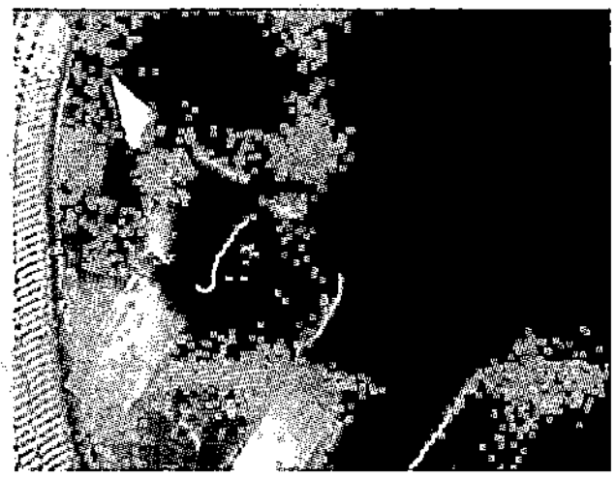	Easily provides humidity Can be used with oxygen (O_2) Vent HMEs can be used with portable ventilators	Should not be used if excessive secretions are present or infant is not being monitored Secretions can be retained in the device and can block air movement Clothing can obstruct the ends Do not obstruct device flow when holding the infant
Trach mask/collar humidity	Used when infant is asleep or awake or when airway secretions are dry Connects to a compressor with a humidified air or oxygen system	Not portable unless accompanied by system
Thermovent O_2	Method of providing O_2 while using the HME	Use only when infant is awake and observed by caregiver
Gauze	If the infant is in room air, an uncut, wet, see-through gauze (single ply, not cotton-filled) can be used to provide moisture if other options are not available	Gauze should not be thick. Use only thin, fine gauze that infant can breathe through easily If mucus is coughed on gauze, the gauze must be changed or infant can no longer breath through the gauze Infant must be monitored
Saline instillation	Should not be necessary if properly humidified Infrequently saline may be necessary if secretions are dry, if secretions cannot be suctioned, or if infant is dehydrated; instilling saline will create a cough and dislodge mucus	

peroxide/water solution and then rinsed with water every 2 to 24 hours, depending on the amount of stoma drainage. Normal saline may be less irritating and can be used if crusted material is not visible. Caregivers should use cotton-tipped applicators, starting close to the stoma and moving outward. The skin should then be completely dried. The ties or tape securing the tube should be changed whenever they appear soiled and at least every few days.[13,14] Maintain one fingerbreadth between the tie and the skin when the infant is in the sitting position or on his or her side; this spacing will prevent both excess pressure and accidental decannulation. Some nebulized medications, such as aerosolized steroids, may affect the integrity of the skin and must be washed off promptly.

A thin, presplit, single-layer 2 inch × 2 inch dressing can be placed under the flanges to keep the

Table 2D-7 Assessment of Secretions

Specific Problem	Possible Cause (Any, Several, or All)
Thick secretions	Diuretic use Decreased intake of fluids Increased sensible water loss Inadequate humidification (e.g., bottle empty) Respiratory infection
Loose secretions	Saliva aspiration Excessive humidification Respiratory infection

skin dry. Use of a hydroabsorbant dressing (e.g., Exu-Dry, Allevyn Foam, or Cutinova) can collect excess secretions and prevent flange pressure on the skin. Avoid displacing the tube anteriorly with bulky dressings. Hand-cut gauze sponges should never be used because microfilaments can enter into the tracheostomy tube.[14]

Skin breakdown is a common complication due to pressure from the tracheostomy tube, flanges, ties, or tracheostomy collar, requiring prompt assessment and treatment. Often, the style of the flange must be changed or perhaps customized to minimize unnecessary pressure. A hydrocolloid dressing (e.g., DuoDerm Extra Thin) can be placed under the flanges to minimize pressure and treat minor skin breakdown.[14] However, this type of dressing may not be prudent in the presence of excessive moisture or secretions. Hydroabsorbant dressings are useful for skin breakdown if excessive secretions are present.

Some clinicians believe that the stoma should be maintained without any type of dressing because it can trap moisture against the skin. Powder should never be used around the tracheostomy site because the powder can be inhaled. Decreasing excess bulkiness of tubing and connectors may minimize pressure on the skin.

Use of an antibacterial cream at the stoma site is controversial, but the cream can be used when there is irritation to prevent exogenous colonization or infection of the lower airways.[15] Silver nitrate can be applied to superficially over granulated tissue by an otolaryngologist. Systemic antibiotics may be necessary if evidence of cellulitis is seen.

Potential Complications

Pediatric mortality rates from tracheostomy tubes range from 0.5% to 3%.[16] These low mortality rates can be attributed to better technology and improved expertise in neonatal and pediatric care. However, complications are common (up to 60%), depending on the age of the patient and the specific study.[17,18] Complications can occur at any time during the immediate postoperative period, late in the recovery phase, and after discharge.

The most common complications in a tracheostomy-dependent child are accidental decannulations and tube occlusions.[1,16] Accidental decannulation must be avoided in the immediate postoperative period. Infants often are sedated and even mechanically ventilated after surgery to prevent movement. If accidental decannulation occurs within the first postoperative week, reinserting the tracheostomy tube may be difficult. Accidental decannulation also can occur after the stoma has healed; an extra tube should always be readily available. This spare tube should have an obturator, similar to a stylette, to guide replacement. The obturator must be removed immediately after the tube is positioned and remain at the bedside in case reinsertion is required. A smaller-sized tube also should be placed at the bedside in case of any difficulty during tracheostomy tube insertion.

Lack of proper humidity can increase the risk for mucus plugs and tube obstruction. If suctioning is ineffective at removing a plug, the tube must be changed emergently. Cuffed tubes should be deflated before removal. Bag-and-mask ventilation over the tracheotomy stoma often does not maintain the airway because creating a seal at the infant's neck usually is difficult, and excessive pressure may be needed. In these circumstances, if the upper airway is functional, a mask can be placed over the nose and mouth while the stoma is occluded. If the same-sized tube cannot be inserted during an emergent recannulation, a smaller tube should be used. An endotracheal tube or a large open-ended suction catheter can be inserted into the stoma during emergent situations.

Other common complications include development of granulation tissue, bleeding, and skin breakdown (Table 2D-8). Aspirations of secretions may occur. The tracheostomy tube may become occluded by the infant's chin, especially if an infant has poor head control or excess skin folds. Rare complications include tracheal stenosis, tracheal erosion, and development of a tracheo-innominate artery fistula.[7] Long-term complications also develop and may include speech delay, problems with phonation, and difficulties with swallowing and/or eating specific foods.

Discharge Teaching

Extensive education of parents and other caregivers will minimize complications in infants with tracheostomy tubes. Educational goals should include training in (1) performing routine tube changes, (2) assessing the airway properly, (3) providing adequate skin care, (4) establishing appropriate humidification, (5) suctioning correctly, (6) using and monitoring the vast amount of mechanical equipment, (7) recannulating in an emergency, and (8) performing cardiopulmonary resuscitation in the tracheotomized infant. Ideally, these objectives should be taught to at least *two* caregivers (Table 2D-9). Teaching aids such as books, dolls, and/or videos may be useful.

After these teaching goals are achieved, a list of supplies is compiled for the family (an example is shown in Table 2D-10). Nursing assistance or respite care should be arranged to allow families to have a reprieve from caregiving. Lack of home services may delay discharge.[17,19-22] Occasionally, discharge to an inpatient pulmonary rehabilitation program is a more viable option than discharge to home.

Table 2D-8 Potential Complications of a Tracheostomy Tube

Common Complications	Cause/ Treatment
Skin breakdown	Skin breakdown can occur if excessive pressure is placed on the skin from the tube flanges, ventilator tubes, or CO_2 monitoring, or from securing ties that are too tight. Excessive humidity can be a contributing factor. Proper cleaning and prevention of excessive moisture and pressure are needed.
Hemorrhage	If proper humidity is not delivered, bleeding can occur from dry mucus membranes. Surgical site itself may bleed. Overly vigorous or excessively deep suctioning often leads to bloody secretions. Humidity and suctioning techniques should be evaluated. Any infant undergoing anticoagulation therapy should be followed closely.
Granuloma (see image below) 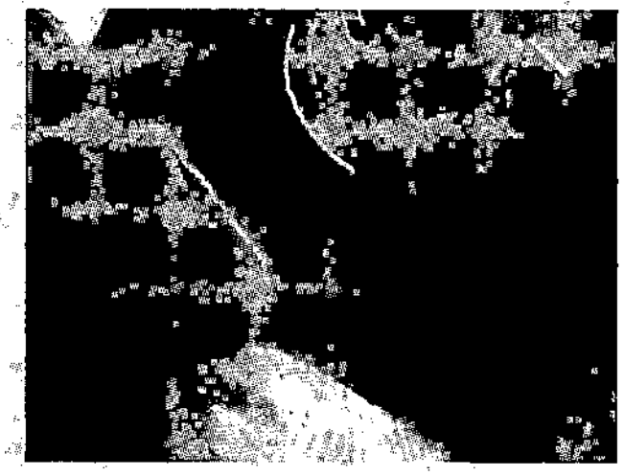	Granulation tissue can develop both internally and externally. Internally, granuloma formation is often the result of overly vigorous suctioning. It can interfere with airway exchange and decannulation. Routine bronchoscopy can diagnose and treat these granulomas. Externally, granuloma formation at the tracheostomy stoma can be caused by irritation, movement, pressure, or secretions. It can be treated with silver nitrate, antibiotic cream, or surgical excision if necessary. Changing the flange that is causing pressure may improve the site.
Tracheostomy tube occluded by chin	Often occurs in infants with poor head control or excess skin folds. An adapter (e.g., Tilson Trach Guard or heat-moisture exchanger) can lengthen the external tip of the tube. Alternatively, a customized tube with a longer proximal length may be needed.

The primary healthcare provider should be comfortable with routine care of patients with tracheostomy tubes. Many resources are available to assist community providers (see the resources listed at the end of this chapter). Companies that design the tracheostomy tubes frequently have free educational materials. A multidisciplinary team approach is ideal. Referral to a local early intervention program should be made early in the postoperative period. The infant should be followed by a pulmonologist as well as an otolaryngologist. Monitoring by a developmental specialist, speech therapist, physical therapist, and occupational therapist also is important. It is essential to notify the local emergency medical service (EMS) response team (police or fire department) and to outline procedures to follow in an emergency. With proper initial teaching and guidance as well as continued care by the primary care provider and specialists, parents should be discharged with the required confidence and skills needed to care for their infant with a tracheostomy tube.

Decannulation (complete removal of the tracheostomy tube)

When a tracheostomy tube is no longer needed, a bronchoscopy can be helpful to determine readiness and decannulation can be considered. Several methods of decannulation can be used. One passive method maintains the same-sized tube as the infant grows, allowing air to flow around the tracheostomy tube. An infant's airway size will increase as the length of the infant increases. The tube can be capped for several hours daily while the infant is observed for any respiratory distress. Over time, the tube is capped for longer periods. If an obstruction is noted, particularly during sleep, a sleep study may be required before decannulation. When the tube can be capped for 24 hours, the child usually is ready for decannulation, which is performed in the hospital setting. Before decannulation, a bronchoscopy is performed in the operating room to assess airway function and patency. If the child has a normal respiratory status and does not have any airway abnormalities, decannulation can occur. Usually, the child is then observed for another 24 hours in the intensive care unit before discharge home.

Another option for decannulation is a gradual reduction in the size of the tracheostomy tube in infants with a history of ventilator dependence or airway obstruction that required a large tracheostomy tube. During this downsizing process, if the infant has a large volume of secretions that cannot be accommodated by a smaller tube, a tube with a larger internal diameter may be necessary. If an

Table 2D-9 Discharge Teaching

Discharge Teaching Goal*	Key Teaching Component(s)
Airway assessment, including signs of respiratory distress	Monitor for signs of occlusion: retractions, apnea, cyanosis, anxious appearance, lethargy, inadequate passage of suction catheter past the tracheostomy tube to length prescribed.
Awareness of potential tracheostomy problems	Describe the clinical findings for granulomas, tracheal stenosis, tracheomalacia, tracheitis, cellulitis, and stoma excoriation.
Skin care	Teach methods to prevent skin breakdown and/or infection.
Appropriate methods of humidification Artificial nose (HME) Oxygen/air with tracheostomy collar	Discuss rationale for humidification. Explain techniques of humidification.
Appropriate suctioning technique and necessary equipment: Gloves Catheters Standby tracheostomy tubes Saline ampules Portable suction Oxygen optional	Suction only slightly past end of tracheostomy (unless otolaryngologist notes otherwise) so that carina is not injured (See image below). 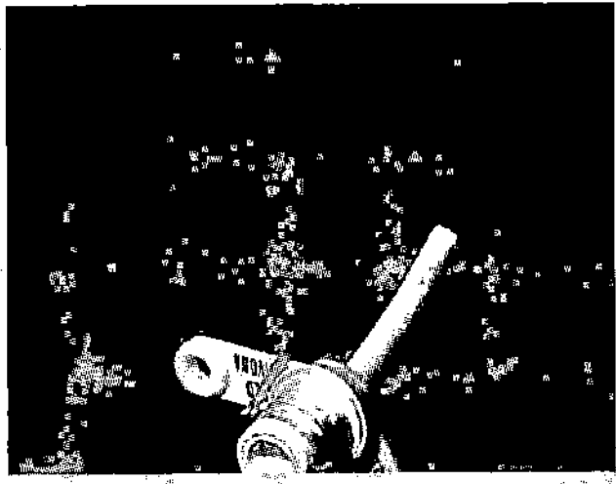
Routine tube changes	Always have standby equipment available: suctioning, extra tracheostomy tubes, oximeter monitor, scissors, Ambu bag with pop-off valve. Critical to maintain one fingerbreadth between the tie and skin. Individualized frequency (varies between weekly and monthly).
Use of mechanical equipment: Ambu bag with popoff valve Suctioning Humidification Oxygen Pulse oximeter with alarms Nebulizer Other: Speaking valves, Tilson Trach Guard, Communication devices	Instruct family about how to use each piece of equipment. Do not use HMEs or speaking valves if infant is left unattended. Ideal to use home care equipment during teaching.
Management of obstruction and emergent recannulation	Know emergency procedures if tracheostomy tube should fall out or become occluded. Discuss management of mucus plugs. Discuss management of vomiting episodes. Discuss management of aspiration.
CPR	Teach CPR to all caretakers.

CPR, Cardiopulmonary resuscitation; *HME,* heat moisture exchanger.
*These teaching goals should be addressed to at least two caregivers. A rooming-in period before discharge should be encouraged. Ideally, decision-making skills should be highlighted; role playing with a doll or mannequin will assist in reinforcing these skills.

obstruction or persistent inability to handle secretions occurs, there may be an anatomic narrowing above or below the tube, possibly from granulation tissue. When the tube size is relatively small, the infant can be admitted to the hospital for bronchoscopy and likely is ready for decannulation.

After decannulation, the stoma usually is closed with Steri-Strips or a Xeroform gauze, covered by an occlusive dressing. Sometimes a stoma does not close, especially if large volumes of secretions are present. This open stoma continues to enable air to pass, further preventing closure. In these

Table 2D-10 Tracheostomy Bedside Supply

Care Needs				
Quantity	**Item Details**			
1/mo	**Trach tube:**	**Type**		**Inner Diameter**
		Size	__ Neonatal _ Pediatric __Adult	__ Custom
2/day	**Split dressings**	**Type**	__Gauze __ Allevyn	__ Exudry __ Other
1/day	**Dale Velcro Trach Ties®**	**Size**	__ Infant#242	__Adult#240 __ Other
24pairs/d	**Gloves**	**Type**	__Non-sterile __Sterile	**Latex allergy?** __Yes __ No
	Peroxide			
10/day	**Applicator sticks**			
give	**Water soluble lubricant**			
give	**Safety edge scissors** (Item #143627)			
	Syringe(s)			
Airway Management				
Quantity	**Item Details**			
1	Self-inflating Ambu® w/ Pop off valve and Swivel Adapter and Mask	**Mask**	__Neonatal __ Pedi __ Adult	
1	Suction machines w/ tubing		__Stationary __Portable	
15/day	Suction catheters	**Size**		**Frequency**
5/day	Saline for instillation	**Package**	__Vial (__ cc/ vial)	__Bottle (__ cc/ bottle)
1	Oximeter	**Use**	__ Continuous __Sleep/Naps only	
		Alarm settings	Heart Rate High O_2 Saturation High__	Heart Rate Low O_2 Saturation Low__
1 of each	Humidification	**Trach Collar Size**	__Pediatric __Adult	__ Portex Thermovent O_2 clip
		Air Compressor	__ Stationary __Tubing/drainage bag	__ Portable ____ Humidification Bottle
		Use	__ Continuous __ Sleep/Naps only	__ PRN
	Oxygen	**Setting**	%	Liters/min
		Type	__ Stationary __ Portable	__ O_2 concentrator
5/day	HME (Heat Moisture Exchanger)(artificial nose):	**Type**	__ Portex Thermovent T	__ Neonatal Giback
Optional Items				
Quantity	**Item Details**			
	Speaking valve	**Type**	__Passy Muir® Purple__ Passy Muir® White __Shiley®__Piling®	
	Tilson Trach Guard (If chin occludes trach)			
	Ointments			
	Other (specify)			
Nursing Home Care Agency:		**VNA:**		
Equipment Vendor:		**Other:**		
Completed by:				

Note: All of this equipment must be at the inpatient's bedside. Created by Mary Horn, RN, MS, RRT.

circumstances, surgical closure may be required after several months.

Oxygen requirements may change after decannulation. Therefore, close monitoring of oxygen saturation, heart rate, and respirations is necessary. The infant should be assessed while awake and while asleep. Usually difficulties arise soon after decannulation, particularly when the child is in deep sleep. In some instances, the tracheostomy tube may have stented the airway open, and clinical evidence of an obstruction may be seen only after decannulation. Indeed, some children fail the decannulation attempt and require reconstructive surgery.

Conclusion

Tracheostomy tube placement in infants has become increasingly more common with a concurrent decrease in pediatric mortality rates. This chapter discussed specific needs of the infant with a tracheostomy. Routine tracheostomy and skin care is critical to ensure stoma patency and minimize complications. Appropriate discharge teaching will maximize the skills and enhance the confidence of the caregivers. Continued external support by the primary care provider, nursing, and the entire health care team is critical to minimize the stress of caring for an infant with a tracheostomy tube and to ensure quality healthcare delivery.

Resources for Families and Clinicians

www.tracheostomy.com

Aaron's Tracheostomy Page is a comprehensive website covering all aspects of care of the child with a tracheostomy tube. This site provides links and a message board with educational materials and is an excellent resource for parents and professionals.

www.trachcare.org.

TrachCare is a nonprofit organization created to provide support and information to parents, caregivers and healthcare providers of children who have a tracheostomy.

http://ajrccm.atsjournals.org/cgi/content/full/161/1/297

This website contains statements adopted by the American Thoracic Society regarding all aspects of care of the child with a tracheostomy tube.

www.omronhealthcare.com

Omron Healthcare manufactures a portable, battery-operated, handheld nebulizer system for humidification.

Often, companies that design tracheostomy tubes have free educational materials.

Families can purchase a tracheostomy tube guide entitled "Just Like You," as well as a book on having a sibling with a tracheostomy. Contact 260-351-3555 for information.

www.nelcor.com

This website offers a free guide, "Parent Guide to Pediatric Homecare."

Acknowledgments

The authors thank Reza Rahbar, DMD, MD, and Sherri Horonjeff, PAC, for critical review of this chapter.

REFERENCES

1. Kremer B, Botos-Kremer AI, Eckel HE, et al: Indications, complications, and surgical techniques for pediatric tracheostomies—an update. *J Pediatr Surg* 37(11): 1556-1562, 2002.
2. Pereira KD, MacGregor AR, McDuffie CM, et al: Tracheostomy in preterm infants: current trends. *Arch Otolaryngol Head Neck Surg* 129(12):1268-1271, 2003.
3. Healy GB: The management of congenital and acquired stenosis of the larynx in infants and children. *Adv Otolaryngol Head Neck Surg* 15:159-170, 1991.
4. Dinwiddie R: Congenital upper airway obstruction. *Paediatr Respir Rev* 5(1):17-24, 2004.
5. Ferraro N: Craniofacial development and the airway during sleep. In Loughlin GM, Carroll JL, Marcus CL, editors: *Sleep and breathing in children: a developmental approach.* New York, 2000, Marcel Dekker.
6. Gupta A, Cotton RT, Rutter MJ: Pediatric suprastomal granuloma: management and treatment. *Otolaryngol Head Neck Surg* 131(1):21-25, 2004.
7. Rozsasi A, Neagos A, Nolte F, et al: Critical analysis of complications and disorders in wound healing after tracheostomy in children. *Laryngorhinootologie* 82(12): 826-832, 2003.
8. Sherman JM, Davis S, Albamonte-Petrick S, et al: Care of the child with a chronic tracheostomy. Official statement of the American Thoracic Society *Am J Respir Crit Care Med* 161:297-308, 2000.
9. Fiske E: Effective strategies to prepare infants and families for home tracheostomy care. *Adv Neonatal Care* 4(1): 42-53, 2004.
10. Kleiber C, Krutzfield N, Rose EF: Acute histologic changes in the tracheobronchial tree associated with different suction catheter insertion techniques. *Heart Lung* 7(1): 10-14, 1988.
11. Schwenker D, Ferrin M, Gift AG: A survey of endotracheal suctioning with instillation of normal saline. *Am J Crit Care* 7(4):255-260, 1998.
12. Bressler K, Coladipietro L, Holinger LD: Protection of the cervical skin in the pediatric patient with a recent tracheostomy. *Otolaryngol Head Neck Surg* 116: 414-415, 1997.
13. Koff PB, Eitzman D, Neu J: *Neonatal and pediatric respiratory care,* ed 2. St Louis, 1993, Mosby-Year Book.
14. Kelleher B: Tracheostomy. In Wise, BV, McKenna C, Garvin G, Harmon BJ, editors: *Nursing care of the general pediatric surgical patient.* Gaithersburg, MD, 2000, Aspen Publishers.
15. Morar P, Makura Z, Jones A, et al: Topical antibiotics on tracheostoma prevents exogenous colonization and infection of lower airways in children. *Chest* 117(2): 513-518, 2000.
16. Czervinske MP, Barnhart SL: *Perinatal and pediatric respiratory care,* ed 2. Philadelphia, 2003, WB Saunders.

17. Schlessel JS, Harper RG, Rappa, H, et al: Tracheostomy: acute and long-term mortality and morbidity in very low birth weight premature infants. *J Pediatr Surg* 28(7): 873-876, 1993.
18. Ilce Z, Celayir S, Tekand GT, et al: Tracheostomy in childhood: 20 years experience from a pediatric surgery clinic. *Pediatr Int* 44(3):306-309, 2002.
19. Buzz-Kelly L, Gordin P: Teaching CPR to parents of children with tracheostomies. *MCN Am J Matern Child Nurs* 18(3):158-162, 1993.
20. Jardine E, O'Toole M, Paton JY, et al: Current status of long term ventilation of children in the United Kingdom: questionnaire survey. *BMJ* 318 (7179):295-299, 1999.
21. O'Brien JE, Dumas HM, Haley SM, et al: Clinical findings and resource use of infants and toddlers dependent on oxygen and ventilators. *Clin Pediatr* 41(3): 155-162, 2002.
22. Edwards EA, O'Toole M, Wallis C: Sending children home on tracheostomy dependent ventilation: pitfalls and outcomes. *Arch Dis Child* 89(3):251-255, 2004.

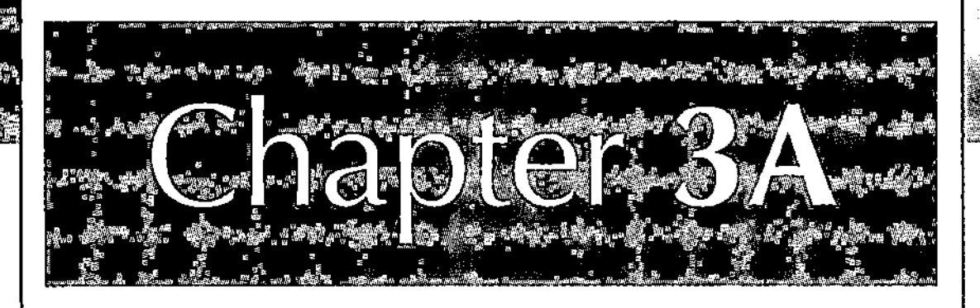

Nutrition and Growth in Primary Care of the Premature Infant

Deirdre M. Ellard, MS, RD/LDN, CNSD

Advances in neonatal care over the past 2 decades have allowed for the increasing survival of infants born smaller, and at younger gestational ages, than ever before. Although improvements in practice have resulted in lower mortality, they also have presented clinicians, both in the hospital and after discharge, with the challenge of reducing the morbidity associated with being born at an extremely low birth weight (ELBW, <1000 g) or at a very low birth weight (VLBW, <1500 g). Enhancing the nutritional care provided to these infants, from birth through hospital discharge, has been a priority. Although research is available to guide care during the initial postnatal period, few data are available regarding what constitutes optimal nutritional management for the older, growing, premature infant during the transition from the neonatal intensive care unit (NICU) to home. This is particularly true for the breastfed infant. The purpose of this chapter is to help identify neonates at greatest risk for nutritional concerns after discharge from the hospital, as well as to review current post-discharge feeding practices.

Postnatal Growth of Premature Infants

The American Academy of Pediatrics (AAP) suggests that the goal of nutritional support for preterm infants is to approximate the rate of growth and body composition of a healthy fetus of the same gestational age while avoiding nutritional excesses or deficiencies.[1] Despite this recommendation, chronic undernutrition and poor growth have been reported widely in the literature. In a large study of infants born weighing 401 g-1500 g, Lemons et al.[2] documented poor postnatal growth as a major cause of morbidity in this population. These researchers determined that 97% of all VLBW infants and 99% of ELBW infants in their study had weights less than the 10th percentile at 36 weeks' postmenstrual gestational age. Poor postnatal growth was the most frequent cause of morbidity seen in VLBW infants. The authors suggested that optimizing nutritional support for this population remains difficult, in part because of the severity of illness frequently encountered and organ immaturity. Lemons et al. also cited a lack of current data and differing attitudes toward nutritional management of these high-risk newborns as potentially contributing to the incidence of poor growth. In addition, Embleton et al.[3] demonstrated that preterm infants accumulate a significant nutrient deficit in the first weeks of life that was not replaced before hospital discharge, even though current recommended dietary intakes (RDIs) were given. RDIs in this study were defined as 120 kcal/kg/day with protein 3 g/kg/day and were based on needs for maintenance and normal growth. No provision for catch-up growth was made. The authors concluded that this nutrient deficit could be related directly to subsequent postnatal growth restriction. Although it has been suggested that elevated nutritional requirements to support catch-up growth should be provided before discharge,[4] Embleton et al. stated that it is unclear whether or not these deficits could be recouped during the hospital stay, especially if infants were fed intakes that were just meeting the RDI.

Ziegler et al.[5] have proposed that, compared with the abundantly nutrient-supplied fetus, the VLBW infant invariably experiences some degree of undernutrition, and that this undernutrition is unphysiologic and undesirable. Furthermore, undernutrition and poor growth may have long-term consequences on neurodevelopmental outcomes. In a randomized trial of early nutrition in preterm infants born weighing <1850 g, Lucas et al.[6] determined that a diet of preterm formula given for an average of 4 weeks after birth was associated with significant improvements in IQ (most notably verbal IQ in boys) at 7½ to 8 years of age when compared with infants who received a diet of term formula. Also, the incidence of cerebral palsy was lower in those infants fed preterm formula compared with those fed term formula. The authors suggested that suboptimal early nutrition in preterm infants could have a permanent effect on their cognitive function. Furthermore, Ehrenkranz et al.[7] determined that growth velocity of ELBW infants during hospitalization exerts a significant, and possibly independent, effect on neurodevelopmental and growth outcomes at 18 to 22 months' corrected age.

Taken together, the evidence strongly suggests that VLBW and ELBW infants invariably incur some degree of nutrient deficits, and that these deficits are not likely to be replaced before discharge from the hospital. However, as Carlson states, not much is known about the nutritional status of these infants postdischarge, and best practice should continue to evolve.[8] Table 3A-1 identifies infants at highest risk for nutritional difficulties after discharge from the NICU.

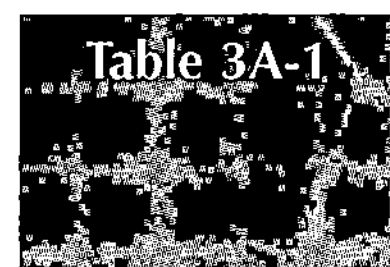

Infants at Highest Risk for Nutritional Concerns after Discharge from the Neonatal Intensive Care Unit

- Very low birth weight (<1500 g at birth) and extremely low birth weight (<1000 g at birth)
- Small for gestational age and intrauterine growth restriction
- Exclusively breastfed infants
- Infants requiring special formulas
- Infants requiring tube feedings at home
- Infants who fail to gain at least 20 g/day before discharge
- Infants with gastrostomies or tracheotomies
- Infants requiring parenteral nutrition for >4 weeks during hospitalization
- Diagnosis of any of the following:
  - Bronchopulmonary dysplasia
  - Chronic renal insufficiency
  - Congenital alimentary tract anomalies
  - Cyanotic congenital heart disease
  - Inborn errors of metabolism
  - Malabsorption
  - Osteopenia of prematurity
  - Poverty or low socioeconomic status
  - Severe neurologic impairment
  - Short bowel syndrome

From: Hovasi Cox J, Doorlag D: Nutritional concerns at transfer or discharge. In Groh-Wargo S, Thompson M, Cox J, et al., editors: *Nutritional care for high-risk newborns*, ed 3. Chicago, 2000, Precept Press.

Postdischarge Nutrition for Premature Infants

Human milk

Because of its many nutritive and nonnutritive benefits, human milk remains the preferred feeding for ELBW and VLBW infants.[1,8-22] However, compared with the feeding of formula to infants, the feeding of unsupplemented human milk to neonates has been associated with slower rates of growth and nutritional deficiencies during their NICU stay and following discharge.[20] As a result, these high-risk newborns typically are fed pumped maternal milk, fortified with calories and other nutrients, via a feeding tube or bottle while they are hospitalized. As readiness for discharge approaches and attempts at breastfeeding progress, the infant's ability to transfer milk effectively during breastfeeding should be evaluated in order to determine the composition and quantity of supplementary/complementary feedings required after discharge.[21] The European Society for Pediatric Gastroenterology, Hepatology, and Nutrition (ESPGHAN) Committee on Nutrition suggests that infants who are discharged with a subnormal weight for postconceptual age should be supplemented to provide adequate nutrient intake, for example with a human milk fortifier.[23] However, the continued use of human milk fortifiers, on ad libitum feedings, beyond the infant's hospital stay has not been studied extensively, and the cost and availability of fortifiers are obstacles to their use after discharge. Moreover, the availability of a nutrient-enriched postdischarge fortifier to meet the unique nutrient requirements of this older, growing, human milk-fed population is lacking.

Facilitating the transition from predominantly bottle feeding calorically enhanced, pumped breast milk to exclusive breastfeeding represents a unique situation and major challenge to the infant, mother, and primary care provider. What is the most favorable strategy to allow for the advancement of exclusive nursing while accommodating the infant's increased needs and/or inability to ingest adequate volume? What is the optimal supplementary/complementary feeding? To date, there are no universally accepted, best practice protocols to support this process. The availability of a nutrient-enriched postdischarge human milk fortifier to meet the unique nutrient requirements of this older, growing, human milk-fed population also is lacking.

Potential discharge strategies used to address this issue include the following:

1. Provide calorically enhanced, pumped breast milk at the energy density the infant had tolerated in the hospital and encourage a gradual increase in exclusive nursing sessions (eliminating approximately one bottle feeding at a time) as the infant "outgrows" the need for the extra calories.
2. Allow the infant to nurse "on demand" but specify a required daily intake of nutrient-enriched postdischarge formula (e.g., the infant must have 2-3 feedings of a postdischarge formula per day). This also offers the infant an enriched source of protein and minerals and may be the preferred option for an infant with a history of osteopenia.

Hindmilk, the fat-rich milk at the end of the feeding, also can be used. However, there is significant within-mother and between-mother variability in the caloric density of these feedings.[22] Further details about transitioning to breastfeeding are provided in Chapter 3B.

Simultaneously decreasing the caloric density of pumped maternal milk and the number of supplemented bottle feeds per day may adversely affect the infant's growth. This process may wean total caloric intake per kilogram too quickly and place too great a demand on the infant to increase volume intake. This is of particular concern in the presence of fluid-sensitive conditions, such as bronchopulmonary dysplasia.[24] However, overfeeding also is undesirable, and continued growth monitoring is required.

The optimal strategy in any given situation should be individualized and is dependent on the unique mother–infant dyad.[19] To facilitate the successful progression to full breastfeeding while allowing for an optimal long-term growth outcome, the primary care provider should refer to the section discussing caloric enhancement, following. Collaboration with a registered dietitian and/or lactation consultant who is familiar with the special needs of this population may be beneficial during this time of transition.

Table 3A-2 Indications for Selected Infant Formulas*

PRETERM
Enfamil Premature LIPIL
Similac Special Care Advance
PRETERM POSTDISCHARGE
EnfaCare LIPIL
NeoSure Advance
TERM
Enfamil LIPIL
Similac Advance
LACTOSE-FREE†
LactoFree LIPIL
Similac Lactose Free Advance
HYPOALLERGENIC†
Nutramigen LIPIL
Pregestimil
Similac Alimentum Advance
EleCare
Neocate
GASTROESOPHAGEAL REFLUX
Standard Formula
Enfamil AR LIPIL†

*Up-to-date nutrient composition data for these formulas are available at: *www.meadjohnson.com*, *www.ross.com*, and *www.shsna.com*

†These products were not designed specifically for the former preterm infant in the postdischarge period. For infants requiring these formulas, the primary care provider should consider micronutrient supplementation based on the formula in use, the infant's history, and the volume ingested. The primary care provider should compare the infant's intake to the enteral recommendations and the infant's estimated requirements.

Nutrient-enriched postdischarge formulas

In the absence of exclusive human milk feeding, nutrient-enriched postdischarge formulas are available for the older, growing, premature infant. Table 3A-2 reviews selected infant formulas. Several clinical trials have investigated the efficacy of postdischarge formulas compared with term infant formulas in this population.

Lucas et al.[25] tested the hypothesis that nutritional intervention in the first 9 months postterm would reverse postdischarge growth deficits and improve neurodevelopment without adverse safety outcomes in infants born preterm weighing <1750 g. A reference group of infants, breastfed until at least 6 weeks' postterm, was included. At 9 months postterm, infants fed the postdischarge formulas were heavier and longer than those fed term formula, and the difference in length persisted at 18 months. The effect of diet was greatest in males. No significant difference was observed in developmental scores at 9 or 18 months, although the infants fed the postdischarge formulas had a 2.8 (-1.3–6.8) point advantage in Bayley motor score scales. At 6 weeks' postterm, the reference group of breastfed infants was lighter and shorter than the postdischarge formula group, and they remained smaller up to 9 months postterm. The authors drew the following conclusions: (1) improving postdischarge nutrition in the first 9 months may alter subsequent growth, particularly for length, until at least 18 months (a follow-up study is planned); (2) the hypothesis that postdischarge nutrition benefits motor development could not be rejected and requires further study; and (3) breastfed, postdischarge preterm infants may require nutritional supplementation (currently under review). No adverse safety outcomes were associated with postdischarge formulas.

Carver et al.[26] reported similar findings. They evaluated the growth of premature infants weighing <1800 g at birth who were fed a postdischarge formula or a term formula from discharge to 12 months' corrected age. Infants were randomized to postdischarge formula or term formula and stratified by gender and birth weight (<1250 g or >1250 g). The authors determined that growth was improved in preterm infants fed a postdischarge formula after discharge to 12 months' corrected age. Beneficial effects were most evident among infants with birth weights <1250 g, particularly for head circumference measurements. In addition, the postdischarge formula seemed more beneficial for the growth of male infants than for female infants.

Currently, the AAP concurs that the use of postdischarge formulas to a postnatal age of 9 months results in greater linear growth, weight gain, and bone mineral content compared with the use of term infant formula.[1] The AAP states that because these formulas are iron and vitamin fortified, no other supplements are needed. However, the average preterm infant taking 150 ml/kg/day may benefit from an additional 1 mg/kg/day iron until 12 months of age.[1]

As with the breastfed neonate, formula-fed former preterm infants frequently are discharged receiving calorically enhanced feedings. Factors to consider when weaning caloric density, while allowing for optimal growth, are reviewed in a later section discussing caloric enhancement. Collaboration with a registered dietitian may assist with the weaning of calorically enhanced feedings. The ESPGHAN Committee on Nutrition suggests that infants discharged with a subnormal weight for postmenstrual age should receive postdischarge formula until a postmenstrual age of at least 40 weeks and possibly until about 52 weeks.[23] Continued growth monitoring is required to adapt feeding choices to the needs of individual infants and to avoid underfeeding or overfeeding.

Other infant formulas

The AAP has several position papers available regarding the use of specific types of infant formulas. These will be reviewed briefly. It is important to note that products intended for use with term infants are not nutritionally equivalent to postdischarge formulas. Preterm infants maintained on term infant formulas in the first months after discharge should be assessed for any necessary vitamin/mineral supplementation, particularly in the setting of low/limited volume intake, as may be seen with bronchopulmonary dysplasia.

It has been determined that providing infants with iron-fortified formula has greatly reduced the incidence of overt iron deficiency, the most common cause of anemia in childhood.[27,28] However, the use of low-iron formulas persists in some pediatric settings. The AAP suggests this may be due to the misconception that iron-fortified formulas cause colic, constipation, diarrhea, or regurgitation. The impression that low-iron formulas are associated with fewer adverse gastrointestinal reactions is not supported. Studies have found no difference in the prevalence of fussiness, cramping, regurgitation, flatus, or colic and no difference in stool characteristics except for color (stools are darker with iron-fortified feedings). Furthermore, the evidence indicates that iron fortification of formulas does not impair the absorption of other minerals to a degree that is nutritionally important, given the levels of zinc and copper in infant formulas. In conclusion, the AAP Committee on Nutrition states that there is no role for the use of low-iron formulas in infant feeding.

Regarding the use of hypoallergenic formulas, the AAP has determined that the development of atopic and other immune-mediated reactions to dietary antigens is both multifaceted and inadequately understood.[28,29] The amount of antigen, age at introduction into the diet, food source, maternal immunity, integrity of the intestinal mucosal barrier, and heredity all contribute to the immune response to the antigen. Human milk, as well as protein hydrolysate formulas, may be useful in the prophylaxis or eradication of symptoms in a sensitized infant. Hydrolysates containing peptides of <1200 molecular weight theoretically have an advantage over other hydrolysates. The AAP further states that there is no evidence to support the routine use of these formulas for the treatment of colic, sleeplessness, or irritability.

Lastly, despite what the AAP considers limited indications, the use of soy protein-based infant formulas doubled during the late 1980s to early 1990s, so that, by 1998, soy protein-based formulas constituted approximately 25% of the market in the United States.[28,30] The conclusions and recommendations of the AAP regarding the use of these formulas are summarized in Table 3A-3. Concerns surrounding the use of soy protein-based infant formulas in preterm infants also are described in this table.

Caloric supplementation

Certain preterm infants may continue to require caloric supplementation above standard dilutions after discharge. Typically, this occurs in the following situations:

1. the infant has a flat or decelerating growth curve pattern;
2. the infant is unable to take enough volume to follow a growth curve; and

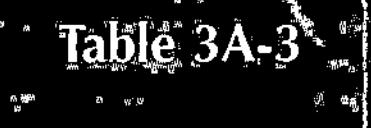

Table 3A-3 Conclusions and Recommendations of the American Academy of Pediatrics Committee on Nutrition on the Use of Soy Protein-Based Infant Formula

The AAP recommends the use of soy formulas for the following:

1. Term infants whose nutritional needs are not met from breast milk. The isolated soy protein-based formulas are safe and nutritionally equivalent alternatives to cow milk-based formula.
2. Term infants with galactosemia or hereditary lactase deficiency.
3. Term infants with documented transient lactase deficiency.
4. Infants with documented immunoglobulin E (IgE)-associated mediated allergy to cow milk (most will tolerate soy protein-based formula).
5. Patients seeking a vegetarian-based diet for a term infant.

The use of soy protein-based formula is not recommended for the following:

1. Preterm infants weighing <1800 g.
2. Prevention of colic or allergy.
3. Infants with cow milk protein-induced enterocolitis or enteropathy.

From American Academy of Pediatrics Committee on Nutrition: Formula feeding of term infants. In Kleinman RE, editor) Pediatric nutrition handbook ed 5. Elk Grove Village, IL, 2004, American Academy of Pediatrics.

3. the infant is volume restricted because of severe lung or cardiac disease and is unable to follow a growth curve.

Although optimal rates of growth in this population have yet to be defined, the guidelines described in Table 3A-4 may be beneficial.[31] Table 3A-5 provides some suggested recipes for the caloric supplementation of breast milk. In addition, Table 3A-6 provides some suggested recipes for formula concentrations above standard dilutions; these recipes should be confirmed at regular intervals with formula manufacturers to ensure continued accuracy. If increased caloric supplementation does not improve the infant's growth pattern, further evaluation by a pediatric endocrinology specialist, gastroenterology specialist, and/or registered dietitian is warranted.

Table 3A-4 Growth Velocity of Preterm Infants from Term to 24 Months*

Age from Term (mo)	Weight (g/day)	Length (cm/mo)	Head Circumference (cm/mo)
1	26–40	3–4.5	1.6–2.5
4	15–25	2.3–3.6	0.8–1.4
8	12–17	1–2	0.3–0.8
12	9–12	0.8–1.5	0.2–0.4
18	4–10	0.7–1.3	0.1–0.4

From Theriot L: Routine nutrition care during follow-up. In Groh-Wargo S, Thompson M, Hovasi Cox J, et al., editors: *Nutritional care for high-risk newborns,* ed 3. Chicago, 2000, Precept Press.
*Range includes ±1 SD.

Strategies for weaning caloric supplementation (reviewed in Table 3A-7), while allowing for continued growth, may include the following:

1. gradual adjustments to caloric density, followed by weight checks;

Table 3A-5 Caloric Supplementation of Breast Milk[1-7]

Caloric Amount	Breast Milk
24 kcal/oz	1 tsp formula powder[8] to 90 ml breast milk[9]
26 kcal/oz	1½ tsp formula powder[8] to 90 ml breast milk

[1]These recipes are approximations and should be confirmed with the formula manufacturers at regular intervals to ensure continued accuracy.
[2]A measured teaspoon should be used for these preparations.
[3]The primary care provider should review these preparations at regular intervals with the family.
[4]The Food and Drug Administration cautions against the use of powdered infant formulas with immunocompromised infants.
[5]Prepared breast milk should be stored in the refrigerator in a covered container and used within 24 hours.
[6]If increased caloric supplementation does not improve the infant's growth pattern, further evaluation by a pediatric endocrinology specialist, gastroenterology specialist, and/or registered dietitian is warranted.
[7]Monitor infant for dietary intolerance (e.g., gastrointestinal symptoms, bloody stools); care should be revised to meet individual needs.
[8]Potential formula powders include the following: EnfaCare LIPIL, NeoSure Advance, Enfamil LIPIL, or Similac Advance.
[9]Certain institutions may add 1 tsp NeoSure Advance powder to 75 ml breast milk to equal 24 kcal/oz.

Table 3A-6 Caloric Supplementation of Formula[1-6]

	EnfaCare LIPIL	NeoSure Advance
24 kcal/oz	For every 2 unpacked, level scoops of powder, add 3.5 fluid oz of water; this will yield 4 oz of formula.	For every 3 unpacked, level scoops of powder, add 5.5 fluid oz of water. This will yield 6.5 oz of formula.
27 kcal/oz	For every 2 unpacked, level scoops of powder, add 3 fluid oz of water; this will yield 3.5 oz of formula.	For every 5 unpacked, level scoops of powder, add 8 fluid oz of water. This will yield 9 oz of formula.

[1]These recipes are approximations and should be confirmed with the formula manufacturers at regular intervals to ensure continued accuracy.
[2]The primary care provider should review these preparations at regular intervals with the family.
[3]The Food and Drug Administration cautions against the use of powdered infant formulas with immunocompromised infants.
[4]Prepared formula should be stored in the refrigerator in a covered container and used within 24 hours.
[5]If increased caloric supplementation does not improve the infant's growth pattern, further evaluation by a pediatric endocrinology specialist, gastroenterology specialist, and/or dietitian is warranted.
[6]Monitor infant for dietary intolerance (e.g., gastrointestinal symptoms, bloody stools). Hydration status should also be monitored, particularly for concentrations greater than 24 kcal/oz. Care should be revised to meet individual needs.

2. serial measurements of growth (adjusting for the infant's prematurity), including assessments of length and head circumference; and
3. *For the breastfed infant:* regular assessments of the infant's ability to transfer sufficient quantities of milk, as well as the adequacy of the mother's milk supply.
4. *For the formula-fed infant:* regular assessments of the infant's volume intake.

If an infant experiences a decline in his or her growth curve subsequent to a change in caloric density, he or she may need to return to the original caloric supplementation and be retried on the lower intake at a later time.

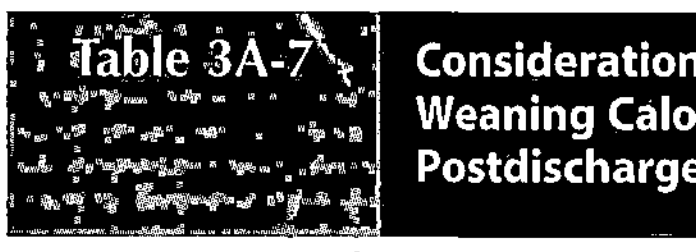

Table 3A-7 Considerations When Weaning Caloric Density Postdischarge*

Breastfed Infants

1. Make gradual changes and follow infant with frequent weight checks.
2. Follow serial measurements of growth (adjusting for the infant's prematurity), including appropriate assessments of length and head circumference.
3. Include regular follow-up assessments of the infant's ability to transfer sufficient quantities of milk as well as the adequacy of the mother's milk supply.

Formula-fed Infants

1. Make gradual changes and follow infant with frequent weight checks.
2. Follow serial measurement of growth (adjusting for the infant's prematurity), including appropriate assessments of length and head circumference.
3. Include regular assessments of the infant's volume intake.

*Further evaluation is required for any infant who is not approaching the lower percentile curve, has a flat curve, or has a decelerating growth curve.

Micronutrient supplementation

To date, there are no commercially available multivitamin/mineral preparations specifically designed for the older, growing, former preterm infant.

Vitamin D

In an effort to prevent rickets and vitamin D deficiency in healthy infants, it is important to ensure that infants are receiving the appropriate amount of Vitamin D (total 200-400 IU/day).[1,32] Acknowledging that it is difficult to determine whether sunlight exposure is adequate, the AAP recommends a supplement of 200 IU vitamin D/ day for the following:

1. all breastfed infants, unless they are weaned to at least 500 ml/day of vitamin D-fortified formula[32] and
2. all nonbreastfed infants who are ingesting <500 ml/day of vitamin D-fortified formula or milk.

However, the Academy of Breastfeeding Medicine recommends continuation of 400 IU/day in breastfed infants born at < 35 weeks' gestation and 200 IU/day supplementation for those born at 35-37 weeks' gestation (late preterm).[33] Most standard multivitamin preparations provide 400 IU of vitamin D/mL. Please refer to Table 3A-8 for recommendations about vitamin D supplementation in premature infants.

Iron

Iron deficiency has been identified as the most common nutritional deficiency in the United States,

Table 3A-8 Iron and Vitamin D Supplementation in the Preterm Infant

Nutrient	Breastfed	Formula fed
Elemental iron[1,2]	2 mg/kg/day iron supplementation starting at 1 month until 12 months[3]	Only iron-fortified formulas are recommended. Because iron-fortified formulas (including postdischarge formulas) supply ≈1.8 mg/kg/day at an intake of 150 mL/kg/day, infants may benefit from an additional 1 mg/kg/day until 12 months of age.
Vitamin D[4]	200 IU/d vitamin D supplementation beginning within the first 2 months of life until 12 months of age[5,6]	If infants are ingesting <500 ml/day of vitamin D-fortified formula or milk, supplement with 200 IU of vitamin D per day.

From Rao R, Georgieff: Microminerals. In Tsang RC, Uauy R, Koletzko B, et al., editors: *Nutrition of the preterm infant: scientific basis and practical guidelines*, ed 3. Cincinnati, 2005, Digital Educational Publishing, and American Academy of Pediatrics (AAP) Committee on Nutrition: Iron deficiency. In Kleinman RE, editor: *Pediatric nutrition handbook*, ed 5. Elk Grove Village, Ill, 2004, American Academy of Pediatrics.

Note that this is a recommended guideline that does not represent a professional standard of care; care should be revised to meet individual patient needs.

[1]Infants who are receiving erythropoietin should receive 6 mg/kg/day iron supplementation.

[2]For infants who are receiving a combination of breast milk and formula, adjust dosages of multivitamins and/or iron as needed.

[3]This is the current American Academy of Pediatrics recommendation, which does not stipulate chronologic vs. corrected age. Tsang et al[10]. continue to recommend a range of 2–4 mg/kg/day.

[4]Note that most standard multivitamin preparations contain 400 IU of vitamin D per milliliter.

[5]If the infant has weaned to at least 500 ml/day of vitamin D-fortified milk or formula, this may be discontinued.

[6]The Academy of Breastfeeding Medicine recommends 400 IU/day in breastfed infants born <35 weeks' gestation and 200 IU/day for those born 35–37 weeks' gestation.[32] The Academy of Breastfeeding Medicine also recommends that strong consideration be given to starting vitamin D supplementation earlier than 2 months of age in all premature infants.

predominantly affecting older infants, young children, and women of childbearing age.[34] Preterm infants are at risk for early iron deficiency because they are born with low iron stores. Adverse neurologic outcomes also have been identified as a consequence of early iron deficiency. At present, the AAP recommends that all breastfed preterm and low-birth-weight infants receive an oral iron supplement (elemental iron), in the form of drops, 2 mg/kg/day, starting at 1 month of age and continuing until 12 months.[1,34] As noted earlier, preterm and postdischarge formulas supply ≈1.8 mg/kg with an average intake ml/kg/day. However, former preterm infants may benefit from an additional 1 mg/kg/day until 12 months of age.[1] Rao and Georgieff[35] state further that the daily enteral iron need in the nonphlebotomized 1000-g preterm infant is 2 mg/kg/day, but that this dose becomes higher when adjusted for noncompensated phlebotomy losses and the number of days that the infant did not receive iron because of feeding intolerance or illness. These authors recommend a range of 2–4 mg/ kg/day supplementation for these ELBW and VLBW infants. Of note, standard pediatric multivitamin with iron preparations frequently contain 10 mg/mL. See Table 3A-8 for recommendations regarding iron supplementation in premature infants. Further information regarding the treatment of anemia can be found in Chapters 3C and 6A.

Calcium and phosphorus

As previously noted, continued use of nutrient-enriched postdischarge formulas in the premature infant until approximately 9 months of age has resulted in improved bone mineral content when compared with infants who received term infant formulas.[1] Because of the lack of a postdischarge human milk fortifier or multivitamin/mineral preparation designed for this population, enhancing the calcium and phosphorus intake of the human milk-fed, former preterm infant presents a greater challenge. As noted earlier, supplementation with 2-3 feedings of a postdischarge formula per day may enhance the infant's mineral intake. For the infant with a history of osteopenia of prematurity, further information may be found in Chapter 7B.

Fluoride

The AAP *Pediatric Nutrition Handbook* provides an in-depth review of the indications for fluoride supplementation in the discussion of nutrition and oral health.[36]

Text continued on page 58

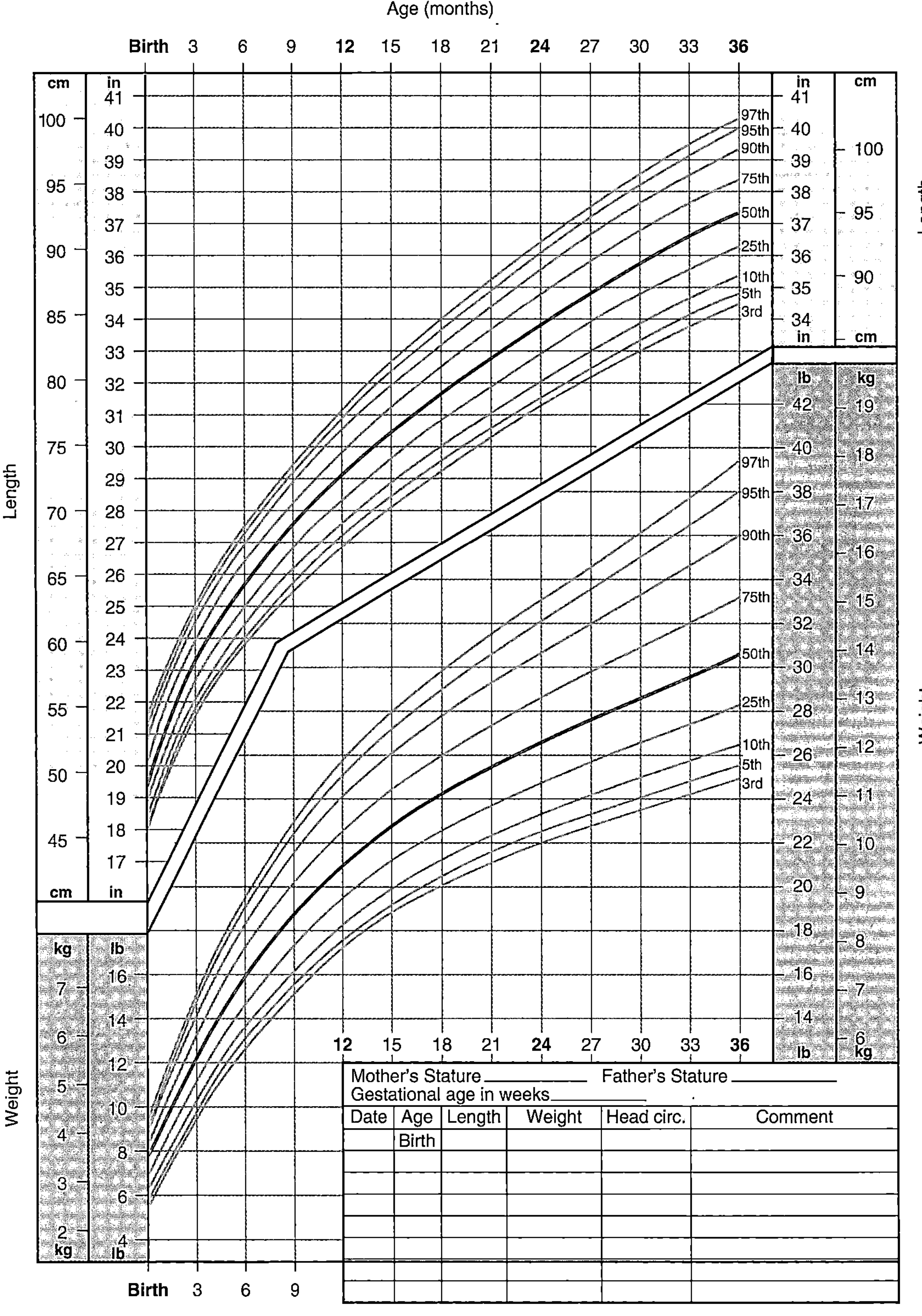

FIGURE 3A-1 This is the CDC US growth chart for the head circumference, length, and weight in girls from birth to age 36 months. A premature infant's growth is plotted by charting for both chronological age and corrected age.

GIRLS: BIRTH TO 36 MONTHS
CDC US GROWTH CHARTS* Name Record #

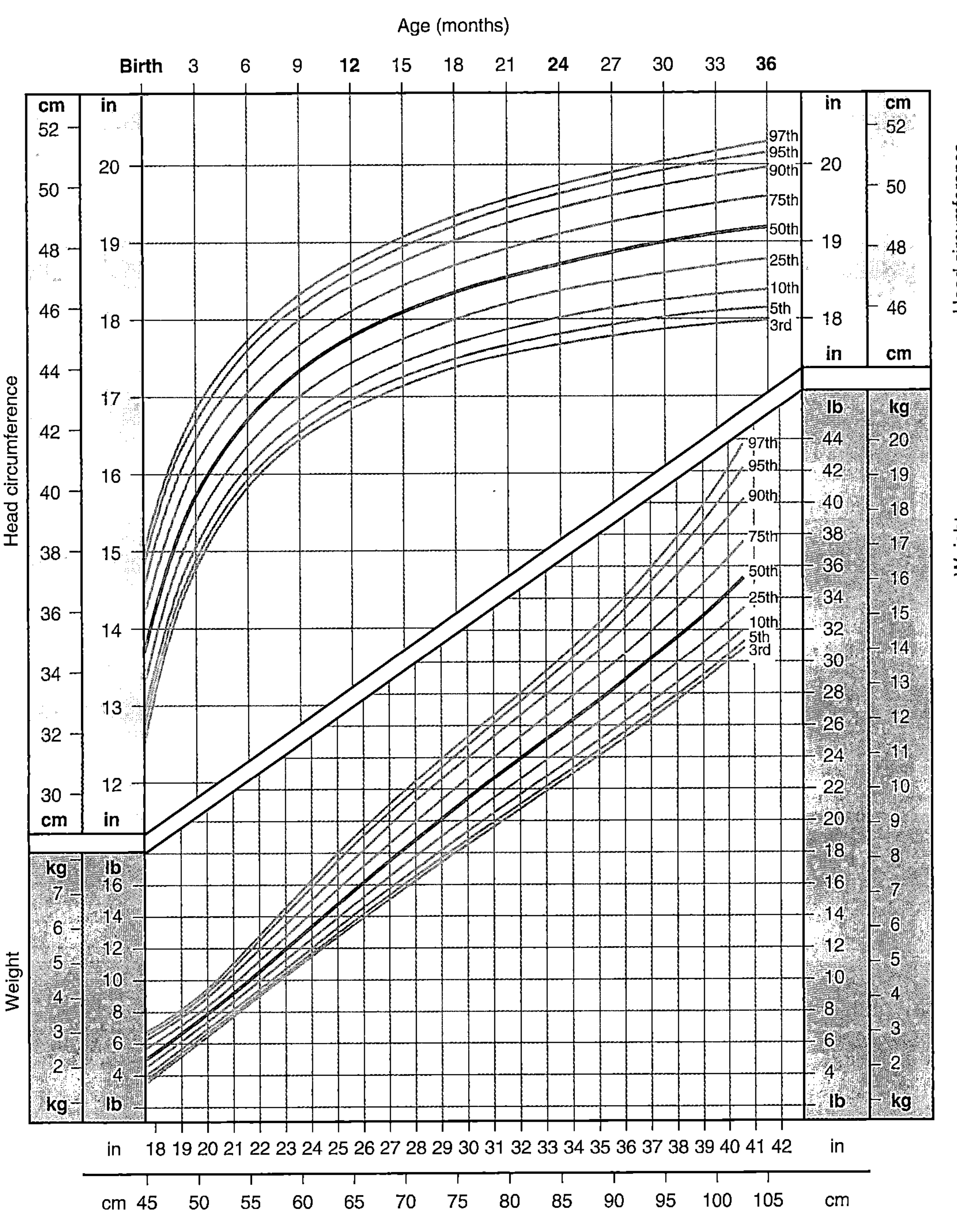

Date	Age	Length	Weight	Head circ.	Comment
	Birth				

FIGURE 3A-1, cont'd

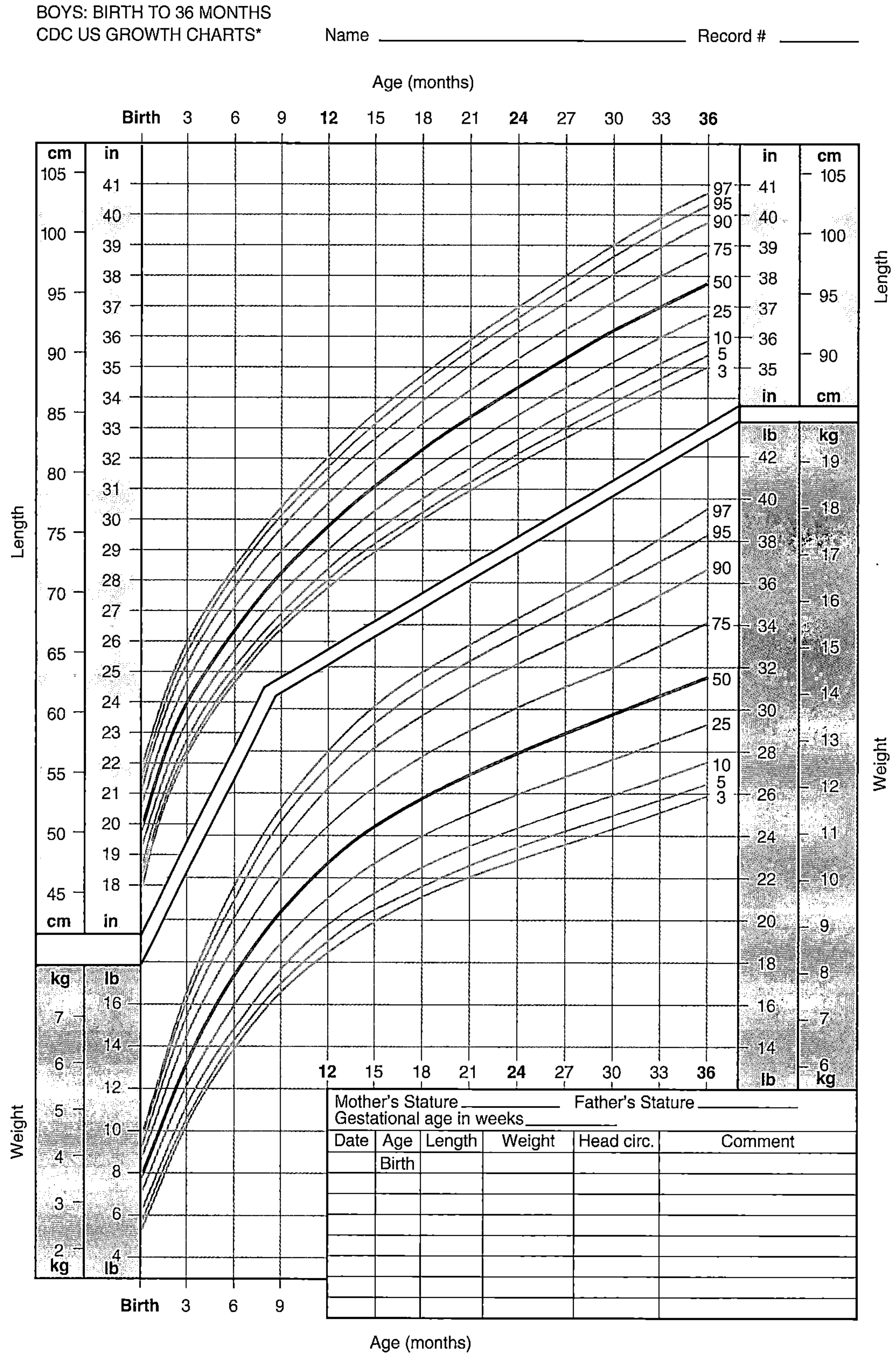

Date	Age	Length	Weight	Head circ.	Comment
	Birth				

FIGURE 3A-2 This is the CDC US growth chart for the head circumference, length, and weight in boys from birth to age 36 months. A premature infant's growth is plotted by charting for both chronological age and corrected age.

BOYS: BIRTH TO 36 MONTHS
CDC US GROWTH CHARTS* Name ______________________ Record # ________

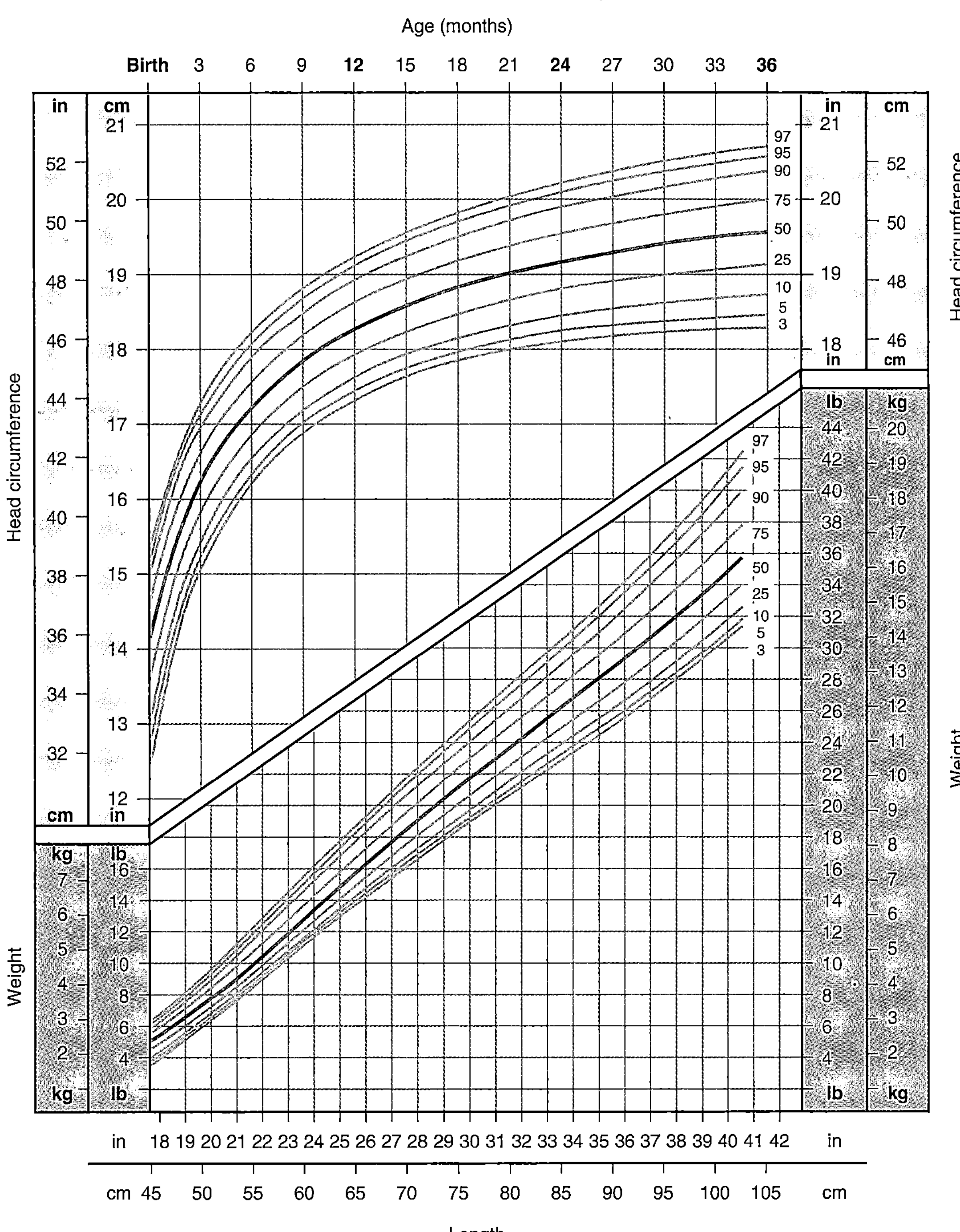

Date	Age	Length	Weight	Head circ.	Comment
	Birth				

FIGURE 3A-2, cont'd

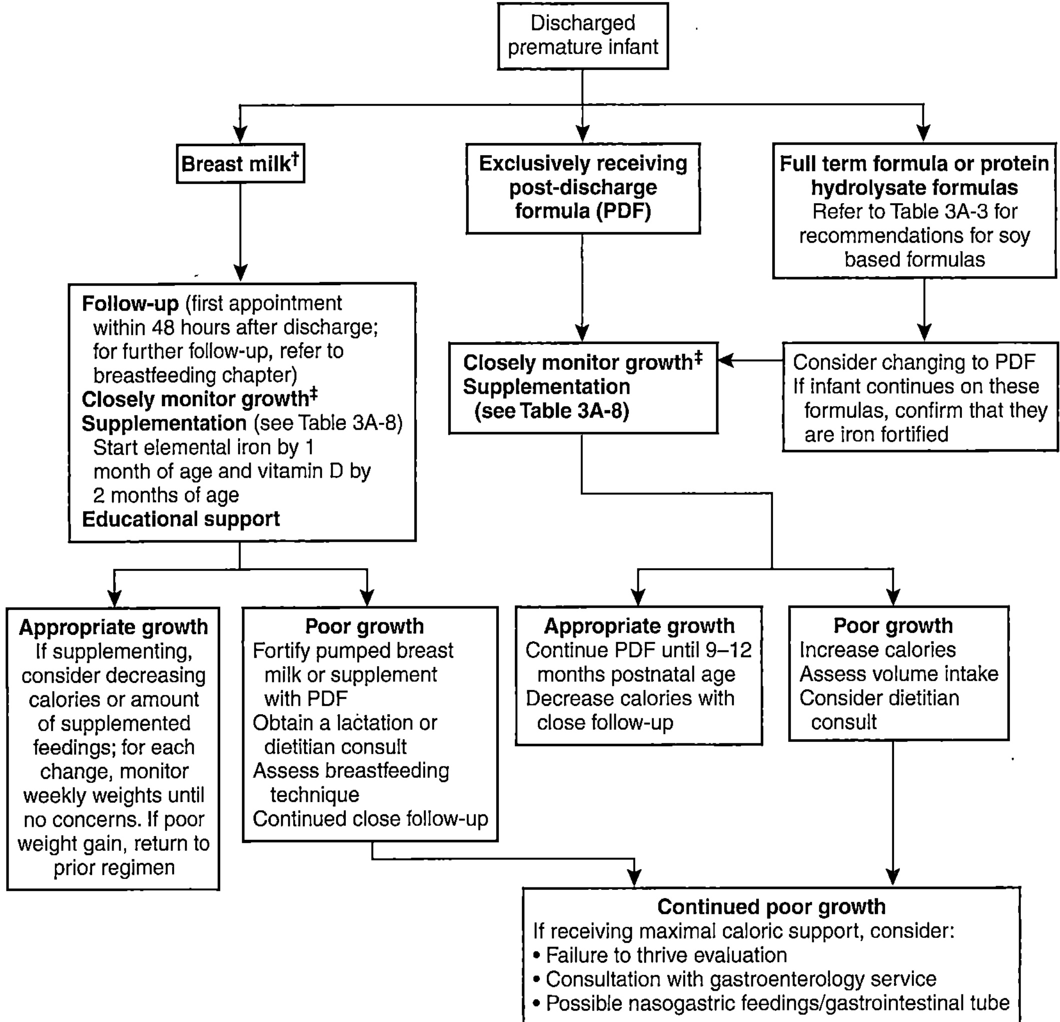

FIGURE 3A-3 This algorithm reviews the outpatient nutritional evaluation of premature infants. *Feeding plan must be individualized; †for details, refer to Figures 3B-1 and 3B-2; ‡when plotting growth, use corrected gestational age. Please note that this is a recommended algorithm that does not represent a professional standard of care; care should be revised to meet individual patient needs.

Growth charts

Two types of growth charts are used with premature infants: intrauterine and postnatal.[37,38] Intrauterine growth charts are desirable because they more closely reflect the ideal growth of the fetus. However, one disadvantage of these charts is that they are based on cross-sectional data. Postnatal growth charts have the advantage of following the same infants over time (i.e., longitudinal data); however, they also represent the actual postnatal growth of preterm infants, which frequently has been shown to be suboptimal. Sherry et al.[39] evaluated the growth references available for VLBW infants in the United States. The authors stated that it was difficult to recommend any one reference. However, they declared that the Infant Health and Development Program (IHDP) graphs were the most useful for comparing the growth of VLBW infants with that of other VLBW babies, and that the Centers for Disease Control and Prevention (CDC) charts were preferable for comparison with the growth of non-VLBW infants (i.e., the neonates' age-adjusted peers) (Figures 3A-1 and 3A-2). Because preterm infants should be striving for rates of growth comparable with those of a healthy population, use of the CDC grids may be more desirable, with the IHDP graphs serving as an adjunct, if necessary.

Regardless of the growth chart used, serial measurements of the infant's weight, length, and head circumference provide the most helpful data from which to assess the infant's overall growth pattern.[31] In clinical practice, the infant's corrected age typically is used for the plotting of anthropometric data until at least 18 months of age. Further evaluation is required for any infant who is not approaching the lower percentile curve, has a flat curve, or has a decelerating growth curve. If enhanced nutritional support does not improve the infant's growth pattern or if an evaluation does not identify an etiology, the primary care provider should obtain a referral from a pediatric endocrinology specialist, gastroenterology specialist, and/or registered dietitian.

Conclusion

The most optimal strategies for the postdischarge nutritional management of ELBW and VLBW infants are unknown. One possible algorithm for the outpatient evaluation of preterm infants is outlined in Figure 3A-3. Additional research is needed to determine the best practice guidelines for transitioning these infants from calorically enhanced discharge feedings to more standard feeding practices, including the progression to full breastfeeding, without compromising growth. In the interim, serial measurements of growth, while appropriate postdischarge feedings are maintained, may offer the most favorable strategy until more specific, universally accepted protocols are established.

Resources for Families and Clinicians

American Dietetic Association
www.eatright.org

The website of the American Dietetic Association provides many resources for clinicians, as well as a method for identifying local dietitians at:

http://www.eatright.org/cps/rde/xchg/ada/hs.xsl/home_fanp_business_ENU_HTML.htm

Growth Charts
http://www.cdc.gov/growthcharts/

The Centers for Disease Control and Prevention provide growth charts along with frequently asked questions, an interactive web-based training module, and a link to Women, Infants and Children (WIC)-specific growth charts.

NASPGHAN: North American Society for Pediatric Gastroenterology, Hepatology and Nutrition
http://www.naspghan.org

This website provides information to families about specific gastrointestinal disorders, including lactose intolerance.

WIC (Women, Infants and Children) Program
www.fns.usda.gov/wic/aboutwic/

WIC is a federally funded program that assists financially eligible pregnant and postpartum mothers and children younger than 5 years with food, nutritional education, and access to healthcare services.

REFERENCES

1. American Academy of Pediatrics (AAP) Committee on Nutrition: Nutritional needs of the preterm infant. In Kleinman RE, editor: *Pediatric nutrition handbook*, ed 5. Elk Grove Village, Ill, 2004, American Academy of Pediatrics.
2. Lemons JA, Bauer CR, Oh W, et al: Very low birth weight outcomes of the national institute of child health and human development neonatal research network, January 1995 through December 1996. NICHD Neonatal Research Network. *Pediatrics* 107:1, 2001.
3. Embleton NE, Pang N, Cooke RJ: Postnatal malnutrition and growth retardation: an inevitable consequence of current recommendations in preterm infants? *Pediatrics* 107:270, 2001.
4. Schulze K, Kashyap S, Ramakrishnan R: Cardiorespiratory costs of growth in low birth weight infants. *J Dev Physiol* 19:85, 1993.
5. Ziegler EE, Thureen PJ, Carlson SJ: Aggressive nutrition of the very low birthweight infant. *Clin Perinatal* 29:225, 2002.
6. Lucas A, Morley R, Cole TJ: Randomised trial of early diet in preterm babies and later intelligence quotient. *BMJ* 317:1481, 1998.
7. Ehrenkranz RA, Dusick AM, Vohr BR, et al: Growth in the neonatal intensive care unit influences neurodevelopmental and growth outcomes of extremely low birth weight infants. *Pediatrics* 117:1253, 2006.
8. Carlson SE: Feeding after discharge: growth, development and long-term effects. In Tsang RC, Uauy R, Koletzko B, et al., editors: *Nutrition of the preterm infant: scientific basis and practical guidelines*, ed 3. Cincinnati, 2005, Digital Educational Publishing.
9. Hovasi Cox J, Doorlag D: Nutritional concerns at transfer or discharge. In Groh-Wargo S, Thompson M, Hovasi Cox J, et al., editors: *Nutritional care for high-risk newborns*, ed 3. Chicago, 2000, Precept Press.
10. Lucas A, Cole TJ: Breastmilk and neonatal necrotizing enterocolitis. *Lancet* 336:1519, 1990.
11. Shulman RJ, Schanler RJ, Lau C, et al: Early feeding, feeding tolerance, and lactase activity in preterm infants. *J Pediatr* 133:645, 1998.
12. Kliegman RM, Pittard WM, Fanaroff AA: Necrotizing enterocolitis in neonates fed human milk. *J Pediatr* 95:450, 1979.
13. Shulman RJ, Schanler RJ, Ou C, et al: Intestinal permeability in the premature infant is related to urinary cortisol excretion. *Gastroenterology* 110:A839, 1996.
14. Fomon SJ, Ziegler EE: Renal solute load and potential renal solute load in infancy. *J Pediatr* 134:11, 1999.
15. Singhal A, Cole TJ, Lucas A: Early nutrition in preterm infants and later blood pressure: two cohorts after randomised trials. *Lancet* 357:413, 2001.
16. Schanler RJ, Shulman RJ, Lau C: Feeding strategies for premature infants: beneficial outcomes of feeding fortified human milk versus preterm formula. *Pediatrics* 103:1150, 1999.

17. Cavell B: Gastric emptying in infants fed human milk or infant formula. *Acta Paediatr Scand* 70:639, 1981.
18. Riordan J: The biological specificity of breastmilk. In Riordan J, editor: *Breastfeeding and human lactation*, ed 3. Sudbury, 2005, Jones and Bartlett.
19. Anderson CH: Human milk feeding. *Pediatr Clin North Am* 32:335, 1985.
20. Schanler RJ, Atkinson SA: Human milk. In Tsang RC, Uauy R, Koletzko B, et al., editors: *Nutrition of the preterm infant: scientific basis and practical guidelines*, ed 3. Cincinnati, 2005, Digital Educational Publishing.
21. Hurst NM, Meier PP: Breastfeeding the preterm infant. In Riordan J, editor: *Breastfeeding and human lactation*, ed 3. Sudbury, 2005, Jones and Bartlett.
22. Valentine CJ, Hurst NM, Schanler RJ: Hindmilk improves weight gain in low birth weight infants fed human milk. *J Pediatr Gastroenterol Nutr* 18:474, 1994.
23. DeCurtis M, Goulet O, Hernell O, et al: Feeding preterm infants after hospital discharge: A commentary by the ESPGHAN Committee on Nutrition. *J Pediatr Gastroenterol Nutr* 42:596-603,2006.
24. Hovasi Cox J: Bronchopulmonary dysplasia. In Groh-Wargo S, Thompson M, Hovasi Cox J, et al., editors: *Nutritional care for high-risk newborns*, ed 3. Chicago, 2000, Precept Press.
25. Lucas A, Fewtrell MS, Morley R, et al: Randomized trial of nutrient-enriched formula versus standard formula for postdischarge preterm infants. *Pediatrics* 108:703, 2001.
26. Carver JD, Wu PYK, Hall RT, et al: Growth of preterm infants fed nutrient-enriched or term formula after hospital discharge. *Pediatrics* 107:683, 2001.
27. American Academy of Pediatrics Committee on Nutrition: Iron-fortified infant formulas. *Pediatrics* 84:1114, 1989.
28. American Academy of Pediatrics Committee on Nutrition: Formula feeding of term infants. In Kleinman RE, editor: *Pediatric nutrition handbook*, ed 5. Elk Grove Village, Ill, 2004, American Academy of Pediatrics.
29. American Academy of Pediatrics Committee on Nutrition: Hypoallergenic infant formulas. *Pediatrics* 83:1068, 1989.
30. American Academy of Pediatrics (AAP) Committee on Nutrition: Soy protein-based formulas: recommendations for use in infant feeding. *Pediatrics* 101:148, 1998.
31. Theriot L: Routine nutrition care during follow-up. In Groh-Wargo S, Thompson M, Hovasi Cox J, et al., editors: *Nutritional care for high-risk newborns*, ed 3. Chicago, 2000, Precept Press.
32. American Academy of Pediatrics Committee on Nutrition: Breastfeeding. In Kleinman RE, editor: *Pediatric nutrition handbook*, ed 5. Elk Grove Village, Ill, 2004, American Academy of Pediatrics.
33. Academy of Breastfeeding Medicine Protocol #12: Transitioning the breastfeeding/breastmilk-fed premature infant from the neonatal intensive care unit to home. Available at: *http://www.bfmed.org/ace-files/protocol/NicuGradProtocol.pdf*
34. American Academy of Pediatrics Committee on Nutrition: Iron deficiency. In Kleinman RE, editor: *Pediatric nutrition handbook*, ed 5. Elk Grove Village, Ill, 2004, American Academy of Pediatrics.
35. Rao R, Georgieff M: Microminerals. In Tsang RC, Uauy R, Koletzko B, et al., editors: *Nutrition of the preterm infant: scientific basis and practical guidelines*, ed 3. Cincinnati, 2005, Digital Educational Publishing.
36. American Academy of Pediatrics Committee on Nutrition: Nutrition and oral health. In Kleinman RE, editor: *Pediatric nutrition handbook*, ed 5. Elk Grove Village, Ill, 2004, American Academy of Pediatrics
37. Anderson DM: Nutritional assessment and therapeutic interventions for the preterm infant. *Clin Perinatol* 29:313, 2002.
38. Ellard D, Olsen IE, Sun Y: Nutrition. In Cloherty JP, Eichenwald EC, Stark AR, editors: *Manual of neonatal care*, ed 5. Philadelphia, 2004, Lippincott Williams & Wilkins.
39. Sherry B, Mei Z, Grummer-Strawn L, et al: Evaluation of and recommendations for growth references for very low birth weight (<1500 grams) infants in the United States. *Pediatrics* 111:750, 2003.

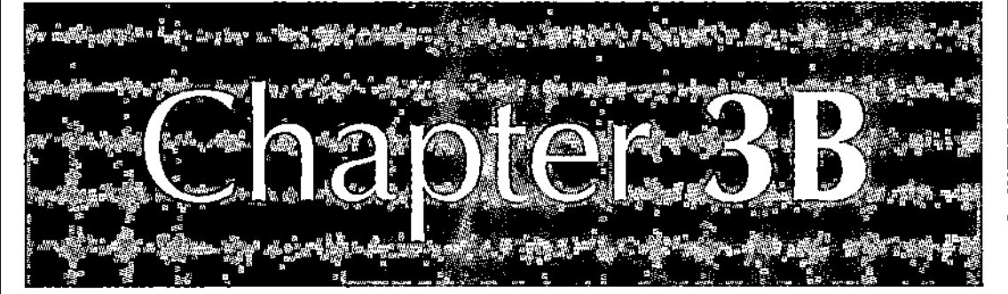

Breastfeeding and the Premature Infant

Kimberly G. Lee, MD, MSc, IBCLC, FABM

When an infant is admitted to the neonatal intensive care unit (NICU), parents lose the opportunity for a "perfect" childbirth experience. Their ability to bond with their child and/or to participate in their child's care often is limited by their infant's condition and by the array of technology involved in supporting a NICU patient. Mothers in this situation may be reassured and empowered by the knowledge that breastfeeding is something important and concrete that only they can do for their babies. Even mothers who did not originally plan to breastfeed often will want to provide milk for their premature infant because of the numerous health benefits. Meier et al.[1] reported in 1993 that mothers ascribed great significance to being able to express milk for their infant's feeding and to breastfeed during and after their child's stay in the NICU, although the failure rate was high.

Although Meier et al.[1] referred to "failure," breastfeeding success may, in fact, have many definitions. Driscoll[2] states that "breastfeeding is a relationship and a method of communication. Breastfeeding success or failure is a personally defined experience that is based on a woman's individual perceptions and self definition." In other words, a woman's personal goals affect her perception of her own success. Primary care providers are uniquely positioned to help the NICU mother redefine her expectations for "breastfeeding success" within the limits imposed by her infant's prematurity and illness severity.

Because most premature infants do not have the strength or maturity to feed exclusively at the breast until close to their due date, giving expressed milk to the infant via gavage is a more realistic initial expectation. However, even this goal involves challenges. Establishing and maintaining a mother's milk supply with a breast pump is more difficult than establishing and maintaining a supply with a vigorous, full-term nursing infant. When the premature infant finally achieves the coordination of sucking, swallowing, and breathing required for oral feeding, learning to feed at the breast may also be a challenging and lengthy process. Professional support from experienced, certified lactation consultants and primary care providers is essential for optimizing breastfeeding in the preterm and late preterm infant. Excellent published resources on breastfeeding are available for healthcare providers.

The purpose of this chapter is to summarize issues involved in breastfeeding the preterm and late preterm infant and to outline the detailed resources that are available to assist providers in supporting these families.

Benefits of Human Milk for Premature Infants

The scientific literature confirms that human milk has several advantages and benefits over formula. Preterm infants need the immunologic and metabolic benefits of their mothers' milk.[3] Although data from randomized controlled trials are extremely limited, premature infants provided with human milk appear to have increased protection from morbidities such as necrotizing enterocolitis and late-onset sepsis.[3] It seems likely that they also receive the numerous benefits identified in the general population: less frequent and/or decreased severity of infections, lower incidence of several chronic illnesses, and possibly better developmental outcomes.[3,4] Milk produced by mothers of preterm infants is different in composition from that of mothers whose infants are born at term. Preterm milk contains more protein and fat and less lactose (thus more caloric density) than term milk for at least the first month after delivery.

Basic Lactation Physiology

Lactation is driven by *demand-and-supply* physiology. In response to infant suckling, mothers produce prolactin (the hormone that stimulates milk production) and oxytocin (the hormone that triggers contraction of myoepithelial cells resulting in the "letdown" reflex). Less familiar but crucial to demand-and-supply physiology is the feedback inhibitor of lactation, which must be removed from the alveoli in order to continue to stimulate milk production.

Because preterm infants tend to be quite "undemanding," their mothers will have to *create a demand* in order to generate a supply. Thus, it is crucial that they

1. Initiate pumping as early as possible, within hours of delivery,
2. Empty their breasts frequently, at least 8 to 10 times per day, and
3. Use a hospital-grade electric pump, "double pumping" both sides at once.

To facilitate oxytocin release, mothers should have

1. Skin-to-skin contact with their infant as early and often as possible (sometimes referred to as "kangaroo care"),
2. A quiet, relaxing and private place in which to pump and/or nurse, and
3. Maximal use of resources for coping with stress.

One study found that mothers randomized to receive a relaxation audiotape produced more than 50% more milk at a subsequent test pumping than did controls.[5] Such recordings now are available commercially.

A mother's milk supply is expected to exceed her premature infant's day-to-day needs by the end of the first 3 weeks postpartum, the period during which prolactin receptors are being upregulated and supply is being established. It is much easier for an infant to "grow into" an already-established milk supply than for the mother to increase her milk supply after the first 3 weeks. Milk production of at least 600 ml in 24 hours is considered optimal, and less than 350 ml in 24 hours is considered low.[6] Mothers of multiples will require higher volumes than mothers of singletons.[7] Table 3B-1 outlines a widely used approach to generate a differential diagnosis for low milk supply. In general, "postglandular" problems, further explained in Table 3B-2, are the most common as well as the most easily ameliorated.

Preterm Infants

Even before the premature infant born at <35 weeks' gestation is ready to begin oral intake, there are several ways to facilitate the transition to the breast:

1. Regular daily practice sessions at the breast during kangaroo care should gradually introduce a fuller breast to the infant.
2. Mothers should be encouraged to pump before kangaroo care so that their infant can practice nuzzling, licking, and eventually latching at a breast that is not completely full.
3. Infants should continue to receive gavage feedings during the session so that they can begin to associate a satiated feeling with nursing.
4. If possible, mothers and staff should avoid introducing bottles until the infant has established success at breastfeeding.

Once a premature infant is beginning to feed at the breast, there are several ways to optimize the transfer of mother's milk to the premature infant:

1. Help the mother learn to provide support for the infant's head and chin.
2. Teach the mother the "alternate massage" technique, in which she compresses her breast during pauses in the infant's sucking to move milk toward the infant and maintain his or her interest.
3. If the infant is unable to latch or effectively transfer milk from the breast, consider using an ultrathin silicone nipple shield.
4. If the infant requires additional calories and volume (i.e., is not gaining weight consistently despite frequent feedings) but does successfully latch and suckle, consider using a supplemental feeder (usually a thin feeding tube connected at one end to a reservoir containing supplement and the other end taped to the mother's nipple).

When possible, unrestricted time at the breast increases volume intake and is an easier and more physiologic solution than is the use of the supplemental feeder.

Prenursing and postnursing weights using a very sensitive scale (e.g., Medela Baby Weigh) can be helpful in quantifying the intake of breast milk. Pumping after practice sessions may also provide mothers with an estimate of the volume of milk taken by the infant. It often is necessary for

Table 3B-1 Understanding Low Milk Supply

Failure of mammogenesis *Presents clinically as a lack of breast growth and development in puberty and pregnancy*	**Preglandular Causes** • Deficiency of mammary growth-stimulating hormones • Hypothalamic destruction or disruption as a result of encephalitis, infiltration of tumour following lymphocytic hypophysitis, or idiopathic etiology • Pituitary space-occupying lesions, hyperplasia, empty sella syndrome, acromegaly, pituitary stalk section • Mammary growth-stimulating hormone deficiency, or antibodies to or biologically inactive lactogenic hormones • Pregnancy-specific mammary nuclear factor may suppress genes involved in mammary gland development **Glandular Causes** • Lack of glandular response to normal lactogens • Polycystic ovarian syndrome with estrogen or prolactin mammary gland receptor deficits • Regulatory factors involved in the development of myoepithelial cells before lactation (not well understood)
Failure of lactogenesis *Presents clinically as lack of colostrum and/or lack of engorgement in first few days postpartum*	**Preglandular Causes** • Intrinsic lack of lactogenic hormones, biologically inactive lactogens, or lactogenic antibodies • Pituitary and hypothalamic pathologies (as described in the preglandular causes for failure of mammogenesis) • Retained placental fragments • Drugs such as bromocriptine **Glandular Causes** • Secondary failure of mammogenesis • Lack of mammary gland responsiveness to lactogenic hormones, including plasma membrane receptor deficits or faulty gene transcription **Postglandular Causes** • Initiation of breastfeeding delayed, lack of hormonal surges • Infrequent early breast stimulation acts as an extrinsic inhibitor of early lactogenic hormone release • Incomplete drainage or unrelieved engorgement leads to accumulation of local inhibitory factors • Outlet obstruction following breast surgical reconstruction • Supplementary infant feedings suppress otherwise vigorous infant's hunger drive
Failure of galactopoiesis *Presents clinically as lack of ongoing copious milk production postpartum*	**Preglandular Causes** • Intrinsic lack of lactogenic hormones • Extrinsic effects of some drugs (e.g., pseudoephedrine, birth control pills), smoking, new pregnancy **Glandular Causes** • Failure of mammogenesis or lactogenesis • Unresponsiveness to lactogenic hormones **Postglandular Causes** • Inadequate ongoing breast stimulation leading to an extrinsic lack of lactogenic hormones • Inadequate regular breast drainage because of inefficient or infrequent breastfeeding, leading to an increase in feedback inhibitor of lactation

Modified from: Morton JA: *Pediatr Ann* 32:308-16, 2003, and Livingstone V. Neonatal insufficient milk syndrome: a classification. Poster presentation, Academy of Breastfeeding Medicine, 2005.

mothers to continue to pump until the infant is able to sufficiently empty the breast (usually at or after term postmenstrual age).

Before discharge, "the team" (i.e., providers, lactation consultant, dieticians, and parents) should develop a feeding plan. The Academy of Breastfeeding Medicine (ABM) has developed a number of protocols to support breastfeeding. Clinical Protocol #12 outlines steps for transitioning the breastfeeding/breast milk-fed premature infant from the NICU to home.[8] Although most premature infants will require caloric supplementation, some infants who are growing without extra calories may have a 1-week trial of ad lib breastfeeding before discharge. During this time, mothers must continue to express milk at least three times per day to maintain their milk supply. This trial period can help the clinician and family identify issues that need to be addressed, such as optimizing the latch, recognizing infant feeding cues, recognizing maternal concerns, and identifying unrealistic expectations. If optimal milk transfer does not occur, the mother may need to pump before feedings in order to facilitate letdown and/or after feedings to

Table 3B-2 Postglandular Reasons for Insufficient Milk and/or Failure to Thrive

Inefficient milk transfer *Presents clinically as small test feed or pump volume with a large residual volume of milk*	**Suboptimal Maternal Breastfeeding Technique** Maternal or infant positioning • Lack of knowledge or physical disability Ineffective latch • Maternal anatomic causes: poorly graspable fixed, retracted, or engorged nipple/ areola **Suboptimal Pumping Technique** Positioning of flange inappropriately Flange inappropriate size for maternal nipple/breast Pump settings (pressure and/or cycles) set inappropriately **Suboptimal Infant Breastfeeding Technique** Ineffective latch and/or suckling • Infant anatomic causes: tongue tie, cleft lip/palate, retrognathia, facial asymmetry • Infant physiologic causes: prematurity, neurologic, respiratory, or cardiac disorders **Inhibited Milk Ejection Reflex** • Temporary inhibition due to adrenalin release if the mother is subjected to unpleasant or painful physical or psychological stimuli, including embarrassment or fear
Inadequate milk intake *Presents clinically as failure to thrive, with near-term infants especially at risk*	**Frequency of Breastfeeds Inadequate** • Prolonged gaps between feeds • Sleepy, ill, jaundiced, "happy to starve" nondemanding infants or overuse of pacifier **Duration of Feeds Inadequate** • Short or interrupted feeds • Early termination of the feed because of misreading cues (e.g., a pause vs sleep)

Modified from: Livingstone V. Neonatal insufficient milk syndrome: a classification. Poster presentation, Academy of Breastfeeding Medicine, 2005.

facilitate emptying. Devices such as nipple shields and/or a supplemental feeding system may be useful when supervised by a trained and certified lactation consultant or knowledgeable healthcare professional. The mother may want to preferentially provide the high-fat milk or "hindmilk," which usually is produced at the end of a feeding or pumping session, to increase caloric density.

Table 3B-3 Discharge Requirements of a Breastfeeding Infant Born <35 Weeks' Gestation

Growth is within normal limits or improving.
- Weight gain >20 g/day
- Length increase >0.5 cm/wk
- Head circumference increase >0.5 cm/wk

Biochemical indices are within normal limits or improving.
- Phosphorus <4.5 mg/dl
- Alkaline phosphatase >450 IU/L
- Blood urea nitrogen <5 mg/dl

Oral intake >120 kcal/kg/day (>180 ml/kg/day of mother's milk without added caloric density). Note that this goal may be less if growth and biochemical indices are appropriate or if the infant is fluid-restricted and growing.

A feeding plan should be provided.

An infant must meet the criteria listed in Table 3B-3 to have an optimal nutritional status before discharge home. If an infant cannot take all feedings orally or takes less than optimal volumes, has inadequate growth (weight gain <20g/day and/or length increase <0.5 cm/week), or has abnormal biochemical indices that are not improving, the infant's nutritional status at discharge is suboptimal. Infants with suboptimal nutritional status should be discharged home taking mother's milk ad lib with at least two to three feedings per day of high-caloric-density formula. The family must be provided with a specific, written feeding plan that includes content, volume, method of supplementation, frequency of supplements per day, and recommended frequency of nursing and pumping. It is critical that mothers of babies whose nutritional status is "suboptimal" continue to express milk at least three times per day to maintain their milk supply.

After discharge, all infants should be monitored closely for adequacy of milk intake as well as for growth. Figure 3B-1 outlines an algorithm for outpatient follow-up *48 hours after discharge and one week after discharge.* If there is evidence of suboptimal nutritional status, the provider should do the following: (1) increase the number of feeds of high-caloric-density formula (up to 30 kcal/oz) per day; (2) ensure

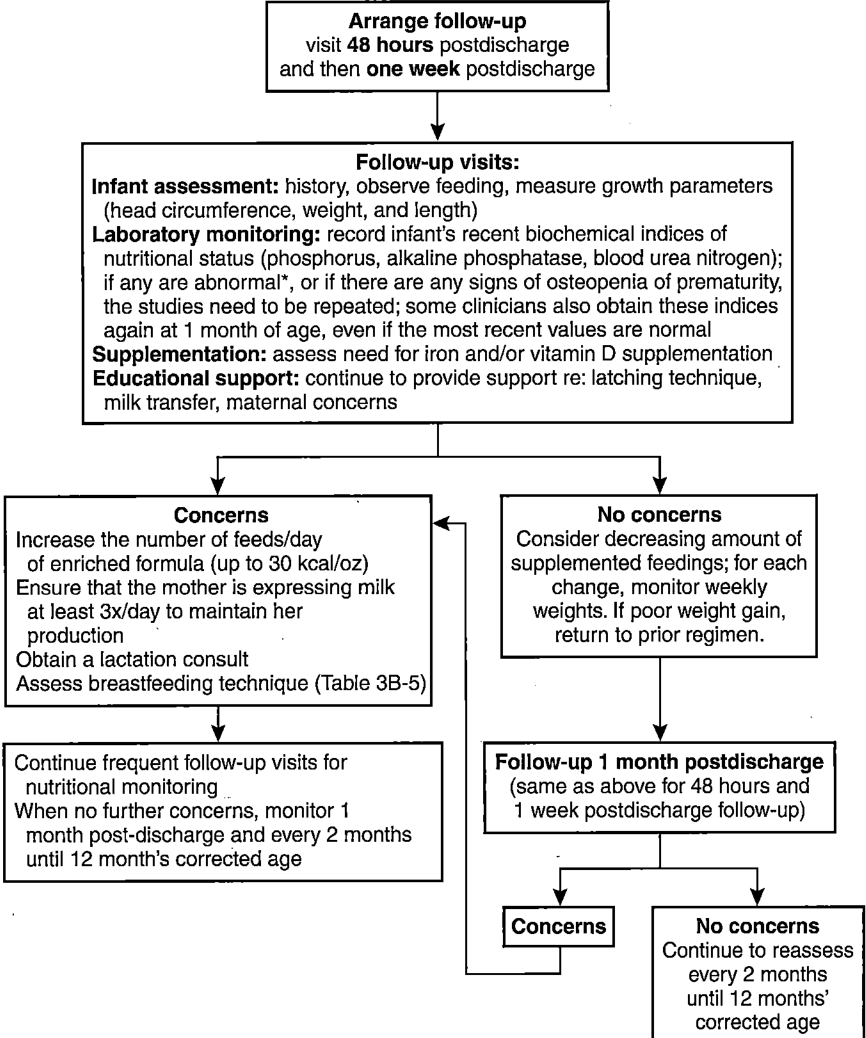

FIGURE 3B-1 Algorithm for Postdischarge Monitoring of a Breastfeeding Preterm Infant (born <35 weeks' gestation)[8]. *Abnormal values if: phosphorus <4.5 mg/dL, alkaline phosphatase >450 IU/L, and/or blood urea nitrogen < 5 mg/dL. Please note that this is a recommended algorithm that does not represent a professional standard of care; care should be revised to meet individual patient needs.

that the mother is expressing milk to maintain her production; and (3) continue frequent primary care follow-up visits for nutritional monitoring.

Late Preterm Infants

Although the "late preterm" infant seems relatively mature and may be admitted directly to a newborn nursery rather than a NICU, such infants often are unable to feed exclusively at the breast. In this chapter, infants born between 35 and 37 weeks' gestation are "late preterm" infants. These "late preterm" infants, if not supported and monitored closely, may tire quickly and thus take in less milk volume than they require to meet their metabolic needs, leading to a "downward spiral" of poor feeding and lethargy. This puts them at high risk for readmission for hyperbilirubinemia, dehydration, and/or significant weight loss. Clinicians and families must maintain realistic expectations for late preterm infants: although they may seem large, they are not yet fully mature.

There are many ways to monitor and maximize breastfeeding success in late preterm infants (Tables 3B-4 and 3B-5). An algorithm for monitoring these infants predischarge and postdischarge

Table 3B-4 Strategies to Maximize Breastfeeding Success Predischarge in the Late Preterm Infant*[4,9]

Maximal mother-to-infant contact
Encourage frequent skin-to-skin contact to prevent hypothermia, promote milk production, and emphasize infant's feeding cues
Teach mother to nurse frequently (at *least* 8 times per 24 hours) based on infant's cues (e.g., rooting, hand-to-mouth movements)
Educate mother that "an awake premie is a hungry premie" (i.e., babies should nurse before being held by other relatives); late preterm infants may need to be awakened to feed
Emphasize provision of breast support and support head/chin as needed
Closely monitor latch and milk transfer
Devices such as nipple shield and/or supplemental nursing system may be useful and should be used under the supervision of a trained lactation consultant or knowledgeable healthcare professional
Carefully monitor weight, urine output, and stool output.* Weights before and after breastfeeding may be helpful
If supplemental feeds are required, ensure that mother pumps after feedings, ideally using a hospital-grade electric pump, until the infant is ≈40 weeks' postmenstrual age and/or is able to completely empty the breasts†
Ensure that if phototherapy is needed, breastfeeding should be disrupted as little as possible because jaundice often is an indicator of inadequate enteral intake and enterohepatic recirculation of bilirubin
Establish a written feeding plan before discharge, including the following‡:
- Frequency, volume, and composition of any supplements
- Method of supplementing most acceptable to mother (cup, fingerfeeding/tube system, bottle)

Determine iron/vitamin supplements that are needed (See Special Topics)
Arrange appropriate follow-up

*Infants may require small volumes of supplemented expressed breast milk or formula (5–10 ml per feed on day 1, 10–30 ml per feed thereafter).
†In this situation, the "triple feeding method" is recommended; first the mother nurses, then the milk expressed after the previous feed is given (this can be done by anyone), followed by pumping.
‡Communicate this feeding plan to the primary care provider; families should maintain a written record of the feeding history.

is outlined in Figure 3B-2. The healthcare professional should revise the breastfeeding plan if there is weight loss >3% of birth weight at 24 hours of age, weight loss >7% of birth weight by 72 hours of age, ineffective milk transfer, or exaggerated jaundice.[9] Once the late preterm infant is discharged to home, the primary care provider will need to follow the infant closely to monitor weight, elimination patterns, and degree of jaundice. The ABM recommends an initial follow-up visit within 48 hours of discharge and weekly weight checks until 40 weeks' postmenstrual age or until the infant is thriving without formula and/or caloric supplements.

Special Topics

Supplements

Although evidence from randomized clinical trials is limited, other evidence suggests that premature infants who are receiving breast milk should be

Table 3B-5 Observational Assessment for Appropriate Breastfeeding Technique

Latch should be asymmetric (more of underside of breast in infant's mouth)
Infant's mouth should be wide open to at least 130- to 150-degree angle, with lips flanged outward
Infant's nose should touch breast
Infant's head, back, and bottom should be aligned in one plane (i.e., neck should not be turned = "nose to breast, chest to chest")
Suck should be rhythmic with pauses for swallowing (at less frequent intervals than suck); latch and position should be maintained throughout feeding
Swallow should be audible as a gulp once lactogenesis II has occurred; audible clicks or smacks are indicative of ineffective latch and require adjustment of position and/or referral to a lactation specialist
Assess mother's breast and appropriate consultations from lactation specialist and/or obstetric provider if:
- Compressed, blanched, bleeding, bruised, blistered, cracked, or otherwise traumatized nipples (indicating problems with latching)
- Engorgement (indicating problems with transfer)
- Mastitis (erythema, fever, systemic symptoms)*

*Treatment of mastitis includes continued breastfeeding with attention to adequate milk transfer and emptying.

ALGORITHM FOR BREASTFEEDING THE LATE PRETERM INFANT

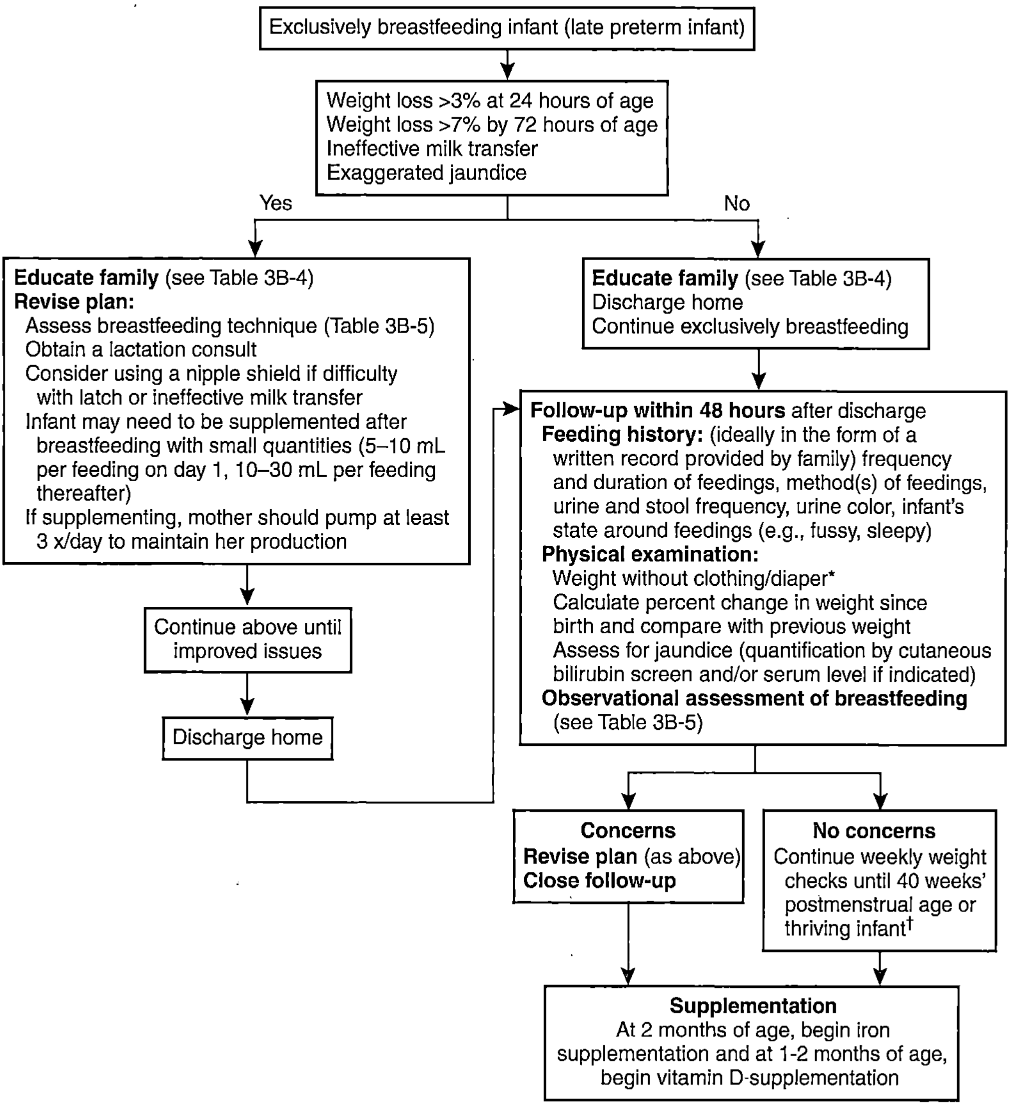

Exclusively breastfeeding infant (late preterm infant)

Weight loss >3% at 24 hours of age
Weight loss >7% by 72 hours of age
Ineffective milk transfer
Exaggerated jaundice

Yes

Educate family (see Table 3B-4)
Revise plan:
Assess breastfeeding technique (Table 3B-5)
Obtain a lactation consult
Consider using a nipple shield if difficulty with latch or ineffective milk transfer
Infant may need to be supplemented after breastfeeding with small quantities (5–10 mL per feeding on day 1, 10–30 mL per feeding thereafter)
If supplementing, mother should pump at least 3 x/day to maintain her production

Continue above until improved issues

Discharge home

No

Educate family (see Table 3B-4)
Discharge home
Continue exclusively breastfeeding

Follow-up within 48 hours after discharge
Feeding history: (ideally in the form of a written record provided by family) frequency and duration of feedings, method(s) of feedings, urine and stool frequency, urine color, infant's state around feedings (e.g., fussy, sleepy)
Physical examination:
Weight without clothing/diaper*
Calculate percent change in weight since birth and compare with previous weight
Assess for jaundice (quantification by cutaneous bilirubin screen and/or serum level if indicated)
Observational assessment of breastfeeding (see Table 3B-5)

Concerns
Revise plan (as above)
Close follow-up

No concerns
Continue weekly weight checks until 40 weeks' postmenstrual age or thriving infant†

Supplementation
At 2 months of age, begin iron supplementation and at 1-2 months of age, begin vitamin D-supplementation

FIGURE 3B-2 Algorithm for Monitoring of an Exclusively Breastfeeding Late Preterm (35-37 weeks' gestation) Premature Infant Predischarge and Postdischarge[9]. *An infant over 4 days of age who is receiving adequate breast milk will have 6-8 voids and 3-4 yellow stools daily, weight loss <7-10% of birth weight, and be satisfied after 20-30 minutes of nursing; †Median weight gain of a healthy late preterm newborn is 26-31 gm/day. Please note that this is a recommended algorithm that does not represent a professional standard of care; care should be revised to meet individual patient needs.

supplemented with iron and/or vitamins after discharge. The American Academy of Pediatrics (AAP) Committee on Nutrition recommends supplementing breastfeeding preterm infants with 2 mg/kg/day of elemental iron between 1 and 12 months of age.[10] For infants receiving ≈50% of intake as formula, the dose should be reduced to 1 mg/kg/day.[10] Infants with anemia of prematurity may require higher amounts of supplemental iron. Please refer to Chapter 3A for more details.

The AAP also recommends a supplement of 200 IU of vitamin D per day for all breastfed infants unless they are weaned to >500 ml/day of vitamin D-fortified formula or milk. This should begin within the first 2 months of age. Most standard infant multivitamin preparations provide 400 IU of vitamin D per milliliter.[10] The ABM recommends that strong consideration be given to starting vitamin D supplementation earlier than 2 months of age in infants born prematurely because they have lower vitamin D stores at birth. Please refer to Chapter 3A for more details.

Maternal medications

Women who are receiving medications after delivery often are concerned about the potential effects on their infant. Indeed, this concern is reported to be one of the major reasons mothers decide to stop breastfeeding. Because drug manufacturers rarely have the resources to test their products in pregnant or lactating women, the standard product information usually advises patients to check with a physician before taking the medication. Thus, it is crucial for physicians to understand the principles of drug transfer into human milk. The history of transplacental exposure to a medication before delivery, specific pharmacologic properties of the medication, and the infant's age (postmenstrual as well as chronologic) are important factors to consider in weighing potential risk(s) to the infant against the known benefits of human milk (Table 3B-6).

Multiples

The majority of multiple births in the United States occur at <37 weeks' gestation. With advances in assisted reproductive technology over the past 2 decades, these preterm multiples have become more numerous. If demand-and-supply physiology were the only consideration for optimal milk production, mothers of multiples would have sufficient supply to meet their infants' increased demand. Although anecdotal experience suggests that this is not the case, large-scale U.S. data are not available. One study noted a significantly shorter duration of breastfeeding for preterm multiples compared with term multiples or preterm singletons.[7] Another study reported that mothers of twins who provided a higher percentage of breast milk feedings by 1 month postpartum were more likely to be providing a high percentage of breast milk feedings at 6 months.[11] These data suggest that it is especially crucial to support mothers of preterm multiples in developing an abundant milk supply in the first few weeks after delivery.

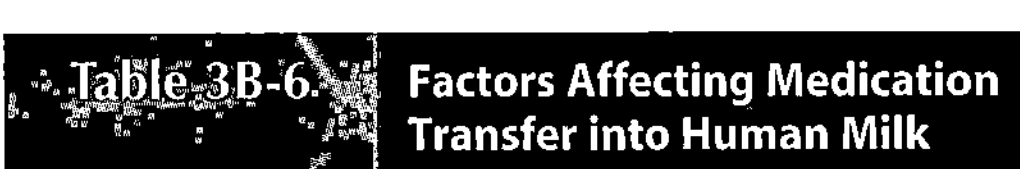
Table 3B-6. Factors Affecting Medication Transfer into Human Milk

Pharmacologic Properties
- Molecular weight (the higher the molecular weight, the less likely medication will enter milk)
- Maternal levels (the lower the level, the less potential for medication to enter milk)
- Lipid solubility (the less lipid soluble, the lower the ability of medication to enter milk)
- pK_a (the more basic the medication [e.g., barbiturates], the more likely the ion form will be trapped in milk)

Age of Infant
- Chronologic age: In the first 4 days postpartum, intracellular gaps persist within mother's alveoli, allowing most medications more access to milk than later
- Gestational age: The more preterm the infant, the less mature the hepatic and renal function and the more likely the infant is to develop higher levels of the medication metabolized by these organs

Cytomegalovirus

Cytomegalovirus (CMV) may be present in human milk and has been reported to cause serious infections in a small number of very premature babies. Because extremely premature infants have not received the transplacental maternal antibodies that might protect against CMV infection, maternal CMV-positive status is a relative contraindication to breastfeeding these infants at younger postmenstrual ages and should be determined on a case-by-case basis. Further data are needed before CMV positivity can be declared a definite contraindication to breastfeeding a preterm infant.[12] Some US centers freeze expressed breast milk from CMV-positive mothers until their infants are older than 28 to 32 weeks' postmenstrual age.

Reimbursement

Because breastfeeding has long-term health benefits, it is imperative that providers support families who choose to breastfeed. Such support can be time-consuming, so providers should become familiar with the appropriate use of diagnostic codes for reimbursement for newborn follow-up visits. Brenner[13] provides guidelines to help clinicians support breastfeeding patients and receive appropriate reimbursement for doing so. For example, coding based on time is appropriate if at least 50% of the time spent during the visit was for counseling and/or coordinating care and is documented as such.

Conclusion

As in most areas of neonatal medicine, breastfeeding support practices for preterm infants vary across individual NICUs and larger geographic regions. For example, in parts of the world where patterns of maternal employment, legislation regarding maternity leave, and reimbursement for such leave differ from those in the United States, the constant presence of mothers in the NICU and exclusive breastfeeding at NICU discharge are the norm. In the United States, however, maternal presence in the NICU often is limited by the demands of employment.

In any case, it is clear that preterm infants benefit at least as much from breastfeeding as do term infants, and that their mothers benefit as well. With appropriate support and monitoring, it is possible for care providers to assist families in meeting the special challenges of making these benefits a reality.

Resources for Families and Clinicians

Academy of Breastfeeding Medicine
www.bfmed.org

This international professional organization of physicians has developed many clinical protocols, including those referenced in this chapter.

American Academy of Pediatrics
www.aap.org/healthtopics/breastfeeding.cfm

This website provides many resources available from the AAP and external organizations to help families initiate and successfully continue breastfeeding.

La Leche League International
www.lalecheleague.org/

This worldwide organization offers mother-to-mother support, education, information, and encouragement to women who want to breastfeed their babies. It aims to promote a better understanding of breastfeeding.

Lactation Consultants

To identify a local consultant, contact the International Board of Lactation Consultant Examiners (*www.iblce.org*) or the International Lactation Consultant Association (*www.ilca.org*).

National Women's Health Information Center
www.womenshealth.gov/breastfeeding

This website provides information about breastfeeding for families. This organization provides a phone number (1-800-994-9662) to answer basic breastfeeding questions.

OTHER SOURCES

Meek JY, editor: *The American Academy of Pediatrics: new mother's guide to breastfeeding,* Elk Grove Village, Ill, 2002, American Academy of Pediatrics.

Hale TW: *Medications and mothers' milk: a manual of lactational* pharmacology, ed 12. Amarillo, Tex, 2006, Pharmasoft Publishing. Also available in a version for downloading to personal digital assistants at: *www.ibreastfeeding.com*

Steube A, Fiuimara K, Lee KG: Principles of medication use during lactation. In Rose BD, editor. *UpToDate.* Wellesley, Mass, 2004, UpToDate. Available at: *www.uptodate.com*

The videotape set "A Premie Needs His Mother" from the Stanford University Breastfeeding Medicine Program is targeted at mothers of preterm infants but is also useful for care providers. Available at: *www.breastmilksolutions.com*

REFERENCES

1. Meier PP, Engstrom JL, Mangurten HH, et al: Breastfeeding support services in the neonatal intensive care unit. *J Obstet Gynecol Neonatal Nurs* 22:338-347, 1993.
2. Driscoll JW: Breastfeeding success and failure: implications for nurses. NAACOGS *Clin Issues Perinat Womens Health Nurs* 3:565-569, 1992.
3. Lang S: The basics of breastfeeding. In Lang S, editor. *Breastfeeding special care babies,* ed 2. Edinburgh, 2002, Bailliere Tindall.
4. Breastfeeding basics. In: *Breastfeeding your premature baby.* Schaumburg, Ill, 2002, La Leche League International.
5. Feher SD, Berger LR, Johnson JD, et al: Increasing breast milk production for premature infants with a relaxation/imagery audiotape. *Pediatrics* 83(1):57-60, 1989.
6. Meier PP: Supporting lactation in mothers with very low birth weight infants. *Pediatr Ann* 32:317-25, 2003.
7. Geraghty SR, Pinney SM, Sethuraman G, et al: Breast milk feeding rates of mothers of multiples compared to mothers of singletons. *Ambul Pediatr* 4(3):226-31, 2004.
8. Academy of Breastfeeding Medicine Protocol #12: Transitioning the breastfeeding/breastmilk-fed premature infant from the neonatal intensive care unit to home, September 2004. Available at: *http://www.bfmed.org/protocol/neonatal.pdf*
9. Academy of Breastfeeding Medicine Protocol #10: Breastfeeding the near-term infant (35 to 37 weeks' gestation). August 2004. Available at: *http://www.bfmed.org/protocol/near_term.pdf*
10. American Academy of Pediatrics (AAP) Committee on Nutrition: Nutritional needs of the preterm infant. In Kleinman RE, editor: *Pediatric nutrition handbook,* ed 5. Elk Grove Village, Ill, 2004, American Academy of Pediatrics.
11. Damato EG, Dowling DA, Madigan EA, et al: Duration of breastfeeding for mothers of twins. *J Obstet Gynecol Neonatal Nurs* 34:201-209, 2005.
12. Bryant P, Morley C, Garland S, et al: Cytomegalovirus transmission from breast milk in premature babies: does it matter? *Arch Dis Child Fetal Neonatal Ed* 87:F75-F77, 2002.
13. Brenner MG: You can provide efficient, effective, and reimbursable breastfeeding support—here's how. *Contemp Pediatr* 22:66-76, 2005.

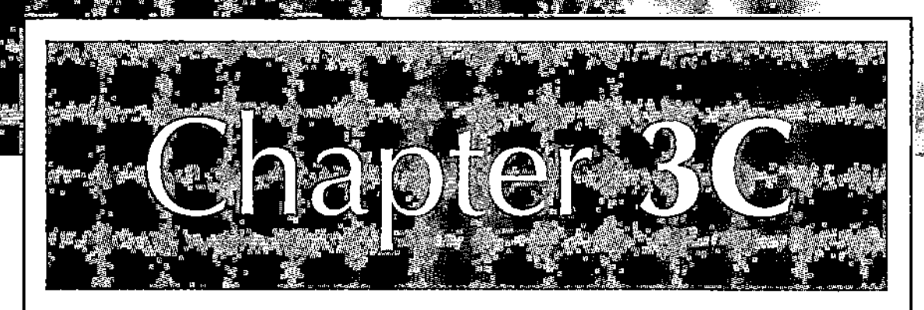

Nutritional Deficiencies

Vincent C. Smith, MD, MPH

Premature infants are at greater risk than term infants for nutritional deficiencies. This chapter focuses on iron, zinc, protein, essential fatty acid, and carnitine deficiencies, with specific emphasis on the premature infant's limitations, clinical signs of deficiency, and recommended supplementations to prevent these deficiencies (Table 3C-1).

Iron Deficiency

Iron metabolism

Iron is an essential component of hemoglobin required for the transport of oxygen to the tissues. Term infants acquire the majority of their iron stores during the third trimester.[1] The total body iron content for the fetus doubles in the last trimester, from 35 to 40 mg at 24 weeks to 75 mg/kg during the last trimester and 225 mg at term.[1] Infants who are born preterm do not have the benefit of developing these iron stores.

After birth, infants obtain most of their iron from their diet. Dietary iron is absorbed from the duodenum and proximal jejunum in two different forms. In the first form, iron forms a complex with porphyrin, referred to as *heme iron*.[2] Heme iron is absorbed directly into the intestinal mucosal cells.[2] Alternatively, the other form of heme is not in a complex and is referred to as *nonheme iron*. The majority of the dietary iron for children is in the nonheme form. The absorption of nonheme iron varies with the infant's overall nutritional status, degree of iron deficiency, and the presence of inhibitors.[2] Infants who are iron replete absorb less, and those who are deficient absorb more. Protein, calcium, phylates (as contained in soy formula), phenol, and tannins all inhibit nonheme iron absorption.[2] Ascorbic acid, citrate, meat, and fish increase the absorption of this type of iron.[2]

After absorption, transferrin transports iron within the body to the transferrin receptor located on the cell surface.[2] The receptor relocates the iron into the cell. If it is a hematopoietic cell, the majority of the iron will be incorporated into hemoglobin. Iron can be stored in a soluble mobile form, ferritin, or an aggregated insoluble form, hemosiderin.[2]

Iron is metabolized in several phases during a preterm infant's life. The first stage involves decreased erythropoiesis. During this phase, the hematocrit will fall and lead to "anemia of prematurity" at approximately 2 to 3 months of age (see Chapter 6A).[3] During the second phase, there is active production of red cells, which requires iron.[3] In the last phase, iron stores are exhausted, and, if the stores are inadequate, "late anemia of prematurity" can develop.[3]

Full-term infants

Iron-fortified infant formulas contain between 6 and 15 mg/L, and "low-iron formulas" have 4.5 mg/L.[1,2] The iron in human milk is more bioavailable; approximately 50% of the iron in human milk is absorbed, compared with 10% to 20% iron absorption in formula.[1]

At birth, appropriate birth weight term infants are able to thrive because they utilize stored or internally recycled iron. They have enough iron stores for the first 4 to 6 months of life.[1] By 3 to 4 months of age, term infants require supplemental exogenous iron.[2] The daily elemental iron requirement for a term infant is 1 to 2 mg/kg/day.[1,4]

At term, the concentration of iron in human milk is low (0.3–0.5 mg/L).[2] Despite this low level, iron deficiency is fairly uncommon in exclusively breastfed term infants during the first 6 months of life.[1] After this time, they have an iron deficiency rate of 20 to 30% unless supplemented at 4 to 6 months of age.[1,5]

Table 3C-1 Nutritional Deficiencies in the Premature Infant

Type of Deficiency	Predisposing Factors for This Deficiency in Premature infants	Clinical Signs of Deficiency	Minimal Enteral Requirement in Premature Infants
Iron	Altered metabolism: After premature infants develop anemia of prematurity caused by decreased erythropoiesis, extremely active production of red blood cells leads to iron deficiency if stores are inadequate to meet the infant's needs Decreased initial iron stores Greater risk for initial iron loss because of phlebotomy Rapid growth rate leading to increased utilization	Pallor, fatigue, irritability, motor developmental delay Possibility of neurodevelopmental sequelae if early and severe iron deficiency	Refer to Chapter 3A for details about iron supplementation
Zinc	Decreased initial zinc stores History of parenteral nutrition without zinc additives Inadequate maternal zinc stores (e.g., from vegetarian diet) and infant exclusively receiving breast milk History of necrotizing enterocolitis requiring surgical repair Diuretic therapy	Growth failure Rash (erythematous, involving perioral, perianal, facial areas) Decreased oral intake, increased irritability, diarrhea, hair loss, impaired wound healing, depressed immune function	1000 µg/kg/day enteral zinc or 833 µg per 100 kcal daily in stable, growing premature infants
Protein	History of necrotizing enterocolitis requiring surgical repair Inadequate stores	Irritability, edema, ascites Skin changes (hyper-pigmentation, hyperkeratosis, desquamation, ulcers) Hair—thin and decreased pigmentation Kwashiorkor syndrome if diet high in carbohydrates with protein deficiency	2.5–3 g per 100 kcal daily in stable, growing premature infants
Essential fatty acid	Inadequate stores Immature ability to synthesize long-chain polyunsaturated fatty acids	Thrombocytopenia Poor growth Skin changes (dry, leathery, desquamative dermatitis) If occurs in infancy, may decrease brain growth Reduced visual acuity	0.44–1.7 g of linoleic acid and 0.11–0.44 g of linolenic acid per 100 kcal daily
Carnitine	Inadequate stores Immature hepatic function cannot easily synthesize carnitine Immature kidneys may not sufficiently reabsorb carnitine	Liver disease Cardiomyopathy Muscle weakness	Carnitine is abundant in breast milk and is supplemented in formulas More likely found in premature infants receiving parenteral nutrition

Preterm infants

During the first 7 weeks of lactation, preterm infants are likely to develop iron deficiency if they are not supplemented adequately. Preterm infants are at greater risk for iron deficiency because of blood loss from phlebotomy and a rapid growth rate.[1] In preterm infants, iron deficiency is also affected by birth weight, initial hematocrit, and blood transfusions.

Clinically, iron deficiency anemia usually manifests itself as pallor, fatigue, irritability, and motor development delay.[5] Early iron deficiency can result in neurodevelopmental sequelae that are immediate and persistent despite correction.[1] One study found that infants who are nutritionally appropriate but deficient in iron performed less well on cognitive function studies than did their peers at 5 to 6 years of age.[2]

In iron deficiency, hemoglobin and/or hematocrit levels will be below normal[2]; mean corpuscular volume (MCV) will be low; free protoporphyrin level will be elevated; transferrin saturation levels will be decreased; and serum ferritin levels will be low.[2]

Because of the lack of prenatally acquired stores, iron supplementation is recommended in preterm infants. The total dose, including dietary intake and supplementation, should approximate 2 to 4 mg/kg/day, depending on birth weight.[1] The American Academy of Pediatrics (AAP) recommends that premature infants should be supplemented with iron between 1 and 12 months of age, as needed. Please refer to Chapter 3A for specific details about iron supplementation in preterm infants.

Zinc Deficiency

Zinc is a vital trace element for development of bone, for the structure and function of transcription factors and steroid receptors, and for its role as a metalloenzyme.[2,6,7] It is essential for regulation of gene expression. Zinc is also required for embryogenesis and fetal growth.[2,7]

During fetal life, most of the zinc stores are amassed during the third trimester of pregnancy. Zinc is stored in the fetal liver and intestinal mucosa in a form called *metallothionein.*[7] During the first week of life, the infant mobilizes metallothionein from the liver to maintain the zinc level.[2,7] Zinc obtained from the diet is absorbed across the intestinal brush border membrane.[2,7] Phylate, fiber, other mineral elements that compete with zinc uptake at the brush border membrane, and exogenous glucocorticoids can inhibit this process.[2,7] At alkaline pH, phylate (found in soy formulas) and calcium form an insoluble complex with zinc that retards its absorption.[2,7] In contrast, amino acids such as histidine and cysteine enhance the uptake of zinc.[2,7]

Homeostasis of endogenous zinc is maintained by altering fecal excretion through bile pancreatic secretions and mucosal sloughing of desquamated cells.[2,7] Zinc acquired via parental nutrition is primarily excreted by the kidneys.[2,7]

Zinc deficiency usually involves either decreased intake or increased loss. Usually zinc intake is adequate if the infant is fed formula or human milk from a mother with adequate zinc stores/consumption.[2,5]

When the infant's mother is zinc replete, infants fed human milk usually have adequate intake of zinc. As long as the mother's intake is adequate, variations in the mother's ingestion do not cause fluctuations in the zinc content in the mother's breast milk. The human milk concentration of zinc precipitously drops naturally from approximately 60 to 22 µmol/L during the first 3 months of lactation.[2,5,7] Because zinc binds to casein (the predominant protein in cow milk), it is better absorbed from human milk than from formula or cow milk.[2,7]

The effect of exclusive human milk versus some formula feeding on the micronutrient status of the infant is unclear.[5] If the mother has inadequate intake of zinc, her breast milk can have lower than expected concentrations of zinc.[7] This could lead to zinc deficiency in the infant. This sometimes happens in mothers on a strict vegetarian diet.

Acquired zinc deficiency is uncommon.[6] Infants who are receiving parenteral nutrition without added zinc are at risk.[6,7] Because they lack zinc stores, infants who are fed parenteral nutrition should have zinc supplementation from the first day after birth to prevent zinc deficiency.[4,6,7] Premature infants who are exclusively breastfed can develop zinc deficiency that becomes apparent by 4 to 5 months of age.[6]

The primary reason for zinc deficiency usually is increased gastrointestinal or nongastrointestinal loss. Gastrointestinal causes include chronic diarrhea, possibly because of malabsorption.[2,3] Zinc metalloproteins are not adequately absorbed because of increased gastrointestinal motility time. This happens in infants after gastric or intestinal surgery.[2] Nongastrointestinal causes of zinc deficiency include high-output renal failure, diuretic therapy, and severe exfoliative dermatoses.[2] If an infant has excessive losses of zinc, zinc supplementation with two to three times the normal intake may be required to achieve a normal zinc level.

Diagnosis of zinc deficiency is primarily based on clinical symptoms. It can result in growth failure, an erythematous skin rash (involving perioral, perianal, and facial areas as well as the extremities), anorexia, and impaired acquisition of sexual characteristics.[2,3,5-7] Infants can have decreased oral intake, increased irritability, diarrhea, hair loss, impaired wound healing, and depressed immune function.[5-7] Laboratory zinc values are less reliable in the diagnosis of zinc deficiency because zinc can be sequestered in tissues during periods of stress, infection, illness, or decreased serum concentration.[2]

Symptomatic zinc deficiency is treated with oral zinc sulfate 0.05 mmol (3 mg)/kg/day until symptoms abate.[2] Premature infants require 500 to 800 µg/kg/day of enteral zinc or 150 µg/ kg/day of parenteral zinc during the transition period (day of life 0–14).[1,4,7] Enteral intake recommendation for stable growing preterm infants is 833 µg/100 kcal/day, or 1000 µg/kg/day.[1,4] If parental zinc is required in a stable or postdischarge preterm infant, the dose is 400 µg/kg/day.[1,4] Toxicity is rare but can be treated with chelation therapy such as desferoxamine.[2]

Protein Deficiency

Mild protein digestion by hydrochloric acid and proteolytic enzymes begins in the stomach.[1] Enterokinase is produced by the duodenal mucosa.[1,2] It activates trypsin, a pancreatic proteolytic enzyme, which in turn activates the remainder of the enzymes facilitating protein digestion.[1] The pancreas releases other proteolytic enzymes into the intestine that continue the digestive process. Peptides in the intestinal lumen may be either transported intact or further degraded to amino acids and then transported across the mucosal cell membrane.[2] Amino acids are transported to the liver via the portal vein for further metabolism.

Infants have gastric hydrochloric acid and pepsin concentrations that are lower than adult levels.[1,2] In preterm infants, these levels are presumably even lower.[1] Despite this situation, intestinal absorption and hepatic metabolism of protein are functionally intact in term and preterm infants.[1]

Although human milk is quantitatively low in protein, it contains appropriate amino acid levels to meet the infant's requirements.[1] Infant formulas receive approximately 10% of their total calories from protein.[1] Human milk is high in whey protein, whereas formula is high in casein protein.[2,3] Both types of protein are well absorbed.[2] Indeed, infants can digest and absorb up to 80% of their protein intake.[2] However, the kidneys are limited in their ability to excrete nitrogen during the first 2 months of life.[2]

Human milk from mothers who deliver preterm is higher in protein, calories, calcium, and sodium compared with term human milk.[1,3] The composition of human milk of mothers who deliver preterm becomes very similar to term human milk after the first month.[1,3]

Clinical symptoms of protein deficiency include irritability, edema, ascites, hypoproteinemia, and hypoalbuminemia.[2] Skin changes such as hyperpigmentation, hyperkeratosis, desquamation, and ulcers may occur.[2] The hair may become thin and lose its pigmentation.[2] The child's cheeks may become round and more prominent.[2] Fat may infiltrate the liver and lead to liver enlargement.[2] Protein deficiency can be associated with severe fat malabsorption and its associated clinical signs.[2]

The serum albumin level is the most frequently monitored laboratory value in infants with a protein deficiency. It more accurately reflects the infant's protein status than do anthropomorphic measurements, which can be skewed because of subcutaneous fat and peripheral edema.[2] Treatment involves management of the associated morbidities, providing adequate dietary intake and treating the underlying problem.

Kwashiorkor is a syndrome associated with infants who receive a diet that is high in carbohydrates but low in protein.[2] It is more common in developing countries. However, it has been reported in up to 35% of at-risk hospitalized infants.[2] The causes in this patient population usually are associated with gastrointestinal disorders or cystic fibrosis.[2] It also can be related to infant feeding practices, for example, feedings of nonstandard, nonnutritionally balanced formula (e.g., homemade), use of standard formulas that are overdiluted, restrictive diets (e.g., vegetarian), and prolonged breastfeeding without appropriate supplementation.[2]

The estimated protein need in term infants during the first month of life is 1.98 g/kg/day.[2] It then declines to 1.18 g/kg/day from 4 to 12 months of life. From birth to approximately 4 months of age, there is an increase in the body protein composition of approximately 3.5 g/day (1 g/kg/day).[2] It then declines to a rate of approximately 3.1 g/day (0.6 g/kg/day).[2] The recommended daily allowance of protein is 2.2 g/kg/day from birth to approximately 6 months of age,[2] declines to 1.6 g/kg/day from 6 to 12 months of life,[2] and finally declines to 1.2 g/kg/day from 1 to 2 years of life.[2]

Enteral intake recommendation for stable, growing preterm infants weighing less than 1 kg is 3.0 to 3.16 g per 100 kcal daily.[5] Enteral intake recommendation for stable, growing preterm infants weighing more than 1 kg is 2.5 to 3.0 g per 100 kcal daily.[5]

Essential Fatty Acid Deficiency

Lipids are a vastly important component of the diet. They are the predominant dietary source of energy for infants and children. From 40% to 55% of the energy provided by human milk and formula is in the form of lipids.[2] Lipids function to slow gastric emptying and intestinal motility, provide essential fatty acids, maintain the structural component of all tissues, and store energy.[2]

Most of the dietary lipids are in the form of triglycerides.[1] They are formed by esterification of three fatty acid moieties to a glycerol backbone. In this form, the majority of fatty acids are stored and transported.[2]

Lipid digestion begins in the stomach and continues in the duodenum with the breakdown of triglycerides into their components.[1,5] Fatty acids are then separated, and phospholipids are hydrolyzed by pancreatic phospholipase.[1] Cholecystokinin is released in response to lipid and protein in the duodenal lumen.[1] It stimulates the release of pancreatic enzymes as well as the release of bile acids from the gallbladder, and facilitates the mixing of digestive juices, lipids, and bile acids.[1] This process is significantly impaired in newborn infants, especially preterm infants, because of relative pancreatic insufficiency.[1]

Lipids with conjugated bile acids form soluble mixed micelles in the duodenum.[5] Bile acids are critical to this process. Without bile acids, only approximately one third of dietary triglycerides, a minimal amount of fatty acids, and a limited amount cholesterol or fat-soluble vitamins are absorbed.[1] Bile acid synthesis in term and preterm infants is limited. Preterm infants also have impaired enterohepatic circulation of bile salts.[1,5] This decreases the preterm infant's ability to form mixed micelles.

Mixed micelles contain fatty acids, monoglycerides, phospholipids, cholesterol, and fat-soluble vitamins.[1] It is in this form that fatty acids can be absorbed by passive diffusion through the mucosa of the intestinal tract.[2] They are then packaged in chylomicrons and secreted into the circulation via the lymphatic system.[2,4,5] Medium-chain triglycerides can be absorbed into enteric cells without being hydrolyzed.[1,5] The peripheral tissues can then uptake the fatty acids that have been hydrolyzed to the endothelial cell–bound lipoprotein lipase.[2,5]

There are several variations of fatty acids: saturated (no double bonds), monounsaturated (one double bond), and polyunsaturated (multiple double bonds).[2] In the unsaturated fatty acids, the position of the double bond is important. The position of this bond is described by its relation to the terminal methyl group (the ω end of the fatty acid). This method of description was chosen because the ω end of the fatty acid is not modified in human metabolism. The other terminal of the fatty acid is the carboxyl end. This is the portion of the fatty acid that is modified in human metabolism.[2] Modifications include elongation or shortening of the chain and/or introduction of double bonds.[2]

The ω-6 and ω-3 fatty acids have their double bonds located on the sixth or third carbon, respectively, from the methyl (ω) end of the fatty acid.[2] Unless oxidation occurs, ω-6 and ω-3 fatty acids remain unchanged in human metabolism.[2] The essential fatty acids ω-6 (linoleic acid) and ω-3 (linolenic acid) have their double bond in the immutable ω-6 and ω-3 position, respectively, and cannot be synthesized endogenously by humans.[5] These fatty acids must be obtained from the diet and are naturally found in many vegetable and some fish oils.[5]

Linoleic acid is critical for formation of the epidermal water barrier.[2] Linoleic and linolenic acids both are required for synthesis of long-chain polyunsaturated fatty acids such as arachidonic acid.[2,5] These types of long-chain polyunsaturated fatty acids contain more than 18 carbons and two or more double bonds.[5] They are a critical component of membrane-rich tissue such as the brain.[2] Whether linoleic and linolenic acids have independent clinical significance other than as precursors for long-chain polyunsaturated fatty acids is unclear.[5]

The fat content of most human milk is 3.5 to 4 g per 100 ml and can approach 55% of the total amount of calories in breast milk.[1,2] Infant formula strives to have a similar composition.[2] Human milk and formula both contain linoleic and linolenic acids as well as fat-soluble vitamins.[2] Human milk contains between 8% and 20% and 0.5% to 1% of the total fatty acid content as linoleic and linolenic acid, respectively.[5] The maternal diet has a dramatic effect on the fatty acid content of breast milk.[5] Women who deliver preterm have a unique fat composition in their milk that allows 95% of the fat content to be absorbed by the infant.[1] Preterm formulas have between 10% and 50% of their fat content in the form of medium-chain triglycerides because of the risk for bile acid deficiencies in this population.[1]

During fetal and early infant life of infants fed human milk, it is not vital that infants be able to endogenously manufacture long-chain polyunsaturated fatty acids because the placenta and human milk can supply them with adequate amounts.[2] Although free long-chain polyunsaturated fatty acids are found in human milk, they are not present in standard infant formulas.[2,3] Instead, formulas commonly manufactured from corn, coconut, soy, safflower alone, high-oleic safflower and sunflower, and palm olein oil usually contain only the precursors.[1,5] Because premature infants may not be able to synthesize long-chain polyunsaturated fatty acids effectively from linoleic and linolenic acids, standard term formulas are inadequate for this population.[1,2] Currently, formulas contain a minimum of 2.7% to 8% and a maximum of 21% to 35% of the total fatty acids as linoleic acid.[5] Formulas provide 1.75% to 4% of the total fatty acids as linolenic acid.[5] Most of the infant formulas in the United States have linoleic acid as approximately 20% and linolenic acid as approximately 2% of total fatty acids.[5] A reasonable balance between linoleic and linolenic acid is between 5:6 and 15:16.[5]

A deficiency in long-chain polyunsaturated fatty acids in premature infants leads to thrombocytopenia, poor growth (failure to thrive), and skin changes (dry, leathery, desquamative dermatitis).[3,5] If the deficiency occurs during infancy, brain growth may be decreased.[8] Linolenic acid-deficient animals may have reduced "electroretinogram responses" and visual acuity in the first month of life.[2] These same clinical symptoms have been observed in human infants who were maintained on parenteral nutrition lacking linolenic acid for several weeks.[5] Although the clinical pictures associated with each essential fatty acid deficiency are distinct, there can be overlap of symptoms between the two entities.[5]

Unfortunately, the exact amount of essential fatty acids required for healthy infants is unknown.[2] Approximately 0.5 g/kg/day of essential fatty acids will prevent deficiency.[3] The minimal intake of linoleic acid recommended for young infants is 2.7% to 4.5% of their nutritional intake.[2] Poor growth and skin changes are seen in infants who receive less than 1% of their nutritional intake as linoleic acid.[2] These skin changes can be corrected with the addition of linoleic acid at a minimum of 1% of their nutritional intake.[2] The enteral intake recommendation for stable, growing preterm infants is 0.44 to 1.7 g of linoleic acid and 0.11 to 0.44 g of linolenic acid per 100 kcal daily.[5]

Carnitine Deficiency

Carnitine is a cofactor involved in the final step in the catabolism of long-chain fatty acids.[3,4] It is formed in the liver from the essential amino acids lysine and methionine.[3,4] Carnitine also transports long-chain fatty acids into the mitochondria for β-oxidation.[3,4] Indeed, carnitine is essential in the transport of many high-energy molecules from one cellular location to another.[4]

An infant acquires carnitine prenatally from his or her mother. At term, infants have adequate stores of carnitine.[3] Preterm infants are at risk for developing carnitine deficiency because their immature hepatic function cannot easily synthesize carnitine. In addition, the kidneys of preterm infants do not sufficiently reabsorb carnitine.[4]

Infants who are carnitine deficient have lower levels of β-hydroxybutyrate and acetoacetate with higher triglyceride and free fatty acid levels.[4]

It is rare for an infant to be carnitine deficient when he or she is receiving enteral feeds. Carnitine is found abundantly in human milk and supplemented in formulas.[1,3] Infants who are receiving parenteral nutrition for more than 3 weeks may become carnitine deficient.[1,4] It is recommended that this population of infants receive supplemental carnitine. Typically, supplementation with 2 to 10 mg/ kg/day can prevent carnitine deficiency.[4] Supplementation should continue in parenterally fed infants until they receive at least half of their volume enterally in order to prevent further deficiency.[4]

Resource for Clinicians and Families

American Academy of Pediatrics

http://www.aap.org/healthtopics/nutrition.cfm

This website provides general information about nutritional issues in infants.

REFERENCES

1. MacDonald MG, Mullett MD, Seshia MMK: *Avery's neonatology: pathophysiology & management of the newborn,* ed 6. Philadelphia, 2005, Lippincott Williams & Wilkins.
2. Tsang RC, Mead Johnson Nutritionals: *Nutrition during infancy: principles and practice.* ed 2. Cincinnati, 1997, Digital Education Publishing.
3. Taeusch HW, Ballard RA, Gleason CA, et al: *Avery's diseases of the newborn,* ed 8. Philadelphia, 2005, WB Saunders.
4. Spitzer AR: *Intensive care of the fetus and neonate,* ed 2. St. Louis, 2005, Mosby.
5. American Academy of Pediatrics Committee on Nutrition, Kleinman RE: *Pediatric nutrition handbook,* ed 5. Elk Grove Village, Ill, 2004, American Academy of Pediatrics.
6. Khoshoo V, Kjarsgaard J, Krafchick B, et al: Zinc deficiency in a full-term breast-fed infant: unusual presentation. *Pediatrics* 89(6 pt 1):1094-1095, 1992.
7. Zlotkin SH, Atkinson S, Lockitch G: Trace elements in nutrition for premature infants. *Clin Perinatol* 22:223-240, 1995.
8. Simmer K, Rao SC: Early introduction of lipids to parenterally-fed preterm infants. *Cochrane Database Syst Rev* (2): CD005256, 2005.

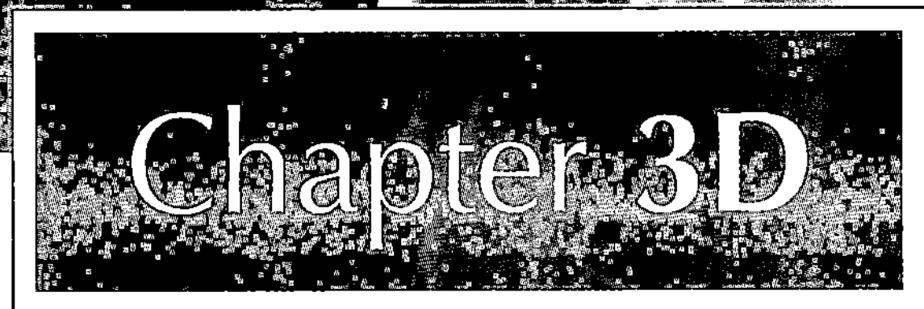

Intrauterine Growth Restriction

Munish Gupta, MD

Fetal growth is determined by a broad array of physiologic and environmental factors, and numerous maternal and fetal conditions can disrupt normal growth. Fetal growth restriction during pregnancy results in significant risks for perinatal morbidity and mortality, and the growth-restricted neonate is at risk for medical complications beginning in the immediate newborn period and potentially extending into childhood and even adulthood. Thus, understanding the long-term consequences of fetal growth restriction is essential for the neonatologist as well as the general pediatric specialist.

Definitions

Intrauterine growth restriction (IUGR) is formally defined as the failure of a pregnancy to reach expected growth of the fetus and manifests as a deviation of fetal growth from normal patterns. The definition of IUGR should be distinguished from that of low birth weight (LBW) and small for gestational age (SGA). *LBW* is a diagnosis based only on birth weight and is most commonly defined as birth weight under 2500 g.[1] *SGA* is a diagnosis based on birth weight of an infant compared with gestational age–specific normal birth weight values. Using a variety of normative curves describing expected birth weights for a given gestational age, newborn infants can be classified as SGA, appropriate for gestational age (AGA), or large for gestational age (LGA). The most commonly used thresholds for defining LGA and SGA are the 90th and 10th percentiles, respectively, although other thresholds, such as the 97th and 3rd percentiles as well as 2 standard deviations (SD) above and below the mean, are occasionally used. Thus, many LBW infants who are delivered prematurely are AGA despite weighing less than 2500 g. A more subtle distinction exists between SGA and IUGR; these terms often are used interchangeably but have important differences. Depending on the thresholds used to define SGA, a certain percent of normally grown infants fall below the threshold and therefore are considered SGA but are not IUGR; these infants are constitutionally small. Similarly, some infants are considered IUGR because their fetal growth sufficiently deviated from their expected growth but still are AGA if their birth weight is above the appropriate threshold.

Epidemiology and Etiology

IUGR is thought to complicate 5% to 8% of all pregnancies.[2,3] Numerous socioeconomic and demographic factors have been associated with an increased risk of IUGR, including lower levels of maternal education,[4] previous delivery of a low birth weight infant,[5] and African-American race.[6]

In the United States, only 40% of cases of IUGR are found to have an identifiable cause.[2] A broad array of factors and conditions can result in fetal growth restriction; these can be categorized as fetal, placental, or maternal in origin. It is important to recognize that IUGR is not a specific disease process but rather a result of complex pathophysiology to which numerous maternal and fetal factors can contribute. Important contributory factors and causes are listed in Table 3D-1.[7] Particularly common causes include excessive maternal smoking, maternal vascular disease including hypertensive disorders, and fetal chromosomal abnormalities.

Diagnosis

The diagnosis of IUGR is made during pregnancy by estimating fetal weight over time and comparing this value with established fetal growth charts. Accurate gestational age dating is essential and is best accomplished by early first-trimester ultrasound in combination with timing of the last menstrual

Table 3D-1 Causes of Intrauterine Growth Restriction[2,3,7]

Fetal	Chromosomal abnormalities Congenital malformations Multiple gestations Fetal infection
Placental	Anatomic abnormalities Small placenta Placental abruption Placenta previa Placental infarcts
Maternal	Low maternal weight Malnutrition Socioeconomic status Hypertension Diabetes Vasculitis Anemia Thrombophilic disorder Maternal infection (especially viral) Uterine malformation or mass Tobacco use Drug use, alcohol use

period.[8] Ultrasonography currently remains the most accurate method for estimating fetal weight throughout pregnancy.[9] Several fetal measurements, including abdominal circumference, head circumference, biparietal diameter, and femur length are used to derive an estimated fetal weight. Expected fetal growth is based on fetal growth charts derived from large population studies.[10,11] Although these are the best available estimates of normal fetal growth, they are inherently limited because they are unable to account for population variances and individual maternal constitutional factors. Notably, growth charts derived from various populations do have important differences.

As discussed earlier, a fetus that is found to be small compared with expected parameters is not necessarily growth restricted. IUGR is most accurately diagnosed by serial ultrasound scans showing absent or poor fetal weight gain compared with expected weight gain as shown on the growth charts. It also can be diagnosed when a single ultrasound scan shows low estimated fetal weight in the presence of other signs of fetal compromise, such as oligohydramnios, congenital anomalies, or fetal distress.[8] A small fetus that shows normal anatomy, normal amniotic fluid volume, and normal intrauterine growth usually grows into a constitutionally small but otherwise normal infant without the physiologic consequences of growth restriction.

IUGR often is classified into two broad categories. In symmetric growth restriction, weight, length, and head circumference all are proportionally reduced. In asymmetric growth restriction, head circumference and often length are spared compared with the reduction in weight. Symmetric growth restriction is thought to result from an insult affecting the fetus early in gestation, such as chromosomal abnormalities, congenital malformations, intrauterine viral infection, or toxin exposure. Asymmetric growth restriction is thought to result from exposures late in gestation, such as maternal hypertension or placental insufficiency. Generally, symmetrically growth-restricted infants tend to have higher risks for associated morbidities, whereas asymmetrically growth-restricted infants tend to have a more favorable prognosis. These differences in outcomes may simply reflect the more severe etiologies associated with symmetric IUGR.[2,7] Other differences between symmetric and asymmetric IUGR are outlined in Table 3D-2.

Table 3D-2 Symmetric and Asymmetric Intrauterine Growth Restriction

	Symmetric IUGR	Asymmetric IUGR
Proportion of IUGR infants	20%–30%	70%–80%
Timing of growth restriction	First or second trimester	Third trimester
Physical appearance	Head size is proportional to small size of body and abdomen	Head size is large relative to size of body and abdomen
Pathophysiology	Impaired cell division Impaired cellular hyperplasia Decreased cell number	Impaired cellular hypertrophy Decreased cell size
Etiology	Chromosomal abnormalities Congenital malformations Drugs Infection Early-onset maternal preeclampsia	Maternal hypertension Placental insufficiency
Outcome	Greater morbidity and mortality	Lower morbidity and mortality

Modified from: Brodsky D, Christou H: *J Intensive Care Med* 19:308, 2004.
IUGR, Intrauterine growth restriction.

Medical Outcomes

IUGR has been well documented to be associated with major perinatal and neonatal complications. Evidence also suggests it may have effects on long-term health extending into childhood and adult life.

Perinatal

Perinatal complications that have been associated with fetal growth restriction include intrauterine fetal demise and perinatal death[12,13]; fetal compromise with perinatal asphyxia, low Apgar scores, neonatal acidosis[14,15]; and premature delivery.[16]

Neonatal

Potential neonatal complications of IUGR are broad and include hypothermia, hypoglycemia, hypocalcemia, thrombocytopenia, neutropenia, polycythemia, hyperbilirubinemia, renal insufficiency, persistent pulmonary hypertension, hypothyroidism, and perinatal depression.[3,17] Numerous physiologic mechanisms contribute to these complications, including intrauterine placental compromise, decreased neonatal glycogen and lipid stores, and neonatal bone marrow suppression. Furthermore, growth-restricted premature infants appear to be at higher risk than normally grown premature infants for neonatal complications such as respiratory distress syndrome, intraventricular hemorrhage, sepsis, necrotizing enterocolitis, and chronic lung disease, although the data are not universally consistent.[3,14,18,19]

Pediatric

Infants born with IUGR generally require further catchup growth beyond the neonatal period. Most of these infants demonstrate increased growth velocity compared with normally sized infants and achieve normal growth parameters by 2 to 3 years of age.[20] Some IUGR infants have persistent delays in catchup growth and have ongoing difficulties, with failure to thrive, growth restriction, and short stature into childhood and adolescence.[20-23] In addition to growth difficulties, neurologic outcomes in childhood appear to be associated with IUGR, with growth-restricted neonates being at higher risk for later developmental and intellectual delays. Even in the absence of other perinatal complications, IUGR has been associated with cerebral palsy, learning disabilities, and behavioral difficulties, although the data are not completely consistent.[2,24-27] Finally, small but significant associations have been reported between IUGR and sudden infant death syndrome in infancy.[28,29]

Long-term and adult disease

It is becoming increasingly established that alterations in fetal growth may affect long-term health. It appears that exposure to intrauterine compromise or stress during a critical period of development results in fetal adaptations and programming that lead to altered physiology lasting into adulthood. Over the past several decades, numerous large epidemiologic studies have shown associations between low birth weight and various long-term outcomes in adults, including cardiovascular disease, hypertension, hyperlipidemia, diabetes, and obesity.[30-33] Several pathways have been postulated to contribute to these associations. The "thrifty phenotype" model suggests that fetal adaptations to intrauterine undernourishment result in alterations in hormonal physiology, which include increased insulin resistance, impaired β-cell function, increased stress response, and growth hormone resistance. When subsequently exposed to adequate nutritional supply, these programmed metabolic changes then predispose to the development of glucose intolerance, obesity, abnormalities of lipid metabolism, and hypertension.[34,35] It also appears that growth-restricted infants have fewer cells in key organs when compared with normally grown infants. This is particularly true in the kidneys, and the discrepancy in cell number is not corrected during postnatal growth.[36,37] These anatomic changes may predispose to later development of hypertension, as it has been shown that adults with primary hypertension have fewer nephrons than those with normal blood pressure.[38]

A growing literature suggests that independent associations exist between fetal growth and later disease development. More recent studies suggest that these associations may be modified by growth in childhood. The greatest risk of later development of cardiovascular disease and diabetes appears to be in those individuals with low birth weight who then have excessive weight gain or obesity during childhood.[33,34,39-41] Additional studies are needed to further define the relationship among birth weight, childhood growth, and long-term outcomes.

Management

Obstetric

Following the intrauterine diagnosis of IUGR, possible causes should be evaluated. Studies may include a full fetal survey, amniocentesis with fetal karyotype, evaluation for infection, and assessment of maternal health and nutritional status. Prenatal interventions focused on maternal health and nutrition have not been shown to alter the course of fetal growth restriction.[42] The challenge for the obstetrician in managing IUGR is determining the optimal time for delivery. Delivery at term or near-term often is indicated for the growth-restricted infant, particularly in the presence of other signs of fetal compromise or significant maternal conditions, such as hypertension. Remote from term, the risks of continuing the pregnancy in a presumably compromised intrauterine environment must be weighed against the risks of prematurity. Management relies on regular assessments of both fetal growth and fetal well-being through methods such as the biophysical profile, nonstress test, amniotic fluid volume measurement, and Doppler velocimetry of fetal vessels.[8] Significantly impaired or absent fetal growth or signs of significant fetal distress, such as abnormalities of umbilical blood flow, are generally considered indications for delivery, but at the extremes of gestational age and prematurity, the balance of risks and benefits is not clear. Antenatal steroids are generally considered to be beneficial before the delivery of growth-restricted infants if premature delivery is required.[7]

Neonatal

Because growth-restricted infants are at risk for perinatal asphyxia and distress, a pediatric specialist or neonatologist skilled in newborn resuscitation should be present at delivery. All growth-restricted infants, regardless of overall appearance, should be monitored for hypothermia and hypoglycemia, with vigilance for other potential complications such as hyperbilirubinemia, hematologic abnormalities, and metabolic disturbances. Term infants who are mild or moderately growth restricted but otherwise well appearing often can be managed in the regular newborn unit, but severely growth-restricted infants, preterm infants, and infants with signs of stress or compromise will require more intensive monitoring and care. Management of growth-restricted premature infants should include particular attention to the potentially increased risks of respiratory distress, chronic lung disease, necrotizing enterocolitis, and intraventricular hemorrhage.

Pediatric

After discharge from the hospital or neonatal intensive care unit, the IUGR infant continues to require focused management from the primary care pediatric specialist (Figure 3D-1). Several areas of the pediatric care of these patients deserve particular attention: (1) assessment of neurologic and intellectual development; (2) monitoring for childhood presentation of potential morbidities and diseases; and (3) maintenance of optimal nutrition and growth.

The known associations between fetal growth restriction and adverse neurologic outcomes and developmental delays warrant regular developmental assessments during infancy and childhood. As with other high-risk populations, early identification of developmental delays and early initiation of interventional programs likely will help to improve the long-term outcomes of these children. Similarly, many of the long-term morbidities and diseases associated with fetal growth restriction can begin to present during childhood, and routine pediatric care should include regular health assessments to evaluate for these complications. Potential morbidities associated with IUGR that could present or be detected in childhood include obesity, hypertension, renal dysfunction, and hyperlipidemia.

Because IUGR infants are at risk for growth difficulties into childhood and adolescence, careful monitoring of growth and appropriate nutritional support is essential. The majority of full-term growth-restricted infants will achieve appropriate catchup growth without particular nutritional supplementation. However, IUGR infants who were born prematurely or with a very low birth weight generally require supplementation with additional calories and minerals to maintain optimal growth. There are limited data on IUGR infants in particular; rather, most studies focus on low birth weight and premature infants in general, many of whom are growth restricted postnatally because of acute illness and prolonged hospitalization. These studies do not, however, yield a clear consensus on nutritional management of these infants. A meta-analysis of randomized trials comparing the use of calorie- and protein-enriched formulas with standard term formulas in the feeding of preterm or LBW infants after hospital discharge found little evidence of a significant impact of the enriched formulas on growth or development.[43] Furthermore, some studies suggest an association between rapid infant growth with the use of enriched formulas and later increased risk of cardiovascular disease.[44]

Despite these concerns, current recommendations overwhelmingly favor the use of enriched formulas or enriched breast milk after discharge for premature and LBW infants. Pending further studies, the preponderance of evidence supports an association between improved growth and improved cognitive outcomes.[44-48] Formulas designed specifically for postdischarge nutrition of preterm and LBW infants (NeoSure by Ross, EnfaCare by Mead-Johnson) provide additional calories (22 kcal per ounce) as well as appropriate mineral and vitamin supplementation. These products also can be used as additives to fortify breast milk and can be further concentrated to provide additional caloric support. Guidelines vary, but in general, the use of enriched formulas is recommended for LBW and premature infants until 6 to 9 months corrected gestational age or until catchup growth is complete, with

ALGORITHM FOR OUTPATIENT MANAGEMENT OF AN IUGR INFANT

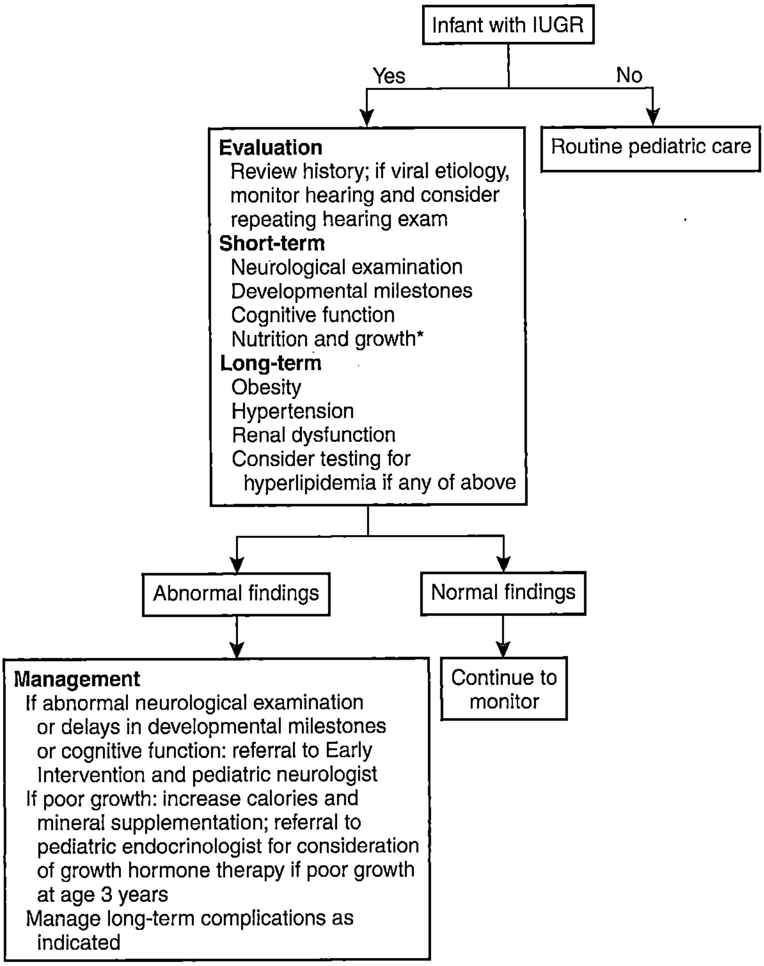

Infant with IUGR

Yes → **Evaluation**
- Review history; if viral etiology, monitor hearing and consider repeating hearing exam

Short-term
- Neurological examination
- Developmental milestones
- Cognitive function
- Nutrition and growth*

Long-term
- Obesity
- Hypertension
- Renal dysfunction
- Consider testing for hyperlipidemia if any of above

No → Routine pediatric care

Abnormal findings → **Management**
- If abnormal neurological examination or delays in developmental milestones or cognitive function: referral to Early Intervention and pediatric neurologist
- If poor growth: increase calories and mineral supplementation; referral to pediatric endocrinologist for consideration of growth hormone therapy if poor growth at age 3 years
- Manage long-term complications as indicated

Normal findings → Continue to monitor

FIGURE 3D-1 *Growth-restricted premature infants usually are discharged from the hospital with specialized formulas (e.g., Neosure by Ross, Enfacare by Mead Johnson) and 22–24 kcal/oz until at least 6–9 months corrected gestational age or until catch-up growth is complete. Please note that this is a recommended algorithm that does not represent a professional standard of care; care should be revised to meet individual patient needs.

supplementation to 24 kcal per ounce until the infant weighs at least 1800 g and then 22 kcal per ounce thereafter.[45,47]

Despite nutritional supplementation, a significant portion of IUGR infants will continue to be growth restricted into childhood. Studies are now investigating the role of growth hormone supplementation in children with a history of fetal growth restriction and persistent short stature. Although still limited, these studies have strongly suggested that treatment with growth hormone results in improvement in growth and final adult height in these patients, without negative side effects and independent of baseline growth hormone levels.[49-52] Growth-restricted infants who remain short in early childhood, such as by age 3, should be referred to a pediatric endocrinology specialist for consideration of growth hormone therapy.[20]

Conclusion

IUGR is a common and important condition affecting the pediatric population. It is heterogeneous in nature, with a multitude of potential contributory causes and pathologic pathways. It carries significant implications for perinatal morbidity and neonatal complications and can have a significant impact on childhood and adult health. Appropriate evaluation and management of IUGR infants requires the participation of the obstetrician, the neonatologist, and the primary care pediatric specialist.

REFERENCES

1. Martin JA, Kochanek KD, Strobino DM, et al: Annual summary of vital statistics—2003. *Pediatrics* 115(3):619-634, 2005.
2. Martinez A, Simmons R: Abnormalities of fetal growth. In Taeusch HW, Ballard RA, Gleason CA, et al., editors: *Avery's diseases of the newborn*, ed 8. Philadelphia, 2005, Elsevier Saunders.
3. Brodsky D, Christou H: Current concepts in intrauterine growth restriction. *J Intensive Care Med* 19(6):307-319, 2004.
4. Clausson B, Cnattingius S, Axelsson O: Preterm and term births of small for gestational age infants: a population-based study of risk factors among nulliparous women. *Br J Obstet Gynaecol* 105(9):1011-1017, 1998.
5. Wang X, Zuckerman B, Coffman GA, et al: Familial aggregation of low birth weight among whites and blacks in the United States. *N Engl J Med* 333(26):1744-1749, 1995.
6. Alexander GR, Kogan MD, Himes JH, et al: Racial differences in birthweight for gestational age and infant mortality in extremely-low-risk US populations. *Paediatr Perinat Epidemiol* 13(2):205-217, 1999.
7. Resnik R: Intrauterine growth restriction. *Obstet Gynecol* 99(3):490-496, 2002.
8. Harkness UF, Mari G: Diagnosis and management of intrauterine growth restriction. *Clin Perinatol* 31(4): 743-764, vi, 2004.
9. ACOG: ACOG Practice Bulletin no. 58: ultrasonography in pregnancy. *Obstet Gynecol* 104(6):1449-1458, 2004.
10. Zhang J, Bowes WA Jr: Birth-weight-for-gestational-age patterns by race, sex, and parity in the United States population. *Obstet Gynecol* 86(2):200-208, 1995.
11. Alexander GR, Himes JH, Kaufman RB, et al: A United States national reference for fetal growth. *Obstet Gynecol* 87(2):163-168, 1996.
12. Cnattingius S, Haglund B, Kramer MS: Differences in late fetal death rates in association with determinants of small for gestational age fetuses: population based cohort study. *BMJ* 316(7143):1483-1487, 1998.
13. Lackman F, Capewell V, Richardson B, et al: The risks of spontaneous preterm delivery and perinatal mortality in relation to size at birth according to fetal versus neonatal growth standards. *Am J Obstet Gynecol* 184(5):946-953, 2001.
14. McIntire DD, Bloom SL, Casey BM, et al: Birth weight in relation to morbidity and mortality among newborn infants. *N Engl J Med* 340(16):1234-1238, 1999.
15. Villar J, de Onis M, Kestler E, et al: The differential neonatal morbidity of the intrauterine growth retardation syndrome. *Am J Obstet Gynecol* 163(1 pt 1):151-157, 1990.
16. Zeitlin J, Ancel PY, Saurel-Cubizolles MJ, et al: The relationship between intrauterine growth restriction and preterm delivery: an empirical approach using data from a European case-control study. *BJOG* 107(6):750-758, 2000.
17. Doctor BA, O'Riordan MA, Kirchner HL, et al: Perinatal correlates and neonatal outcomes of small for gestational age infants born at term gestation. *Am J Obstet Gynecol* 185(3):652-659, 2001.
18. Simchen MJ, Beiner ME, Strauss-Liviathan N, et al: Neonatal outcome in growth-restricted versus appropriately grown preterm infants. *Am J Perinatol* 17(4):187-192, 2000.
19. Bernstein IM, Horbar JD, Badger GJ, et al: Morbidity and mortality among very-low-birth-weight neonates with intrauterine growth restriction. The Vermont Oxford Network. *Am J Obstet Gynecol* 182(1 pt 1):198-206, 2000.
20. Lee PA, Chernausek SD, Hokken-Koelega AC, et al: International Small for Gestational Age Advisory Board consensus development conference statement: management of short children born small for gestational age, April 24-October 1, 2001. *Pediatrics* 111(6 pt 1):1253-1261, 2003.
21. Karlberg J, Albertsson-Wikland K: Growth in full-term small-for-gestational-age infants: from birth to final height. *Pediatr Res* 38(5):733-739, 1995.
22. Botero D, Lifshitz F: Intrauterine growth retardation and long-term effects on growth. *Curr Opin Pediatr* 11(4): 340-347, 1999.
23. Strauss RS, Dietz WH: Effects of intrauterine growth retardation in premature infants on early childhood growth. *J Pediatr* 130(1):95-102, 1997.
24. Paz I, Laor A, Gale R, et al: Term infants with fetal growth restriction are not at increased risk for low intelligence scores at age 17 years. *J Pediatr* 138(1):87-91, 2001.
25. Strauss RS: Adult functional outcome of those born small for gestational age: twenty-six-year follow-up of the 1970 British Birth Cohort. *JAMA* 283(5):625-632, 2000.
26. Jarvis S, Glinianaia SV, Torrioli MG, et al: Cerebral palsy and intrauterine growth in single births: European collaborative study. *Lancet* 362(9390):1106-1111, 2003.
27. Ellenberg JH, Nelson KB: Birth weight and gestational age in children with cerebral palsy or seizure disorders. *Am J Dis Child* 133(10):1044-1048, 1979.
28. Buck GM, Cookfair DL, Michalek AM, et al: Intrauterine growth retardation and risk of sudden infant death syndrome (SIDS). *Am J Epidemiol* 129(5):874-884, 1989.
29. Getahun D, Amre D, Rhoads GG, et al: Maternal and obstetric risk factors for sudden infant death syndrome in the United States. *Obstet Gynecol* 103(4):646-652, 2004.
30. Barker DJ, Fall CH: Fetal and infant origins of cardiovascular disease. *Arch Dis Child* 68(6):797-799, 1993.
31. Barker DJ, Hales CN, Fall CH, et al: Type 2 (non-insulin-dependent) diabetes mellitus, hypertension and hyperlipidaemia (syndrome X): relation to reduced fetal growth. *Diabetologia* 36(1):62-67, 1993.
32. Curhan GC, Willett WC, Rimm EB, et al: Birth weight and adult hypertension, diabetes mellitus, and obesity in US men. *Circulation* 94(12):3246-3250, 1996.
33. Rich-Edwards JW, Colditz GA, Stampfer MJ, et al: Birthweight and the risk for type 2 diabetes mellitus in adult women. *Ann Intern Med* 130(4 pt 1):278-284, 1999.
34. Barker DJ: The developmental origins of well-being. *Philos Trans R Soc Lond B Biol Sci* 359(1449):1359-1366, 2004.
35. Barker DJ: Fetal nutrition and cardiovascular disease in later life. *Br Med Bull* 53(1):96-108, 1997.
36. Hinchliffe SA, Lynch MR, Sargent PH, et al: The effect of intrauterine growth retardation on the development of renal nephrons. *Br J Obstet Gynaecol* 99(4):296-301, 1992.
37. Manalich R, Reyes L, Herrera M, et al: Relationship between weight at birth and the number and size of renal glomeruli in humans: a histomorphometric study. *Kidney Int* 58(2): 770-773, 2000.
38. Keller G, Zimmer G, Mall G, et al: Nephron number in patients with primary hypertension. *N Engl J Med* 348(2): 101-108, 2003.
39. Eriksson J, Forsen T, Tuomilehto J, et al: Fetal and childhood growth and hypertension in adult life. *Hypertension* 36(5):790-794, 2000.
40. Eriksson JG, Forsen T, Tuomilehto J, et al: Early growth and coronary heart disease in later life: longitudinal study. *BMJ* 322(7292):949-953, 2001.
41. Forsen T, Eriksson J, Tuomilehto J, et al: The fetal and childhood growth of persons who develop type 2 diabetes. *Ann Intern Med* 133(3):176-182, 2000.
42. Gulmezoglu M, de Onis M, Villar J: Effectiveness of interventions to prevent or treat impaired fetal growth. *Obstet Gynecol Surv* 52(2):139-149, 1997.
43. Henderson G, Fahey T, McGuire W: Calorie and protein-enriched formula versus standard term formula for improving

growth and development in preterm or low birth weight infants following hospital discharge. *Cochrane Database Syst Rev* (2):CD004696, 2005.

44. Lucas A: Long-term programming effects of early nutrition—implications for the preterm infant. *J Perinatol* 25(suppl 2):S2-S6, 2005.
45. Bhatia J: Post-discharge nutrition of preterm infants. *J Perinatol* 25(suppl 2):S15-S16; discussion S17-S18, 2005.
46. Carver JD: Nutrition for preterm infants after hospital discharge. *Adv Pediatr* 52:23-47, 2005.
47. Groh-Wargo S, Thompson M, Cox JH: *Nutritional care for high-risk newborns*, rev ed 3. Chicago, Ill, 2000, Precept Press.
48. Kleinman RE, American Academy of Pediatrics Committee on Nutrition: *Pediatric nutrition handbook*, ed 5. Washington, DC, 2004, American Academy of Pediatrics.
49. Dahlgren J, Wikland KA: Final height in short children born small for gestational age treated with growth hormone. *Pediatr Res* 57(2):216-222, 2005.
50. Czernichow P: Growth hormone treatment strategy for short children born small for gestational age. *Horm Res* 62(suppl 3):137-140, 2004.
51. Rosilio M, Carel JC, Ecosse E, et al: Adult height of prepubertal short children born small for gestational age treated with GH. *Eur J Endocrinol* 152(6):835-843, 2005.
52. Van Pareren Y, Mulder P, Houdijk M, et al: Adult height after long-term, continuous growth hormone (GH) treatment in short children born small for gestational age: results of a randomized, double-blind, dose-response GH trial. *J Clin Endocrinol Metab* 88(8):3584-3590, 2003.

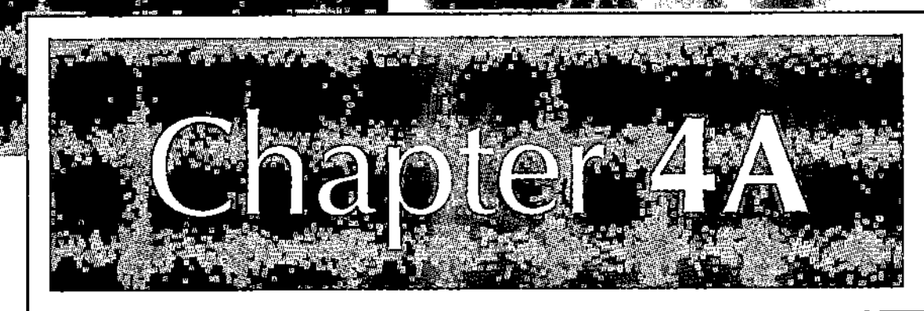

Gastroesophageal Reflux in the Premature Infant

Dara Brodsky, MD

Gastroesophageal reflux (GER) is the retrograde involuntary movement of gastric contents into the esophagus and areas above. The gastric contents can include acidic gastric juices, formula, or bile. Although the incidence of reflux is extremely high in infants born prematurely, the primary care provider must differentiate between physiologic or functional (i.e., regurgitation) and pathophysiologic (i.e., GER disease) reflux in order to determine which infants require treatment. Reflux can be characterized by degrees, with mild GER being a physiologic developmental process that resolves with maturation, and moderate to severe GER being pathologic.

Unfortunately, the majority of recommendations about the diagnosis and treatment of GER in premature infants have been extrapolated from studies conducted in full-term infants, children, and adults. This chapter focuses on the occurrence of reflux in premature infants, differentiating physiologic from pathophysiologic causes, with an emphasis on clinical presentation and therapeutic options.

Incidence

Mild GER has been reported in 40% to 65% of healthy infants born at term.[1] The natural history of physiologic GER is spontaneous improvement over time, as evidenced by a disappearance of symptoms in 55% of term infants by 10 months of age, in 81% by 18 months of age, and in 98% by 2 years of age.[2] Although most clinicians believe that mild reflux is more common in premature than full-term infants,[3] Jeffery and Page[4] found that the frequency and duration of mild reflux is less in preterm infants born between 24 and 32 weeks' gestation at term postmenstrual age compared with matched full-term infants, and Kohelet et al.[5] reported similar findings.

The reported prevalence of pathologic GER in infants is 6% to 7% of infants born at term and, similarly ≈3% to 10% of premature infants born weighing less than 1500 g.[1,6,7] Most infants with pathologic reflux receive some treatment, ≈1% to 2% undergo diagnostic evaluation, and ≤1% undergo antireflux surgery.[7,8] Reflux disease is more common in infants who have the risk factors listed in Table 4A-1. Premature infants who are receiving methylxanthine or β-mimetic therapy are more likely to have GER disease.[9] Infants with neurologic impairment, such as cerebral palsy, also are at greater risk for reflux because of abnormal gastrointestinal motility.[10] Data about the association of bronchopulmonary dysplasia and GER disease are conflicting.[6,11-15] Independent from lung disease, prolonged endotracheal intubation can exacerbate the degree of reflux, probably by causing damage to the superficial afferent nerve endings that stimulate swallowing.[4]

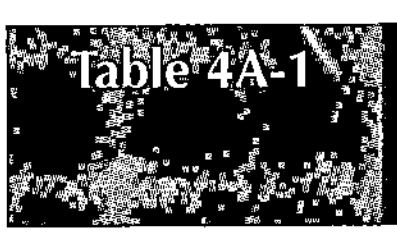

Table 4A-1 Risk Factors for Gastroesophageal Reflux Disease in Infants

- Prematurity
  - Medications (e.g., methylxanthines, β-mimetics)
  - Prolonged intubation
  - Bronchopulmonary dysplasia (inconsistent association)
  - Orogastric/nasogastric feeding tube
- Perinatal depression
- Neonatal sepsis
- Congenital anomalies (e.g., status post repair of esophageal atresia)
- Neurological impairment and/or delay (e.g., cerebral palsy)
- History of extracorporeal membrane oxygenation

Table 4A-2 Potential Mechanisms of Reflux in Premature Infants

Mechanisms	Relationship with Prematurity
Relaxation of lower esophageal sphincter (most common)[23]	Most common mechanism in premature infants Pressure is even less in infants fed through orogastric/nasogastric tubes Based on studies in full-term infants, probably worse in the supine position and slumped in car seat
Sluggish esophageal motility	Nonperistaltic motor patterns in the esophagus of a premature infant occur more often than peristalsis[17]
Central nervous system disorder (e.g., cerebral palsy)	Probably from esophageal dysmotility[10]
Increased intra-abdominal pressure (leading to elevated gastric pressure)	Contributor of reflux in premature infants with respiratory disorders such as bronchopulmonary dysplasia caused by altered balance of intrathoracic and intra-abdominal pressures
Decreased gastric compliance	Leads to lower esophageal sphincter relaxation at lower intragastric volumes; greater role in infants compared with older children; uncertain whether greater role in premature infants compared with full-term infants
Anatomic	All infants have a less acute angle of indentation of the esophagus into the stomach
Abnormal diaphragmatic activity[94]	Not specific for premature infants; common cause of reflux in infants with congenital diaphragmatic hernia
Delayed gastric emptying	Not very significant in premature infants[23]

Pathophysiology

The mechanisms that lead to pathologic reflux in premature infants are multifactorial (Table 4A-2).[16] At baseline, mean lower esophageal sphincter (LES) tone measurements in older infants are lower (≈5–20 mm Hg) than adult levels (20–30 mm Hg).[17-19] Although initial studies found that premature infants have lower average LES pressures compared with term infants,[3] later studies demonstrate that premature infants can generate LES pressures that are higher than intragastric pressures.[17,19] The most significant mechanism of GER in premature infants probably is *transient* and inappropriate relaxations of the LES.[20,21] LES relaxations are most common immediately postprandially and decrease in frequency after 1 hour.[20] Premature infants requiring orogastric/nasogastric tubes or methylxanthine therapy will have reduced LES pressure.[22] Sluggish esophageal motility is more common in preterm infants.[17] It can delay clearance of refluxed gastric contents and place premature infants at greater risk for esophageal mucosal damage. Delayed gastric emptying does not seem to have a significant impact on reflux in premature infants.[21,23]

Clinical Presentation

Infants with physiologic reflux (usually manifested as regurgitation of gastric contents into the mouth) thrive and do not manifest any of the stigmatas associated with pathologic GER. A study of full-term infants reported that at least one episode of regurgitation occurred per day in ≈50% of infants 0 to 3 months old, 67% of infants 4 months old, 21% of infants 6 to 7 months old, and in only 5% of infants 10 to 12 months old.[24] Infants born prematurely display similar clinical findings, which usually resolve by 1 to 2 years of age, corresponding with developmental maturity.

It is critical to distinguish functional GER from GER disease (Table 4A-3). Severe or pathologic reflux (i.e., GER disease) is associated with poor weight gain; feeding difficulties, with frequent emesis; sleeping difficulties; chronic respiratory problems; and esophagitis. Infants may have excessive irritability or oral aversion (see Chapter 4C) because of associated pain from exposure of the esophagus to acidic gastric fluids. Older infants and children with a prolonged course of severe reflux may develop esophageal strictures and/or failure to thrive. Infants may have an atypical presentation of GER disease in which they present with failure to thrive without any gastrointestinal symptoms. This "silent GER disease" occurs in a subset of infants who have significant reflux, as evidenced by esophageal pH monitoring.[25]

In infants with atypical symptoms and signs of GER disease (Table 4A-4), the primary care provider should consider other causes, such as inborn errors of metabolism (urea cycle defects); isolated metabolic abnormalities (e.g., renal tubular acidosis, hypocalcemia); central nervous system disease (hydrocephalus, meningitis); partial gastrointestinal obstruction (e.g., pyloric stenosis, hiatal hernia, pyloric or antral webs, malrotation); nutrient intolerance; infectious causes (e.g., viral

Table 4A-3 Comparison of Mild Gastroesophageal Reflux and Moderate-to-Severe Gastroesophageal Reflux

Mild Gastroesophageal Reflux	Moderate-to-Severe Gastroesophageal Reflux
= Reflux	= Gastroesophageal Reflux Disease
Physiologic or functional	Pathologic
Limited episodes of emesis per day (≈1–2 per day)	Excessive daily episodes of emesis
Regurgitation/emesis with appropriate weight gain	Regurgitation/emesis with poor weight gain
No other symptoms besides regurgitation	Other symptoms, such as hoarseness, sleep disturbances
No evidence of esophagitis	Evidence of esophagitis:
	Persistent irritability (especially postprandial)
	Hematemesis, iron deficiency anemia
No significant respiratory symptoms	Evidence of respiratory symptoms:
	Wheezing
	Recurrent aspiration pneumonia
	Chronic cough
	Stridor
No neurobehavioral symptoms	Evidence of neurobehavioral symptoms:
	Sandifer syndrome: arching of back, torsion of the neck, lifting up of the chin
No long-term effects	Long-term effects:
	Oral aversion
	Esophageal stricture
	Failure to thrive

Modified from: Jung AD: *Am Fam Physician* 64:1854, 2001.

gastroenteritis, hepatitis, urinary tract infection); and toxin exposure.

Potential Clinical Associations

Although apnea of prematurity has been thought to be associated with reflux, studies have not demonstrated any temporal relationship.[26-30] Peter et al.[29] studied 19 premature infants (median gestational age 30 weeks, median postnatal age 26 days), recording breathing movements, nasal airflows, oxygen saturations, electrocardiographic (ECG) findings, and heart rates over a 6-hour period. They compared these cardiorespiratory findings with reflux episodes measured by multiple intraluminal impedance. The frequency of any cardiorespiratory event occurring within 20 seconds before or after a reflux episode was not significantly different from the number occurring during reflux-free periods. Indeed, only 3.5% of apneic episodes were associated with a reflux event that reached the pharyngeal level, with most of these apneas occurring after rather than before the reflux. To further support the nontemporal association of reflux and apnea, a retrospective study found that antireflux medications (cisapride and metoclopramide) did not reduce the incidence of apnea in premature infants.[30] Similarly, a study showed that GER does not prolong apnea duration and does not exacerbate the decrease in heart rate or oxygen saturation level during the apneic event.[31]

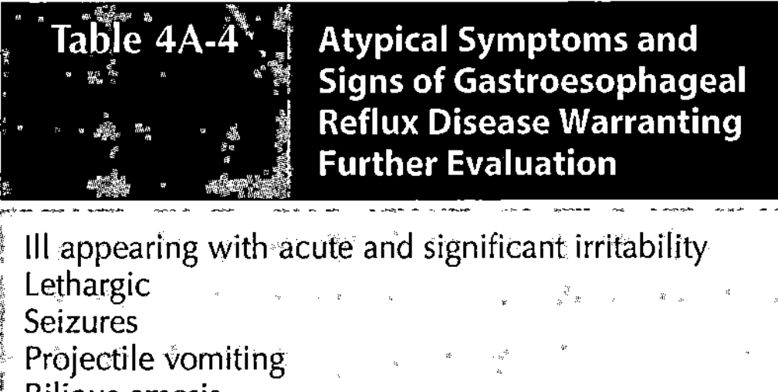

Table 4A-4 Atypical Symptoms and Signs of Gastroesophageal Reflux Disease Warranting Further Evaluation

Ill appearing with acute and significant irritability
Lethargic
Seizures
Projectile vomiting
Bilious emesis
Hematemesis
Abdominal distention
Abnormal bowel sounds
Respiratory distress
Jaundice, hepatosplenomegaly
Diarrhea
Dehydration

Modified from: Orenstein SR: *Am J Med* 103:117s, 1997.

Whether severe GER contributes to the occurrence of apparent life-threatening events (ALTEs) or sudden infant death syndrome (SIDS) is unclear. Some studies suggest that severe GER is associated with these events.[32,33] However, even these reports propose that severe GER probably is not the only precipitant. One possible mechanism is stimulation of laryngeal chemoreceptors when reflux occurs to the level of the pharynx. If the infant's swallowing is impaired or if the infant has depressed arousal (attributable to prone sleeping, prematurity, sedatives, seizures, or upper respiratory tract infections), there can be a potentially fatal outcome.[34] In contrast, other studies have not found any association between severe GER and SIDS or ALTE.[35-37]

Diagnosis

Diagnostic tools to evaluate reflux in infants are limited because of technical difficulties and inconsistent interpretations. When reflux is suspected clinically, physicians often administer an empiric trial of medications before an extensive evaluation is undertaken; this may or may not be in consultation with a gastroenterology specialist. If symptoms resolve after the medication trial, further diagnostic testing may not be needed. For infants who do not respond to empiric pharmacotherapy, those who display severe symptoms/signs (e.g., recurrent aspiration pneumonia, persistent excessive vomiting, ALTE, and/or failure to thrive), and infants with atypical or inconsistent symptoms of reflux (Table 4A-4), diagnostic testing, in consultation with a gastroenterology specialist, usually is warranted. The specific diagnostic approach will depend upon the infant's symptoms and their severity. Unfortunately, in most cases, no single test definitively diagnoses GER disease.[38]

A comparison of the available diagnostic tools in GER disease is provided in Table 4A-5. The 24-hour esophageal pH probe is the mainstay quantitative diagnostic evaluation in infants with acid reflux. Calibrated electrodes placed in the distal esophagus record the number and duration of acid reflux (pH <4) episodes.[39] This monitoring is particularly useful to determine any temporal association between reflux and other clinical findings, such as apnea or bradycardia. A pH probe study also is useful for assessing the effect on gastric pH following acid suppressive medical therapy.[40] For infants with nonacid reflux, the pH probe contributes little to the evaluation. It is important to note that normal values in infants born prematurely have not been established.[38]

Although an upper gastrointestinal series lacks adequate sensitivity and specificity to diagnose reflux, it can help to rule out congenital partial or intermittent gastrointestinal obstructions, such as pyloric stenosis, malrotation, and annular pancreas.[41] For infants with respiratory symptoms that suggest aspiration, a modified barium swallow, typically conducted in collaboration with a speech or occupational therapist, might be helpful. Upper endoscopic study typically is reserved for infants with persistent or worsening symptoms in the context of adequate medical therapy. In these cases, an endoscopic study can help to assess for the presence of mucosal disease (esophagitis) and to determine whether the reflux is primarily the result of acid/peptic versus allergic or infectious (e.g., yeast) processes. In some cases, endoscopy may be useful for identifying antral and duodenal webs or esophageal strictures that may be difficult to demonstrate radiographically.

Management

For infants with mild reflux, conservative therapy is preferred. Pharmacologic therapy is reserved for infants with moderate-to-severe symptoms, such as weight loss, severe feeding or sleeping difficulties, chronic respiratory problems, esophagitis, and oral aversion. Whether medical therapy should be initiated before or after a diagnostic evaluation is debatable. In our institution, medical therapy usually is started before diagnostic testing in infants with classic symptoms of GER disease. Infants with atypical symptoms/signs of GER disease warrant diagnostic testing before a medical regimen is started. The primary care provider should regularly reassess the infant's clinical symptoms to determine whether a different approach is warranted. In addition, a gastroenterology specialist should monitor all infants who have persistent severe symptoms, are unresponsive to pharmacotherapy, and/or require diagnostic testing. A proposed algorithm for managing infants with reflux is given in Figure 4A-1.

Conservative therapy

Some data suggest that *positioning* the infant in a flat prone position after feeding can decrease the number of reflux episodes, improve gastric emptying, and decrease the risk of aspiration.[42,43] However, because of the risk of SIDS associated with the prone position, this posture should be considered only when the risk of death and complications from reflux outweighs the risk of SIDS.[41] Prolonged positioning in a car safety seat is not recommended (especially postprandially) because of a greater risk for reflux associated with a higher intra-abdominal pressure, particularly because the premature infant is likely to slump.[44] Although data do not support elevating the head of the crib in the supine position for treating reflux in infants,[45] placing the infant in the upright position for 30 minutes postprandially might lessen the symptoms of mild reflux. Although the right lateral position has been shown to decrease the emptying time, it seems to lead to greater episodes of reflux.[21]

The effect of *dietary alterations* on the degree of reflux varies. Potential changes include smaller volumes with more frequent feedings as well as thickened feedings. Although smaller feeding volumes (often with increased calories/oz in premature infants) may help to minimize gastric distention, the need for frequent feedings may actually exacerbate GER because reflux is more common postprandially.[16] Some term infants with severe regurgitant reflux may benefit from thickened feedings (rice cereal, carob flour, or sodium alginate).[46-49]

Table 4A-5 Diagnostic Tools

Tool	Description	Advantages	Disadvantages
Empiric medical therapy	Treat with acid suppressant and monitor infant	Simple Inexpensive Noninvasive Low risk if conservative regimen	Limited data about effects of medications in premature infants
Extended esophageal pH probe monitoring (most common)	Probe is positioned in the esophagus and pH is monitored over 24 hours; number, duration, and severity of acid reflux episodes are quantified "Reflux index" is calculated as the percentage of total time that esophageal pH <4 and estimates cumulative esophageal acid exposure	Simple Minimal risks Can be combined with a pneumogram Quantifies acid reflux Provides a temporal relationship with other symptoms Helpful to assess the degree of acid suppression after medical treatment	Degree of calculated acid reflux dependent on position of the probe Does not evaluate nonacid reflux Milk intake may buffer the degree of acidosis for up to 2 hours postprandially Altered by infant position† Usually requires overnight hospital stay Must discontinue acid suppressants for 2–4 days before testing
Upper gastrointestinal series with small bowel follow through	Contrast is visualized under fluoroscopy as it enters the infant's esophagus, stomach, and small intestine	Evaluates the anatomy of the upper gastrointestinal tract strictures, pyloric stenosis, webs, malrotation Can assess esophageal motility	Nonphysiologic conditions (infant often supine in a cold room) Brief period of fluoroscopic examination and thus lower specificity for assessing for reflux Risk of aspirating the contrast Operator dependent
Modified barium swallow	= Esophagram Study observes the quality of the infant's swallowing under fluoroscopy when infant is given different consistencies of milk Usually in conjunction with speech pathology specialist or occupational therapy specialist	Assesses for aspiration	Not helpful if infant is unable to feed by mouth
Esophageal endoscopy ± biopsy	Provides direct visualization and histopathologic evaluation of the esophageal mucosa	Assesses anatomy of the gastrointestinal tract Visualizes the mucosa for diagnosis of ulcers, strictures Useful for diagnosing esophagitis and esophageal strictures	Invasive Requires sedation
Nuclear (technetium) scintigraphy	Technetium-labeled milk is ingested and then the infant is scanned to detect isotope distribution in the esophagus, stomach, and lungs	Useful for determining the rate of gastric emptying Identifies nonacidic refluxate that a pH probe would not be able to detect Less radiation exposure compared with upper gastrointestinal series	Variable sensitivity because of differences in technique
Multiple intraluminal impedance	Detects reflux by measuring changes in impedance caused by a bolus of liquid entering the esophagus retrogradely	Independent of changes in pH and thus can detect acid and nonacid reflux Can quantify the reflux volume‡	Insufficient studies to establish normative data in infants Analysis is extremely time consuming
Esophageal manometry	Measures changes in pressures within upper gastrointestinal tract	Useful for assessing esophageal motility and LES function	Technical limitations

Modified from: Berseth CL: Gastroesophageal reflux in premature infants. Available at: *www.uptodate.com*, and Jadcherla SR, Rudolph CD: *NeoReviews* 6:e91, 2005.
†From: Hampton FJ, MacFadyen UM, Simpson H: *Arch Dis Child* 65:1249-1254, 1990.
‡From: Wenzl TG, Moroder C, Tachterna M, et al: *J Pediatr Gastroenterol Nutr* 34:519-523, 2002.

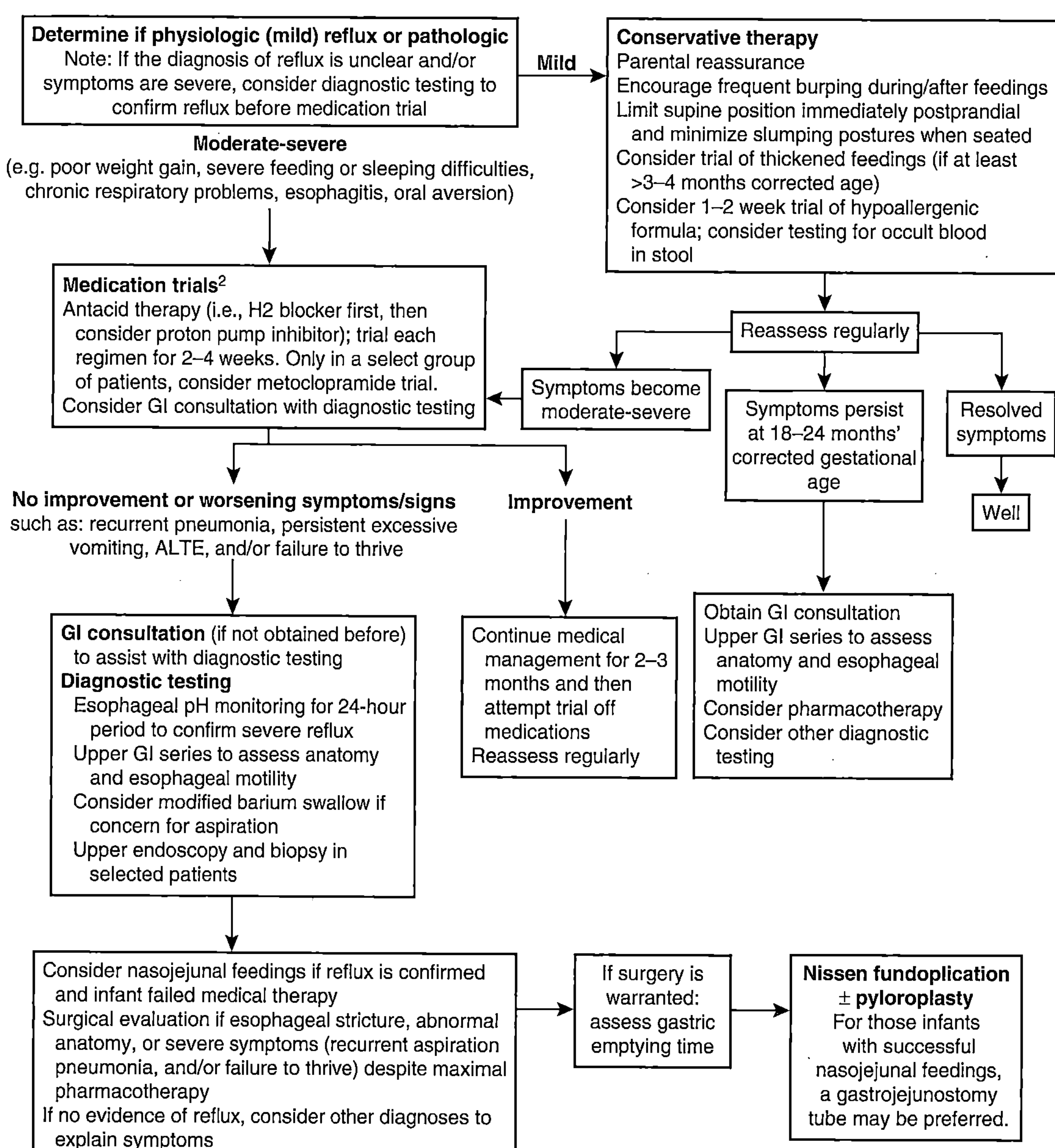

FIGURE 4A-1 [1]Modified from: Lifschitz CH. Clinical manifestations and diagnosis of gastroesophageal reflux disease in infants and children. Accessible: *www.uptodate.com* and from: Rudolph CD, Mazure LJ, Liptak GS, et al: Guidelines for evaluation and treatment for GER in infants and children. J Pedatr Gastroenterol and Nutr 2001; 32:S1–31. [2]Due to limited data on efficacy and adverse effects in infants born prematurely, usage of these medications in this group must be balanced with the degree of GER disease. GI = gastrointestihnal; ALTE = apparent life-threatening event Please note that this is a recommended algorithm that does not represent a professional standard of care; care should be revised to meet individual patient needs.

Recent antiregurgitant formulas (e.g., Enfamil AR), which contain starches that become thick in an acidic gastric environment, also can be given a trial.[38,50] Although reflux index scores do not usually change in term infants receiving thickened feedings,[47,51] these feedings have been shown to decrease the amount of emesis, lessen the crying time, and increase postprandial sleeping periods.[45,46,50] Thickened feedings offer the added benefit of increasing daily caloric intake. When a trial of thickened feedings is initiated, the infant should not be receiving acid suppressants because this dietary change is most effective in an acidic environment.[50] Despite potential benefits, thickened feedings must be used judiciously because they might increase the risk of coughing,[52] and studies suggest a possible association with type I diabetes–associated autoantibodies in infants exposed to cereal when they are younger than 3 months.[53,54] In infants born prematurely, thickened feedings have not been systematically evaluated for efficacy or safety.

Other dietary alterations also may be considered. The primary care provider should recommend that families eliminate clear liquids such as water and juice from the infant's diet because these are easy to regurgitate. Frequent burping during feedings is recommended. Although human milk has been shown to lead to subtle improvements in reflux episodes, reports have not found a clear benefit of human milk over formula.[55]

Studies suggest that nearly 50% of infants with GER may have an associated cow milk allergy.[56-58] As such, primary care providers could consider a 1- to 2-week trial of hypoallergenic (protein hydrolysate) formula (e.g., Alimentum, Nutramigen, Carnation Good Start) in formula-fed infants with frequent emesis and/or regurgitation.[41,56] Some infants also are allergic to hydrolysate and will respond only to an amino acid–based formula.[58,59] Of note, a transition to soy formula may not relieve the infant's symptoms, as at least 20% of allergic infants are sensitive to both cow milk and soy.[7] Presently, no elemental formulas are tailored to infants born prematurely. Thus, when managing premature infants, the potential nutritional imbalance of using currently available elemental formulas must be weighed against the concern for cow milk allergy.[38] Infants born prematurely who are changed from transitional premature infant formula to elemental formula should receive extra vitamin and/or calcium supplementation, depending on the contents in the new formula compared with the original formula.

Families should be advised to minimize the infant's exposure to smoke because second-hand smoking is likely to worsen the reflux.[60] In addition, primary care providers should educate families about the widespread prevalence of GER in infants and reassure families that symptoms are likely to resolve with time.

Pharmacotherapy

Currently there is no standard approach to the medical management of infants with GER. The decision about which specific agent to use is based on the patient's age, the type and severity of symptoms, and the risk/benefit ratio of the medication. The advantages and disadvantages of potential pharmacotherapeutic agents are summarized in Table 4A-6. Data about drug metabolism, adverse effects, or dosing range of the potential antireflux medications are lacking for infants born prematurely, and use of these drugs must be balanced with unknown risks.

Acid suppression is one of the main goals of medical therapy, especially if there is evidence of esophagitis. *Histamine-2 (H_2) antagonists* (e.g., ranitidine, cimetidine, famotidine, nizatidine) increase gastric pH by blocking histamine receptors in the gastric parietal cells. Studies in infants and children demonstrate potential efficacy with nonserious side effects such as increased irritability.[61-63] Although the pharmacokinetics of ranitidine has been evaluated in preterm infants and shows that premature infants should receive lower and less frequent doses,[64] the pharmacokinetics of the other H_2 antagonists has not been evaluated in this population. None of these agents have been evaluated for efficacy in infants born prematurely.

Proton pump inhibitors (omeprazole, lansoprazole, rabeprazole) are more potent acid suppressants that decrease gastric acid secretion by irreversibly binding to and inhibiting the parietal cell H^+/K^+-ATPase pump. Multiple studies in adults have demonstrated efficacy of these pump inhibitors in improving reflux disease, and some document an advantage of these agents over H_2 blockers.[65] Omeprazole has been the most studied proton pump inhibitor in term infants. Similar information is not yet available from studies conducted in preterm infants. Children (age 6 months to 13 years) with severe esophagitis showed significant improvement in symptoms and gastric acid pH after treatment with omeprazole.[66] Similar results were found in infants (age 3 to 12 months) who had reduced esophageal acid after treatment with omeprazole.[67] Ten-year follow-up data have found that omeprazole is generally safe in children, although prolonged administration may increase the risk of enteric infections and vitamin B_{12} malabsorption.[67] There is theoretical concern that gastric acid suppression in preterm infants may lead to negative consequences, such as (1) overgrowth of small intestinal bacteria, (2) elevated serum gastrin levels with an associated risk of

Table 4A-6 Medications for Managing Moderate-to-Severe Gastroesophageal Reflux

Pharmaco-therapeutic Agent	Mode of Action	Advantages	Disadvantages
Histamine (H_2) Receptor Antagonists (e.g., Cimetidine/Tagamet, Ranitidine/Zantac)	Lowers gastric pH by inhibiting H_2 receptors of gastric parietal cells	Pharmacokinetics of ranitidine has been studied in preterm infants May improve esophagitis	Efficacy has not been evaluated in preterm infants Cimetidine may increase serum levels of theophylline, warfarin, phenytoin, antiarrhythmic agents
Omeprazole (Prilosec) *Note:* Lansoprazole (Prevacid) is a proton pump inhibitor that is available in a liquid form for children	Proton pump inhibitor—decreases gastric acid secretion by inhibiting the parietal cell H^+/K^+-ATPase pump	Most effective acid suppressant in adults and older children	Efficacy, safety, and pharmacokinetics have not been evaluated in premature infants More costly than H_2 antagonists May increase toxicity of warfarin, digoxin, and phenytoin May decrease effects of ketoconazole
Metoclopramide (Reglan)	Prokinetic—dopamine antagonist with potential to increase gastric emptying and/or esophageal sphincter tone	Pharmacokinetics has been evaluated in infants born >31 weeks' gestation May increase peristalsis, gastric emptying, and lower esophageal sphincter tone in some infants	Uncertain efficacy in infants born prematurely or at term[69,70] Use with caution when administered at >0.3 mg/kg per dose because of possible central nervous system disturbances such as dystonic reactions and extrapyramidal movements
Erythromycin	Prokinetic—acts on neural motilin receptors and stimulates antral contractions[71]	Some evidence of improved gastroduodenal contractility in preterm infants >33 weeks' postmenstrual age May improve gastric emptying	High-dose therapy may be associated with hypertrophic pyloric stenosis
Cisapride	Prokinetic—noncholinergic nondopaminergic agent that increases gastrointestinal motility by releasing acetylcholine and functioning as a serotonin receptor agonist	Improves esophageal peristalsis and increases lower esophageal sphincter pressure	Use in infants is not approved by Food and Drug Administration because of small risk of cardiac toxicity (prolongs QTc) No longer marketed in the United States

developing hypertrophic pyloric stenosis, and (3) decreased acid-dependent enzyme activity leading to ineffective digestion.[38] Because of these possible adverse effects, the minimal data on efficacy and long-term safety in preterm infants, and their substantial acid suppression, proton pump inhibitors should be reserved for infants born prematurely who are not responsive to H_2 blockers.[38]

Although *prokinetic agents* are the second-line approach to treating GER disease in infants born at term and children, their efficacy in infants born prematurely has not been evaluated. Because premature infants usually do not have delayed gastric emptying time, these agents might not be as beneficial for treating reflux in this group. Metoclopramide (Reglan) is a prokinetic agent that functions as a dopamine antagonist, stimulates cholinergic receptors of gastric smooth muscle cells, and increases acetylcholine release. These actions enable metoclopramide to improve gastric emptying with some effect on increasing LES pressure and enhancing esophageal peristalsis. Some trials in children younger than 2 years found that metoclopramide lessens daily reflux symptoms and reduces the reflux index, but these benefits must be weighed against possible side effects.[45,68] Specifically, infants must be monitored for dystonic reactions and extrapyramidal movements. Other studies in infants showed no clear benefit of metoclopramide compared with placebo,[69] and one study actually found symptoms were worse with metoclopramide.[70]

Studies have suggested that low-dose erythromycin, acting as a prokinetic agent by binding to neural motilin receptors and stimulating antral contractions, may decrease symptoms of reflux in some premature infants.[71-73] Jadcherla and Berseth[74] demonstrated improved gastroduodenal contractility in preterm infants older than 33 weeks' postmenstrual age but no effect on LES tone or esophageal motility. However, because reports of erythromycin therapy suggest an association with hypertrophic pyloric stenosis[75,76] as well as the potential to induce cardiac arrhythmias or septicemia from multiresistant organisms, this treatment is not used routinely.[59,77]

Previously, cisapride had been used as a prokinetic agent. Even though it was effective at improving GER disease, it is no longer marketed in the United States because of the small but fatal risk of cardiac arrhythmias.

Medical therapy for infants with moderate-to-severe GER disease usually begins with an H_2 receptor antagonist. For infants without any change in symptoms after 2 to 4 weeks, 24-hour esophageal pH testing can be considered to determine whether the agent was effective at suppressing gastric pH. If the initial acid suppressant was ineffective at the maximal recommended dose for age, a 2- to 4-week trial with a proton pump inhibitor can be considered. Because pH testing often requires hospitalization, this testing may be deferred, and the second acid suppressant can be given a trial. The prokinetic agent metoclopramide can be added to either antacid, but, because of potential side effects, therapy should be limited to a select group of patients and to a 2- to 4-week trial. If the infant does not improve or has worsening symptoms despite medical therapy, a consultation with a gastroenterology specialist and diagnostic testing are recommended.

Transpyloric feedings

Nasojejunal feedings can be considered in infants with transient severe GER disease. In the neonatal intensive care unit, this feeding regimen may transiently provide enteral nutrition to premature infants who demonstrate signs of aspiration associated with their reflux disease and are not yet feeding orally. As the infant matures, these feedings possibly can be discontinued.

At present, no data address the risks and benefits of continuous transpyloric feedings in older infants born prematurely. Because a nasogastric tube has been shown to increase the number of reflux episodes in preterm infants,[78] using a chronic nasojejunal tube may actually worsen GER disease.[38] Because of their lack of documented efficacy and their complication risks, nasojejunal tubes are not often used in the community setting.

Surgical therapy

Surgical therapy is required in only a small number of infants with GER disease. Currently, infants with diagnostic evidence of reflux and severe symptoms (recurrent aspiration pneumonia, presence of esophageal stricture/ulceration, and/or failure to thrive) despite maximal pharmacotherapy may benefit from surgical intervention. Studies have attempted to identify infants who are more likely to require surgery. Da Dalt et al.[79] reported minimal success with medical management of GER in infants having 24-hour pH probe evidence of more than 20 reflux episodes lasting longer than 5 minutes or a reflux index >27%. Some reports found that prolonged reflux during sleep correlates with a favorable response to surgery in a large majority of children.[80] However, normal pH probe studies have also been found in children who had esophagitis and responded to surgical intervention.[81] Infants with major neurologic morbidity who require a feeding gastrostomy tube often require surgical repair of their reflux.[82]

A Nissen fundoplication is the procedure of choice for surgical repair of GER disease.[83] Historically, this technique involves wrapping the gastric fundus around the back of the lower esophagus.[84] Since that original description, many variations have been described, with modifications in the approach, the looseness of the wrap, and the portion of the stomach used. Experience with a laparoscopic approach is limited in infants. Because of the high reported incidence of delayed gastric emptying in infants requiring a fundoplication, providers should consider whether a concurrent pyloroplasty to improve gastric emptying is indicated.[85] This can be assessed by a technetium gastric emptying study or milk scan.

Most outcome studies following a fundoplication are based on data from studies in children. Symptomatic relief has been observed in ≈60% to 90% of children,[86,87] and studies in infants have found similar results.[88,89] Although surgery has a low mortality risk (0%–5%), complications occur in 2% to 45%.[41,89] Potential complications following a Nissen fundoplication include delayed gastric emptying, esophageal obstruction caused by tight wrap, dislodgement of the wrap, prolapse of the fundoplication into the mediastinum, small intestinal obstruction, and infection.[90-92] Some of these morbidities may lead to recurrent reflux disease, with reoperation required in 3% to 19%.[89,92]

For infants who benefited from nasojejunal feedings, a jejunostomy feeding tube can be placed percutaneously and may provide another alternative to fundoplication.[93] Particularly, infants with dysmotility syndromes as determined by swallowing studies may benefit from a jejunostomy tube.[93]

Conclusion

The majority of clinical, diagnostic, and therapeutic recommendations about GER in premature infants have been extrapolated from studies conducted in full-term infants, children, and adults. Primary care providers should differentiate between physiologic or functional (i.e., regurgitation) and pathophysiologic (i.e., GER disease) reflux in order to determine which infants require treatment. Severe or pathologic reflux is associated with weight loss; feeding difficulties, with frequent emesis; sleeping difficulties; chronic respiratory problems; esophagitis; and/or oral aversion. Although infants with mild reflux can be managed conservatively, infants with severe symptoms/signs should receive medical therapy. The decision about which specific agent to use is based on the patient's age, the type and severity of symptoms, and the risk/benefit ratio of the medication. Acid suppressive therapy with H_2 antagonists is the preferred first-line approach to infants born prematurely with GER disease. For infants who continue to have severe symptoms despite maximal medical therapy, a diagnostic evaluation under the guidance of a gastroenterology specialist is warranted. A small number of infants with diagnostic evidence of reflux and persistent severe symptoms (recurrent aspiration pneumonia, presence of esophageal stricture/ulceration, and/or failure to thrive) despite maximal pharmacotherapy may benefit from surgical intervention. Because many aspects of GER disease in infants born prematurely remain incompletely understood, evaluating and managing this disease remains a challenge to neonatologists, gastroenterology specialists, and primary care providers. Randomized controlled trials to evaluate appropriate and effective therapies are warranted.

Resources for Families and Clinicians

Children's Digestive Health and Nutrition Foundation
www.CDHNF.org

This website provides educational information (including videos) about GER disease for families and clinicians.

www.KIDSACIDREFLUX.org

Cartoon sponsored by the Children's Digestive Health and Nutrition Foundation that explains reflux to children.

National Digestive Disease Information Clearinghouse (NDDIC)
http://digestive.niddk.nih.gov/ddiseases/pubs/gerdinfant/

Review of physiologic and pathologic reflux for families.

The North American Society for Pediatric Gastroenterology, Hepatology and Nutrition
www.NASPGHAN.org

Pediatric/Adolescent Gastroesophageal Reflux Association (PAGER)
www.reflux.org

This website of a national parent support group provides information regarding reflux/medication/testing; site is available in Spanish.

Acknowledgment

The author thanks Paul A. Rufo, MD, MMSc, for extremely thorough review of this chapter.

REFERENCES

1. Hart JJ: Pediatric gastroesophageal reflux. *Am Fam Physician* 54:2463-2472, 1996.
2. Shepherd RW, Wren J, Evans S, et al: Gastroesophageal reflux in children. Clinical profile, course and outcome with active therapy in 126 cases. *Clin Pediatr* 26:55-60, 1987.
3. Newell SJ, Booth IW, Morgan ME, et al: Gastro-oesophageal reflux in preterm infants. *Arch Dis Child* 64:780-786, 1989.
4. Jeffery HE, Page M: Developmental maturation of gastro-oesophageal reflux in preterm infants. *Acta Paediatr* 1995;84:245-2450.
5. Kohelet D, Boaz M, Serour F, et al: Esophageal pH study and symptomatology of gastroesophageal reflux in newborn infants. *Am J Perinatol* 21:85-91, 2004.
6. Hrabsovsky EE, Mullett MD: Gastroesophageal reflux and the premature infant. *J Pediatr Surg* 21:583-587, 1986.
7. Orenstein SR: Infantile reflux: Different from adult reflux. *Am J Med* 103:114S-119S, 1997.
8. Dhillon AS, Ewer AK: Diagnosis and management of gastro-oesophageal reflux in preterm infants in neonatal intensive care units. *Acta Paediatr* 93:88-93, 2004.
9. Vandenplas Y, De Wolf D, Sacre L: Influence of xanthines on gastroesophageal reflux in infants at risk for sudden infant death syndrome. *Pediatrics* 77:807-810, 1986.
10. Del Giudice E, Staiano A, Capano G, et al: Gastrointestinal manifestations in children with cerebral palsy. *Brain Dev* 21:307-311, 1999.
11. Akinola E, Rosenkrantz TS, Pappagallo M, et al: Gastroesophageal reflux in infants <32 weeks gestational age at birth: lack of relationship to chronic lung disease. *Am J Perinatol* 21:57-62, 2004.
12. Fuloria M, Hiatt D, Dillard RG, et al: Gastroesophageal reflux in very low birth weight infants: association with chronic lung disease and outcomes through 1 year of age. *J Perinatol* 20:235-239, 2000.
13. Sindel BD, Maiesels MJ, Ballantine TV: Gastroesophageal reflux to the proximal esophagus in infants with bronchopulmonary dysplasia. *Am J Dis Child* 143:1103-1106, 1989.
14. Glassman M, George D, Grill B: Gastroesophageal reflux in children. Clinical manifestations, diagnosis, and therapy. *Gastroenterol Clin North Am* 24:71-98, 1995.
15. Khalaf MN, Porat R, Brodsky NL, et al: Clinical correlations in infants in the neonatal intensive care unit with varying severity of gastroesophageal reflux. *J Pediatr Gastroenterol Nutr* 32:45-49, 2001.
16. Berseth CL: Gastroesophageal reflux in premature infants. Accessible at: *www.uptodate.com*
17. Omari TI, Miki K, Fraser R et al: Esophageal body and lower esophageal sphincter function in healthy premature infants. *Gastroenterology* 109:1757-1764, 1995.

18. Dodds WJ, Dent J, Hogan WJ, et al: Mechanisms of gastroesophageal reflux in patients with reflux esophagitis. *N Engl J Med* 307:1547-1552, 1982.
19. Omari TI, Benninga MA, Barnett CP et al: Characterization of esophageal body and lower esophageal sphincter motor function in the very premature neonate. *J Pediatr* 135:517-521, 1999.
20. Omari TI, Barnett CP, Benninga MA, et al: Mechanisms of gastro-oesophageal reflux in preterm and term infants with reflux disease. *Gut* 51:475-479, 2002.
21. Omari TI, Rommel N, Staunton E, et al: Paradoxical impact of body positioning on gastroesophageal reflux and gastric emptying in the premature infant. *J Pediatr* 145:194-200, 2004.
22. Newell SJ, Sarkar PK, Durbin GM, et al: Maturation of the lower oesophageal sphincter in the preterm baby. *Gut* 29:167-172, 1988.
23. Ewer AK, Durbin GM, Morgan ME et al: Gastric emptying and gastro-oesophageal reflux in preterm infants. *Arch Dis Child Fetal Neonatal Ed* 75:F117-F121, 1996.
24. Nelson SP, Chen EH, Syniar GM, et al: Prevalence of symptoms of gastroesophageal reflux during infancy. A pediatric practice-based survey. Pediatric Practice Research Group. *Arch Pediatr Adolesc Med* 151:569-572, 1997.
25. Hyman PE: Gastroesophageal reflux: one reason why baby won't eat. *J Pediatr* 125:S103-S109, 1994.
26. Barrington KJ, Tan K, Rich W: Apnea at discharge and gastroesophageal reflux in the preterm infant. *J Perinatol* 22:8, 2002.
27. de Ajuriaguerra M, Radvanyi-Bouvet MF, Huon C, et al: Gastroesophageal reflux and apnea in prematurely born infants during wakefulness and sleep. *Am J Dis Child* 145:1132-1136, 1991.
28. Molloy EJ, Di Fiore JM, Martin RJ: Does gastroesophageal reflux cause apnea in preterm infants? *Biol Neonate* 87:254-261, 2005.
29. Peter CS, Sprodowski N, Bohnhorst B, et al: Gastroesophageal reflux and apnea of prematurity: no temporal relationship. *Pediatrics* 109:8-11, 2002.
30. Kimball AL, Carlton DP: Gastroesophageal reflux medications in the treatment of apnea of premature infants. *J Pediatr* 138:355-360, 2001.
31. Di Fiore JM, Arko M, Whitehouse M, et al: Apnea is not prolonged by acid gastroesophageal reflux in preterm infants. *Pediatrics* 116:1059-1063, 2005.
32. Veereman-Wauters G, Bochner A, Van Caillie-Bertrand M: Gastroesophageal reflux in infants with a history of near-miss sudden infant death. *J Pediatr Gastroenterol Nutr* 12:319-323, 1991.
33. Thack BT: Sudden infant death syndrome: can gastroesophageal reflux cause sudden infant death? *Am J Med* 108(suppl 4a):144S-148S, 2000.
34. Page M, Jeffery H: The role of gastro-oesophageal reflux in the aetiology of SIDS. *Early Hum Dev* 59:127-149, 2000.
35. Arad-Cohen N, Cohen A, Tirosh E: The relationship between gastroesophageal reflux and apnea in infants. *J Pediatr* 137:321-326, 2000.
36. Vandenplas Y, Hauser B: Gastro-oesophageal reflux, sleep pattern, apparent life threatening event and sudden infant death. The point of view of a gastro-enterologist. *Eur J Pediatr* 159:726-729, 2000.
37. Kahn A, Rebuffat E, Sottiaux, et al: Sleep apneas and esophageal reflux in control infants and in infants with an apparent life-threatening event. *Biol Neonate* 57:144-149, 1990.
38. Jadcherla SR, Rudolph CD: Gastroesophageal reflux in the preterm neonate. *NeoReviews* 6:e87-e98, 2005.
39. Jung AD: Gastroesophageal reflux in infants and children. *Am Fam Physician* 64:1853-1860, 2001.
40. Colletti R, Christie D, Orenstein S: Indications for pediatric esophageal pH monitoring: statement of the North American Society for Pediatric Gastroenterology and Nutrition. *J Pediatr Gastroenterol Nutr* 21:253-262, 1995.
41. Rudolph CD, Mazur LJ, Liptak GS, et al: Guidelines for evaluation and treatment of GER in infants and children. *J Pedatr Gastroenterol and Nutr* 32:S1-S31, 2001.
42. Meyers WF, Herbst JJ: Effectiveness of positioning therapy for gastroesophageal reflux. *Pediatrics* 69:768-772, 1982.
43. Vandenplas Y, Sacre-Smits L: Seventeen-hour continuous esophageal pH monitoring in the newborn: evaluation of the influence of position in asymptomatic and symptomatic babies. *J Pediatr Gastroenterol Nutr* 4:356-361, 1985.
44. Orenstein SR, Whitington PF, Orenstein DM: The infant seat as treatment for gastroesophageal reflux. *N Engl J Med* 209:760-763, 1983.
45. Craig WR, Hanlon-Dearman A, Sinclair C, et al: Metoclopramide, thickened feedings, and positioning for gastro-oesophageal reflux in children under 2 years. *Cochrane Database Syst Rev* 18:CD003502, 2004.
46. Orenstein SR, Magill HL, Brooks P: Thickening of infant feedings for therapy of gastroesophageal reflux. *J Pediatr* 110:181-186, 1987.
47. Vandenplas Y, Sacre L: Milk-thickening agents as a treatment for gastroesophageal reflux. *Clin Pediatr* 26:66-68, 1987.
48. Wenzyl TG, Schneider S, Scheele F, et al: Effects of thickened feeding on gastroesophageal reflux in infants: a placebo-controlled crossover study using intraluminal impedance. *Pediatrics* 111:e355-e359, 2003.
49. Buts JP, Barudi C, Otte JB: Double blind controlled study on the efficacy of sodium alginate (Gaviscon) in reducing gastroesophageal reflux assessed by 24 hour continuous pH monitoring in infants and children. *Eur J Pediatr* 146:156-158, 10987.
50. Vanderhoof JA, Moran JR, Harris CL, et al: Efficacy of a pre-thickened infant formula: a multicenter, double-blind, randomized, placebo-controlled parallel group trial in 104 infants with symptomatic gastroesophageal reflux. *Clin Pediatr* 42:483-495, 2003.
51. Bailey DJ, Andros JM, Danek GE, et al: Lack of efficacy of thickened feeding as treatment for gastroesophageal reflux. *J Pediatr* 110:187-189, 1987.
52. Orenstein SR, Shalaby TM, Putman PE: Thickened feedings as a cause of increased coughing when used as a therapy for gastroesophageal reflux in infants. *J Pediatr* 121:913-915, 1992.
53. Norris JM, Barriga K, Klingensmith G, et al: Timing of initial cereal exposure in infancy and risk of islet autoimmunity. *JAMA* 290:1713-1720, 2003.
54. Ziegler AG, Schmid S, Huber D, et al: Early infant feeding and risk of developing type 1 diabetes-associated autoantibodies. *JAMA* 290:1721-1728, 2003.
55. Heacock HJ, Jeffery HE, Baker JL, et al: Influence of breast versus formula milk on physiological gastroesophageal reflux in healthy, newborn infants. *J Pediatr Gastroenterol Nutr* 14:41-46, 1992.
56. Salvatore S, Vandenplas Y: Gastroesophageal reflux and cow milk allergy: is there a link? *Pediatrics* 110:972-984, 2002.
57. Cavataio F, Carroccio A, Iacono G: Milk-induced reflux in infants less than one year of age. *J Pediatr Gastroenterol Nutr* 30(suppl):S36-S44, 2000.
58. D'Netto MA, Herson VC, Hussain N, et al: Allergic gastroenteropathy in preterm infants. *J Pediatr* 137:480-486, 2000.
59. Poets CF: Gastroesophageal reflux: a critical review of its role in preterm infants. *Pediatrics* 113:e128-e132, 2004.
60. Shabib S, Cutz E, Sherman P: Passive smoking is a risk factor for esophagitis in children. *J Pediatr* 127:435-437, 1995.
61. Hallerback B, Glise H, Johanssen B, et al: Gastro-oesophageal reflux symptoms—clinical findings and effect of ranitidine treatment. *Eur J Surg Suppl* 53:61-13, 1998.
62. Cucchiara S, Gobio-Casali L, Balli F, et al: Cimetidine treatment of reflux esophagitis in children: an Italian multicenter study. *J Pediatr Gastroenterol Nutr* 8:150-156, 1989.

63. Orenstein SR, Shalaby TM, Devandry SN, et al: Famotidine for infant gastro-oesophageal reflux: a multi-centre, randomized, placebo-controlled, withdrawal trial. *Aliment Pharmacol Ther* 17:1097-107, 2003.
64. Kuusela Al, Ruuska T, Karikoski R, et al: A randomized, controlled study of prophylactic ranitidine in preventing stress-induced gastric mucosal lesions in neonatal intensive care unit patients. *Crit Care Med* 25:346-351, 1997.
65. Chiba N, De Gara CJ, Wilkinson JM, et al: Speed of healing and symptom relief in grade II to IV gastroesophageal reflux disease: a meta-analysis. *Gastroenterology* 112:1798-1810, 1997.
66. Cucchiara S, Minella R, Iervolino C, et al: Omeprazole and high dose ranitidine in the treatment of refractory reflux oesophagitis. *Arch Dis Child* 69:655-9, 1993.
67. Moore DJ, Tao BS, Lines DR, et al: Double-blind placebo-controlled trial of omeprazole in irritable infants with gastroesophageal reflux. *J Pediatr* 143:219-223, 2003.
68. Tolia V, Calhoun J, Kuhns L, et al: Randomized, prospective double-blind trial of metoclopramide and placebo for gastroesophageal reflux in infants. *J Pediatr* 115:141-135, 1989.
69. Bellissant E, Duhamel JF, Guillot M, et al: The triangular test to assess the efficacy of metoclopramide in gastroesophageal reflux. *Clin Pharmacol Ther* 61:377-384, 1997.
70. Machida HM, Forbes DA, Gall DG, et al: Metoclopramide in gastroesophageal reflux of infancy. *J Pediatr* 112:483-487, 1988.
71. Kaul A: Erythromycin as a prokinetic agent. *J Pediatr Gastroenterol Nutr* 34:13-15, 2002.
72. Costalos C, Gavrili V, Skouteri V: The effect of low-dose erythromycin on whole gastrointestinal transit time of preterm infants. *Early Hum Dev* 65:91-96, 2001.
73. Oei J, Lui K: A placebo-controlled trial of low-dose erythromycin to promote feed tolerance in preterm infants. *Acta Paediatr* 90:904-908, 2001.
74. Jadcherla SR, Berseth CL: Effect of erythromycin on gastroduodenal contractile activity in developing neonates. *J Pediatr Gastroenterol Nutr* 34:16-22, 2002.
75. Hauben M, Amsden GW: The association of erythromycin and infantile hypertrophic pyloric stenosis: causal or coincidental? *Drug Saf* 25:929-942, 2002.
76. Cooper WO, Griffin MR, Arbogast P, et al: Very early exposure to erythromycin and infantile hypertrophic pyloric stenosis. *Arch Pediatr Adolesc Med* 156:647-650, 2002.
77. Ng PC, So KW, Fung KSC, et al: Randomised controlled study of oral erythromycin for treatment of gastrointestinal dysmotility in preterm infants. *Arch Dis Child Fetal Neonatal Ed* 84:F177-182, 2001.
78. Peter CS, Wiechers C, Bohnhorst B, et al: Influence of nasogastric tubes on gastroesophageal reflux in preterm infants: a multiple intraluminal impedance study. *J Pediatr* 141:277-279, 2002.
79. Da Dalt L, Mazzoleni S, Montini G, et al: Diagnostic accuracy of pH monitoring in gastro-oesophageal reflux. *Arch Dis Child* 64:1421-1426, 1989.
80. Eizaguirre I, Tovar JA: Predicting preoperatively the outcome of respiratory symptoms of gastroesophageal reflux. *J Pediatr Surg* 27:848-51, 1992.
81. Tovar JA, Angulo JA, Gorostiaga L, et al: Surgery for gastroesophageal reflux in children with normal pH studies. *J Pediatr Surg* 26:541-545, 1991.
82. Wilkinson JD, Dudgeon DL, Sondheimer JM: A comparison of medical and surgical treatment of gastroesophageal reflux in severely retarded children. *J Pediatr* 99:202-520, 1981.
83. Barnes N, Robertson N, Lakhoo K: Anti-reflux surgery for the neonatal intensive care-dependent infant. *Early Hum Dev* 75:71-78, 2003.
84. Nissen R: Gastropexy and "fundoplication" in surgical treatment of hiatus hernia. *Am J Dig Dis* 6:954-961, 1961.
85. Bustorff-Silva J, Fonkalsrud EW, Perez CA, et al: Gastric emptying procedures decrease the risk of postoperative recurrent reflux in children with delayed gastric emptying. *J Pediatr Surg* 34:79-82, 1999.
86. Dedinsky GK, Vane DW, Black T, et al: Complications and reoperation after Nissen fundoplication in childhood. *Am J Surg* 153:177-183, 1987.
87. Opie JC, Chaye H, Fraser GC: Fundoplication and pediatric esophageal manometry: Actuarial analysis over 7 years. *J Pediatr Surg* 22:935-938, 1987.
88. Fonkalsrud EW, Bustorff-Silva J, Perez CA, et al: Antireflux surgery in children under 3 months of age. *J Pediatr Surg* 34:527-531, 1999.
89. Fonkalsrud EW, Ashcraft KW, Coran AG, et al: Surgical treatment of gastroesophageal reflux in children: a combined hospital study of 7467 patients. *Pediatrics* 101: 419-422, 1998.
90. Spitz L, Kirtane J: Results and complications of surgery for gastro-oesophageal reflux. *Arch Dis Child* 60:743-747 1985.
91. Hanimann B, Sacher P, Stauffer UG: Complications and long-term results of the Nissen fundoplication. *Eur J Pediatr Surg* 3:12-14, 1993.
92. Lifschitz CH. Management of gastroesophageal reflux disease in infants and children. 12/04; Accessible at: *www.uptodate.com*
93. Albanese CT, Towbin RB, Ulman I, et al: Percutaneous gastrojejunostomy versus Nissen fundoplication for enteral feeding of the neurologically impaired child with gastroesophageal reflux. *J Pediatr* 123:371-375, 1993.
94. Fasching G, Huber A, Uray E, et al: Gastroesophageal reflux and diaphragmatic motility after repair of congenital diaphragmatic hernia. *Eur J Pediatr Surg* 10:360-364, 2000.

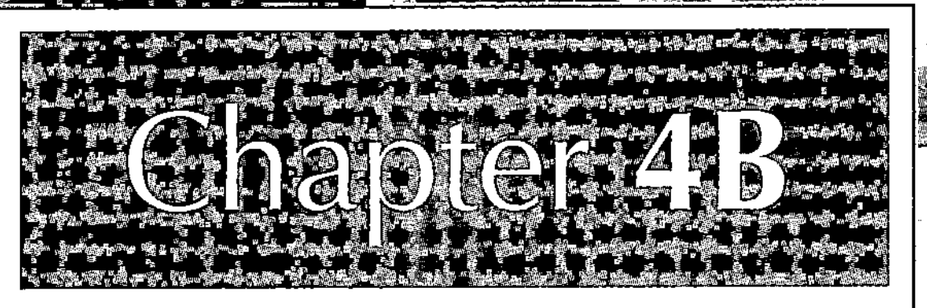

Chapter 4B

Colic

Jill S. Fischer, MD

Colic consists of crying episodes that typically begin in full-term infants at approximately 2 weeks of age and continue until approximately 4 months of age. It is thought to occur in 5% to 25% of infants.[1,2] The most commonly used definition describes crying periods that last for 3 hours, occur more than 3 days per week, and endure for more than 3 weeks.[3] Crying most commonly begins in the evening.[4] During the crying episodes, the baby is inconsolable, with clenched fists and flexed legs. The abdomen may be firm, and the baby may pass gas. A baby with colic is often described by a parent to "look as if he or she is in pain." The crying episodes are unpredictable and often occur without any obvious stimulus.[5]

Studies of colic are challenging because all babies experience fussy periods, generally with an evening onset.[5] In western societies, normal babies cry for up to 2 hours per day at 2 weeks of age and up to 3 hours per day at 6 weeks of age. Periods of crying, which peak at approximately 2 months of age, have been described in African and Asian babies. Colicky babies experience the same frequency of crying *episodes* as do noncolicky babies, but the duration of the episodes is longer. This has led some authors to suggest that colic is best described as "primary excessive crying."[3] Although the cries of colicky babies are traditionally thought to differ from those of noncolicky babies, studies have not found this to be the case.[3] It has been noted, however, that the quality of a premature infant's cry is unique and "may be perceived as more irritable."[6]

Premature babies have been noted to have a crying pattern similar to that of full-term infants, beginning shortly after the expected due date, peaking at approximately 6 weeks' corrected age and ending at 3 to 4 months' corrected age.[3,4] Although data are limited, this pattern probably is not related to postnatal medical complications.[5] One study found no difference in the incidence of colic between premature and term populations of infants.[7]

Differential Diagnosis

The diagnosis of colic can be challenging because all babies experience crying episodes. It is important to distinguish excessive crying from normal crying that is merely poorly tolerated by the parents.[3] A variety of disease processes can present with crying,[5] but organic disease is thought to cause less than 5% of excessive crying.[1,5] Some organic causes of unusual crying are listed in Table 4B-1. It is important to note that the definition of colic does not include poor weight gain[4]; thus, the evaluation of infants with crying and failure to thrive is different from the assessment of infants with crying and adequate weight gain. Similarly, gastroesophageal reflux (see Chapter 4A) may present with crying but should be addressed as a syndrome separate from colic.[4]

Etiology

Colic traditionally has been described as related to intestinal cramping, and parents often believe that their infant is suffering from dietary intolerance, abdominal cramping, or even intestinal blockage. Studies do not support the theory that infants with colic have any gastrointestinal pathology. Drawing up the legs, popularly thought to represent a response to abdominal pain, can occur in response to "a variety of noxious stimuli."[3] Air swallowed during crying episodes conceivably can lead to gassiness and abdominal distention, but these represent sequelae, rather than causes of, excessive crying. Other studies do not support previously held theories that colic results from parental inexperience or anxiety.[4] This is an important point to emphasize when counseling parents of colicky babies.

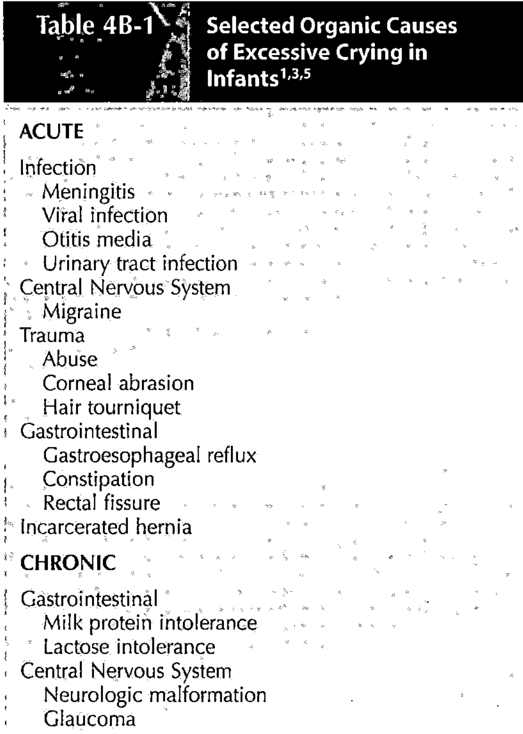

Table 4B-1 Selected Organic Causes of Excessive Crying in Infants[1,3,5]

Causes
ACUTE
Infection
Meningitis
Viral infection
Otitis media
Urinary tract infection
Central Nervous System
Migraine
Trauma
Abuse
Corneal abrasion
Hair tourniquet
Gastrointestinal
Gastroesophageal reflux
Constipation
Rectal fissure
Incarcerated hernia
CHRONIC
Gastrointestinal
Milk protein intolerance
Lactose intolerance
Central Nervous System
Neurologic malformation
Glaucoma

Current theories focus on the temperament and regulatory capability of the colicky infant. One theory suggests that infants with colic react appropriately to stimuli but show a relative inability to self-regulate, that is, an inability to regulate their response to a noxious stimulus. This would explain why infants with colic have the same frequency of crying episodes but have bouts with longer duration.[5] This theory may be particularly applicable to premature infants, whose hypertonicity can make self-soothing more difficult.[6]

Evaluation

Evaluation of the colicky baby should begin with a description by the parent or caregiver of the crying. This can be done with a written diary or with a verbal recounting of a typical day.[3] It is helpful to elicit not only the times and intensity of crying but also the parent's response to the crying infant, as well as a description of which interventions, if any, are successful in lessening the crying. A complete medical history is important to rule out potential organic etiologies. Family and social history are particularly helpful and important for eliciting particular parental anxieties.[3] A careful physical examination is essential, both to exclude possible medical problems and to reassure parents that their infant is not ill. If the history and physical examination are not concerning for organic pathology, laboratory testing and imaging generally may be deferred.

Management

The sequelae of colic can include maternal anxiety, premature weaning, and even child abuse.[5] Therefore, it is important to address symptoms of colic in the primary care setting. It also is essential to establish realistic expectations for treatment. Because all babies experience episodes of crying, no treatment will completely eliminate fussiness and irritability.[4]

Unfortunately, there are no proven methods for treating colic. It is difficult to make conclusions from clinical studies because they do not use a consistent definition of colic. In addition, many studies include only referred patient populations, which may not be representative of the population as a whole.[3]

Management can be separated into behavioral interventions and pharmacologic methods. Although carrying an infant may be a helpful modality in a fussy, noncolicky baby, studies in which parents of babies with colic are instructed to spend more time carrying their infants do not show a significant improvement in infant symptoms.[3] This is thought to represent an inability on the part of the colicky infant to regulate his or her behavior using the contact pathway.[5] Massage and chiropractic therapies have not been shown to be effective.[1] Car ride simulators, vibrating devices that attach to cribs, are not believed to be effective, although it is notably difficult to include them in a double-blinded study.[2] Of existing behavioral modalities, decreasing stimulation of the infant has been shown to have a significant effect; however, the study that demonstrated this effect used a subjective definition of colic and was not double-blinded.[2] Intensive parent training in "parent–infant communication skills" has been suggested to be helpful but requires a significant investment of time and resources by both the parent and the primary care provider.[2]

Pharmacologic and dietary interventions have been of limited help overall in the treatment of colic. Some are to be strictly avoided because of potentially serious or even fatal side effects. Hyoscyamine (Levsin) can lead to irritability and tachycardia.[8] A mixture containing scopolamine and dimenhydrinate (Dramamine) has been associated with apparent life-threatening events in eight infants.[9] Dicyclomine (Bentyl) is thought to have a positive effect on colic symptoms but can cause seizures, coma, and death and is not indicated for use in infants.[2] Gripe water is a commonly available herbal formula but has not been conclusively demonstrated to be an effective therapy. In addition, one case of *Pseudomonas* septic shock has been reported in association with contaminated gripe water.[10]

Some interventions are without significant side effects but also without proven clinical benefit. These include simethicone and addition of fiber or lactase to formula or breast milk. Sucrose solution has a calming effect but lasts for fewer than 30 minutes.[2] One author warns that caution must be taken even with harmless interventions as "the inevitable failure to eliminate colicky crying reinforces the parental perception that something is fundamentally unhealthy in the child, themselves, or both."[4]

Some interventions require further study. Both hypoallergenic diets (without wheat, egg, nuts, or cow milk) and hydrolysate formulas have been suggested to be helpful. It is possible that milk-free diets are effective in a subset of infants who suffer from milk protein allergy rather than colic, but these can be difficult to distinguish. Herbal teas containing chamomile, vervain, licorice, fennel, and balm mint have been effective, but when studied they were given in doses up to 32 ml/kg/day. This amount obviously could have a dramatic negative impact on caloric intake, especially in premature infants.[2]

Because no clear remedy for colic is known, it is difficult for primary care providers to counsel parents of colicky infants. It is essential to educate parents that their baby is not ill. Optimism regarding the infant's health may result in better morale for the parents and "calmer handling" of the child.[4] Parents can be educated about normal patterns of infant crying.[3] Some parents need reassurance that picking up their crying baby will not "spoil" him or her. Prompt responsiveness to distressed infants is actually thought to reduce crying at 1 year of age.[4] Some parents need to be encouraged to allow their baby to cry for a short period; they must be educated that fatigue can be a cause of crying. All parents must be encouraged to take a break from their infant occasionally and to enlist the help of friends or relatives. On rare occasions, infants are admitted to the hospital for respite care.

Prognosis

There is no clear evidence that colicky infants are temperamentally different from other infants once their colic resolves. They are, however, susceptible to vulnerable child syndrome, in which the parents mistakenly perceive their child to be ill or prone to illness.[3] Some authors also caution that the experience of parenting a baby with colic can "damage family dynamics,"[1] which may already be at risk in the household of a premature infant. Although there are no known methods for preventing colic, primary care providers are well advised to counsel new and even prospective parents about normal infant crying patterns, as well as methods of soothing infants.[3]

A greater understanding of normal infant behavior and development will empower parents to cope better with their colicky infant.

Resource for Families and Clinicians

NASPGHAN (North American Society for Pediatric Gastroenterology, Hepatology and Nutrition)
http://www.naspghan.org

This website provides information to families about specific gastrointestinal disorders, including colic. For handouts about colic in English, Spanish or French, click on "public information" then "disease information" and then "colic."

REFERENCES

1. Roberts DM, Ostapchuk M, O'Brien J: Infantile colic. *Am Fam Physician* 70:735, 2004.
2. Garrison MM, Christakis DA: A systematic review of treatments for infant colic. *Pediatrics* 106:184, 2000.
3. Carey WB: "Colic": prolonged or excessive crying in young infants. In Levine MD, Carey WB, Crocker AC, editors: *Developmental-behavioral pediatrics.* Philadelphia, 1999, WB Saunders.
4. Weissbluth M: Colic. In Burg F, Ingelfinger J, editors: *Gellis & Kagan's current pediatric therapy.* Philadelphia, 2002, WB Saunders.
5. Barr RG: Colic and crying syndromes in infants. *Pediatrics* 102:1282, 1998.
6. Bernbaum J: *Primary care of the premature infant.* St. Louis, 1991, Mosby.
7. Oberklaid F, Prior M, Sanson A: Temperament of preterm versus full-term infants. *J Dev Behav Pediatr* 7:159, 1986.
8. Myers JH, Moro-Sutherland D, Shook JE: Anticholinergic poisoning in colicky infants treated with hyoscyamine sulfate. *Am J Emerg Med* 15:532, 1997.
9. Hardoin RA, Henslee JA, Christenson CP, et al: Colic medication and apparent life-threatening events. *Clin Pediatr* 30:281, 1991.
10. Sas DO, Enrione MA, Schwartz RH: Pseudomonas aeruginosa septic shock secondary to "gripe water" ingestion. *Pediatr Infect Dis J* 23:176, 2004.

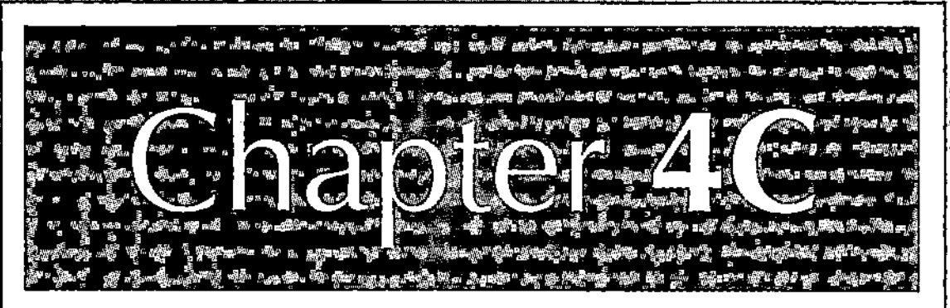

Oral Aversion

Mary Quinn, NNP, IBCLC

Premature infants with a prolonged neonatal intensive unit (NICU) hospitalization are at increased risk for developing oral aversion, which is a sensory-based feeding disorder. Premature infants are particularly susceptible to oral aversion as a result of multiple noxious oral experiences, including intubation, suctioning, placement of orogastric or nasogastric tubes, and vigorously pursued oral feedings in the presence of stress signals. In a manner similar to that in the premature infant, oral aversion may develop in full-term infants with a history of neurodevelopmental disorders, chronic medical conditions, gastrointestinal disorders, genetic and metabolic diseases, sensory defects, dysphagia, or anatomic abnormalities. Infants with these organic conditions may have persistent feeding difficulties as a result of a behavioral response.[1]

Infants with oral aversion may have learned that discomfort or pain is associated with oral experiences and feeding. As a protective response to these negative associations, an oral aversion ensues. In addition to a learned response, oral aversion may be associated with altered sensation and/or impaired swallowing. Previous trauma to the oral and pharyngeal region, as well as prior orogastric or nasogastric tube placement, may alter sensory perception, decreasing sensitivity to that region.[2] Aversive stimulation to the nasal and pharyngeal region may lead to an infant's reluctance to swallow, known as "conditioned dysphagia." This may result in avoidance behaviors, such as refusal of food, arching or turning away, gagging, refusing to swallow, vomiting, or physically expelling food.[2]

Clinically significant gastroesophageal reflux (GER) may contribute to oral aversion as a result of visceral hyperalgesia. This occurs when a prior experience alters sensory nerves so that previously innocuous stimuli are perceived as painful.[3] In addition, infants with GER who experience actual pain from luminal distention or acid reflux are at greater risk for developing oral aversion.

Oral aversion typically is not manifested at the time of discharge from the NICU. This is primarily because the primitive suck swallow reflex remains intact until approximately 3 to 4 months. After that age, this reflex disappears, feeding becomes more deliberate or volitional, and aversive behaviors may become apparent.

Diagnosis

Oral aversion or sensory-based feeding problems are challenging to recognize and usually are diagnosed by exclusion. Often, patients undergo extensive medical evaluations that do not yield any definitive diagnosis. If neurologic findings and oral–motor dysfunctions are absent, the problem often is deduced to be sensory in nature. Table 4C-1 summarizes the broad clinical manifestations of a sensory-based feeding disorder.[3,4]

The development of oral aversion can be subtle and can surprise parents, especially if the infant had been feeding well in the NICU. Oral aversion can occur at any time but typically becomes apparent during feeding transitions. The first period of transition arises at approximately 3 months of age as anatomic changes occur and feeding shifts from reflexive to volitional.

Oral aversion may manifest in several ways. An aversion may develop to a particular feeding method. For example, an infant may not drink from a bottle yet be interested in taking pureed food from a spoon or cup. Other infants may be resistant to particular foods or specific textures. In addition, some infants may be unwilling to accept a new consistency, such as moving from liquids to purees or from purees to solid foods.

Management

A multidisciplinary treatment approach to infants/children with sensory-based feeding

Table 4C-1 Manifestations of a Sensory-Based Feeding Disorder*

BIRTH–3 MONTHS

Unable to sustain a nutritive sucking pattern
Feeds better in a less than alert or sleep state with eyes closed, usually at night
Does not easily transition between bottle and breast feeding
Poor oral intake, falls off growth curve
Strong adverse reaction to change of taste from the nipple

OLDER THAN 3 MONTHS

Poor oral intake, inadequate weight gain
Able to swallow liquids, particularly water, but demonstrates difficulty with textures (water is most similar to saliva and, therefore, most easily tolerated)
Tolerates only own fingers in mouth
Does not appear hungry or is not interested in feeding
Avoids touching food
Tongue retracts in response to touch
Hypersensitive gag with or without emesis
Volitional open mouth posture occurs when food is placed in the mouth
Holds food under tongue or in buccal cavity to avoid swallowing
Able to sort out small pieces of solids from sauces and gravies, expels solid food pieces while swallowing liquids
Able to bite and chew solids in mouth but unable to do so in the oropharyngeal area
Adverse reaction to brushing the teeth
Persistent drooling (Several theories are available on why drooling persists in children after the irritation of erupting dentition has passed. It may be a fine motor issue or related to a decrease in the sensory awareness of the usual cues that trigger swallowing.[4])

Modified from Hyman PE: *J Pediatr* 125(6 pt 2): S103-S109, 1994.
**Note:* Normal oral motor patterns typically are present.

disorders is ideal.[1,5,6] Intervention needs to be collaborative to address nutritional, medical, psychosocial, and developmental needs. An immediate evaluation by a qualified feeding specialist is essential. This specialist may be a speech language pathologist (SLP) or an occupational therapist (OT), depending on the region. Because an infant's reluctance to become an oral feeder or tolerate feeding transitions may be due to decreased sensory perception in the pharynx, management of infants with oral/sensory feeding disorders must be targeted to the pharynx.[2] The feeding specialist should assess the child's feeding skills, overall development, consistency preference, and communicative/interactive feeding behavior.

In general, management strategies should emphasize (1) altering one variable at a time, (2) making small incremental changes, (3) introducing unfamiliar food with preferred choices, and (4) encouraging chewing behavior if age appropriate.[7] In an infant older than 3 months with a volitional suck, the utensil or feeding volumes can be changed (see Table 4C-2 for possible interventions).[8] Majorie Palmer and others (e.g., Kay Toomey) have published separate recommendations for transitioning infants/children with sensory-based feeding disorders from liquids to purees to solids, and these might be helpful guidelines for families.[9] Feeding specialists (SLPs/OTs) should provide recommendations for grading, which is the introduction of solids and textures in small incremental changes. Specialists and primary care providers should emphasize positive oral stimulation and introduce food play at the appropriate developmental stage. The environment can be altered to provide positive associations.

Referral to gastrointestinal or surgical consultants may be necessary if a gastrostomy tube (GT) placement is indicated. The decision for GT placement should be based on the infant's overall growth, feeding patterns, and status of swallowing function. In addition, because prolonged feeding periods are common in infants with oral aversion, one of the most important questions to ask the family is, "How long does it take to feed your baby?"[10] Parents should realize that a GT is a temporary and supplemental measure and does not preclude oral feedings unless airway safety is an issue. Once the tube is placed, the pressure of attaining specific oral volume intake is removed, paving the way for improving the social/emotional environment surrounding feeding. It is important to remind families that infants still can eat by mouth while receiving supplemental tube feedings.

Table 4C-2 Interventions for Infants Older than Three Months with Volitional Suck

Alternative utensils for intake of liquids: cup, spoon, syringe, dropper
Alternative utensils for intake of pureed food: open cup, spout cup, Infa-Feeder,* syringe, dropper, spoon feeder
Alternative bolus size
Alternative placement of bolus: lower lip, under tongue, buccal cheek cavity

*The Infa-Feeder is a wide spoon that can be purchased from NUTURCARE, PO Box 6050, Monroe, LA 71211. Product #1551, UPC #0-48526-01551-1, available from *www.Luvncare.com*
Modified from Palmer MM: Diagnostic-based intervention for the infant with feeding problems. In *Evaluation and treatment of oral feeding disorders conference booklet.* Sponsored by Therapeutic Media, California, 2002, p. 44.

Table 4C-3 Transitioning from Gastrostomy Tube to Oral Feedings[11]

Possible Question	Comments
What is the status of tube feeding (type and schedule), and how long has the child been on tube feedings?	Provides information to establish the child's baseline.
How does the child manage his or her own secretions?	Although management with glycopyrrolate (Robinul) might be helpful, the child must be managed closely because of the possibility of causing thicker secretions that may lead to an obstructed airway.
Would an imaging study be helpful?	Assessing for aspiration is essential. Consider an upper gastrointestinal study and/or modified barium swallow study.
Does the child have any current medical conditions or dietary restrictions?	These conditions/restrictions may dictate which foods can be used.
Does the child manage solids, semi-solids, or liquid foods in different ways?	Begin with the consistency that the child tolerates best and then introduce new textures in small incremental changes.
Does positioning aid oral feeding in any way?	If so, use that technique when beginning oral feeds.
Are there any abnormal oral–motor patterns and/or orofacial tone?	A speech/occupational therapist can recommend a specific feeding utensil/nipple.
Is the child defensive around the mouth because of hyposensitivity or hypersensitivity; is the sensitivity different in front or in the back of mouth, lips, or tongue?	This sensitivity may guide the way feedings are given and which feeding utensil/nipple is used.
How motivated is the primary care provider?	Success depends on the primary caretaker having oral feeding as a goal.
What are the primary care provider's feeding goals for the child?	List these goals for the family.

Infants who are ready for the transition from GT to oral feedings require close evaluation. Consider the questions and suggestions outlined in Table 4C-3 before beginning the transition.[11] Once a decision has been made to transition from GT to oral feedings, one can utilize the principles outlined in Table 4C-4.[12] The SLP/OT should provide guidance to parents when their child appears ready to transition to oral feedings. It is not necessary for a child to be eating solid foods before stopping gastrostomy feedings; adequate intake of one consistency, such as pureed, is sufficient. Establishing drinking skills also is beneficial to facilitate the weaning process. The Palmer Protocol for Sensory-Based Weaning describes a comprehensive method for gradually weaning from gastrostomy feedings to oral feeds that some families might find useful.[12] The website New Visions (*www.new-vis.com*) provides other protocols for this transition. Regardless of the specific method, a collaborative approach with parents, the primary care provider, and all involved specialists is essential.

Parental Support

Parental support and education during the evaluation and treatment of feeding disorders is extremely critical. Parents report extreme stress when confronted with an infant who has a feeding disorder. Because feeding is central to the nurturing process, parents feel that they have failed because their child does not feed appropriately.[6] Feeding disorders disrupt the parent–child relationship and alter the family dynamics, often with negative consequences to the family. Family life becomes centered around the feeding of this particular child. Parents report that health professionals do not listen or take their concerns seriously, thus prolonging the time until adequate management strategies are undertaken.[6] Behavioral intervention sometimes is necessary. Parent training to establish positive mealtime interactions is especially important.

Conclusion

This chapter discusses the concepts of oral aversion in premature infants. Infants and children with oral aversion are more likely to have a successful outcome if the primary care provider (1) maintains an awareness of the disorder, (2) provides an early diagnosis, (3) establishes collaborative therapeutic strategies, and (4) provides extensive family support.

Resources for Families and Clinicians

Kids with Tubes
www.kidswithtubes.org

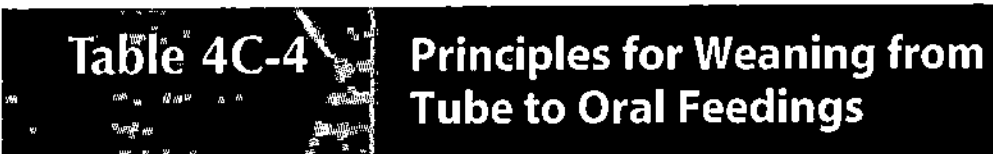

Table 4C-4 Principles for Weaning from Tube to Oral Feedings

1. Discontinue all nighttime continuous drip feedings.
2. Discontinue all continuous drip feedings by day.
3. Develop age-appropriate mealtime schedule for daytime bolus feeds.
4. Transition from predigested formula containing enzymes (e.g., Nutramigen, Pregestimil, Vivonex) to standard stock formula.*
5. Introduce oral activities and feeding as part of the total mealtime, just before tube feeding.
6. Use primitive reflexes as a foundation in infants.
7. Approach the "oral sensorium" from the buccal cheek cavity; to prevent gagging, avoid the tongue, which is sensitive to touch pressure stimuli.
8. Practice nasal breathing and active closing of the lips in infants.
9. Use "mealtime toy bag" as a distraction for toddlers.
10. Be sure the child is receiving sufficient calories to grow and that weight is adequate before beginning the program.
11. Modify only one variable for oral feeding at a time, that is, texture, utensil, placement.
12. Duration of tube feeding should approximate the length of the oral feed.
13. Liquid/food fed orally should be equal to 30 calories per ounce.†
14. Once oral feeding is established, a direct subtraction from gastrostomy tube feeding may begin.
15. Discuss "60-hour wean" with family and physician.‡
16. Successful weaning is dependent upon good candidate selection.

From Palmer MM: *Pediatr Nurs* 23(5):476, 1998.
*Consider flavoring the formula.
†Caloric intake should be determined after consultation with a nutritionist.
‡Refer to original source (Palmer, above) for details.

This organization is run by parents and offers a variety of support services for caregivers of tube-fed (nasogastric, gastric, or jejunal) children.

New Visions
www.new-vis.com

Provides resources for working with infants and children with feeding, swallowing, oral–motor, and prespeech problems.

Pediatric/Adolescent Gastroesophageal Reflux Association (GERD)
www.reflux.org

Information regarding reflux/medication/testing. Site is available in Spanish.

Small Wonders Preemie Place
Members.aol.com/_ht_a/Lmwill262/index.html

Resource page, list serve, and bulletin board for feeding issues in babies and young children.

Acknowledgment

The author thanks Kara Fletcher, MS, SLP-CCC, for critical review of this chapter.

REFERENCES

1. Byars KC, Burklow KA, Ferguson K, et al: A multicomponent behavioral program for oral aversion in children dependent on gastrostomy feedings. *J Pediatr Gastroenterol Nutr* 37:473-480, 2003.
2. Palmer MM, Heyman MB: Assessment and treatment of sensory-versus motor based feeding problems in very young children. *Infants Young Child* 6:67-73, 1993.
3. Hyman PE: Gastroesophageal reflux: one reason why baby won't eat. *J Pediatr* 125(6 pt 2):S103-S109, 1994.
4. Palmer MM, Heyman MB: The effect of sensory-based treatment of drooling in children: a preliminary study physical and occupational therapy in pediatrics. *Phys Occup Ther Pediatr* 18(3/4):85-95, 1998.
5. Rommel N, De Meyer AM, Feenstra L, et al: The complexity of feeding problems in 700 infants and young children presenting to a tertiary care institution. *J Pediatr Gastroenterol Nutr* 37(1):75-84, 2003.
6. Strudwick S: Gastro-oesophageal reflux and feeding: the speech and language therapist's perspective. *Int J Pediatr Otorhinolaryngol* 67(suppl 1):S101-S102, 2003.
7. Palmer MM: Sensory-based feeding disorders: feeding aversion, delayed development of chewing and difficulty with transition to solid food. In *Evaluation and treatment of oral feeding disorders conference booklet.* Sponsored by Therapeutic Media, California, 2002, p. 83.
8. Palmer MM: Diagnostic-based intervention for the infant with feeding problems. From *Evaluation and treatment of oral feeding disorders conference booklet.* Sponsored by Therapeutic Media, California, 2002, p. 44.
9. Palmer MM: Feeding transitions and intervention strategies for sensory-based oral feeding disorders in children who are oral feeders. In *Evaluation and treatment of oral feeding disorders conference booklet.* Sponsored by Therapeutic Media, California, 2002, p. 82.
10. Bousvaros A, Puder M: Feeding tubes. In Hansen A, Puder M, editors: *Manual of neonatal surgical intensive care.* New York, 2003, BC Decker.
11. Palmer MM: The non-oral feeder: determining readiness for feeding therapy. In *Evaluation and treatment of oral feeding disorders conference booklet.* Sponsored by Therapeutic Media, California, 2002, p.103.
12. Palmer MM: Weaning from gastrostomy tube feeding: commentary on oral aversion. *Pediatr Nurs* 23(5):475-478, 1998.

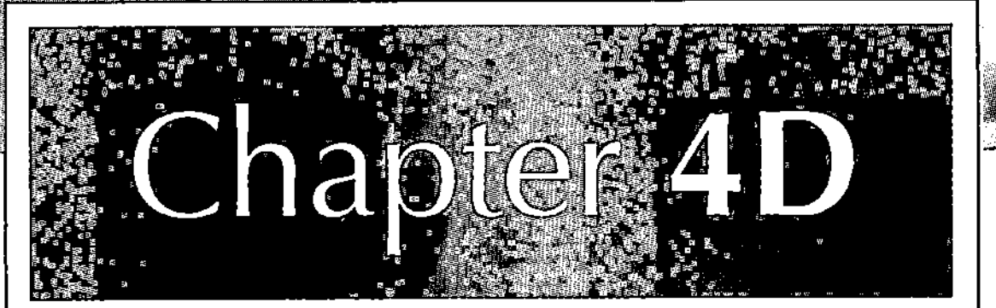

Constipation

Jill S. Fischer, MD

"Constipation" is a common concern for parents of premature infants. To ensure that a parent's definition of constipation is accurate and truly reflects an infant's abnormal stooling pattern, a detailed history is necessary. Infrequent stooling is not necessarily pathologic. Although frequent stools (two to three per day) are common in the immediate postnatal period, some infants pass only one soft stool per week with no ill effects.[1] Many parents believe their infant to be constipated when he or she is actually experiencing infant dyschezia. "Dyschezia" is defined as "at least 10 minutes of straining and crying before successful passage of soft stools in an otherwise healthy infant less than 6 months of age."[2] Dyschezia is thought to result from imperfect coordination of abdominal and pelvic floor muscles and in most cases resolves spontaneously. Accordingly, intervention for constipation is best reserved for infants whose stools are consistently hard and difficult to pass.

Differential Diagnosis

Constipation in infants often has no clear etiology. However, several important causes must be eliminated before constipation is considered to be idiopathic (Table 4D-1).

Diet may contribute to constipation in three ways. First, premature infants may be consuming concentrated formulas, which are limited in free water content.[3] Second, an infant who is having difficulty breastfeeding may have limited fluid intake, which may change stool consistency. Third, some studies suggest that formulas based on cow's milk protein may contribute to constipation in certain infants.[4]

Anatomy also can contribute to constipation. It is thought that an anteriorly placed anus leads to constipation because of malalignment of the (normally functioning) interior sphincter and the anal canal. Congenital intestinal strictures can cause constipation, as can strictures acquired after necrotizing enterocolitis.[1]

Metabolic disorders, such as hypothyroidism, celiac disease, and cystic fibrosis, are well known to cause constipation. In addition, cerebral palsy or any neuromuscular disorder leading to decreased abdominal muscle tone will cause difficulties with evacuation. Use of medications, such as calcium channel blockers or opiates, may result in excessively hard stools.

A history of infrequent or difficult stooling should always lead to the consideration of Hirschsprung disease. Infants with Hirschsprung disease are lacking innervation within an intestinal segment and consequently are less able to pass stools normally. Ninety-eight percent of babies will pass meconium within the first 48 hours of life;[5] a history of delayed initial stooling should raise the question of

Table 4D-1 Differential Diagnosis of Constipation

- Idiopathic
- Diet
  - Concentrated formulas (low free water content)
  - Difficulty breastfeeding (limited fluid intake)
  - Cow's milk protein formula (some cases)
- Anatomy
  - Anteriorly placed anus
  - Intestinal strictures
    - Congenital
    - Acquired after necrotizing enterocolitis
  - Hirschsprung disease
- Metabolic
  - Hypothyroidism
  - Celiac disease
  - Cystic fibrosis
- Neurologic
  - Cerebral palsy
  - Neuromuscular disorder
- Medications
  - Calcium channel blockers
  - Opiates

Hirschsprung disease in a constipated child. Referral may then be warranted to a subspecialist for further evaluation and treatment. One potential complication of Hirschsprung disease is toxic megacolon, an enterocolitis that is associated with a mortality rate of 20%.[6]

Evaluation

To address the potential etiologies of constipation, a thorough evaluation should be performed. It is helpful to record as accurately as possible the time of first passage of stool after birth. It also is important to note the duration and onset of the current symptoms, as well as any previous history of constipation. Past and present diets should be documented. A complete list of medications must be reviewed. Intercurrent illnesses should be considered.

On physical examination, one should assess for dysmorphic features, as various genetic syndromes are associated with anal problems and constipation.[1] Weight should be plotted on an appropriate growth chart. Special attention should be paid to hydration status. A careful abdominal examination will note any distention, abnormal or absent bowel sounds, masses, or tenderness. The back should be examined for sacral abnormalities, which might be associated with abnormal innervation of the gut. The skin should be examined for eczema, which may be a sign of milk protein intolerance. Anal fissures may be seen; these can result from hard stools and perpetuate the stooling difficulty because some children will withhold stools in order to avoid pain associated with the fissure.

If the history is benign and the results of physical examination are not of concern, therapy can be initiated. Imaging is rarely necessary on initial presentation but is reserved for infants in whom initial therapies are ineffective. Similarly, laboratory testing often is deferred until after an initial trial of therapy.

Management

There are no formal guidelines for treatment of the constipated premature infant. The North American Society for Pediatric Gastroenterology and Nutrition has published a comprehensive algorithm for the management of constipation;[6] however, they excluded neonates younger than 72 hours and premature infants less than 37 weeks' gestation. Nonetheless, premature infants may be treated for constipation with many of the same therapies used in full-term infants once organic causes have been ruled out.

Some infants who have hard stools with a milk-based formula diet will have softer stools once the diet is changed to soy or hydrolysate formulas. For parents who are reluctant to use medications or for whom adding more medications to their infant's regimen is challenging, this is sometimes a helpful approach. For infants who are not candidates for a change in formula(s) or for those who do not respond, several other choices are available (Table 4D-2). Of note, treatment with mineral oil is contraindicated because it carries a risk for lung damage if aspirated. Enemas and stimulant laxatives are not recommended.[6]

Table 4D-2 Management Options for Constipation in the Premature Infant[6,7]

Management	Dose	Side Effects	Other
Fruit juice	Not standardized		Prune, pear, or apple juice can be used
Corn syrup	Not standardized: many authors advise giving one tablespoon PO QD		Not considered a significant source of *Clostridium botulinum* spores
Sorbitol (70% solution)	1–3 ml/kg/day in divided doses	Diarrhea, abdominal discomfort	Less expensive than lactulose
Lactulose syrup (10 g per 15 ml)	1–3 ml/kg/day in divided doses	Diarrhea, abdominal discomfort	Expensive
Malt extract (16 g per 15 ml)	2–10 ml PO in formula or juice	Diarrhea, abdominal discomfort	Distinctive odor may be unpleasant
Glycerin suppository	One infant suppository PR		Onset of action is approximately 15–30 min Only for occasional use to avoid dependence
Mineral oil	Not applicable		**Contraindicated** in infants because of pneumonitis that could result from aspiration

Follow-up and Prognosis

Establishment of a therapeutic regimen for constipation in infants initially may require weekly phone contact or office visits in order to discuss the effects of dietary changes or medications. Parents should be encouraged to titrate therapy to achieve regular passage of soft stools. Once an effective regimen is found, follow-up may be limited to routine well-child visits. For infants in whom the initial therapies listed are not effective, laboratory testing may help to guide further evaluation and possible referral to a subspecialist. Recommended tests include levels of thyroid-stimulating hormone, thyroxine (T_4), and calcium as well as evaluation for celiac disease and testing for cystic fibrosis.

Unfortunately, no well-described prognostic factors can predict whether the constipation will persist or resolve. Long-term follow-up of a group of extremely-low-birth-weight infants showed the prevalence of constipation was 13%, but this occurred mostly in neurologically impaired children.[8] Determining which infants will continue to have constipation requires careful follow-up and re-evaluation by the primary care provider.

Resource for Families and Clinicians

NASPGHAN (North American Society for Pediatric Gastroenterology, Hepatology and Nutrition)
http://www.naspghan.org

This website provides information to families about specific gastrointestinal disorders, including colic. For handouts about constipation in English, Spanish, or French, click on "public information" then "disease information" and then "constipation."

REFERENCES

1. Murphy M: Constipation. In Walker W, Durie P, editors: *Pediatric gastrointestinal disease.* St. Louis, 1996, Mosby.
2. Rasquin-Weber A, Hyman PE, Cucchiara S, et al: Childhood functional gastrointestinal disorders. *Gut* 45(suppl II):II60, 1999.
3. Bernbaum J: *Primary care of the premature infant.* St. Louis, 1991, Mosby.
4. Sicherer SH: Clinical aspects of gastrointestinal food allergy in childhood. *Pediatrics* 111(6 pt 3):1609, 2003.
5. Broderick A, Kleinman R: Constipation. In Burg F, Ingelfinger J, editors: *Gellis & Kagan's current pediatric therapy.* Philadelphia, 2002, WB Saunders.
6. Baker SS, Liptak GS, Colletti RB, et al: Constipation in infants and children: evaluation and treatment. A medical position statement of the North American Society for Gastroenterology and Nutrition. *J Pediatr Gastroenterol Nutr* 29:612, 1999.
7. Taketomo CK, Hodding JH, Kraus DM: *Pediatric dosage handbook.* Hudson, Ohio, 2003, Lexi-Comp.
8. Hack M, Taylor G, Klein N, et al: Functional limitations and special health care needs of 10- to 14- year old children weighing less than 750 grams at birth. *Pediatrics* 106:554, 2000.

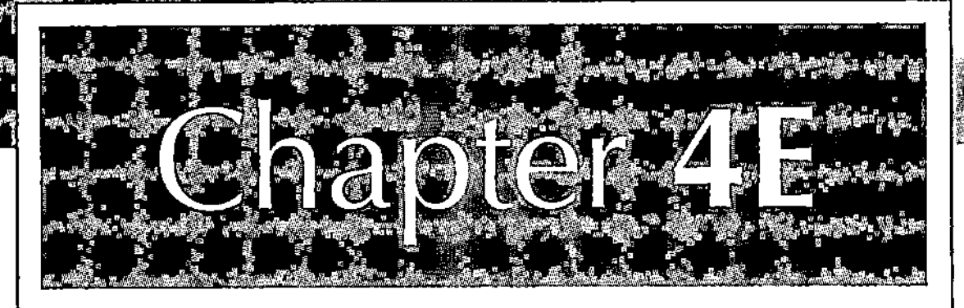

Enteral Tubes: Care and Management

Sandy Quigley, MS, CWOCN, CPNP, and Julie Iglesias, RN, MS, CPNP

Premature infants may require enteral feedings if they are temporarily or permanently unable to swallow or consume adequate nutrients to meet their nutritional requirements. Enteral support is the preferred modality for premature infants because it is more physiologic and is safer to administer than parenteral nutrition. Delivery of nutrients to the intestine minimizes gut atrophy and decreases the risk of bacterial translocation.

Because suboptimal nutrition in children may correlate with long-term consequences, a growing percentage of premature infants are being discharged from the hospital receiving nutritional support via an enteral tube. This chapter reviews the route of enteral feedings, modes of delivery, methods for tube placement, and enteral tube care and management.

Route of Enteral Feedings

Enteral feeding routes can be divided into two major categories: those entering the gastrointestinal tract *through the oral or nasal cavity* (oroenteric, nasoenteric, nasojejunal tubes) and those entering *through the abdominal wall* (transabdominal), including gastrostomy, duodenostomy, and jejunostomy tubes.

There are many indications for placing an oroenteric, nasoenteric, or nasojejunal tube. In general, many practitioners recommend a nasoenteric/oroenteric feeding tube if the anticipated time of supplemental feedings is short term (i.e., no longer than 1–3 months). Because premature infants have a poorly coordinated suck-and-swallow sequence, they require nasal/oral enteral feedings until this reflex is mature (usually ≈34 weeks' gestation) and are able to ingest their feedings orally. Full-term infants with short-term medical issues (e.g., ventilator support) also may require nasal/oral enteric feedings. In addition to supplying nutritional needs, the nasoenteric/oroenteric tube can be used for gastric decompression and/or administration of medication. A nasojejunal tube can be used in infants with a depressed gag reflex, delayed gastric emptying, severe gastroesophageal reflux, and severe bronchospasm and in those at high risk for aspiration.

Some premature infants will continue to require prolonged enteric feedings and may need placement of a *transabdominal* enteral feeding tube. More commonly, the transabdominal feeding tube is placed in full-term infants with chronic conditions, such as congenital anomalies of the mouth, mandible, pharynx, gastrointestinal tract, and/or airway (e.g., tracheoesophageal fistula, cleft lip and palate, intestinal atresia, and abdominal wall defects) or neurologic disease. Infants with genetic syndromes or chronic illnesses, such as cerebral palsy, cystic fibrosis, solid organ transplants, or congenital heart defects also may require long-term enteral supplementation if their oral intake is not sufficient to meet their nutritional needs.

The two common transabdominal options are a gastrostomy tube and a transpyloric jejunostomy. The *gastrostomy tube* is appropriate for children who have an intact gag and cough reflex with adequate gastric emptying. A gastrostomy tube offers many more advantages than a transpyloric jejunostomy tube. The gastric route allows the normal digestive process to continue and is fundamental in supporting intestinal immunity, an important defense system for the premature infant. In addition to the bactericidal effects of stomach acid, the gastric route is easier to manage, and feedings can be administered in boluses. Gastric feedings can provide large osmotic loads with less frequent cramping, distention, or diarrhea and a decreased risk of dumping syndrome.

Transpyloric feeding tubes may be indicated in patients at high risk for aspiration, such as those with a depressed gag reflex, delayed gastric emptying, and severe gastroesophageal reflux. Gastric outlet obstruction and proximal bowel fistulas are additional indications for bypassing the stomach and feeding into the small intestine. Transpyloric feedings ensure delivery of enteral feedings to the main sites of nutrient absorption and have the theoretical advantage of decreasing the risk of esophageal reflux and aspiration into the lungs because of their distal administration. However, feeding by the transpyloric route is associated with potential problems. Because the gastric phase of the digestion process is bypassed, the secretion of intestinal hormones and growth factors may be impaired. There also is the risk that potentially pathogenic organisms that would have been removed in the acidic environment of the stomach will be delivered directly into the small bowel. Furthermore, transpyloric feeding tubes are difficult to place and may migrate back into the stomach.

A comparison of transpyloric and gastric tube feedings in preterm infants was conducted to determine which route improved feeding tolerance, as well as growth and development, without increasing adverse events. No evidence of benefit was found, but potentially harmful differences were observed in premature infants who received transpyloric feedings. Specifically, gastrointestinal disturbances, such as abdominal distention, gastric bleeding, and bilious vomiting, were more common in the group receiving transpyloric feedings.[1]

Mode of Delivery

Enteral feedings can be administered by either bolus or continuous drip. A bolus feeding delivers milk over a time period similar to that of an oral feeding (i.e., <30 minutes). This technique is relatively simple and allows the infant an opportunity to be equipment free for long periods. Intolerance of this method is evidenced by large gastric residuals, malabsorption, dumping syndrome, aspiration, and persistent regurgitation.

Bolus feedings may not be well tolerated distal to the pylorus because of the inability of the small bowel to buffer osmotic loads effectively. For the transpyloric approach, continuous infusion via a feeding pump is beneficial because milk is delivered in an evenly distributed infusion, thus avoiding the problems associated with an uneven administration rate (e.g., milk coagulation and tube occlusion).

Methods of Tube Placement

Oroenteric/nasoenteric/nasojejunal tubes

Nasogastric/orogastric tubes should be placed by healthcare providers and parents who have been properly trained. Some children may have intermittent tube placement to minimize inadvertent dislodgment and social pressure of tube presence. Nasogastric tubes that are composed of polyurethane and silicone rubber are soft and pliable and can be left in place for up to 1 month or in accordance with the protocol of the facility that placed the tube. Because polyvinyl chloride tubes become stiff and nonpliable when left in place for more than a few days, this material may be better suited for tubes that are placed intermittently.

The size of the nasogastric tube depends on the size of the nares and nasal cavity lumen; a 5- or 8-French tube is appropriate for most neonates. Once the size of the tube is determined, the nasogastric tube is inserted according to the recommendations given in Table 4E-1. The infant may cough or gag during insertion, but this should stop once the tube is in the correct place. If the infant develops severe coughing, cyanosis, difficulty breathing, or vomiting, *the tube should be removed immediately.*

Many methods can be used to confirm appropriate placement of the nasogastric tube. Many centers recommend auscultation over the stomach after insufflation of air as an initial stop to verify proper tube position. Appropriate placement also can be checked by observing for bubbling from the distal end of the tube when it is placed under water. However, limited published research supports these conventional methods for verifying nasogastric/orogastric tube placement. Indeed, differentiating from among gastric, pulmonary, esophageal, and intestinal placement cannot be accomplished by auscultation alone.[2] Tubes can be inappropriately placed in the lung, into the pleural cavity after a lung perforation, or coiled in the esophagus, and they may be mistakenly determined to be in proper position by the aforementioned bedside auscultation techniques. Excluding radiographic confirmation, *the most reliable and safest indicator of gastric feeding tube placement is testing the pH of the gastric aspirate.* A pH ≤5 is consistent with gastric placement. Testing with pHydrion Vivid 0-9 is a relatively simple procedure to teach families how to properly assess nasogastric/orogastric tube placement. Table 4E-1 provides more details about testing the gastric pH.

Some polyurethane or silicone rubber feeding tubes have a weight at the tip that makes them useful for duodenal or jejunal feedings. Nasojejunal tubes are not used often in the community setting because of their complication risk. The lumens of these tubes are much smaller than the lumens of gastric tubes and are prone to clogging; only liquids should be administered through a nasojejunal tube. These tubes require frequent flushing (every 4 hours). Jejunal tubes never should be checked for residual content because they are a poor indicator of small

Table 4E-1 Nasogastric Tube Insertion Procedure

1. Elevate the infant's head to an angle of at least 30 degrees.
2. Measure the nasogastric tube for the distance it will be inserted:
   A. Hold the tip of the tube at the end of the child's nose.
   B. Extend the tube to the child's earlobe.
   C. Extend the tube to the bottom of the child's xyphoid process.
   D. Mark the length measured with a piece of tape or an indelible marker on the tube.
3. Inspect the tube for any defects, such as rough edges or a partially closed lumen.
4. Some tubes have a hydromer coating with a water-activated lubricant on the tip (e.g., CORPAK). Always check the product insert to verify whether it is water activated. If it is, then activate the hydromer lubricant by submersing the tip in water for 5 seconds. If the tube does not have a hydromer coating, lubricate the end of the tube sparingly with water-soluble jelly before insertion.
5. The tube may contain a wire (stylet), which helps guide the tube. Be sure the stylet is securely placed in the tube before putting it into the child's nose. Instill approximately 2–3 ml of water into the end of the stylet. This facilitates removal of the stylet. **Never insert the stylet when the tube is in the child.**
6. Gently insert the tube into one nostril with a steady motion. Direct the tube up and back. Tube insertion can be facilitated by slightly flexing the patient's head (unless medically contraindicated), lubricating the tube, and rotating the tube as it is advanced. DO NOT force the tube. You may need to try the other nostril if the tube does not go in easily. *Note:* the child is likely to gag during tube insertion. **REMOVE the tube immediately** if the child has severe coughing, develops cyanosis or difficulty breathing, or vomits.
7. Insert the tube until the mark is reached, then securely tape the tube without tension at the nares.
8. Confirm nasogastric tube placement before using the tube. Use a 30- to 60-ml syringe to aspirate stomach contents. Withdraw the plunger slowly. If unable to aspirate back, reposition the infant on his or her side and wait a few minutes. This position may help the tube to fall below the fluid level in the stomach. Check the pH of the stomach contents by applying one to two drops of gastric contents onto pH paper. A pH of 0–5 indicates that the tube most likely is in the proper position in the stomach. If gastric residual cannot be obtained or if pH >5, contact with a gastroenterology specialist and/or the physician (MD) from the referring hospital may be necessary to determine whether the child should undergo radiography to confirm placement. A patient receiving gastric acid-blocking medications (e.g., proton pump inhibitors, H_2 blockers, antacids) may have a gastric pH >5. If a child is receiving these medications, families should be instructed to check the pH just before giving these medications.
9. Gently remove stylet (if tube has one) after placement is confirmed.
10. Measure the external length of the tube (or note mark printed on tube) for documentation. Instruct family to always check that the length is the same before each feeding or before giving medication.

bowel residual content. A transabdominal tube often is required later in life because of the high complication rate of nasojejunal tubes.

Nasojejunal tube placement should be performed only by skilled practitioners. Nasojejunal tubes can be placed using endoscopic or fluoroscopic guidance. Typically, the tube length is based on the measurement from the child's nose to ear to xiphoid process to right midaxillary line. Based on the age and size of the child, an additional length is added (5 cm in infants, 7 cm in toddlers, 10 cm in children). The tube length from the nares to the distal tip should be documented in the medical record for future placements. If the exit marker migrates or the accuracy of placement is in question, the position of the nasojejunal tube must be confirmed radiographically. Tube displacement may be evidenced by respiratory distress, vomiting, or abdominal distention.

Transabdominal tubes

A variety of transabdominal tubes are available in the United States. These tubes have three components: an internal portion on the anterior stomach wall, an external portion that is visible on the abdominal surface, and the feeding access port. The internal portion is either a balloon or a non-balloon tip that has a mushroom-shaped dome or a collapsible port. The external portion can be a tube that either extends out from the skin or can be a skin-level device. Several common types of gastrostomy and gastrojejunal tubes are available for infants (Table 4E-2). The method of insertion and the type of gastrostomy tube depend on the infant's clinical condition and the specific indications for the tube. The techniques for creating the gastrostomy tract include percutaneous endoscopic gastrostomy or via surgical or radiographic placement (Table 4E-3). Most patients can be submerged in a bath 7 days after tube placement unless there is a specific contraindication, such as a wound infection.

Care and Management

The care and management of a child with an enteral tube focuses on four primary issues: (1) ensuring that the child is receiving the appropriate volume of feedings; (2) tube patency; (3) appropriate skin care; and (4) tube stabilization. In addition, maintenance fluid needs must be calculated and free water intake must be maintained,

Text continued on page 116

Table 4E-2 Enteral Feeding Tube Type Reference Tool

Note: These materials reflect the author's knowledge and experience at the time of writing. Practitioners should double check for improvements and options that may not have existed at that time. These are examples, and their inclusion here is not intended as an endorsement of any particular product © Children's Hospital, Boston, 2007. All rights reserved. Prepared by Sandy Quigley, RN, CWOCN, CPNP and Lori Hartigan, RN, BSN.

MIC-KEY® Skin Level Gastrostomy Tube

Description/Use
Skin level silicone device with a side access port to insert a syringe to inflate/deflate the balloon that holds the tube in place. There is an anti-reflux valve located inside the MIC-KEY feeding tube that prevents gastric leakage from the lumen of tube.

Accessories
Feeding Tube Extension sets

- For **continuous feeding** with a formula pump use MIC-KEY® SECUR-LOK extension set (90-degree angle). See Figure 3.
- For **bolus feedings or venting** use MIC-KEY® bolus extension set which is straight and the lumen is larger than SECUR-LOK set.

To attach, open "flip" tab and align the black line on the extension set with the black line on the MIC-KEY feeding tube port. Gently push in and rotate it quarter turn clockwise. Then, attach to feeding bag connector with a firm push and twist.

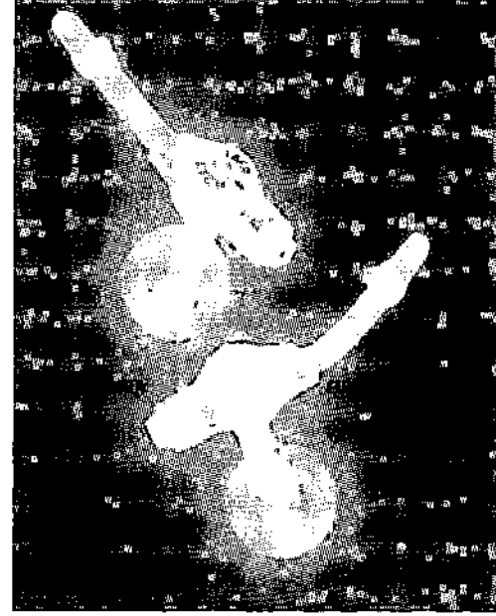

FIGURE 1 MIC-KEY Gastrostomy Tube

Comment
This technique is necessary to provide a secure connection and avoid disconnection resulting in leakage of formula.
The extension set "swivels" with movement and allows infant to change position during feeding.
Tube should be stabilized securely on abdominal surface with tape for the first 6 weeks post-op to avoid inadvertent dislodgement and/or tract enlargement. See Figures 2 and 3 below.

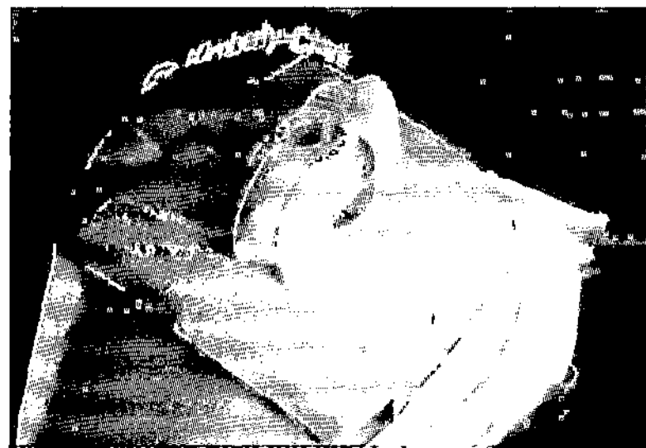

FIGURE 2 MIC-KEY Gastrostomy tube flip tab closed

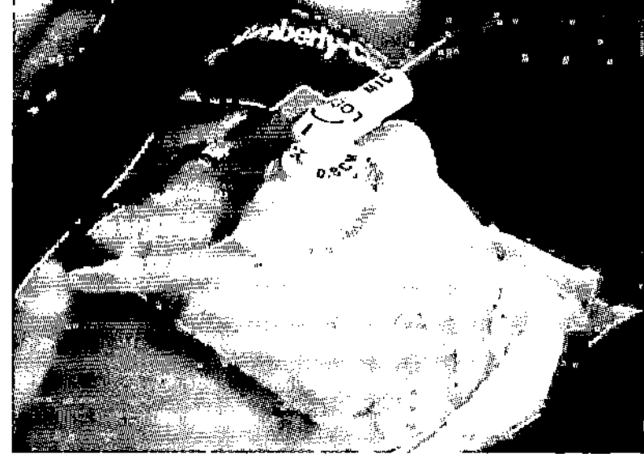

FIGURE 3 MIC-KEY Gastrostomy tube with connector (stablized)

MIC™ "G" Gastrostomy Tubes

Description/Use
Non-skin level device (~7 inches long) made of silicone with 3 ports: feeding, medication, and balloon access to inflate/deflate balloon that holds the tube in place. A round flange ("disk") is movable along tube length and can accomodate variety of abdominal girths. Often used when infants require venting or continuous gastric decompression.
Can be attached directly to feeding bag connector with a firm push and twist.

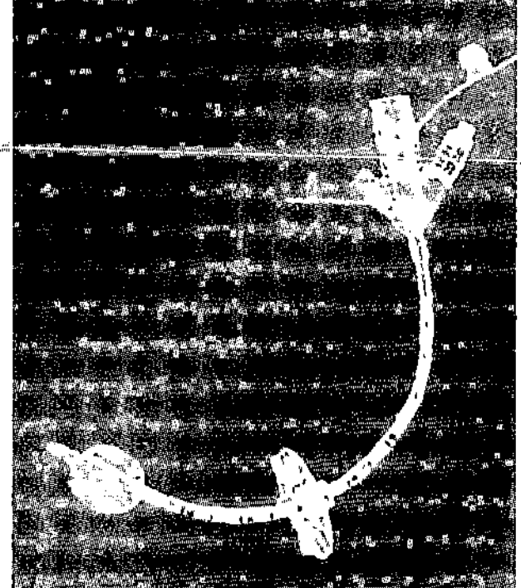

FIGURE 4 MIC Gastrostomy Tube

Table 4E-2 Enteral Feeding Tube Type Reference Tool—cont'd

Comment	Tube should be stabilized securely on abdominal surface with tape for the first 6 weeks post-op to avoid inadvertent dislodgement and/or tract enlargement due to weight of tube. See Figure 5. Also stabilizing will avoid inadvertent tube dislodgement from infant pulling and causing traction on the tube.

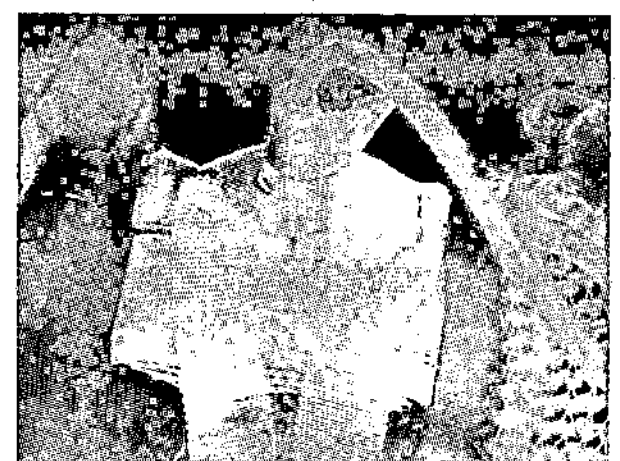

FIGURE 5 MIC Gastrostomy Tube inserted and stabilized

MIC™ "G-J" Tubes

Description/Use	Non-skin-level device made of silicone with 3 ports: gastric, jejunal, and balloon access to inflate/deflate balloon that holds the tube in place. A round flange ("disk") is movable along tube length and can accommodate variety of abdominal girths. Radiopaque stripe to help aid in catheter visualization during radiographic studies. Most often placed in Interventional Radiology through an existing gastrostomy site.
Comment	Separate gastric and jejunal ports for simultaneous access. See Figure 6. Radiopaque jejunal lumen facilitates verification of tube placement with x-ray study. Tube should be stabilized securely on abdominal surface with tape for the first 6 weeks post-op to avoid tract enlargement due to weight of tube. See Figure 7. Also stabilizing will avoid inadvertent tube dislodgement from infant pulling and causing traction on the tube.

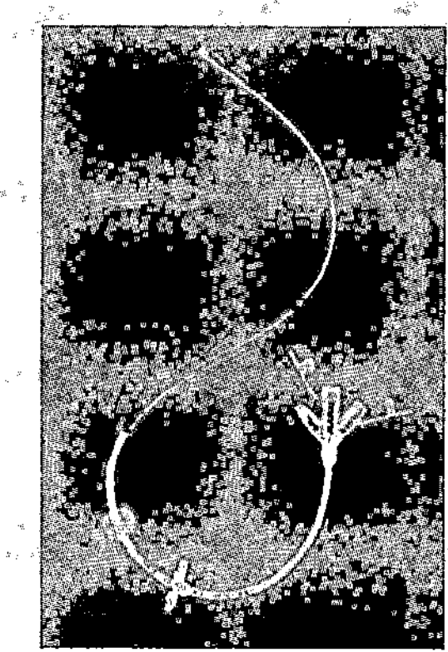

FIGURE 6 MIC G-J™ Tube

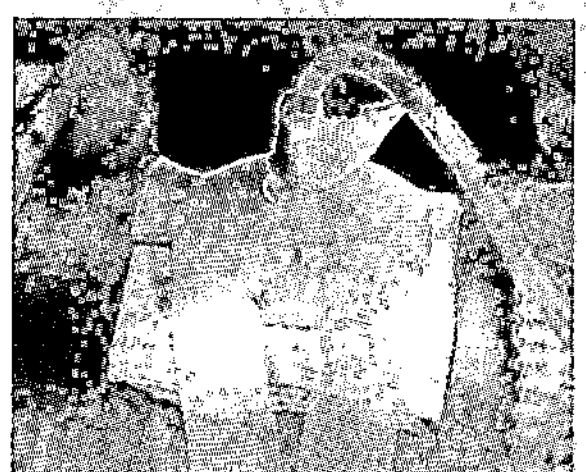

FIGURE 7 MIC G-J tube stabilized

MIC-KEY® "G-J" Tube Skin Level Gastrostomy-Jejunal Tube

Description/Use	Skin level silicone device with a side access port to insert a syringe to inflate/deflate the balloon that holds the tube in place against wall of stomach. **There are separate jejunal and gastric ports.** See Figures 8-10. There are anti-reflux valves located inside the gastric and jejunal ports that prevent leakage from the lumens of the tube. Radiopaque stripe to help aid in catheter visualization during radiographic studies. Most often placed in Interventional Radiology through an existing gastrostomy site.
Accessories	**Feeding Tube Extension sets** • For **continuous feeding into jejunal port** with a formula pump use MIC-KEY® SECUR-LOK extension set (90-degree angle). See Figure 10. • For **bolus feedings or venting into gastric port** use MIC-KEY® bolus extension set which is straight and the lumen is larger than SECUR-LOK set. See Figure 10.

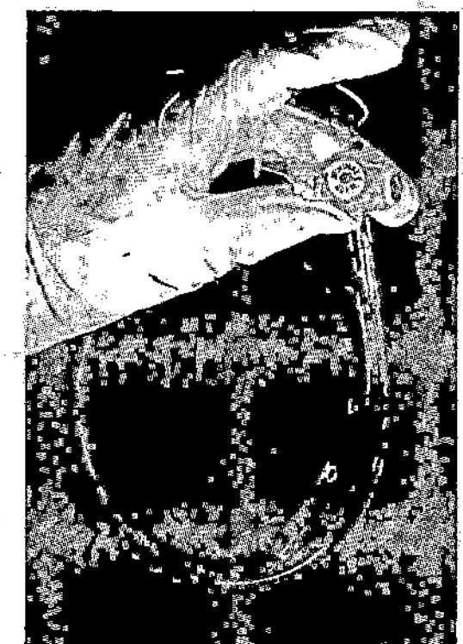

FIGURE 8 MIC-KEY G-J Tube

Continued

Table 4E-2 Enteral Feeding Tube Type Reference Tool—cont'd

	To attach, open "flip" tab and align the black line on the extension set with the black line on the MIC-KEY feeding tube port. Gently push in and rotate it quarter turn clockwise. Then, attach to feeding bag connector with a firm push and twist.
Comment	**The tube is designed for infants who may need simultaneous jejunal feeding and/or gastric decompression.** It has multiple jejunal exit ports to improve flow and minimize risk of clogging. Tube should be stabilized securely on abdominal surface with tape for the first 6 weeks post-op to avoid inadvertent dislodgement and/or tract enlargement
	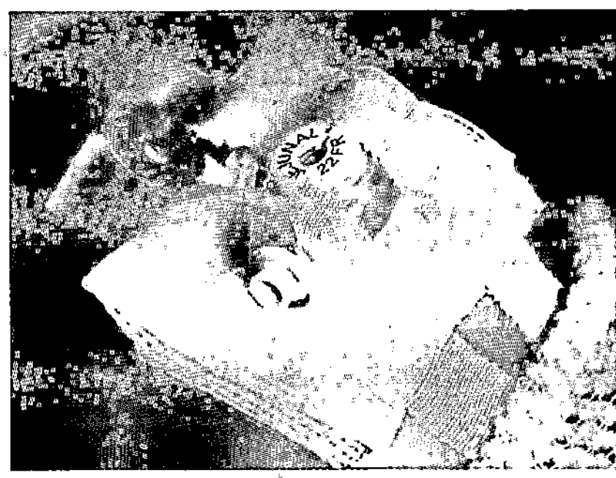 **FIGURE 9** MIC-KEY G-J Tube open and stabilized 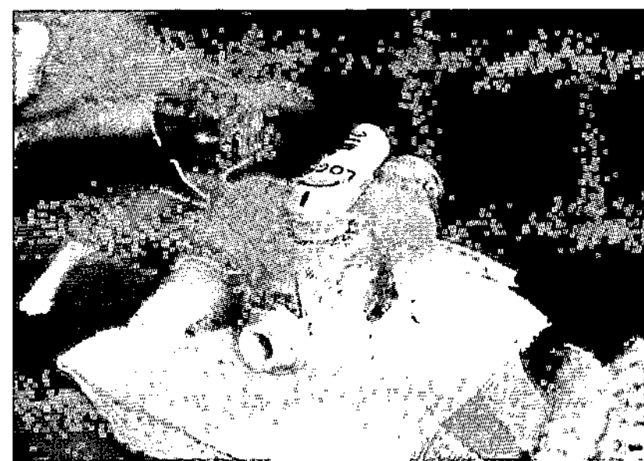 **FIGURE 10** MIC-KEY G-J Tube with connectors (*gastric port on side* with straight connector inserted; *jejunal port on top* with right-angle connector inserted. [balloon access port not connected]
Bard Button™	
Description/Use	Skin level silicone device with soft radiopaque retention dome that holds the tube in place (see Figure 11). There is an anti-reflux valve located inside the Button™ that prevents gastric leakage from the lumen of tube. 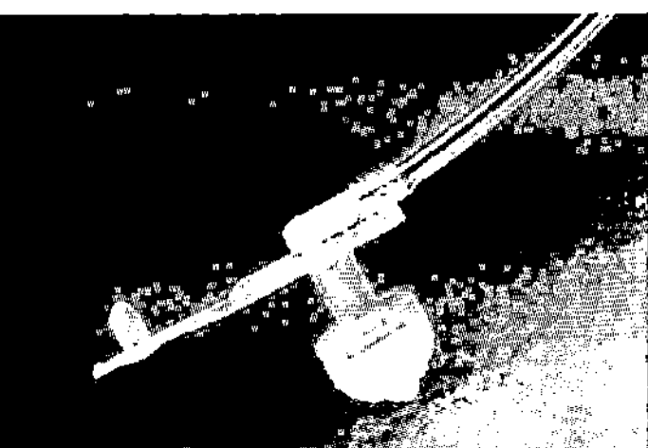 **FIGURE 11** Bard Button™ with right-angle extension set inserted
Accessories	**Feeding Tube Extension sets** For ***continuous feeding*** with a formula pump use: Bard Button™ right-angle extension set (90-degree angle). For ***bolus feedings*** use: Bard Button™ straight angle extension set is straight and the lumen is larger than right angle set. To attach, open "flip" tab and insert extension set into the lumen of the tube. Then, attach to feeding bag connector with a firm push and twist. The extension set "swivels" with movement and allows patient to change position during feeding.
Decompression Tube	There is also a decompression extension set available to aspirate, "vent" or empty to gravity drainage set (see Figures 12 and 13). Length of decompression tube **must** match centimeter length of tube, refer to size embossed on "flip tab" of tube.
Comments	When inserting feeding set push in the plastic notch into skin level opening.
	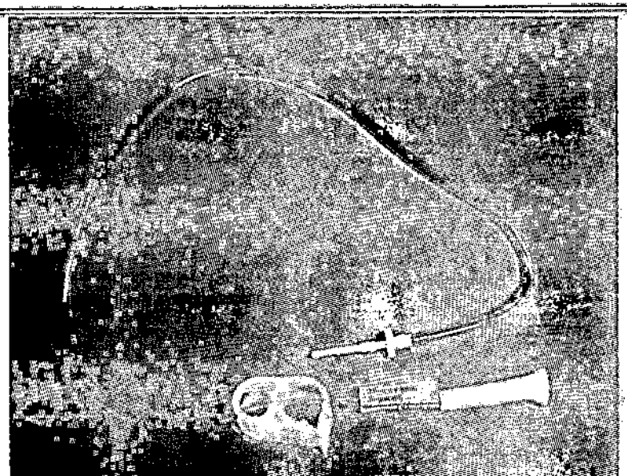 **FIGURE 12** Decompression extension set 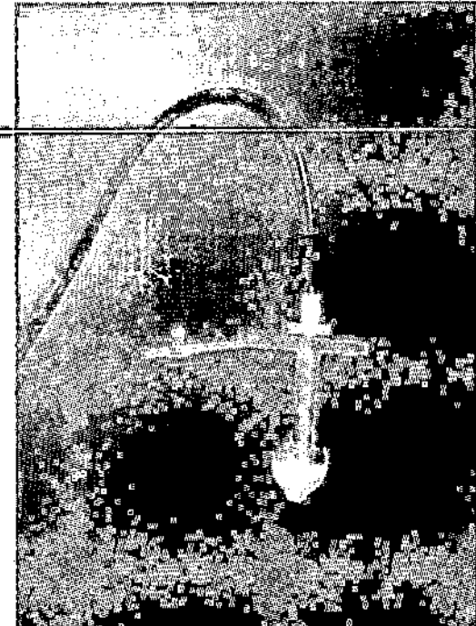 **FIGURE 13** Bard Button™ with decompression tube inserted

Table 4E-2 Enteral Feeding Tube Type Reference Tool—cont'd

PEG (Percutaneous Endoscopic Gastrostomy) Tube

Description/Use	CORPAK CORFLO® PEG Tubes are the type most commonly placed at our institution. This polyurethane tube is inserted under endoscopic guidance (Figure 14). On the proximal end of the PEG there is an internal bolster that resembles a "sponge with an air sac" stabilizing the tube on the anterior stomach wall. The distal end of the PEG tube is brought out through the abdominal wall and is then stabilized with cross-bar bolster on the abdominal surface (Figure 15). At the end of the procedure a Y-connector is threaded and secured with an adaptor to the distal end of the PEG tube for feeding and/or medication administration.
Comment	This adapter is necessary to provide access for feeding and/or medication administration. Then, attach to feeding bag connector with a firm push and twist. Otherwise leaking and disconnection will occur.

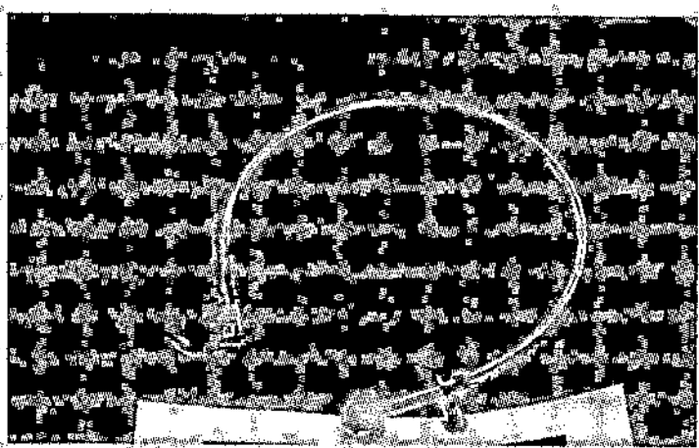

FIGURE 14 CORPAK CORFLO®-PEG Tube

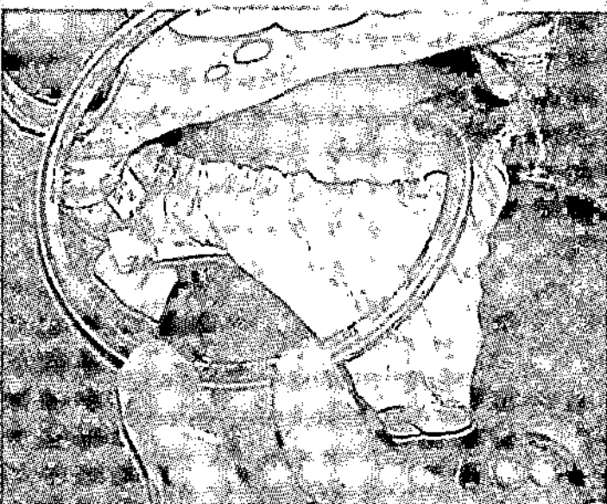

FIGURE 15 CORPAK CORFLO®-PEG Tube inserted and stabilized on model

Foley Catheter Tube

Description/Use	A non-skin level tube inserted into a gastrostomy site. There is a feeding and/or venting port and a balloon access port to inflate/deflate balloon that holds the tube in place (Figure 16).
Comments	This tube is available in latex and latex free varieties. Latex free indwelling foley catheters are most commonly used for enteral access. It is **imperative to stabilize securely** to avoid inadvertent dislodgement or migration of tube which, may result in gastric outlet obstruction. Often a temporary tube which is replaced after 6-12 weeks with a MIC g-tube™ or MIC-KEY™ tube.

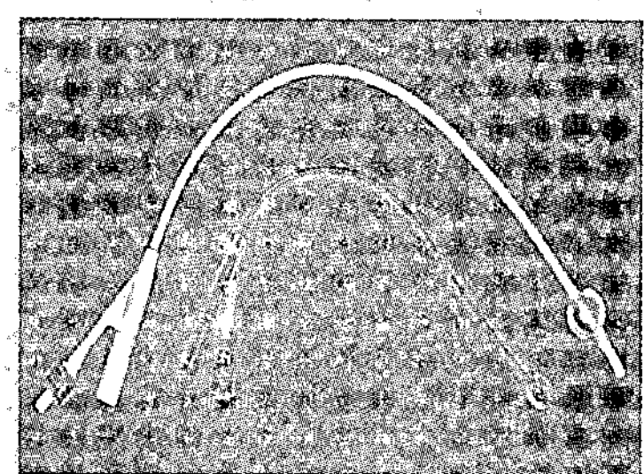

FIGURE 16 Foley Catheter Tubes

Malecot Tube

Description/Use	This tube has a soft bulb that looks like a tiny, open weaved basket holding it inside the stomach as an internal anchor (see Figure 17). The open weave allows fluids to enter and exit the stomach. However, it may pull out easily with any tension.
Comment	This tube is available in latex and latex free varieties. Latex free indwelling Foley catheters are most commonly used for enteral access. It is **imperative to stabilize securely** to avoid inadvertent dislodgement or migration of tube, which may result in gastric outlet obstruction. Often a temporary tube which is replaced after 6-12 weeks with a MIC g-tube™ or MIC-KEY™ tube.

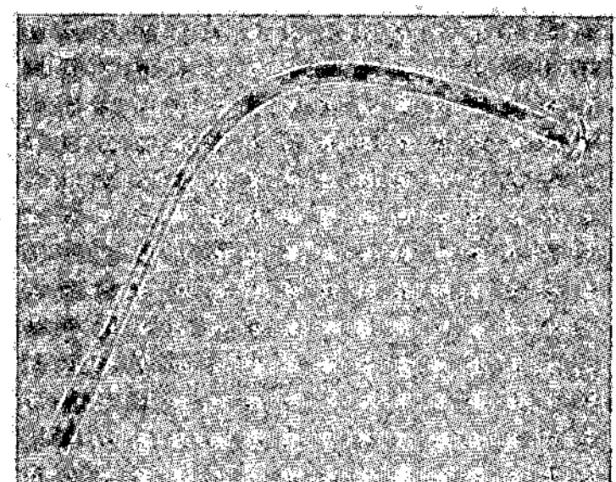

FIGURE 17 Malecot

Table 4E-3 Methods to Create a Gastrostomy Tract

Term	Technique
Percutaneous Endoscopic Gastrostomy (PEG)	Flexible, fiberoptic scope is advanced via the oral cavity into the stomach, where an appropriate location in the gastric mucosa is chosen for tube placement.
	Small incision is made on the abdominal surface, and a needle and angiocatheter are advanced into the stomach through the skin.
	Guidewire is inserted through the abdominal incision, snared by the endoscope, and exited from the mouth.
	PEG tube is attached to the guidewire and passed from the mouth, down the esophagus, and into the stomach.
Surgical	Technique involves a midline incision or laparoscopic assistance through a small incision on the abdomen.
	Appropriate site on the anterior stomach wall is chosen for insertion of the gastrostomy tube (G tube).
	Pursestring suture is placed on the gastric wall, and opening is made into the lumen of the stomach. The opening is dilated, and an appropriately sized G tube is inserted into the stomach.
	Multiple sutures are placed into the stomach and secured to the abdominal wall to create a permanent connection and prevent leakage of feeds and gastric contents into the peritoneal cavity.
	Separate site in the left upper quadrant is selected for exit of the G tube. G tube is grasped and brought through the abdominal wall and can be secured to the skin with sutures and tape.
	Primary incision is closed in layers using absorbable sutures.
Radiographic Approach	G tube is positioned correctly on the anterior stomach wall using fluoroscopic guidance.
	In neonates, transpyloric tubes can be placed endoscopically through existing gastrostomies. This approach can be used to verify placement of an inadvertently dislodged G tube.

particularly during periods of increased water loss, such as fever, vomiting, or diarrhea.

Ensuring appropriate volume of feedings

Routinely checking the flow rate of the infused feed is one simple and effective way of monitoring whether a child is receiving the appropriate amount.

Maintaining tube patency

It is essential to prevent tube occlusion. The flow rate should be fast enough to prevent blockage but not too rapid to cause reflux. Pump-assisted infusion of milk is recommended over gravity deliverance. The slight degree of pump-assisted pressure delivers the milk in a continuous, even infusion. This method can minimize residuals clinging to the inner lumen of the tube that can accumulate and eventually clog the tube. In addition, this method can prevent coagulation, a complication of calorically dense milk.

Routinely flush enteral tubes every 4 to 6 hours with an irrigant such as water to prevent clogging and to restore the patency of partially obstructed tubes.[3] Routinely flushing tubes before and after each feeding and/or medication can minimize pharmacokinetic incompatibilities between medications and enteral feedings. To maintain patency, a gastrostomy tube should be flushed before and after feedings, after medications, and twice daily if not in use. The typical flush volume to maintain patency is ≈2 ml for premature infants, ≈3 ml for full-term infants, and ≈1 ml per year of age for children. Children older than 10 years require a volume of 10 to 30 ml.

Physicians should be aware of potential tube occlusion caused by medications. To minimize tube occlusion, prioritize medications first in the form of a solution, secondarily as suspension, and then lastly in crushable pill form. Consult with a pharmacist to obtain liquid forms for as many medications as possible. Acidic liquid medications such as elixirs tend to clump in enteral formulas, whereas liquid medications with sweeteners that contain sorbitol can act as cathartics. Sustained-action capsules, enteric-coated tablets, and sustained-release tablets are not recommended for tube administration.

If the feeding tube is occluded, attempt to flush it with warm water or normal saline and attempt to "milk" the tubing. Carbonated beverages and cranberry juice seldom are effective and actually may cause obstruction by promoting formula coagulation. To relieve the obstruction, follow the recommended protocol given in Table 4E-4.

Skin care

Families and primary healthcare providers should monitor the tube insertion site regularly for signs of infection. For *nasally placed* tubes, routine daily inspection of the nares for mucosal irritation, skin breakdown, erythema, and distortion is important.

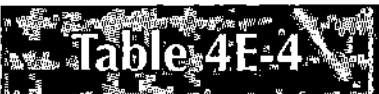

Enteral Feeding Gastrostomy Tube Troubleshooting Reference Tool*

Action	Rationale/Comments
Leakage (may be due to ineffective intragastric seal, e.g., inadequate balloon volume, excess transabdominal length, or migration of tube, or inadequate stabilization)	
• If **ineffective intragastric seal** results from ***inadequate balloon volume*** in balloon-inflated device (e.g., Foley, MIC, MIC-KEY), check fluid volume and add normal saline or sterile water (not air) PRN. Position the balloon against the stomach wall by very gently pulling the tube until mild resistance is met. Apply split gauze or foam dressing for absorption and stabilize securely with tape onto abdominal surface. If leakage persists, there may be a leak in the balloon. Assess peristomal skin integrity and, if compromised, refer to treatment recommendations outlined below.	Ensures effective intragastric seal. Volume dependent on patient's size: 2 ml for premature infant, 3 ml for full-term infant, and ≈1 ml per year of age for children. A balloon that is leaking fluid may need to be replaced. Notify primary service MD/NP at facility where tube was placed.
• If **ineffective intragastric seal** results from ***excess transabdominal tube length***, assess transabdominal segment length of tube. If shaft length is too long, may need to use one or more split gauze or foam dressings under abdominal flange to prevent tube migrating in/out of track, resulting in ineffective intragastric seal. May need to "bolster" up external flange to improve intragastric seal. Apply split gauze(s) or foam dressing (i.e., Allevyn) until adequately stabilized, then secure with tape onto abdominal surface. If MIC tube, may need to slide down clear circular external flange or "disk" along tube to improve intragastric seal.	If tube (i.e., MIC, MIC-KEY, Bard Button, or Foley catheter) can be moved through abdominal tract with gentle up-and-down traction, consider the intragastric seal to be ineffective. Poor tube stabilization and subsequent movement may result in formation of granulation tissue.
• If **ineffective intragastric seal** results from ***migration of mushroom tipped tube*** (i.e., Malecot or Bard Button), very ***gently*** pull the tube up until mild resistance met. Now the mushroom-shaped dome is positioned against the stomach wall. Apply split gauze or foam dressing for absorption and stabilize tube securely with tape onto abdominal surface to prevent movement. If leakage persists, notify primary service MD/NP at facility where tube was placed.	May need to change to balloon-inflated device if leakage persists and the tract is well healed, in order to obtain more effective intragastric seal.
• If leakage results from **inadequate stabilization**, assess tube. Be certain that tape stabilizes the tube, as well as the dressing onto abdominal skin to prevent movement of tube in the tract. Do not tape PEG tube on abdominal surface unless approved by the gastrointestinal (GI) service that placed tube.	A tube that is inadequately stabilized will move from side to side, as well as in/out of the track, resulting in stoma tract enlargement and potential tube dislodgment. Because of possible edema from procedure at insertion site, need to allow for some external flange movement.
• Regardless of cause of leakage, must assess for peristomal skin compromise (refer to treatment recommendations outlined below).	Leakage may have resulted in irritated peristomal skin.
Dislodgment	
• If the gastrostomy tube is dislodged, **never** attempt to reinsert the tube. Rather, cover the site with gauze.	Because of risk of tract disruption, enteral tubes must be replaced by an appropriately trained person. This is particularly critical during the first 6 weeks after the procedure. Gauze will absorb leakage from the site.
• Identify creation date of tract, method of insertion (surgically or via PEG), and specialist who created tract.	It is important that general surgery or GI services be notified.
• ***Immediately*** notify the primary service MD or emergency room triage MD at the facility where the tube was placed. Up to first 12 weeks postoperatively, only a surgeon can attempt to replace a dislodged surgical tube (in our hospital).	Tracts less than 6 weeks postprocedure may close within a few hours. Because of risk of tract disruption (e.g., perforation), only specially trained personnel should replace gastrostomy tubes.

*These guidelines have been created in the context of the specific care environment of Children's Hospital, Boston and may or may not be suitable for use in other care environments. Clinicians should consider carefully how to adapt these guidelines to their own environment and to exercise their own clinical judgment in applying them to actual clinical situations. These guidelines are not suitable for distribution to patients because clinical judgment is required.

Continued

Table 4E-4 Enteral Feeding Gastrostomy Tube Troubleshooting Reference Tool—cont'd

Intervention	Rationale
Dislodgment—cont'd	
After 12 weeks postoperatively, in many facilities a specially trained nurse practitioner (NP)/nurse can replace the tube.	
• Once the tube is replaced, the gastrostomy tube must ***never*** be used unless placement is confirmed by aspiration of gastric secretions or, if this is not possible, by x-ray film. This is the responsibility of the MD or specially trained NP/nurse who replaced the tube.	Because of risk of tract disruption or false passage creation during tube replacement, tube replacement must be confirmed.
Occlusion (unable to instill feedings or medication)	
• Slowly flush with 5–10 ml warm water or normal saline (unless child is volume restricted), attempt "milking" tubing, remove any kinks. Revaluate patency of the tube. Never attempt to push an object into the tube to unclog it.	Carbonated beverages, cranberry juice, or other "sticky" syrup-based products are seldom effective and may increase risk of the tube lumen adhering to itself.
• If patency is restored, review the potential risk factors for obstructions: flush volume and frequency, inadequately crushed medications, thickened formulas, physical or pharmokinetic incompatibilities.	Primary intervention in each of these circumstances is routine irrigation of the enteral tube before and after medications and feedings unless the child is volume sensitive. Consult a pharmacist about availability of liquid dosage form or alternative dosage equivalents, instead of administering crushing tablets.
• If water or normal saline fails to clear the tube, contact the MD from the facility where the tube was placed to determine whether the tube needs to be replaced. Some hospitals use an enzymatic solution (derived from Cotazyme capsule or Viocase tablet) from the pharmacy to manage obstruction before considering tube replacement.	This must be done ASAP to increase the likelihood of enzymatic activity unclogging the tube.
Peristomal Skin Compromise (caused by contact with gastric or jejunal contents)	
• Identifying the cause of leakage (e.g., ineffective gastric seal or inadequate stabilization) is of primary importance. Apply absorbent topical powder (e.g., Stomahesive powder), followed by split gauze or foam dressing (i.e., Allevyn) for additional absorption. Then stabilize securely with tape onto abdominal surface.	Need to identify etiology of leakage to decrease moist environment.
• Identify whether a candidal/monilial rash is present. It is characterized by an erythematous rash with satellite papules and pustules and often is associated with pruritis. If present, need to treat with ***topical antifungal ointment***.	Candidal rash will resolve only with medication.
• Consider Aveeno soaks or colloidal oatmeal in attempt to relieve irritated, itchy skin that often is present with candidal/monilial rashes.	Provides relief of inflamed skin conditions.
• If open, denuded skin, consider Domeboro soaks (combine one packet Domeboro with 6 oz water to make a 1:20 solution). This is an astringent, indicated for relief of inflammatory skin conditions, that will promote "drying out" of denuded, weepy skin.	Not uncommon for epidermis to be compromised when macerated with gastric or jejunal contents.
Bleeding from Stoma Site	
• Assess whether blood originates from center of stoma or from stoma itself. If bleeding is from stoma site itself, assess for presence of granulation tissue around tube insertion site.	Attempt to identify site of bleeding. Granulation tissue may bleed with tube movement in tract.
• Apply gauze with pressure and determine whether bleeding is slight, moderate, or excessive. Apply direct pressure for 5 minutes.	Attempt to stop bleeding.
• Identify any high-risk clinical scenarios that may place patient at risk for stomal bleeding.	Certain underlying disease processes (e.g., anticoagulation therapy, gastritis) may result in excessive bleeding from stoma site.
• Determine whether tube's moving in/out of tract is causing mucosal irritation. If so, stabilize securely with tape onto abdominal surface.	Continuous tube movement and friction may result in mucosal tissue bleeding.
Granulation Tissue (caused by growth of excess, moist pink red tissue that protrudes from the stoma site, representing overgrowth of new capillaries that may bleed easily)	
• Identify the presence of granulation tissue, which secretes a clear, serous, or brown exudate. Granulation tissue often is "friable."	Monitor for bleeding.

Table 4E-4 Enteral Feeding Gastrostomy Tube Troubleshooting Reference Tool—cont'd

• Stabilize the tube securely to prevent movement of tube in stoma. If excess shaft length, need to accommodate.	Stabilizing the tube can help prevent granulation tissue from increasing in size.
• Consider one of the following **treatment options** for excess granulation tissue:	
• ***Cauterize with silver nitrate*** applicator sticks daily until tissue flat. Need to apply petrolatum-based topical ointment to surrounding peristomal skin to silver nitrate. Cauterized granulation tissue will turn gray or black for 24–48 hours after application, then return to moist pink-red.	Silver nitrate will decrease proliferation of granulation tissue by coagulating cellular protein to form an eschar-like layer on the protect from caustic surface.
• ***Application of triamcinolone cream*** 0.5% TID for 7–10 days.	May decrease proliferation of granulation tissue.
Tube Breakage	
• Identify type of enteral feeding tube and area of damage on tube. May refer to manufacturer website and/or notify primary service at facility where tube was placed to determine repair plan. Specific repairs include:	
• If **"flip tab" from MIC-KEY or Bard Button tube is broken**, securely tape in place until tube can be replaced to decrease potential patient aspiration risk. If clinically determined that patient can remove tape, remove broken flip tab and tape over tube until replaced. Tube also can be clamped or a "plug" can be inserted to prevent gastric contents from leaking out.	"Flip tab" may pose aspiration risk if not taped securely in place until tube is changed.
• If **CORPAK PEG or MIC tubing is cracked**, CORPAK Y-Adaptor repair kits may work if breakage occurs where tube meets the Y-connector.	Step-by step instructions on repair technique included in package insert.
Connector Misfit	
• Determine whether extension or connector matches the type of tube (i.e., same manufacturer of product).	If the connection between the bag and tube is loose, firmly push the tube into the connection and confirm that the connection is secure. Wrap the connection with tape to decrease risk of disconnection.

If skin irritation is present at the nares, clean with water and apply a small amount of bacitracin ointment to decrease friction and promote lubrication. Secure the tube with tape above the upper lip and on the cheek to prevent pressure on the nares. If skin irritation is observed where the tube is secured, apply a small piece of hydrocolloid dressing (e.g., DuoDERM Extra Thin, ConvaTec) to serve as an anchor and stabilize the tape onto this dressing.

For *transabdominally placed* tubes, routine daily skin care of the abdominal tube insertion site includes cleaning with water and allowing the site to dry completely. A small amount of drainage around the tube is normal. If dry, crusted exudates are present, a solution of ¼-strength hydrogen peroxide and normal saline or water (one part peroxide to three parts normal saline or water) followed by a water rinse will help to remove the exudate gently and effectively. Consider using a thin layer of bacitracin ointment at the site to promote lubrication. If leakage occurs, it is important to determine the cause and to alleviate the leak as soon as possible before significant irritant contact dermatitis occurs (Table 4E-4). Place a split gauze or foam dressing around the site to facilitate absorption of the drainage and prevent peristomal skin compromise.

Fever, erythema, induration, foul odor, and/or pain at the insertion site may indicate infection. Treatment may include systemic and topical antibiotics. If there is excessive drainage from the site, a methylcellulose-based powder (Stomahesive powder, ConvaTec) may aid in increasing moisture absorption. The child may benefit from local application of colloidal oatmeal soaks (i.e., Aveeno) one to two times per day for 5 to 10 minutes to soothe the inflamed skin. If the epidermis is denuded, then local application of an astringent (i.e., Domeboro) one to two times per day for 5 to 10 minutes will vasoconstrict the capillaries and promote drying out of the area. If the site is erythematous with characteristic pinpoint satellite papules and pustules consistent with candidal infection, apply a thin layer of topical antifungal ointment two to three times per day. Evaluate the child for oral candidiasis and simultaneously treat with oral antifungal solution. Also inspect the perianal area for a coexisting candidal rash.

Stabilization

To prevent inadvertent tube dislodgment, the nasoenteric tube should be secured above the upper lip and on the cheek with tape. A small strip of DuoDERM Extra Thin dressing may be applied to protect the skin before the tape is applied. Another anchoring device commonly used is the Tender Grip). Longer tubes also can be secured to clothing to prevent inadvertent dislodgment. It is imperative to anchor transabdominal enteral tubes securely to prevent dislodgment, tract enlargement, internal migration into the gastrointestinal tract, and formation of granulation tissue. Tape should be applied *across* the tube flange and the dressing and then placed on the abdominal skin to stabilize the tube. The tape and dressing should be changed daily and PRN. A skin barrier wafer can be applied to the skin prophylactically to prevent contact dermatitis from the tape. Application of a skin sealant, such as 3M Cavilon No Sting Barrier Film, may be necessary to provide a protective layer to the skin surface before tape application. Other tapes or products can be used in accordance with the child's specific allergies. Skin-level tubes may not require tape stabilization once the stoma and track are well healed. Granulation tissue may develop if there is persistent leakage, poor stabilization, or improper fit (see Table 4E-4 for management options). This tissue may bleed easily when the dressing or tube is manipulated.

If the transabdominal tube has a balloon-inflated device, it is necessary to check the amount of fluid in the balloon to ensure an adequate seal on the anterior stomach wall. This should be checked once per week to ensure proper inflation and to minimize the risk of inadvertent tube dislodgment. Ideally, the check should be performed on the same day each week. The balloon should be inflated with either normal saline or sterile water.

Complications

The primary care provider should be aware of the potential complications of feeding tube use. Specific gastrointestinal problems and metabolic abnormalities are discussed in this section.

Gastrointestinal

Gastrointestinal problems (e.g., diarrhea) are one of the most common complications associated with enteral nutrition. The complications usually arise from the feeding regimen but may have other causes, such as antibiotic usage. Some clinicians prescribe lactobacilli with oral antibiotics to minimize stool frequency. The enteral feeding infusion rate and formula osmolality may contribute to gastrointestinal rapid transit. To prevent some of the complications, parents and caregivers should attempt to minimize enteral formula contamination by cleaning and changing the enteral delivery set every 24 hours.

Metabolic

Numerous metabolic complications may occur, most commonly during an acute illness. Some of these metabolic derangements can be prevented by providing the child with the appropriate recommended daily nutritional requirements and ensuring that the child receives the total volume that is prescribed.

Hyperglycemia caused by reduced circulating insulin may be predictive of impending sepsis. Hypoglycemia may occur much more quickly than hyperglycemia, especially if the child has diabetes, has liver or metabolic disease, or is receiving steroids. Hypernatremia may occur if the child becomes dehydrated, is severely fluid restricted, receives large amounts of sodium bicarbonate, or develops renal dysfunction. Hyponatremia may occur when the child is overhydrated or if the child has gastrointestinal losses with inadequate replacement. Hyperkalemia often is the result of metabolic acidosis in combination with renal insufficiency. Hypokalemia may result from diarrhea or large amounts of diuretics. Hyperphosphatemia may be associated with renal dysfunction.

Conclusion

This chapter discussed enteral feeding tubes in the pediatric population. Knowledge of care and management of enteral tubes can positively influence outcomes by providing appropriate assessment, prevention, treatment, and evaluation. Coordination between the acute care and community services for effective discharge planning is essential and provides the additional benefits of uniting families sooner and reducing healthcare costs. Primary care clinicians and families must continue to monitor for potential complications of enteral feedings. Premature infants who have a complex medical course and a longer transition to oral feedings are more likely to develop a feeding disorder, so instituting an oral motor stimulation program is essential to avoid oral aversion (see Chapter 4C). For children with gastrostomy tubes, regular assessment for potential leakage, dislodgment, occlusion, skin compromise, and granulation tissue formation is essential.

It is important to remind families that placement of an enteral feeding tube in premature infants usually is a temporary solution, as many children with adequate gastrointestinal absorptive capacity ultimately will be able to transition to oral nutritional intake over time. Optimal nutritional intake is imperative to minimize morbidity and mortality in children.

Resources for Families and Clinicians

Kids with Tubes
http://www.kidswithtubes.org/

Kids with Tubes is an organization operated by parents that offers a variety of support services for parents and caregivers of tube-fed children. Its mission is to provide forums for sharing information and mutual support. This organization aims to bring together families whose children have feeding tubes (nasogastric, gastric, gastrojejunal, jejunal, and/or nasojejunal tubes) without regard to the children's underlying diagnoses.

Mealtime Notions
http://www.mealtimenotions.com/

Mealtime Notions LLC was created to provide mealtime support for parents and professionals who feed infants and young children with special feeding challenges. The organization serves children who have difficulties coordinating the process of sucking, swallowing, and breathing; handling the sensory aspects of mealtimes; and consuming sufficient calories for growth. Many of these children require a supplemental tube feeding to help with nutrition. This organization provides educational opportunities with workshops, therapy consultation, and shared information, as well as favorite mealtime resources and materials.

New Visions
http://www.new-vis.com/

New Visions provides continuing education and therapy services to professionals and parents working with infants and children with feeding, swallowing, oral–motor, and prespeech problems.

The Oley Foundation
http://www.oley.org

The Oley Foundation is a national, independent, nonprofit organization that provides up-to-date information, outreach services, conference activities, and emotional support for home parenteral or enteral nutrition support consumers, their families, caregivers, and professionals.

REFERENCES

1. McGuire W, McEwan P: Systemic review of transpyloric versus gastric tube feeding for preterm infants. *Arch Dis Child Fetal Neonatal Ed* 89(3):F245-F248, 2004.
2. Huffman S, Pieper P, Jarczyk KS, et al: Methods to confirm feeding tube placement: application of research in practice. *Pediatr Nurs* 30:10-13, 2004.
3. Methany N, Eisenberg P, McSweeney M: Effect of feeding tube properties and three irrigants on clogging rates. *Nurs Res* 37(3):165-169, 1988.

BIBLIOGRAPHY

Abad-Sinden A, Sutphen J: Enteral nutrition. In Walker WA, Goulet O, Kleinman R, et al., editors: *Pediatric gastrointestinal disease vol. 2*, ed 4. Hamilton, Ontario, Canada, 2004, BC Decker.

Beckwith MC, Barton RG, Graves CA: A guide to drug therapy in patients with enteral feeding tubes: dosage form selection and administration methods. *Hosp Pharm* 32:57-64, 1997.

Borkowski S: Pediatric stomas, tubes, and appliances. *Pediatr Clin North Am* 45(6):1419-1435, 1998.

Burd A, Burd RS: The who, what, why, and how-to guide for gastrostomy tube placement in infants. *Adv Neonatal Care* 3(4):197-205, 2003.

Cirgin M, Croffie J, Cohen M, et al: Gastric tube placement in young children. *Clin Nurs Res* 14(3):238-252, 2005.

Krupp KB, Heximer B: Going with the flow. How to prevent feeding tubes from clogging. *Nursing* 28(4):54-55, 1998.

Marcuard SP, Stegall KL, Trogdon S. Clearing obstructed feeding tubes. *J Parenter Enteral Nutr* 13:81-3:1989.

Methany N, Wehrle MA, Wiersema L, et al: Testing feeding tube placement: auscultation vs. pH method [Erratum in: *Am J Nurs* 98(8):1289, 1998]. *Am J Nurs* 98(5):37-42, 1998.

Shiao SY, Novotny DL: The features of different gastric tubes used in nurseries. *Neonatal Netw* 17(4):78-9, 1998.

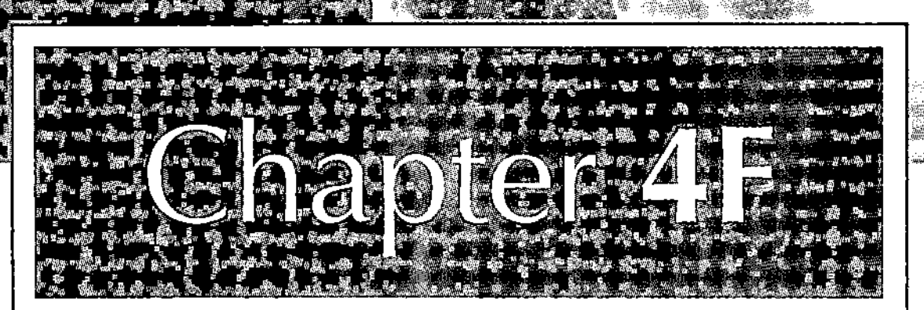

Necrotizing Enterocolitis and Short Bowel Syndrome

Camilia R. Martin, MD, MS

PART I: NECROTIZING ENTEROCOLITIS

Introduction

Necrotizing enterocolitis (NEC) is the most common neonatal gastrointestinal emergency[1,2] predominantly affecting low-birth-weight, premature infants.[1-5] NEC is characterized by disruption of intestinal mucosal integrity, leading to an acute clinical presentation of feeding intolerance, bloody stools, cardiorespiratory compromise, and severe hemodynamic instability. Despite extensive study, the etiology and pathophysiology of NEC are not fully understood. This is a devastating disease with a mortality rate of 10% to 50%.[1,3,4,6] Morbid sequelae among survivors include impaired growth, short bowel syndrome, prolonged neonatal hospitalization, repeated hospitalizations, and poor long-term neurodevelopment.[4,7,8]

General Epidemiology

The overall incidence of NEC for all births is approximately 1–3/1,000. From 1% to 7.7% of all infants admitted to the neonatal intensive care unit (NICU) develop NEC.[6] The epidemiologic literature examining the historical and clinical risk factors for development of NEC is extensive; however, the understanding about the precise risk factors and pathogenesis of the disorder is limited. Although numerous risk factors have been identified, many of them are nonspecific and are shared by a vast majority of sick preterm infants in the NICU. Only a selected few have been reliably reproduced from study to study.

Infant risk factors

Prematurity and low birth weight consistently have been found to be risk factors for NEC.[1-3,9-14] Ninety percent of NEC cases occur in preterm infants, with the greatest risk in the smaller, more premature infants. Compared with an overall incidence rate of 1% to 7.7%, up to 7% to 14% of very-low-birth-weight infants (VLBW, <1500 g)[10,11,15-18] are diagnosed with NEC.

The evidence associating intrauterine growth restriction[14,19-21] and race (increased risk for black infants)[10,22] with the development of NEC is increasingly strong.

Infection appears to play an important role in the evolution of this disease. Bacterial organisms are often, but not always, isolated from the blood and/or peritoneal fluid of the infant with NEC. Commonly isolated species include *Klebsiella* spp., *Enterobacter* spp., *Escherichia coli, Bacteroides* spp., and *Staphylococcus epidermidis.*[23-27] The clinical presentation of NEC is, at times, similar to that of sepsis. This similarity and the tendency for cluster outbreaks suggest an infectious process.[28]

Other infant risk factors whose contribution to NEC is more controversial include the timing, type, and volume of enteral feedings; the presence of indwelling central catheters; concomitant illnesses or conditions, such as patent ductus arteriosis; and medical treatments, including indomethacin and phototherapy.[1-3,29,30]

Although the preterm infant may have many potential coexisting risk factors that contribute to some extent to the development of NEC, the full-term infant is more likely to a have a single predominating risk factor. Approximately 10% of all infants with NEC are term (≥37 weeks' gestation), and significant risk factors in this population include intrauterine growth restriction, congenital heart disease, congenital intestinal anomalies, asphyxia, and a previous exchange transfusion.[31-34]

Maternal risk factors

The current epidemiologic literature has identified potential maternal risk factors and the later development of NEC in their offspring; however, these risk factors are not consistent across studies. Risk factors that may be important by reducing overall fetal mesenteric blood flow include preeclampsia/toxemia, maternal hemorrhage, and placental abruption.[10,35-38]

In the literature there is an emerging hypothesis of altered gastrointestinal susceptibility resulting from inflammatory stimuli and its associated modulation by maternal and fetal inflammatory responses. Maternal and fetal cytokine mediators have been detected in the amniotic fluid and fetal plasma in pregnancies complicated by chorioamnionitis, preterm labor, and prolonged premature rupture of membranes. Cytokine mediators released during the fetal inflammatory response may be responsible for initiating preterm delivery[39-41]and for subsequent neonatal morbidity, including NEC.[39-47] Supporting evidence for the role of maternal/fetal inflammation and the development of NEC include the findings of increased NEC with duration of ruptured membranes and maternal chorioamnionitis.[7,10,48-50] The role of antenatal glucocorticoids in the risk of NEC remains unclear. A study has shown an increased risk for development of NEC after receipt of antenatal corticosteroids[51]; however, a larger number of studies have shown a reduced risk.[1,3,52-56]

Hospital and practice variations

Hospital variation in the incidence of neonatal morbidities, including NEC, is well established. In two large cohort studies of VLBW infants in multiple NICUs, the incidence of NEC varied from 0% to 22%.[17,18] This is a testament to the likely existence of amenable practice parameters that need further study,[10] with the hope of identifying effective clinical management strategies to reduce the occurrence of NEC.

Pathophysiology

As evident by the preceding discussion, a multifactorial process most likely contributes to the development of NEC. Many risk factors are shared by ill, preterm infants; however, only a fraction of infants are diagnosed with NEC. The vulnerability of an infant for the development of NEC appears to be modulated by (1) degree of prematurity, (2) intestinal integrity and function, (3) bacterial colonization, (4) enteral feedings, (5) maturity of immune defenses, including local mucosal defenses and regulation of systemic inflammatory responses, and (6) genetic susceptibility. Current literature supports the theory that these various factors likely interact with one another and have a final common inflammatory pathway leading to bowel injury and the clinical syndrome of NEC.[1,57,58]

Clinical Presentation and Diagnosis

The diagnosis of NEC is made from a combination of clinical signs and symptoms coupled with specific radiologic findings. NEC can present in a variety of ways, from a subtle, insidious onset to a more fulminant presentation with precipitous cardiorespiratory and hemodynamic compromise. Signs and symptoms can be specific to the gastrointestinal system or be more generalized or systemic, reflecting the infant's overall instability (Table 4F-1).

The average age at presentation for all infants in the NICU is approximately between 2 and 3 weeks of life. However, the age at presentation varies on the basis of gestational age at birth, with the more immature infants presenting at a later day of life (Table 4F-2).

Laboratory abnormalities include leukopenia (more common than leukocytosis), neutropenia, thrombocytopenia, hyponatremia, hypokalemia, metabolic acidosis, disseminated intravascular coagulopathy (DIC), and glucose instability.

The clinical diagnosis is supported by abnormal radiographs. Plain abdominal radiographs (preferably two views: prone with lateral or decubitus) may reveal pneumatosis intestinalis (intramural gas), dilated loops of bowel, fixed loops of bowel, thickened bowel wall (edema), ileus, air–fluid levels, ascites, pneumoperitoneum, and portal venous air. The most common areas of involvement are the distal ileum and colon.[59,60] NEC is staged according to clinical and radiographic findings and correlates with illness severity (Table 4F-3). NEC staging can be helpful in prognosticating short- and long-term outcomes. It also is useful in the research setting, where accurate disease classification is necessary for proper study.

Treatment

Most infants can be managed medically; however, surgical intervention may be necessary if specific complications arise (23–50%).[8,22,61] All infants will require a period of bowel rest with nothing by

Table 4F-1 Signs and Symptoms Associated with Necrotizing Enterocolitis

Gastrointestinal	Systemic
Abdominal distention	Lethargy
Abdominal tenderness	Apnea or respiratory distress
Feeding intolerance	Temperature instability
Delayed gastric emptying (usually represented by high gastric residuals before the next enteral feeding)	"Not right"
Vomiting	Acidosis (metabolic and/or respiratory)
Occult or gross blood in stool	Glucose instability
Change in stool pattern or diarrhea	Poor perfusion or shock
Abdominal mass	Disseminated intravascular coagulopathy
Abdominal wall erythema	Positive blood culture results

From: Kanto WP Jr, Hunter JE, Stoll BJ: *Clin Perinatol* 21(2):336, 1994.

mouth (NPO) and abdominal decompression. To maintain appropriate hydration and nutrition, the infant will require parenteral nutrition (PN). Broad-spectrum antibiotics typically are provided to treat concomitant sepsis and/or to prevent the potential for nosocomial infection by opportunistic organisms. The initial broad-spectrum coverage typically is provided with ampicillin and gentamicin. Clindamycin is considered for additional anaerobic coverage, especially in the presence of pneumatosis or pneumoperitoneum. However, the decision to add clindamycin should be considered carefully because of possible increased risk for late intestinal strictures with its use.[62] Vancomycin is considered if methicillin-resistant *Staphylococcus* sp. is a concern. Additional medical care is tailored to the specific clinical presentation and medical support required to ensure cardiorespiratory stability. Frequent serial laboratory assessments (for electrolyte imbalance, DIC, metabolic acidosis) and radiologic monitoring are necessary to monitor for NEC progression and resolution. A surgical consultation should be requested for all infants with NEC in case progression of the disease warrants surgical intervention.

Table 4F-2 Average Age at Onset of Necrotizing Enterocolitis by Gestational Age

Gestational Age at Birth (wk)	Average Age at Onset (days)
≤30	20.2
31–33	13.8
≤34	5.4

Data from: Stoll BJ, Kanto WP, Glass RI, et al: *J Pediatr* 96:447, 1980.

Surgical intervention is necessary or strongly considered under specific clinical circumstances. The presence of free intra-abdominal air is a definite surgical indication and is the most common reason for surgery (42%).[63] Other clinical conditions in which surgical intervention should be strongly considered include a fixed loop of bowel, portal venous air, abdominal mass, abdominal wall erythema, and severe illness or clinical deterioration manifested by intractable metabolic acidosis, persistent thrombocytopenia or coagulopathy, and recurrent positive blood cultures.[59,64] In the infant weighing more than 1500 g, surgical management typically consists of exploratory laparotomy with resection of the diseased bowel and formation of an enterostomy and stoma. The most optimal surgical approach for the VLBW infant is unknown. Some centers use the same strategy as used for bigger infants, whereas other centers perform primary peritoneal drainage, where the abdominal cavity is irrigated through a small incision and a Penrose drain is placed. A later explorative laparotomy may or may not be necessary, depending on the clinical course of the VLBW infant. A randomized trial is currently ongoing to help determine the best surgical strategy in the VLBW infant.[65] Infants who require surgery are at risk for postoperative complications, such as sepsis, wound infection, intra-abdominal abscess, intestinal strictures, and short bowel syndrome.[63] Enterostomy closure is targeted at 4 weeks postoperatively to 4 months of age. Benefits associated with early closure include fewer metabolic derangements, reduced risk for cholestatic liver disease, and improved growth.[59,66]

Outcomes

Acutely, infants with NEC are at risk for *electrolyte derangements*, *DIC*, *cardiorespiratory collapse*, *sepsis*, and gastrointestinal compromise requiring

Table 4F-3 Modified Bell Staging Criteria for Necrotizing Enterocolitis

		Signs		
	Stage	Systemic	Intestinal	Radiographic
I	Suspected	Temperature instability, apnea, bradycardia	Elevated gastric residuals, mild abdominal distention, occult Blood in stool	Normal or mild ileus
IIA	Mild	Similar to stage I	Prominent abdominal distention ± tenderness, absent bowel sounds, grossly bloody stools	Ileus, dilated bowel loops, focal pneumatosis
IIB	Moderate	Mild acidosis, thrombocytopenia	Abdominal wall edema and tenderness, ± palpable mass	Extensive pneumatosis, early ascites, ± portal venous gas
IIIA	Advanced	Respiratory and metabolic acidosis, mechanical ventilation, hypotension, oliguria, disseminated coagulopathy	Worsening wall edema and erythema with induration	Prominent ascites, persistent bowel loop, no free air
IIIB	Advanced	Vital signs and laboratory evidence of deterioration, shock	Evidence of perforation	Pneumoperitoneum

From: Kleigman RM, Walsh MC: *Curr Prob Pediatr* 17:213, 1987.

surgical intervention. The clinical deterioration often seen with NEC typically results in a *longer period of intubation* and *prolonged hospitalization.*[15]

During the period of medical management, usually up to 14 days, plus during the gradual process of reinitiating enteral feedings, the infant can be solely or mostly dependent on PN for a minimum of 2 weeks. During this time, it is not unusual to see evidence of *PN-induced cholestasis* with elevation of liver function tests and direct hyperbilirubinemia. Typically, this process is reversible once enteral feedings are re-established, and symptoms resolve in 1 to 3 months.[8]

Convalescing infants with NEC are at increased risk for *intestinal strictures,* which occur in approximately 10% to 35% of infants[8,22,59,61,63,67-69] and most often in the colonic region.[67] Careful attention to feeding intolerance and monitoring for signs of intestinal obstruction are necessary once feedings are restarted. The mean age at presentation of intestinal strictures is 49 days after resolution of NEC for infants treated medically and 80 days from the initial surgical intervention for infants requiring surgery.[67] In an unusual case report, a child presented with obstruction at age 11 years, presumably from a previously unrecognized NEC stricture.[70]

Mortality from NEC has been reported from 10% to as high as 50%,[15,60,61,71] with the smaller, more premature infants at greatest risk.[63] Clinical factors associated with a greater risk of mortality include advanced NEC stage, multisystem organ failure, capillary leak syndrome, intrauterine growth restriction, diffuse bowel involvement, presence of portal venous air, and thrombocytopenia.[72-77]

Once the infant is discharged from the NICU, the primary healthcare provider must manage potential long-term sequelae, which include *short bowel syndrome, impaired growth,* and *poor neurodevelopment.* Short bowel syndrome is discussed in detail in Part II of this chapter. Growth and neurodevelopmental outcomes are discussed here.

Growth

Infants diagnosed with NEC demonstrate decreased weight gain velocity during their stay in the NICU. At discharge from the NICU, they are more likely to have growth measurements (weight, height, and head circumference) less than the tenth percentile for corrected age.[78,79] Limited studies have documented the long-term growth outcomes in infants who had NEC during their NICU course. Most of existing literature report studies that followed very small cohorts, some of which demonstrated good catch-up growth,[79,80] whereas others demonstrated persistent growth failure.[15,60,61,81-83] Infants who had advanced stages of NEC or who underwent bowel resection appear at greatest risk.[7,81,84] Of most concern are the long-term studies demonstrating subnormal head circumferences, as head circumference has been shown to correlate with long-term neurodevelopmental outcomes.[8,15,81,85]

Preterm growth velocity varies by hospital and practice style[86] and may account for the differences in growth outcomes seen for infants with NEC. This variation in practice raises the possibility of amenable nutritional practices both in the NICU and after discharge to optimize growth in former preterm infants who had NEC.

Long-term neurodevelopment

NEC is increasingly shown to be an important contributor and independent risk factor for poor long-term neurodevelopment in premature infants. In cohorts of premature infants followed through 18 to 22 months' corrected age, NEC was shown to be a major contributor to poor neurodevelopmental outcomes.[87,88] In studies that specifically examined the relationship of NEC and long-term neurodevelopment, infants with NEC consistently demonstrated poor neurodevelopment, especially within the psychomotor domain, compared with their gestational age and/or birth weight–matched controls.[15,61,79,81] This relationship is strongest among the more ill infants, as demonstrated by an advanced stage of NEC or need for surgical intervention.[7,81,89]

The pathogenesis of NEC on long-term neurodevelopment remains to be elucidated. Whether poor neurodevelopment is a primary consequence of NEC or is a secondary consequence from comorbidities associated with NEC is unclear. Such comorbidities include prolonged intubation and increased risk for chronic lung disease, nosocomial sepsis, prolonged and repeated hospitalizations with limited social interaction, and poor overall growth, including subnormal head circumference.[8] All of these comorbidities have been shown to be potential risk factors for poor long-term neurodevelopment; however, even after accounting for these associated risks, NEC remains an important contributor to neurodevelopment.

PART II: SHORT BOWEL SYNDROME

Clinical Presentation

Under certain clinical scenarios, surgical intervention is necessary for the management of NEC. A major goal during surgery is to leave as much bowel behind as possible to preserve the infant's ability to process enteral nutrients in a normal fashion. However, at times, excessive loss of intestine is necessary but results in significant reduction of mucosal surface area and increased enteral transit times. When this occurs, the infant may demonstrate malabsorption of enteral nutrients, leading to diarrhea and poor growth. This clinical state is called *short bowel syndrome* (SBS). Although in this chapter SBS is discussed as a consequence of NEC, SBS can be seen after loss of bowel from other gastrointestinal disorders, including intestinal atresias, gastroschisis, and volvulus. After intestinal resection, SBS occurs in approximately 7% to 25% of infants.[22,61,63,65,90] Mortality rates for SBS from 8% to 22% have been reported. The majority of deaths are related to PN-associated liver failure.[90,91]

The severity of symptoms seen with SBS depends on length of bowel removed, location of resected bowel, and whether the ileocecal valve was left intact. This becomes evident when one considers the physiologic function of each component of the gastrointestinal system (Table 4F-4).[91,92]

Treatment

One of the most important goals is to transition the infant or child to enteral feedings as soon as possible. This will reduce the amount of dependency on PN and its associated complications (discussed later). However, some children may require lifelong PN and, ultimately, small bowel transplantation.

Factors that have been associated with the increased likelihood of transitioning to all enteral feedings include the following:

- *Length of residual small bowel.* The remaining bowel length is inversely correlated with the duration of PN.
- *Functional capacity of the remaining small bowel.* The ileum possesses the adaptive ability to assume the absorptive roles of the jejunum. The jejunum is less likely to adapt to the large loss of ileal tissue. A large loss of small bowel and colon has a less favorable prognosis.
- *Intact ileocecal valve.*
- *Intact colon.*
- *Successful intestinal adaptation.* Intestinal adaptation relies on the adaptive ability of the remaining bowel to assume the role of the lost bowel and the ability of the remaining bowel to lengthen and increase its absorptive surface area.

Table 4F-4 Physiologic Function of the Gastrointestinal System and Clinical Significance

Component	Physiologic Function	Clinical Presentation with Loss or Absence
Duodenum	• Mineral reabsorption	• Iron deficiency • Folate deficiency • Calcium malabsorption

Jejunum	• Primary location for digestion and absorption of nutrients
	  ○ Large surface area for absorptive function
	  ○ High concentration of digestive enzyme
	• Location of many transport proteins
	• Unable to adapt and assume the role of the ileum in case of large loss of ileal tissue
		• Reduction in efficiency of digestion and absorption of nutrients
		• However, this usually is transient because the ileum will adapt and compensate for loss of jejunal tissue

Ileum	• Reabsorption from jejunum of luminal contents consisting of water and electrolytes • Vitamin B_{12} absorption in terminal ileum • Bile acid absorption	• Electrolytes losses • Fluid losses • Vitamin B_{12} deficiency • Poor absorption of fat, including fat-soluble vitamins • Secretory diarrhea • Hyperoxaluria and kidney stones
Ileocecal valve	• Regulates flow of luminal contents from small bowel to colon to allow transit times most suitable for proper absorption. • Prevent backward flow of contents and colonic bacteria	• Increased transit time and therefore reduced absorption • Bacterial overgrowth of small bowel with subsequent inflammation, worsening malabsorption, diarrhea, and colitis
Colon	• Primarily responsible for absorption of water and electrolytes	• Electrolyte losses • Fluid losses

This adaptive response begins within 24 hours after bowel resection. Intestinal adaptation is less likely with smaller amounts of remaining small bowel, absence of the ileocecal valve, significant or complete colonic resection, and the inability to successfully perform a primary anastomosis. Intestinal adaptation usually occurs by age 3 years. If intestinal adaptation has not occurred by age 3 years, it is unlikely to do so.[93,94]

Prevent dehydration and electrolyte imbalance

To prevent dehydration and electrolyte imbalances, careful monitoring of fluid losses and adherence to an electrolyte and fluid replacement protocol for stoma and fecal losses will be necessary (see Table 4F-5 for approximate electrolyte losses for specific fluid types). Losses in sodium chloride content typically are high. Excessive diarrhea as a result of bile salt malabsorption may respond to cholestyramine.

Establish enteral feedings and promote intestinal adaptation

For successful intestinal adaptation to occur, enterocytes must be exposed to intraluminal nutritional contents. It will be important to provide early enteral feedings and to taper PN as early and as aggressively as possible. Steady, but cautious, advancement in enteral volumes can be made by closely monitoring total enteral losses and the presence of stool-reducing substances (Table 4F-6).

Table 4F-5 Electrolyte Composition of Various Body Fluids

Fluid	Na^+ (mEq/L)	K^+ (mEq/L)	CL^- (mEq/L)
Gastric	20–80	5–20	100–150
Pancreatic	120–140	5–15	90–120
Small bowel	100–140	5–15	90–130
Bile	120–140	5–15	80–120
Ileostomy	45–135	3–15	20–115
Diarrhea	10–90	10–80	10–110

From: Gunn VL, Nechyba C, editors: *The Harriet Lane handbook*, ed 16. Philadelphia, 2002, Mosby.

Table 4F-6 Suggested Guidelines for Enteral Feeding Advancement in the Infant with Short Bowel Syndrome

FEEDING ADVANCEMENT PRINCIPLES

- Quantify feeding intolerance primarily by stool or ostomy output and secondarily by reducing substances. Reducing substances should be measured twice daily.
- Assess tolerance no more than twice per 24 hours. Advance no more than once per 24-hour period.
- Ultimate goals: 130–200 ml/kg/day and/or 100–140 kcal/kg/day
- If ostomy/stool output precludes advancement at 20 cal per ounce for 7 days, then caloric density of the formula can be increased.
- As feedings are advanced, parenteral nutrition should be isocalorically reduced.

GUIDELINES FOR FEEDING ADVANCEMENT

Clinical Parameter	Amount	Enteral Adjustment
Stool output	<10 g/kg/day or <10 stools/day	Advance rate by 10–20 ml/kg/day
	10–20 g/kg/day or 10–12 stools/day	No change
	>20 g/kg/day or >12 stools/day	Reduce rate or hold feeds*
Ostomy output	<2 g/kg/hr	Advance rate by 10–20 ml/kg/day
	2–3 g/kg/hr	No change
	>3 g/kg/hr	Reduce rate or hold feeds*
Stool-reducing substances	<1%	Advance feeds per stool or ostomy output
	=1%	No change
	>1%	Reduce rate or hold feeds*
Signs of dehydration	Absent	Advance feeds per stool or ostomy output
	Present	Reduce rate or hold feeds*
Gastric aspirates	<4 times previous hour's infusion	Advance feeds
	>4 times previous hour's infusion	Reduce rate or hold feeds*

From: Utter SL, Jaksic T, Duggan C: In Hansen AR, Puder M, editors: *Manual of neonatal surgical intensive care*. Hamilton, Ontario, Canada, 2003, BC Decker.
*Feeds generally should be held for 8 hours and then restarted at 75% of the previous rate.

Reduce osmotic load

Diets low in carbohydrate content and high in fat composition reduce the overall osmotic load of feedings and are better tolerated. Although protein hydrolysate formulas are generally well tolerated, it has been demonstrated that breast milk and amino acid-based formulas may be more effective in promoting intestinal adaptation.[66] Continuous feedings or small-volume feedings will also reduce overall osmotic load.

Optimize growth and prevent nutritional deficiencies

To achieve optimal growth, additional calories may be necessary to overcome losses from malabsorption. Monitoring of serum levels of calcium, magnesium, zinc, selenium, and vitamins A, D, E, and K (fat-soluble vitamins) at least every 3 months is recommended.[90,93] Supplemental vitamins and minerals should be considered. Vitamin B_{12} is recommended if the distal ileum is absent.

Monitor for and treat associated medical complications of short bowel syndrome[95]

Bacterial overgrowth may worsen malabsorption and incite an inflammatory response that can lead to colitis. Diagnosis can be made by jejunal aspirate culture or breath testing. Treatment options include antibiotics, anti-inflammatory agents, and salicylate.

Complications secondary to prolonged PN include *cholestatic liver disease* and *catheter-related complications* such as line sepsis. PN-associated cholestatic liver disease is a major cause of death in children with SBS. Liver disease can range from transient elevation of liver transaminases and conjugated bilirubin to cirrhosis and portal hypertension and ultimately liver failure. Factors that are positively associated with the development of cholestatic liver disease include duration of amino acid infusion, delayed enteral feedings, sepsis, bacterial overgrowth, prolonged period with diverting ostomy, low birth weight, and degree of prematurity.[91] Management strategies for reducing the risk of cholestasis are outlined in Table 4F-7.

Cholecystokinin has shown promise for the prevention and treatment of cholestasis, and ursodeoxycholic acid has been shown to be effective in normalizing liver function tests.

Increased oxalate absorption and urinary oxalate excretion result in *hyperoxaluria and the development of renal stones*. This is best managed by reducing overall oxalate absorption, i.e., following a

Table 4F-7 Steps for Reducing the Risk of Cholestasis Associated with Parenteral Nutrition

Method	Comments
Avoid overfeeding	90–100 kcal/kg average parenteral energy requirement
Cycle parenteral nutrition off at least 2–6 hr/day	Promotes cyclic release of gastrointestinal hormones
Aggressively treat and prevent infection	Meticulous central line care; treat bacterial overgrowth of the small bowel
Encourage enteral nutrition	Promotes intestinal adaptation; transition to all enteral feedings is the ultimate goal of therapy

From: Utter SL, Jaksic T, Duggan C: Short-bowel syndrome. In Hansen AR, Puder M, editors: *Manual of neonatal surgical intensive care*. Hamilton, Ontario, Canada, 2003, BC Decker.

low oxalate diet, increasing daily fluid intake, and providing potassium citrate for metabolic acidosis.

D-Lactic acidosis results from the accumulation of D-lactate, a by-product of colonic metabolism of unabsorbed carbohydrates by gram-positive anaerobes. Symptomatology is rarely present. Potential symptoms include metabolic acidosis, confusion, cerebellar ataxia, and slurred speech. Treatment consists of correcting the metabolic acidosis with sodium bicarbonate, administering antimicrobials to reduce D-lactate–producing organisms, and reducing the amount of unabsorbed carbohydrates presented to the colon with a low-carbohydrate diet.

Despite meticulous attention and aggressive enteral feeding regimens, some children will be unable to achieve full enteral feedings and will be dependent on PN. These children may be eligible for intestinal lengthening procedures. If significant clinical complications arise from PN dependency, they also may be eligible for intestinal transplantation. *Intestinal lengthening procedures* can be considered as early as 6 months of age if the child is still dependent on PN. Two intestinal lengthening procedures currently are available, the Bianchi procedure and the STEP procedure, both aimed at increasing intestinal length and surface area. The indications for isolated *intestinal transplantation* include "intractable symptoms necessitating recurrent hospitalization and patients with recurrent catheter sepsis who have lost critical central venous access." Combined liver/small bowel transplantation is considered with "irreversible PN-induced liver disease in patients who are likely to die in the subsequent two years."[93]

Table 4F-8 Postdischarge Care of the Neonatal Intensive Care Unit Graduate with History of Necrotizing Enterocolitis

Outcome	General Care Recommendations
Late intestinal stricture	• Monitor for signs and symptoms of bowel obstruction • If concerns, radiologic evaluation for bowel obstruction • Surgical consultation
Growth and nutrition	• Optimize volume and caloric density in enteral feedings for adequate growth • Regular assessments of anthropometric measurements • If concerns, consultation with pediatric nutritionist
Neurodevelopment	• Involvement with local early intervention program • Regular assessments with the neonatal intensive care unit's follow-up program
Short bowel syndrome	• Provide care in concert with surgery, gastroenterology, and nutritional services • Monitor for dehydration and electrolyte imbalance • Establish enteral feedings and promote intestinal adaptation • Optimize volume and caloric density in enteral feedings for adequate growth • Frequent monitoring of vitamin and mineral deficiencies • Regular assessments of anthropometric measurements • Assess for associated complications: ○ Bacterial overgrowth ○ Parenteral nutrition-induced cholestatic liver disease ○ Catheter-related complications ○ Hyperoxaluria and renal stones ○ D-lactic acidosis

Conclusion

All former premature infants require comprehensive discharge planning, including parent teaching and thorough communication with the intended primary care physician. Former premature infants present unique challenges to the primary care physician. These infants are at risk for ongoing medical and developmental concerns that may affect their overall quality of life. Close monitoring of these issues by parents and physicians is essential to optimize outcomes. The former premature infant who had NEC is at risk for long-term sequelae even after the acute episode is successfully treated and resolved. The family should be apprised of these issues before discharge from the NICU, and the primary care physician should help to monitor these issues and provide extended care as needed. A summary of these issues and recommendations for follow-up care is outlined in Table 4F-8.

Resources for Families and Clinicians

Parent resources

Insurance considerations
http://www.aetna.com/cpb/data/CPBA0605.html
Insurance payment guidelines for intestinal failure.

The Oley Foundation
http://c4isr.com/oley/; 1-800-776-OLEY

Founded in 1983, the Oley Foundation is a national organization providing information and psychosocial support to individuals requiring long-term parenteral nutrition and tube-fed enteral nutrition. All services are free of charge. Many members include children with short bowel syndrome as a result of NEC.

Physician resources

American Gastrointestinal Association
www.guideline.gov/summary/summary.aspx?ss=15&doc_id=3795&nbr=3021

Provides technical review of short bowel syndrome and intestinal transplantation.

North American Society for Pediatric Gastroenterology, Hepatology and Nutrition
http://www.naspghan.org/

Includes parent information handouts of short bowel syndrome in several languages including English, Spanish, and French.

Review of Short Bowel Syndrome
http://www.emedicine.com/med/topic2746.htm

REFERENCES

1. Neu J: Necrotizing enterocolitis: the search for a unifying pathogenic theory leading to prevention. *Pediatr Clin North Am* 43(2):409-432, 1996.
2. Stoll BJ: Epidemiology of necrotizing enterocolitis. *Clin Perinatol* 21(2):205-218, 1994.
3. Kliegman RM, Walker WA, Yolken RH: Necrotizing enterocolitis: research agenda for a disease of unknown etiology and pathogenesis. *Pediatr Res* 34(6):701-708, 1993.
4. Kliegman RM: Models of the pathogenesis of necrotizing enterocolitis. *J Pediatr* 117(1 pt 2):S2-S5, 1990.
5. Kliegman RM: Neonatal necrotizing enterocolitis: bridging the basic science with the clinical disease. *J Pediatr* 117(5): 833-835, 1990.
6. Kosloske AM: Epidemiology of necrotizing enterocolitis. *Acta Paediatr Suppl* 396:2-7, 1994.
7. Hintz SR, Kendrick DE, Stoll BJ, et al: Neurodevelopmental and growth outcomes of extremely low birth weight infants after necrotizing enterocolitis. *Pediatrics* 115(3):696-703, 2005.
8. Simon NP: Follow-up for infants with necrotizing enterocolitis. *Clin Perinatol* 21(2):411-424, 1994.
9. Holman RC, Stoll BJ, Clarke MJ, et al: The epidemiology of necrotizing enterocolitis infant mortality in the United States. *Am J Public Health* 87(12):2026-2031, 1997.
10. Uauy RD, Fanaroff AA, Korones SB, et al: Necrotizing enterocolitis in very low birth weight infants: biodemographic and clinical correlates. National Institute of Child Health and Human Development Neonatal Research Network. *J Pediatr* 119(4):630-638, 1991.
11. Yu VY, Joseph R, Bajuk B, et al: Necrotizing enterocolitis in very low birthweight infants: a four-year experience. *Aust Paediatr J* 20(1):29-33, 1984.
12. Blond MH, Chavet MS, Lecuyer AI, et al: [Necrotizing enterocolitis and apnoeas: bradycardias of the preterm newborn]. *Arch Pediatr* 10(2):102-9, 2003.
13. Bhatt AB, Tank PD, Barmade KB, et al: Abnormal Doppler flow velocimetry in the growth restricted foetus as a predictor for necrotising enterocolitis. *J Postgrad Med* 48(3):182-185, 2005; discussion 48(3):185, 2002.
14. Bernstein IM, Horbar JD, Badger GJ, et al: Morbidity and mortality among very-low-birth-weight neonates with intrauterine growth restriction. The Vermont Oxford Network. *Am J Obstet Gynecol* 182(1 pt 1):198-206, 2000.
15. Salhab WA, Perlman JM, Silver L, et al: Necrotizing enterocolitis and neurodevelopmental outcome in extremely low birth weight infants <1000 g. *J Perinatol* 24(9):534-540, 2004.
16. El-Metwally D, Vohr B, Tucker R: Survival and neonatal morbidity at the limits of viability in the mid 1990s: 22 to 25 weeks. *J Pediatr* 137(5):616-622, 2000.
17. Lee SK, McMillan DD, Ohlsson A, et al: Variations in practice and outcomes in the Canadian NICU network: 1996-1997. *Pediatrics* 106(5):1070-1079, 2000.
18. Lemons JA, Bauer CR, Oh W, et al: Very low birth weight outcomes of the National Institute of Child Health and Human Development neonatal research network, January 1995 through December 1996. NICHD Neonatal Research Network. *Pediatrics* 107(1):E1, 2001.
19. Gilbert WM, Danielsen B: Pregnancy outcomes associated with intrauterine growth restriction. *Am J Obstet Gynecol* 188(6):1596-1599, 2003; discussion 9-601, 2003.
20. Aucott SW, Donohue PK, Northington FJ: Increased morbidity in severe early intrauterine growth restriction. *J Perinatol* 24(7):435-440, 2004.
21. Zaw W, Gagnon R, da Silva O: The risks of adverse neonatal outcome among preterm small for gestational age infants according to neonatal versus fetal growth standards. *Pediatrics* 111(6 pt 1):1273-1277, 2003.
22. Llanos AR, Moss ME, Pinzon MC, et al: Epidemiology of neonatal necrotising enterocolitis: a population-based study. *Paediatr Perinat Epidemiol* 16(4):342-349, 2002.
23. Bell MJ, Ternberg JL, Bower RJ: The microbial flora and antimicrobial therapy of neonatal peritonitis. *J Pediatr Surg* 15(4):569-573, 1980.

24. Boccia D, Stolfi I, Lana S, et al: Nosocomial necrotising enterocolitis outbreaks: epidemiology and control measures. *Eur J Pediatr* 160(6):385-391, 2001.
25. Hoy CM, Wood CM, Hawkey PM, et al: Duodenal microflora in very-low-birth-weight neonates and relation to necrotizing enterocolitis. *J Clin Microbiol* 38(12):4539-4547, 2000.
26. Mollitt DL, Tepas JJ, 3rd, Talbert JL: The microbiology of neonatal peritonitis. *Arch Surg* 123(2):176-179, 1988.
27. Mollitt DL, Tepas JJ, Talbert JL: The role of coagulase-negative Staphylococcus in neonatal necrotizing enterocolitis. *J Pediatr Surg* 23(1 pt 2):60-63, 1988.
28. Willoughby RE Jr, Pickering LK: Necrotizing enterocolitis and infection. *Clin Perinatol* 21(2):307-315, 1994.
29. Yu VY, Joseph R, Bajuk B, et al: Perinatal risk factors for necrotizing enterocolitis. *Arch Dis Child* 59(5):430-434, 1984.
30. Yao AC, Martinussen M, Johansen OJ, et al: Phototherapy-associated changes in mesenteric blood flow response to feeding in term neonates. *J Pediatr* 124(2):309-312, 1994.
31. Kanto WP Jr, Hunter JE, Stoll BJ: Recognition and medical management of necrotizing enterocolitis. *Clin Perinatol* 21(2):335-346, 1994.
32. Ostlie DJ, Spilde TL, St Peter SD, et al: Necrotizing enterocolitis in full-term infants. J *Pediatr Surg* 38(7):1039-1042, 2003.
33. Polin RA, Pollack PF, Barlow B, et al: Necrotizing enterocolitis in term infants. *J Pediatr* 89(3):460-462, 1976.
34. Wiswell TE, Robertson CF, Jones TA, et al: Necrotizing enterocolitis in full-term infants. A case-control study. *Am J Dis Child* 142(5):532-535, 1988.
35. Kliegman RM, Hack M, Jones P, et al: Epidemiologic study of necrotizing enterocolitis among low-birth-weight infants. Absence of identifiable risk factors. *J Pediatr* 100(3):440-444, 1982.
36. Kanto WP Jr, Wilson R, Breart GL, et al: Perinatal events and necrotizing enterocolitis in premature infants. *Am J Dis Child* 141(2):167-169, 1987.
37. Harms K, Rath W, Herting E, et al: Maternal hemolysis, elevated liver enzymes, low platelet count, and neonatal outcome. *Am J Perinatol* 12(1):1-6, 1995.
38. Bashiri A, Zmora E, Sheiner E, et al: Maternal hypertensive disorders are an independent risk factor for the development of necrotizing enterocolitis in very low birth weight infants. *Fetal Diagn Ther* 18(6):404-407, 2003.
39. Dudley DJ, Trautman MS, Mitchell MD: Inflammatory mediators regulate interleukin-8 production by cultured gestational tissues: evidence for a cytokine network at the chorio-decidual interface. *J Clin Endocrinol Metab* 76(2):404-410, 1993.
40. Dudley DJ: Pre-term labor: an intra-uterine inflammatory response syndrome? *J Reprod Immunol* 36(1-2):93-109, 1997.
41. Romero R, Gomez R, Ghezzi F, et al: A fetal systemic inflammatory response is followed by the spontaneous onset of preterm parturition. *Am J Obstet Gynecol* 179(1):186-193, 1998.
42. Yoon BH, Romero R, Kim KS, et al: A systemic fetal inflammatory response and the development of bronchopulmonary dysplasia. *Am J Obstet Gynecol* 181(4):773-779, 1999.
43. Yoon BH, Romero R, Park JS, et al: Fetal exposure to an intra-amniotic inflammation and the development of cerebral palsy at the age of three years. *Am J Obstet Gynecol* 182(3):675-681, 2000.
44. Yoon BH, Romero R, Yang SH, et al: Interleukin-6 concentrations in umbilical cord plasma are elevated in neonates with white matter lesions associated with periventricular leukomalacia. *Am J Obstet Gynecol* 174(5):1433-1440, 1996.
45. Leviton A, Paneth N, Reuss ML, et al: Maternal infection, fetal inflammatory response, and brain damage in very low birth weight infants. Developmental Epidemiology Network Investigators. *Pediatr Res* 6(5):566-575, 1999.
46. Gomez R, Romero R, Ghezzi F, et al: The fetal inflammatory response syndrome. *Am J Obstet Gynecol* 179(1):194-202, 1998.
47. Dammann O, Leviton A: Role of the fetus in perinatal infection and neonatal brain damage. *Curr Opin Pediatr* 12(2):99-104, 2000.
48. Ruangtrakool R, Laohapensang M, Sathornkich C, et al: Necrotizing enterocolitis: a comparison between full-term and pre-term neonates. *J Med Assoc Thai* 84(3):323-331, 2001.
49. Bracci R, Buonocore G: Chorioamnionitis: a risk factor for fetal and neonatal morbidity. *Biol Neonate* 83(2):85-96, 2003.
50. Martinez-Tallo E, Claure N, Bancalari E: Necrotizing enterocolitis in full-term or near-term infants: risk factors. *Biol Neonate* 71(5):292-298, 1997.
51. Guthrie SO, Gordon PV, Thomas V, et al: Necrotizing enterocolitis among neonates in the United States. *J Perinatol* 23(4):278-285, 2003.
52. Bauer CR, Morrison JC, Poole WK, et al: A decreased incidence of necrotizing enterocolitis after prenatal glucocorticoid therapy. *Pediatrics* 73(5):682-688, 1984.
53. Crowley P, Chalmers I, Keirse MJ: The effects of corticosteroid administration before preterm delivery: an overview of the evidence from controlled trials [see comments]. *Br J Obstet Gynaecol* 97(1):11-25, 1990.
54. Halac E, Halac J, Begue EF, et al: Prenatal and postnatal corticosteroid therapy to prevent neonatal necrotizing enterocolitis: a controlled trial. *J Pediatr* 117(1 pt 1):132-138, 1990.
55. Qublan HS, Malkawi HY, Hiasat MS, et al: The effect of antenatal corticosteroid therapy on pregnancies complicated by premature rupture of membranes. *Clin Exp Obstet Gynecol* 28(3):183-186, 2001.
56. Vasan U, Gotoff SP: Prevention of neonatal necrotizing enterocolitis. *Clin Perinatol* 21(2):425-435, 1994.
57. Caplan M, Jilling T: The pathophysiology of necrotizing enterocolitis. *NeoReviews* 2(5):c103-c108, 2001.
58. Treszl A, Heninger E, Kalman A, et al: Lower prevalence of IL-4 receptor alpha-chain gene G variant in very-low-birth-weight infants with necrotizing enterocolitis. *J Pediatr Surg* 38(9):1374-1378, 2003.
59. Kosloske AM, Musemeche CA: Necrotizing enterocolitis of the neonate. *Clin Perinatol* 16(1):97-111, 1989.
60. Kurscheid T, Holschneider AM: Necrotizing enterocolitis (NEC): mortality and long-term results. *Eur J Pediatr Surg* 3(3):139-143, 1993.
61. Yeh TC, Chang JH, Kao HA, et al: Necrotizing enterocolitis in infants: clinical outcome and influence on growth and neurodevelopment. J *Formos Med Assoc* 103(10):761-766, 2004.
62. Faix RG, Polley TZ, Grasela TH: A randomized, controlled trial of parenteral clindamycin in neonatal necrotizing enterocolitis. *J Pediatr* 112(2):271-277, 1988.
63. Horwitz JR, Lally KP, Cheu HW, et al: Complications after surgical intervention for necrotizing enterocolitis: a multicenter review. *J Pediatr Surg* 30(7):994-998; discussion 8-9, 1995.
64. Hansen AR, Sena L, Jaksic T: Necrotizing enterocolitis. In Hansen A, Puder M, editors: *Manual of neonatal surgical intensive care.* Hamilton, Ontario, Canada, 2003, BC Decker.
65. Dimmitt R, Moss R: Clinical management of necrotizing enterocolitis. *NeoReviews* 2(5):c110-c116, 2001.
66. Andorsky DJ, Lund DP, Lillehei CW, et al: Nutritional and other postoperative management of neonates with short bowel syndrome correlates with clinical outcomes. *J Pediatr* 139(1):27-33, 2001.
67. Schimpl G, Hollwarth ME, Fotter R, et al: Late intestinal strictures following successful treatment of necrotizing enterocolitis. *Acta Paediatr Suppl* 396:80-83, 1994.

68. Lemelle JL, Schmitt M, de Miscault G, et al: Neonatal necrotizing enterocolitis: a retrospective and multicentric review of 331 cases. *Acta Paediatr Suppl* 396:70-73, 1994.
69. Radhakrishnan J, Blechman G, Shrader C, et al: Colonic strictures following successful medical management of necrotizing enterocolitis: a prospective study evaluating early gastrointestinal contrast studies. *J Pediatr Surg* 26(9):1043-1046, 1991.
70. Goettler CE, Stallion A, Grisoni ER, et al: An unusual late complication of necrotizing enterocolitis. *J Pediatr Surg* 36(12):1853-1854, 2001.
71. Stanford A, Upperman JS, Boyle P, et al: Long-term follow-up of patients with necrotizing enterocolitis. *J Pediatr Surg* 37(7):1048-1050; discussion 1050, 2002.
72. Sonntag J, Wagner MH, Waldschmidt J, et al: Multisystem organ failure and capillary leak syndrome in severe necrotizing enterocolitis of very low birth weight infants. *J Pediatr Surg* 33(3):481-484, 1998.
73. de Souza JC, da Motta UI, Ketzer CR: Prognostic factors of mortality in newborns with necrotizing enterocolitis submitted to exploratory laparotomy. *J Pediatr Surg* 36(3):482-486, 2001.
74. Kenton AB, O'Donovan D, Cass DL, et al: Severe thrombocytopenia predicts outcome in neonates with necrotizing enterocolitis. *J Perinatol* 25(1):14-20, 2005.
75. Molik KA, West KW, Rescorla FJ, et al: Portal venous air: the poor prognosis persists. *J Pediatr Surg* 36(8):1143-1145, 2001.
76. Cikrit D, Mastandrea J, West KW, et al: Necrotizing enterocolitis: factors affecting mortality in 101 surgical cases. *Surgery* 96(4):648-655, 1984.
77. Kosloske AM, Musemeche CA, Ball WS Jr, et al: Necrotizing enterocolitis: value of radiographic findings to predict outcome. *AJR Am J Roentgenol* 151(4):771-774, 1988.
78. Clark RH, Thomas P, Peabody J: Extrauterine growth restriction remains a serious problem in prematurely born neonates. *Pediatrics* 111(5 pt 1):986-990, 2003.
79. Sonntag J, Grimmer I, Scholz T, et al: Growth and neurodevelopmental outcome of very low birthweight infants with necrotizing enterocolitis. *Acta Paediatr* 89(5):528-532, 2000.
80. Stevenson DK, Kerner JA, Malachowski N, et al: Late morbidity among survivors of necrotizing enterocolitis. *Pediatrics* 66(6):925-927, 1980.
81. Walsh MC, Kliegman RM, Hack M: Severity of necrotizing enterocolitis: influence on outcome at 2 years of age. *Pediatrics* 84(5):808-814, 1989.
82. Whiteman L, Wuethrich M, Egan E: Infants who survive necrotizing enterocolitis. *Matern Child Nurs J* 14(2):123-133, 1985.
83. Cikrit D, West KW, Schreiner R, et al: Long-term follow-up after surgical management of necrotizing enterocolitis: sixty-three cases. *J Pediatr Surg* 21(6):533-535, 1986.
84. Tejani A, Dobias B, Nangia BS, et al: Growth, health, and development after neonatal gut surgery: a long-term follow-up. *Pediatrics* 61(5):685-693, 1978.
85. Hack M, Breslau N, Weissman B, et al: Effect of very low birth weight and subnormal head size on cognitive abilities at school age. *N Engl J Med* 325(4):231-237, 1991.
86. Olsen IE, Richardson DK, Schmid CH, et al: Intersite differences in weight growth velocity of extremely premature infants. *Pediatrics* 110(6):1125-1132, 2002.
87. Ambalavanan N, Nelson KG, Alexander G, et al: Prediction of neurologic morbidity in extremely low birth weight infants. *J Perinatol* 20(8 pt 1):496-503, 2000.
88. Vohr BR, Wright LL, Dusick AM, et al: Neurodevelopmental and functional outcomes of extremely low birth weight infants in the National Institute of Child Health and Human Development Neonatal Research Network, 1993-1994. *Pediatrics* 105(6):1216-1226, 2000.
89. Tobiansky R, Lui K, Roberts S, et al: Neurodevelopmental outcome in very low birthweight infants with necrotizing enterocolitis requiring surgery. *J Paediatr Child Health* 31(3):233-236, 1995.
90. Ricketts RR: Surgical treatment of necrotizing enterocolitis and the short bowel syndrome. *Clin Perinatol* 21(2):365-387, 1994.
91. Utter SL, Jaksic T, Duggan C: Short-bowel syndrome. In Hansen A, Puder M, editors: *Manual of neonatal surgical care.* Hamilton, Ontario, Canada, 2003, BC Decker.
92. Vanderhoof JA, Young RJ: Pathophysiology of the short bowel syndrome in children. In Rose BD, editor: *UpToDate.* Wellesley, Mass, 2004, UpToDate.
93. Vanderhoof JA, Young RJ: Management of the short bowel syndrome in children. In Rose BD, editor: *UpToDate.* Wellesley, Mass, 2004, UpToDate.
94. Quiros-Tejeira RE, Ament ME, Reyen L, et al: Long-term parenteral nutritional support and intestinal adaptation in children with short bowel syndrome: a 25-year experience. *J Pediatr* 145(2):157-163, 2004.
95. Vanderhoof JA, Young RJ: Chronic complications of the short bowel syndrome in children. In Rose BD, editor: *UpToDate.* Wellesley, Mass, 2004, UpToDate.

Chapter 4G

Direct Hyperbilirubinemia

Kristen E. Lindamood, RNC, MS, NNP, and Dara Brodsky, MD

Approximately one in 2500 infants is affected by direct (conjugated) hyperbilirubinemia, or cholestasis.[1,2] Early detection of cholestasis by the primary care provider is critical. With the assistance of a pediatric gastroenterology specialist, the clinician can focus on distinguishing from among transient liver dysfunction, an underlying disease process, and primary liver disease. By identifying the etiology in a timely manner, the clinician will be able to effectively treat infants with direct hyperbilirubinemia and potentially minimize the associated morbidity and/or mortality.[3,4] This chapter provides an overview of how to evaluate and manage an infant with cholestasis, with an emphasis on premature infants.

Etiology

Cholestasis is attributable to reduced bile formation, impairment of bile flow, or the failure to excrete conjugated bilirubin from the hepatocyte into the duodenum. The etiology can be grouped into an obstructive (Table 4G-1) or a hepatocellular (Table 4G-2) pathway. Biliary atresia and neonatal hepatitis are the two most common causes of neonatal cholestasis in full-term infants, accounting for 70% to 80% of cases.[5] Biliary atresia is due to bile duct inflammation that leads to progressive obliteration of the extrahepatic biliary tract.[6] α_1-Antitrypsin deficiency accounts for approximately 5% to 15% of full-term infants with cholestasis.[1,2] Premature infants usually develop cholestasis as a result of prolonged total parenteral nutrition or sepsis. Biliary atresia is rarely the cause of cholestasis in premature infants.

Presentation in the neonatal period can be multifactorial, with infectious, metabolic, anatomic, and/or toxic etiologic factors causing liver cell injury or obstruction to bile flow, which then causes congestion, obstruction, inflammation, and/or infiltration.[3,4,7] This can be caused by viral, bacterial, parasitic, or fungal infections, accumulation of storage products from fats, metals, abnormal proteins, or glycogen, and/or infiltration of primary malignant or benign tumors. The ill neonate who presents with acute cholestasis is more likely to have a primary illness, such as sepsis (particularly a urinary tract infection), with a secondary cholestasis. In the latter situation, cholestasis usually resolves after treatment of the underlying disease process.

Because premature infants have a relative physiologic and developmental immaturity to the structure and function of the liver and biliary tree, they are at higher risk for exaggerated physiologic cholestasis. This physiologic cholestasis may be compounded by perinatal depression, sepsis, an underlying intestinal disease process such as necrotizing enterocolitis, late onset of enteral feedings, prolonged parenteral nutrition for more than 3 weeks, or preexisting liver disease.[8,9]

Table 4G-1 Obstructive Causes of Neonatal Cholestasis

Alagille syndrome
Biliary atresia
Choledochal cyst
Cholelithiasis
Congenital hepatic fibrosis/Caroli disease
Cystic fibrosis
Gallstones or biliary sludge
Hemolytic disease
Hepatic or biliary hemangioma
Inspissated bile
Intrahepatic/extrahepatic tumors
Neonatal sclerosing cholangitis

Note: This list is not all inclusive.
Modified from: Askin DF, Diehl-Jones WL: *Neonatal Netw* 22:7-8, 2003, D'Agata ID, Balistreri WF: *Pediatr Rev* 20:378, 1999, Moyer V, Freese DK, Whitington PF, et al: North American Society for Pediatric Gastroenterology, Hepatology and Nutrition: *J Pediatr Gastroenterol Nutr* 39(2):116, 2004.

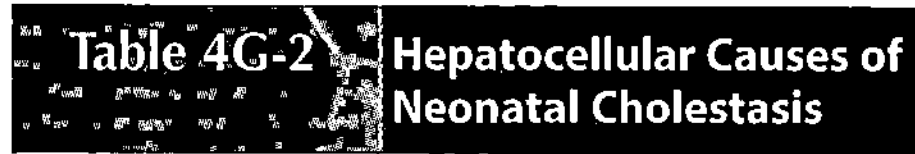

Table 4G-2 Hepatocellular Causes of Neonatal Cholestasis

ASSOCIATED MEDICAL/SURGICAL CONDITIONS

Gastroschisis
Ruptured omphalocele
Necrotizing enterocolitis

BACTERIAL/VIRAL INFECTIONS

Adenovirus
Cytomegalovirus
Epstein-Barr virus
Enterovirus
Hepatitis A, B, or C
Herpes simplex virus
Human herpesvirus 6
Human immunodeficiency virus
Parvovirus B19
Rotavirus
Reovirus type 3
Rubella
Sepsis
Syphilis
Toxoplasmosis
Urinary tract infection

GENETIC/STORAGE AND METABOLIC DISORDERS

α_1-Antitrypsin deficiency
Arginase deficiency
Cystic fibrosis
Disorders of bile acid metabolism
Fructosemia
Galactosemia
Gaucher disease
Glycogen storage disease type IV
Hemochromatosis
Hypothyroidism
Mitochondrial disorders
Panhypopituitarism
Progressive familial intrahepatic cholestasis
Niemann-Pick type C
Tyrosinemia
Wolman disease
Zellweger syndrome

MISCELLANEOUS

Parenteral nutrition
Perinatal hypoxia
Previous umbilical catheter
Shock/hypoperfusion

Note: This list is not all inclusive.
Modified from: Askin DF, Diehl-Jones WL: *Neonatal Netw* 22:7-8, 2003, D'Agata ID, Balistreri WF: *Pediatr Rev* 20:378, 1999, Moyer V, Freese DK, Whitington PF, et al: North American Society for Pediatric Gastroenterology, Hepatology and Nutrition: *J Pediatr Gastroenterol Nutr* 39(2):116, 2004.

Premature infants with short bowel syndrome following intestinal resection are at high risk for cholestasis. This cholestasis is the result of multiple potential factors, including sepsis, bacterial overgrowth, mucosal atrophy or a diverting ostomy, delayed enteral feedings, and use of parenteral nutrition.[10] Direct hyperbilirubinemia is further compounded by the already reduced rate of bile flow in the neonate.[11]

Evaluation

Clinical practice guidelines have been developed by the North American Society for Pediatric Gastroenterology, Hepatology and Nutrition (NASPGHAN) to recognize and improve the timely diagnosis and treatment of cholestasis in the neonatal period.[3] Any infant with clinical jaundice at age 2 weeks should be evaluated for cholestasis by measuring serum total and direct bilirubin levels. Primary care providers may delay these initial blood tests in jaundiced infants who are breastfeeding and appear well, without pale stools or dark urine, until age 3 weeks. However, if close follow-up will be difficult and/or delayed until the routine 2-month visit, immediate evaluation is required because of the narrow window for therapy for some causes of cholestasis. Premature infants with a known history of cholestasis must undergo further evaluation if the cholestasis becomes more severe without an explanation or if the cholestasis persists after 2 to 3 months' corrected gestational age. This re-evaluation should assess for metabolic causes of hepatic injury.

Neonatal cholestasis is an elevated serum direct bilirubin level >1.0 mg/dl if the total serum bilirubin level is <5 mg/dl, or >20% of the total serum bilirubin measurement if the total bilirubin level is >5 mg/dl.[3] Once the diagnosis of cholestasis is made, immediate evaluation is warranted. Evidence suggests that early diagnosis and surgical repair (by 45–60 days of life) may improve outcomes of infants with biliary atresia.[12] In addition, early diagnosis and treatment of other causes of cholestasis may improve outcomes by preventing complications of liver disease. The initial evaluation of an infant who presents with cholestasis as an outpatient is outlined in Figure 4G-1.

To assess for an inherited disorder, one should obtain a family history for cholestasis and any unexplained fetal or neonatal deaths. Maternal history should include prenatal maternal infections, blood transfusions, prescription or illicit drug use, and maternal cholestasis. The clinician should document prenatal ultrasound results to assess for choledochal cysts or bowel anomalies. One should obtain an infant history and assess for infections, surgeries, polycythemia, abnormal bleeding, and/or umbilical venous catheter placement. In addition, one should determine whether there was a history of isoimmune hemolysis, as 3% of infants with severe isoimmune hemolysis may have elevated direct bilirubin levels until age 2 weeks.[13]

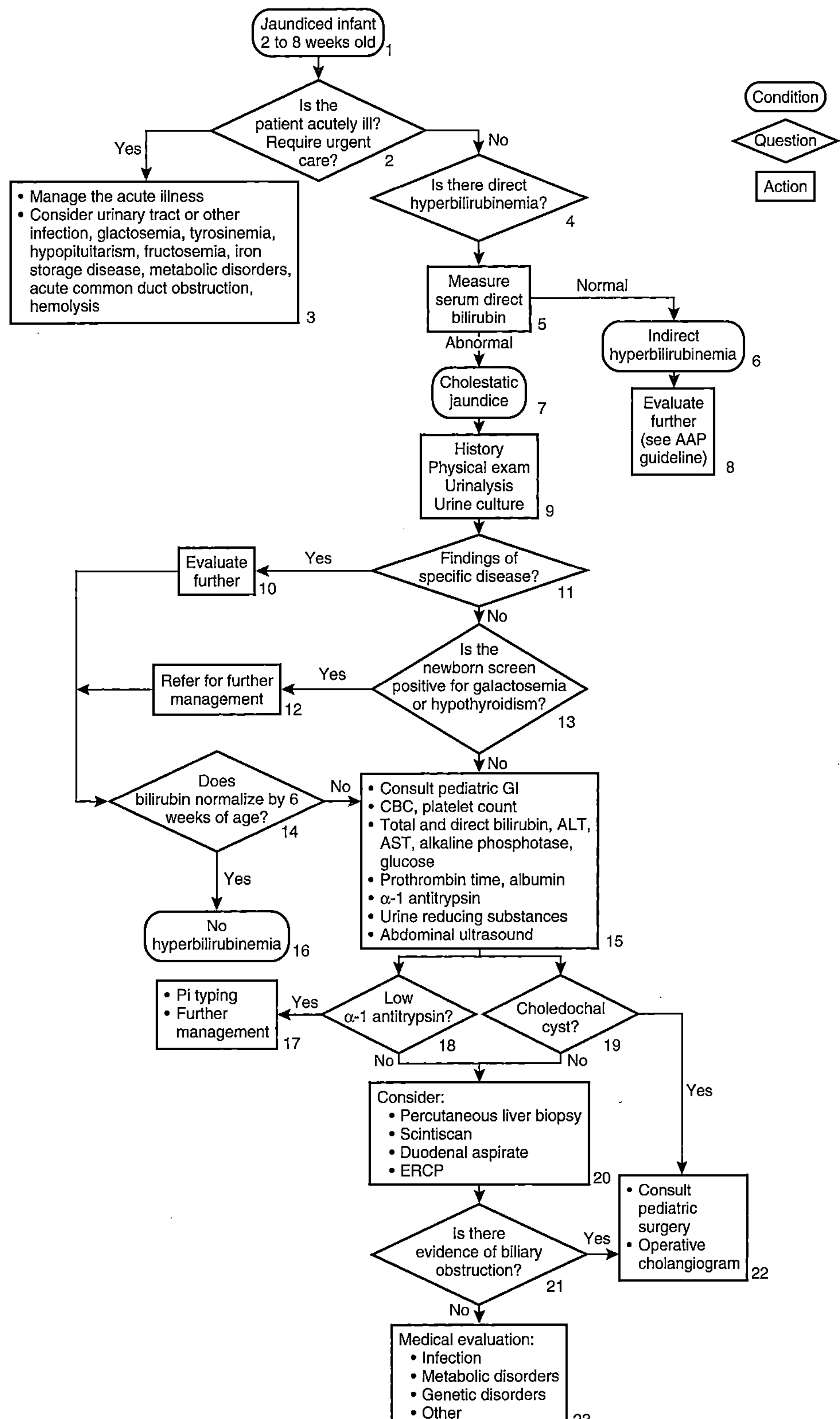

FIGURE 4G-1 Algorithm for neonatal cholestasis practice recommendations and guideline. From Moyer V, Freese DK, Whitington PF, et al: North American Society for Pediatric Gastroenterology, Hepatology and Nutrition: *J Pediatr Gastroenterol Nutr* 39(2):188, 2004. *AAP,* American Academy of Pediatrics; *ALT,* alanine transaminase; *AST,* aspartate transaminase; *CBC,* complete blood count; *ERCP,* endoscopic retrograde cholangiopancreatography; *GI,* gastroenterologist.

One should obtain results of the newborn state screen to assess for metabolic causes, such as galactosemia and hypothyroidism. The clinician should assess the infant's growth and nutrition, documenting the infant's current amount and type of feedings, stooling and urinary pattern, history of emesis, and weight gain since birth.

The physical examination should include a general assessment of wellness, neurologic findings, and nutritional status. The most common associated findings in infants with cholestasis are persistent jaundice, pale stools, and/or dark urine. Although most infants appear healthy, some infants fail to thrive. The clinician should assess for abdominal distention, ascites, hepatomegaly, splenomegaly, and abdominal masses. In addition to these nonspecific examination findings, some clinical features are associated with specific causes of cholestasis. Examples include cutaneous hemangiomas and hepatic or biliary hemangiomas; situs inversus and extrahepatic biliary atresia; purpura, chorioretinitis, myocarditis, and viral infections; cataracts and galactosemia; and facial characteristics (e.g., broad nasal bridge, triangular facies, and deep-set eyes), butterfly vertebrae, cardiac defects, and Alagille syndrome.

Laboratory and radiographic testing can help to differentiate cholestasis caused by hepatocellular versus obstructive disorders. Depending on the type of disorder, medical and/or surgical management may be indicated. To assist with the evaluation, referral to a pediatric gastroenterology specialist should be considered at this time.

The initial laboratory testing should include synthetic liver function tests by obtaining levels of serum albumin, coagulation factors, and serum ammonia. Aminotransferases and lactic dehydrogenase levels can determine hepatocyte integrity, whereas alkaline phosphatase and γ-glutamyl transpeptidase (GGTP) levels determine obstructive cholestasis secondary to metabolic or anatomic causes. The serum GGTP level may be helpful because elevated levels may signify biliary atresia or damage to the bile ducts.[14,15] Low GGTP levels might suggest a transport defect, such as progressive familial intrahepatic cholestasis, or a bile acid synthetic defect.[16,17] If the infant appears clinically ill, one should obtain blood, urine, and cerebrospinal fluid to identify a bacterial or viral etiology. If the newborn state screen does not test for galactosemia, one should test the urine for reducing substances. Specific laboratory testing, such as thyroid function tests, viral serologies, urine organic acid levels, serum amino acid levels, chloride sweat test, and α_1-antitrypsin testing, may be warranted, depending on the infant's history and physical examination.

Radiographic imaging is the next diagnostic step in identifying whether the underlying cause of cholestasis is hepatocellular inflammation or obstruction. Timely identification of cholestasis secondary to biliary atresia is warranted because surgical intervention will be necessary with a Kasai portoenterostomy, which is most effective if performed before 45 to 60 days of age. Because of their small size and likely exposure to parenteral nutrition, premature infants with cholestasis usually undergo initial abdominal ultrasound screening, and further radiographic imaging is deferred until the infant has reached a postmenstrual age of 40 weeks or weight >2000 g.[3,9] If resolution of cholestasis has not occurred by then, further radiographic imaging is indicated.[3]

Radiographic studies include abdominal ultrasonography, hepatobiliary scintigraphy, computed tomography, magnetic resonance cholangiopancreatography, and endoscopic retrograde cholangiopancreatography. These studies have potential limitations, such as limited availability at nontertiary centers, limited expertise, and cost/benefit ratios with high false-positive and false-negative results. After a review of the literature, NASPGHAN concludes that the hepatobiliary radionuclide scan and liver biopsy are the most valuable tools for determining whether surgical or medical management is preferable, with liver biopsy having the greatest accuracy to date.[3]

Abdominal ultrasound is an easy first test that is readily available and noninvasive. One can identify the size and texture of the liver, detect choledochal cysts, and identify structural abnormalities of the hepatobiliary tract. The study can assist in the diagnosis of biliary atresia; an inability to visualize the gallbladder or the presence of the triangular cord sign, described as a triangular-shaped periportal echogenic density, can be diagnostic.[18]

Hepatobiliary scintigraphy is another evaluative technique for infants with cholestasis. It is performed by injecting radioactive isotope and visualizing the radioactivity within the intestines 24 hours after the initial injection. Appropriate uptake of isotope but lack of excretion by 24 hours can indicate biliary obstruction (e.g., biliary atresia), whereas slow uptake of isotope with normal excretion can diagnose hepatocellular dysfunction and eliminate biliary atresia as a cause.[19] The scan is time consuming and expensive, with some false-positive and false-negative results. Hepatobiliary scintigraphy is not routinely recommended but may be useful if other tests to assess for biliary obstruction are not available.[3]

Computed tomography scans are useful in the detection and characterization of liver masses and may help to distinguish deposits of glycogen, lipid, and iron within the liver parenchyma. However, computed tomography is expensive and exposes the infant to radiation. Similarly, magnetic resonance cholangiopancreatography can identify masses or chemical deposits. However, magnetic resonance cholangiopancreatography usually involves deep sedation or anesthesia. Although this type of study may help to diagnose biliary atresia without the radioactive exposure of hepatobiliary scintigraphy or use of contrast, it is not currently recommended because of limited data.

Endoscopic retrograde cholangiopancreatography (ERCP) is used to detect biliary obstruction. It usually requires general anesthesia and clinical expertise in specialized centers because of the technical difficulty of the procedure. The technique involves injection of contrast through a catheter threaded endoscopically within the biliary and pancreatic ducts using a duodenoscope. ERCP is recommended before surgery only if liver biopsy results are equivocal.[3,18]

Percutaneous liver biopsy remains the single most definitive diagnostic procedure for the evaluation of cholestasis and can be performed on infants at age 1 week. It is recommended that this procedure be performed in most infants with cholestasis of unknown etiology before surgical intervention.[3,18] The tissue sample provides histologic and biochemical information used to identify metabolic, storage, or parenchymal disease. Accurate biopsy interpretation is dependent on the skill of the pathology specialist. The results of the biopsy may vary by the stage of the disease process; for example, infants in the early phase of biliary atresia may have liver biopsy results similar to those of hepatitis. Thus, infants with an equivocal biopsy result may require a repeat procedure.[3,18]

Management

The management of an infant with cholestasis depends on the underlying cause and should be coordinated with a gastroenterology specialist. If the infant's oral intake is inadequate to allow for weight gain, one should consider increasing calories, supplementing with nasogastric night feedings, and/or placing a gastrostomy tube. Increased caloric intake up to 125% of recommended daily requirements may be indicated because of rapid transit from short bowel or malabsorption.[9] The clinician should consider changing the infant to specialized formula preparations (e.g., Pregestimil, Alimentum), which contain medium-chain triglycerides that are more easily absorbed.[9] One should provide two to four times the recommended daily allowances of fat-soluble vitamins A, D, E, and K because these vitamins are poorly absorbed without the presence of bile acids in the intestine.[9] One should continue this supplementation for at least 3 months after the cholestasis resolves. A liquid form of vitamin E (vitamin E-TPGS, D-α-tocopheryl polyethylene glycol) often is used because it is absorbed more readily.[20] For infants who are receiving parenteral nutrition, one should consider cycling off parenteral nutrition for 4 to 6 hours each day while monitoring for hypoglycemia in an attempt to reduce the severity of the cholestasis.[8] Parenteral nutrition that provides amino acid preparations with TrophAmine appears less toxic to the liver.[8] Further adjustments in parenteral nutrition might include supplementation with taurine and glutamine, alteration of mineral concentrations of copper and magnesium to minimize mineral accumulation, and limiting intake of lipids.[8] One should initiate enteral feedings as soon as possible to stimulate bile flow.[8]

Medical management is limited and believed to be purely supportive. Drug therapy can be considered, especially if the cholestasis is attributable to inflammation instead of obstruction, but is not routinely recommended. Phenobarbital increases conjugation and excretion of bilirubin by inducing hepatic microsomal enzymes and enhancing bile acid synthesis. Phenobarbital is not routinely recommended because it has sedating effects, may have long-term implications for the undeveloped nervous system, and may increase the risk for rickets.[8,9] Ursodeoxycholic acid is a hydrophilic acid, which functions by altering the bile pool and replacing toxic bile acids. There are anecdotal concerns of potential adverse outcomes if ursodeoxycholic acid is administered, including the risk for gram-negative sepsis and necrotizing enterocolitis.[8] Furthermore, the efficacy of ursodeoxycholic acid has not been confirmed.

Other potential therapies that are not well studied include (1) cholecystokinin-octapeptide (a gastrointestinal hormone that induces the gallbladder to contract, thus stimulating intrahepatic bile flow); (2) cholestyramine (an anion exchange resin that binds bile acids in the intestinal lumen, blocking the circulation of bile acids and increasing excretion; may lead to a metabolic acidosis); and (3) rifampin (an antibiotic that induces hepatic microsomal enzymes and inhibits bile acid uptake by the hepatocyte; may lead to rickets, particularly in premature infants).[9] Ongoing trials are investigating other medical approaches for treatment of cholestasis, including increasing the supplementation of specific fatty acids.

Surgical management includes the Kasai porto enterostomy in infants with biliary atresia. This procedure increases the chance of re-establishing bile flow and prolongs survival if performed before 45 to 60 days of life.[12,21-23] Because of a guarded long-term prognosis following the Kasai procedure, liver transplantation may be necessary.[10] Infants with an obstruction, such as a choledochal cyst, also require surgical intervention.

Specific Management Issues in a Premature Infant with Cholestasis

Many premature infants are discharged from the hospital with persistent cholestasis. If these infants are otherwise well, the primary care provider should ensure that the infants are receiving adequate amounts of fat-soluble vitamins. Infants should be followed regularly during the first year of life to ensure that there are no signs of portal hypertension or persistent hepatic injury. Cholestasis will resolve in the majority of premature infants. If cholestasis worsens or persists 2 to 3 months after discharge, further evaluation is warranted to assess for continuing hepatic injury.

Conclusion

Although the presentation of cholestatic jaundice in an infant is an uncommon issue for primary caregivers, the clinician must be aware of the appropriate evaluation and management. Referral to a pediatric gastroenterology specialist for further laboratory and radiographic testing will ensure timely diagnosis and treatment as well as limit further liver injury. Rapid diagnosis and management of the infant with cholestasis are of utmost importance in improving outcomes.

Resources for Families and Clinicians

NASPGHAN: North American Society for Pediatric Gastroenterology, Hepatology and Nutrition
http://www.naspghan.org

This website provides information to families about specific gastrointestinal disorders. For handouts about biliary atresia in English, Spanish or French, click on "public information" then "disease information" and then "biliary atresia."

http://www.naspghan.org/PDF/PositionPapers/CholestaticJaundiceInInfants.pdf

This website provides the NASPGHAN guidelines for management of cholestasis.

Acknowledgment

The authors thank Jon Watkins, MD, for critical review of this chapter.

REFERENCES

1. Dick MC, Mowat AP: Hepatitis syndrome in infancy: an epidemiologic survey with 10-year follow up. *Arch Dis Child* 60:512-516, 1985.
2. Balistreri WF: Neonatal cholestasis. *J Pediatr* 106:171-184, 1985.
3. Moyer V, Freese DK, Whitington PF, et al: North American Society for Pediatric Gastroenterology, Hepatology and Nutrition: Guideline for the evaluation of cholestatic jaundice in infants: recommendations of the North American Society for Pediatric Gastroenterology, Hepatology and Nutrition. *J Pediatr Gastroenterol Nutr* 39(2):115-128, 2004.
4. Askin DF, Diehl-Jones WL: The neonatal liver: Part III: pathophysiology of liver dysfunction. *Neonatal Netw* 22: 5-15, 2003.
5. el-Youssef M, Whitington PF: Diagnostic approach to the child with hepatobiliary disease. *Semin Liver Dis* 18:195-202, 1998.
6. Bates MD, Bucuvalas JC, Alonso MH, et al: Biliary atresia: pathogenesis and treatment. *Semin Liver Dis* 18:281-293, 1998.
7. D'Agata ID, Balistreri WF: Evaluation of liver disease in the pediatric patient. *Pediatr Rev* 20:376-398, 1999.
8. Hansen AR, Cloherty J: Pathological consequences and management of cholestasis. *Clinical Working Group*, October 2003 at Children's Hospital, Department of Neonatology, Boston, MA.
9. Venigalla S, Gourley GR: Neonatal cholestasis. *Semin Perinatol* 28(5):348-355, 2004.
10. Abrams SH, Shulman RJ: Causes of neonatal cholestasis. *UpToDate.* Available at: *uptodate.com.*
11. Teitelbaum DH: Parenteral nutrition-associated cholestasis. *Curr Opin Pediatr* 9:270-275, 1997.
12. Chardot C, Carton M, Spire-Benelac N, et al: Is the Kasai operation still indicated in children older than 3 months diagnosed with biliary atresia? *J Pediatr* 138:224-228, 2001.
13. Sivan Y, Merlob P, Nutman J, et al: Direct hyperbilirubinemia complicating ABO hemolytic disease of the newborn. *Clin Pediatr* 22:537-538, 1983.
14. Wright K, Christie DL: Use of gamma-glutamyl transpeptidase in the diagnosis of extrahepatic biliary atresia. *Am J Dis Child* 135:134-136, 1981.
15. Maggiore G, Bernard O, Hadchouel M, et al: Diagnostic value of serum gamma-glutamyl transpeptidase activity in liver diseases in children. *J Pediatr Gastroenterol Nutr* 12:21-26, 1991.
16. Bezerra J, Shneider BL: Genetic modifiers of cholestatic liver disease: evolving field. *J Pediatr Gastroenterol Nutr* 42(1):7-8, 2006.
17. Hermeziu B, Sanlaville D, Girard M, et al: Heterozygous bile salt export pump deficiency: a possible genetic predisposition to transient neonatal cholestasis. *J Pediatr Gastroenterol Nutr* 42(1):114-116, 2006.
18. Abrams SH, Shulman RJ: Approach to neonatal cholestasis. *UpToDate.* Available at: *uptodate.com.*
19. McLin VA, Balisteri WF: Approach to neonatal cholestasis. In Walker WA, Golet O, Kleinman RE, et al., editors: *Pediatric gastrointestinal disease: pathopsychology, diagnosis, management*, ed 4. Hamilton, Ontario, Canada, 2004, BC Decker.
20. Sokol RJ, Heubi JE, Butler-Simon N, et al: Treatment of vitamin E deficiency during chronic childhood cholestasis with oral d-alpha-tocopheryl polyethylene glycol-1000 succinate. *Gastroenterology* 93(5):975-985, 1987.
21. Mieli-Vergani G, Howard ER, Portman B, et al: Late referral for biliary atresia-missed opportunities for effective surgery. *Lancet* 1:421-422, 1989.
22. Altman RP, Lilly JR, Greenfeld J, et al: A multivariable risk factor analysis of the portoenterostomy (Kasai) procedure for biliary atresia: *Ann Surg* 226:348-353, 1997.
23. Mowat AP, Davidson LL, Dick MC: Earlier identification of biliary atresia and hepatobiliary disease: selective screening in the third week of life. *Arch Dis Child* 72:90-92, 1995.

GENERAL REFERENCES

Bisgard LD: Visual diagnosis: a 10-week old infant who has jaundice. *Pediatr Rev* 22(12):408-412, 2001.

Chen CY, Tsao PN, Chen HL, et al: Ursodeoxycholic acid (UDCA) therapy in very-low-birth-weight infants with parenteral nutrition-associated cholestasis. *J Pediatr* 145(3):317-321, 2004.

Diehl-Jones WL, Askin DF: The neonatal liver: part II: assessment and diagnosis of liver dysfunction. *Neonatal Netw* 22(2):7-15, 2003.

Diehl-Jones WL, Askin DF: The neonatal liver: part I: embryology, anatomy, and physiology. *Neonatal Netw* 21(2):5-12, 2002.

Ferenchak AP, Ramirez RO, Sokol RJ: Medical and nutritional management of cholestasis. In Suchy FJ, Sokol RJ, Balistreri WF, editors: *Liver disease in children,* ed 2. Philadelphia, 2002, Lippincott Williams & Wilkins.

Hengst JM: Direct hyperbilirubinemia: a case study of parenteral nutrition-induced cholestatic jaundice. *Neonatal Netw.* 21(4):57-69, 2002.

Karpen SJ: Update on the etiologies and management of neonatal cholestasis. *Clin Perinatol* 29(1):159-180, 2002.

Pratt CA, Garcia MG, Kerner JA: Nutritional management of neonatal and infant liver disease. *NeoReviews* 2:e215-e222, 2001.

Suchy FJ: Neonatal cholestasis. *Pediatr Rev* 25(11):388-396, 2004.

Suchy FJ: Approach to the infant with cholestasis. In Suchy FJ, Sokol RJ, Balistreri WF, editors: *Liver disease in children,* ed 2. Philadelphia, 2001, Lippincott Williams & Wilkins.

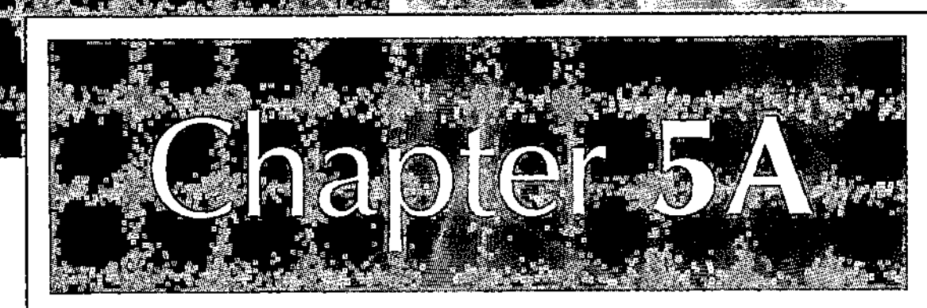

Intraventricular Hemorrhage and Posthemorrhagic Hydrocephalus

Vincent C. Smith, MD, MPH

Intraventricular Hemorrhage

Intraventricular hemorrhage (IVH) occurs in approximately 35% to 40% of infants born less than 35 weeks' gestation.[1,2] The incidence of IVH increases with earlier gestational age and lower birth weight.[3] Improvement in obstetric and neonatal medical management as well as a greater understanding of neonatal pathophysiology has decreased the overall incidence of IVH.[4] These same advances in care ensure the survival of more very-low-birth-weight (VLBW) premature infants, thus guaranteeing the persistence of IVH and its complication—posthemorrhagic hydrocephalus (PHH).[3]

Clinical presentation

The timing and spectrum of the clinical presentation of IVH vary. The occurrence of IVH within the first 6 hours of birth varies between 25% and 70%.[5] Clinical symptoms may not be present for hours to weeks after the initial incident. Symptoms range from silent incidental findings to cataclysmic deterioration.[3] In half of the silent cases, a sudden drop in the infant's hematocrit level is the only clinical sign of IVH.[3]

In intermediate cases, there can be any compilation of the following symptoms: bulging anterior fontanel, a change in muscular tone and/or activity, seizures, apnea, respiratory distress, abnormal eye findings (staring, persistent vertical or horizontal nystagmus, anisocoria, lack of pupillary reaction to light in infants older than 29 weeks' gestational age, and/or lack of an oculovestibular response), and tight popliteal angle.[3,6-9]

Severe cases usually result from an acute, rapidly evolving hemorrhage. These infants can progress quickly from normal to decerebrate posturing and coma.[3] Infants also may have symptoms that progress in a staggered pattern over several days. Regardless of the rate of clinical progression in these severe cases, the outcome is poor.

Etiology

The precise etiology of IVH is not completely understood. It is, however, primarily associated with premature birth. Several factors about the premature brain make it more susceptible to IVH. First, premature infants have a germinal matrix, which is located below the ventricular lining at the level of the head of the caudate nucleus. This region is thought to be the place of origin of most cases of IVH in premature infants.[6] The germinal matrix is a site of neuronal and glial proliferation. It becomes very cellular and gives rise to a fragile group of blood vessels beginning at approximately 10 weeks' gestation.[6] The germinal matrix disappears by term gestational age.[6] This highly vascular area is exquisitely sensitive to hypoxia and dramatic fluctuations in the systemic or cerebral circulation, making it prone to rupture and hemorrhage.[3,10,11] Experimental studies in premature baboons show that rapid restoration of blood pressure after acute hypotension results in a supernormal increase in blood flow to the regions of maximum perfusion, including the brain.[12] Similarly, stressed infants who receive blood or albumin respond to the increased circulating volume by increasing cerebral blood flow out of proportion to the increase in mean arterial blood pressure.[12] The combination of a maximally dilated cerebrovascular bed after volume expansion and immature vessels in a poorly supported matrix may lead to capillary overdistention and leakage of blood.[12]

The premature infant also is at greater risk for IVH because cerebral perfusion in a stressed premature infant is pressure passive.[6] Specifically, cerebral blood flow varies directly with arterial blood pressure. Therefore, fluctuations in arterial blood pressure may lead to decreased cerebral perfusion followed by excessive reperfusion, which may lead to hemorrhage.[3,6,13,14] Oxygen free radical production after perfusion[14] and aggressive local fibrinolytic activity also may contribute to the initial injury. [3]

Risk factors

The infants at highest risk are born at an earlier gestational age, have a greater need for resuscitation in the delivery room (1-minute Apgar score <5), require higher positive inspiratory pressure and inspired oxygen concentration, and have higher partial pressure of carbon dioxide.[15,16] Stable preterm infants who have intact cerebrovascular regulation are at low risk for IVH.[5]

A persistent patent ductus arteriosus and rapid volume expansion are associated with fluctuations in cerebral blood flow and increase the risk for IVH.[5] Rapid infusion of hypertonic solutions, such as sodium bicarbonate, also has been implicated in the development of IVH.[9] Intubated premature infants are especially at risk for IVH because mechanical ventilation can cause fluctuations in arterial blood pressure.[13] Depending on the type of ventilation, there also can be impedance of venous return, further increasing the infant's chance of developing IVH.[13] In addition, a high inspired oxygen concentration during the first 24 hours of life increases the possibility of IVH.[4] An obstructed endotracheal tube and a pneumothorax are additional risk factors for the development of IVH.[6] In all of these scenarios, it is not clear whether it is the intervention or the *need* for the intervention that increases the likelihood of developing IVH.

Finally, some evidence indicates that the conditions of conception and birth play a role in the formation of IVH. Fertility treatments (particularly in vitro fertilization) may be associated with an increased risk of severe IVH.[4]

Diagnosis

Ultrasound has replaced computed tomography as the modality of choice for the diagnosis of IVH and PHH.[2,11] It has the advantage of being portable, accurate, fast, and safe.[11] Once IVH is diagnosed, a neonatologist usually obtains weekly ultrasounds to monitor for progression of the hemorrhage and development of PHH.[2,11] For infants who have rapidly progressive hemorrhage or ventricular dilatation, more frequent monitoring is needed. Signs of increased intracranial pressure (ICP), such as occipital–frontal head circumference expansion greater 2 cm/wk, merit more frequent monitoring.[11]

Grading system

The system established by Papile et al.[7] traditionally has been used to grade IVH:

1. Grade I is a hemorrhage confined to the germinal matrix.
2. Grade II is a hemorrhage within the germinal matrix and intraventricular regions without ventricular dilatation.
3. Grade III is IVH with ventricular dilatation.
4. Grade IV is IVH with ventricular enlargement and a parenchymal hemorrhage extending beyond the germinal matrix.[3,7]

Figure 5A-1 shows images corresponding to these grades. Because this type of classification may oversimplify or misrepresent the actual findings, classification using a more descriptive staging is preferred (e.g., moderate left IVH with mild ventricular dilatation).[17]

Management and follow-up

See section on posthemorrhagic hydrocephalus.

Prevention

The ideal method for preventing IVH would be to eliminate premature births; unfortunately, this is not currently possible. Treating pregnant women in preterm labor with antenatal steroids currently is the only strategy that consistently has been shown to lower the risk of IVH.[4] Although some studies have demonstrated prevention of IVH by prophylactic indomethacin treatment,[18-21] improvements in long-term morbidity have not been demonstrated.[22-24] Some studies suggest that infants born by cesarian section are at lower risk for IVH,[16,25] but this has not been supported by other studies.[15] Other unproven pharmacologic interventions that might decrease the incidence of IVH include muscle paralysis (to stabilize cerebral blood flow), phenobarbital, vitamin E, and ethamsylate.[10] Similar to indomethacin prophylaxis, these interventions still may not be able to reduce mortality or disability.[10]

Posthemorrhagic Hydrocephalus

Etiology

PHH is a complication of IVH that can occur in up to 25% to 35% of VLBW infants with IVH.[3,11,26] PHH primarily results from an increase in ICP resulting from an imbalance between cerebrospinal fluid (CSF) absorption and production. The imbalance can be due to an obstruction by clots or other debris, which impedes circulation and reabsorption of CSF.[2,3,10,11,27,28] An inflammatory response to

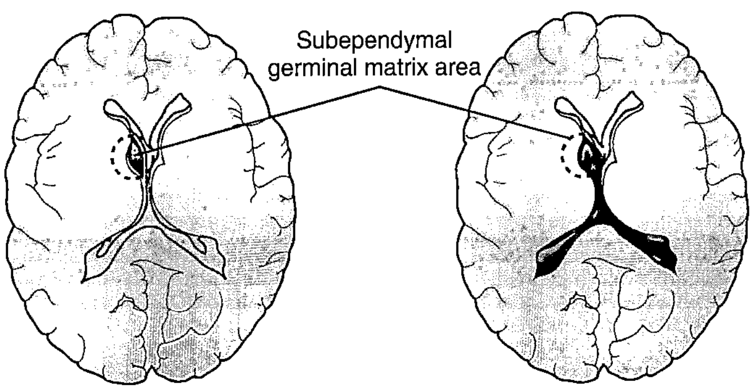

Grade I–subependymal hemorrhage only

Grade II–intraventricular hemorrhage without ventricular dilation

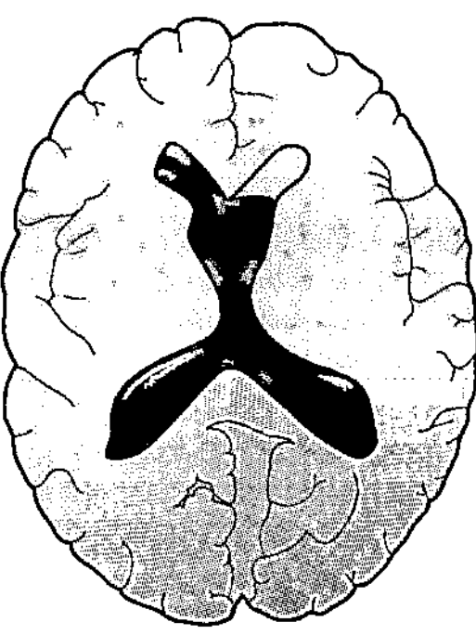

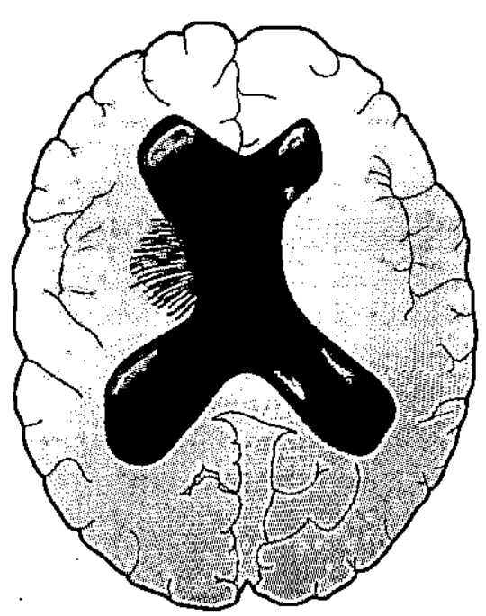

Grade III–intraventricular hemorrhage with ventricular dilation

Grade IV–intraventricular hemorrhage with parenchymal hemorrhage

FIGURE 5A-1 Grading system. (From Rozmus C: *Matern Child Nurs* 17:79,1992.)

blood can lead to an adhesive arachnoiditis within the basilar cisterns, posterior fossa, and arachnoid granulations.[3] This arachnoiditis can cause obliteration, principally affecting the posterior fossa, and lead to ventricular dilatation.[2,11,27]

Clinical signs

Generally, ventricular dilatation is subacute, occurring 1 to 3 weeks after IVH.[3,11] Once observed, dilatation may progress along several paths:

1. Resolve spontaneously,
2. Stabilize but remain dilated without symptoms, or
3. Progressively expand the ventricular size, causing symptomatic increased ICP.[11]

The clinical signs in the third type of ventricular dilatation usually are attributed to the increase in ICP[11] and usually occur days to weeks following IVH.[2] Classic findings include a bulging anterior fontanel, widely separated cranial sutures, and an inappropriate increase in the occipital–frontal head circumference (>2 cm/wk).[2,11] Other symptoms of PHH often are mild and nonspecific, such as lethargy, poor feeding, or increased frequency or severity of apnea and bradycardia.[11]

It is important to note that PHH is not always associated with abnormal head growth.[6] This is because the preterm infant brain has a paucity of myelin, increased water content, and large subarachnoid spaces.[3] These factors can prevent an increase in ICP even though the ventricles are dilated.[3] However, infants with ventricular dilatation alone may still be at risk for neurologic deficits.[3]

It is important to distinguish ex vacuo ventricular dilatation from PHH. The former is due to atrophy of brain matter usually caused by perinatal asphyxia.[3,11] The time course is different for these two entities. Whereas PHH occurs 1 to 3 weeks after the IVH, ex vacuo ventricular dilatation occurs several months after the incident.[3]

Risk factors

The risk factors for PHH are similar to the risk factors for IVH. Infants born less than 32 weeks' gestation or have birth weight less than 1500 g are at greatest risk. The strongest predictor of progressive ventricular dilatation is the severity of IVH.[26] Eighty percent of infants who have parenchymal involvement will develop PHH.[3]

Predictors of ventricular dilatation in VLBW infants with IVH include smaller, more immature, infants who are extremely ill during the first 12 hours of life, especially those requiring inotropic support.[26] Ventricular enlargement has been shown to be a more significant predictor of having IQ less than 70 compared with birth weight, gestational age, Apgar score less than 5, bronchopulmonary dysplasia, sepsis, grade of IVH, presence of periventricular leukomalacia, and maternal education.[29]

Inpatient management of PHH

The literature reports that approximately 19% to 65% of infants with progressive ventricular dilatation have spontaneous arrest of ventricular dilatation without medical treatment within 1 month of onset.[11,26] In these cases, ICP has remained at an acceptable level of less than 80 to 100 mm H_2O.[11] Any signs of increased ICP are indications for therapeutic intervention.[1,11] Management also should be considered if rapid ventricular dilatation is detected on ultrasound or if the ventricular diameter exceeds 1.5 cm.[1]

PHH remains a serious problem without adequate treatment.[28,30] The two basic strategies for temporary treatment are (1) reducing CSF production and (2) increasing CSF elimination. Management can include serial lumbar punctures;[1,11,31] medications to halt CSF production (including carbonic anhydrase inhibitors, adenosine, triphosphate inhibitors, osmotic agents, and diuretics);[2,3,11,28,32,33] and/or placement of surgical shunts.[1,11,31] Because no definitive treatment is available, treatment choices should be based on the pros and cons of each intervention.[3] Currently, no management strategy has proven to be uniformly efficacious.[11]

Serial lumbar punctures (LPs) are often the first-line treatment of PHH. However, in order for LPs to be effective, both communication between the ventricles and the lumbar subarachnoid space and removal of 10 to 15 ml/kg of CSF must be achieved with each LP.[3,11,28] LPs should be repeated when signs of increased ICP occur. The timing of LPs ranges from every 24 hours to weekly, depending on the return of symptoms.[11] This procedure generally is well tolerated and is without complications. However, with serial LPs, achieving an adequate volume of CSF removal each time occasionally is difficult.[28] In addition, some evidence indicates that this form of treatment increases the risk for CSF infection.[30] The rate of infection (including epidural abscess, vertebral osteomyelitis, and arachnoiditis) associated with multiple LPs is 9% to 27%.[3,11,28] Other possible complications include hyponatremia, chordoma, and intraspinal epidermoid tumor.[11] When LPs are compared with conservative therapy, the relative risk for shunt placement, death, a disability, and multiple disabilities is close to 1.0 with no statistically significant effect.[28,30] Although serial LPs have been shown to decrease the rate of ventricular expansion, they have not been shown to change the natural history of PHH.[3] Often the aqueduct of Sylvius becomes blocked with clots and debris, preventing use of serial LPs as a viable therapy.

Medications that decrease CSF production (e.g., acetazolamide and furosemide) when used together can produce almost complete cessation of CSF production.[3] Potential complications associated with their use include metabolic acidosis, electrolyte imbalance, dehydration, and hypercalciuria.[3,28] Nephrocalcinosis also has been reported.[3,28,32] A meta-analysis showed that use of diuretic therapy did not reduce the risk for placement of a ventriculoperitoneal (VP) shunt.[32] A slight increase in risk for motor impairment at age 1 year in infants treated with acetazolamide and furosemide has been suggested.[32] Currently, diuretic therapy is not recommended as a safe or effective treatment of PHH.[3,32] Other osmotic agents, such as glycerol and isosorbide, have been used to reduce CSF production by increasing the serum osmolarity.[3] Emesis and diarrhea are common side effects.[3]

Phenobarbital has been suggested as a safe prophylactic treatment to stabilize blood pressure and reduce the risk of IVH; however meta-analysis does not support this suggestion and has actually shown an increased risk for mechanical ventilation.[14] Phenobarbital currently is not recommended in the management of IVH.[5] Fibrinolytic therapy also has been used to treat IVH. However, intraventricular streptokinase after IVH is *not* recommended over conservative approaches (such as serial LPs and VP shunt) to drain CSF.[32]

Serial percutaneous ventricular punctures can be used to temporarily treat PHH.[28] However, this practice has been associated with subdural or parenchymal hemorrhage.[28] Areas of encephalomalacia and porencephaly can develop along the needle tracts, especially in the presence of hydrocephalus.[3,28] The risk for complications makes this an unacceptable long-term treatment.[3]

External ventricular drains are easy to insert and will control the ICP and ventricular dilatation in the short term.[3] However, there is significant risk for infection (reported 11%–60%) with these devices.[3] The longer the device is in place, the higher the risk for infection. These devices can become occluded or dislodged.[3] Placement of these drains is not an effective treatment of PHH if the devices are expected to be in place for more than a few weeks.[3]

Ventriculosubgaleal shunts have been used as temporizing measures until an infant can receive a VP shunt.[33] This type of shunt drains CSF into a surgically created subgaleal pocket.[3] Ventriculosubgaleal shunts have been used for more than 100 years for temporary CSF diversion.[33] Tubbs et al.[34] reported that the survival time of these primary shunts is 32.2 days and that the shunts can last for approximately 2.5 months with intermittent subgaleal shunt revisions.[35]

Complications with ventriculosubgaleal shunts include infection, intracranial hemorrhage, and wound leakage.[33] Hudgins[3] reported a 17% incidence of a second ventriculosubgaleal placement, 10% infection rate, and 90% incidence of permanent shunt placement. Ventriculosubgaleal shunts offer a simple, effective, and relatively safe means of temporizing hydrocephalus.[33,34,36]

The definitive treatment for progressive PHH is placement of a VP shunt[11] (see Chapter 5B for further details).

Outpatient management of PHH or intraparenchymal hemorrhage

Currently, neonatologists usually order a head ultrasound for all infants who are born less than 32 weeks' gestation or are born weighing less than 1500 g. If IVH is identified, the neonatologist will monitor for progression with weekly ultrasounds; surgical management may be required before discharge. Regardless of the neonatal management, the primary care provider must continue to closely follow infants with a grade III IVH, PHH, or white matter injury (see Figure 5A-2 for a suggested algorithm). This monitoring includes regular neurologic examinations, measuring head circumferences, and assessing the infant's developmental milestones and cognitive function. All of these infants require early intervention and infant follow-up clinic (if available). The provider also can consider referral to a pediatric neurology specialist. If the infant remains stable, continued *monthly* monitoring by either the neurology specialist or the primary care provider is recommended for 12 months. Infants with abnormal findings should be referred to a pediatric neurology specialist. In addition, brain magnetic resonance imaging is recommended to assess for (or assess extent of) white matter injury 3 to 6 months after discharge.

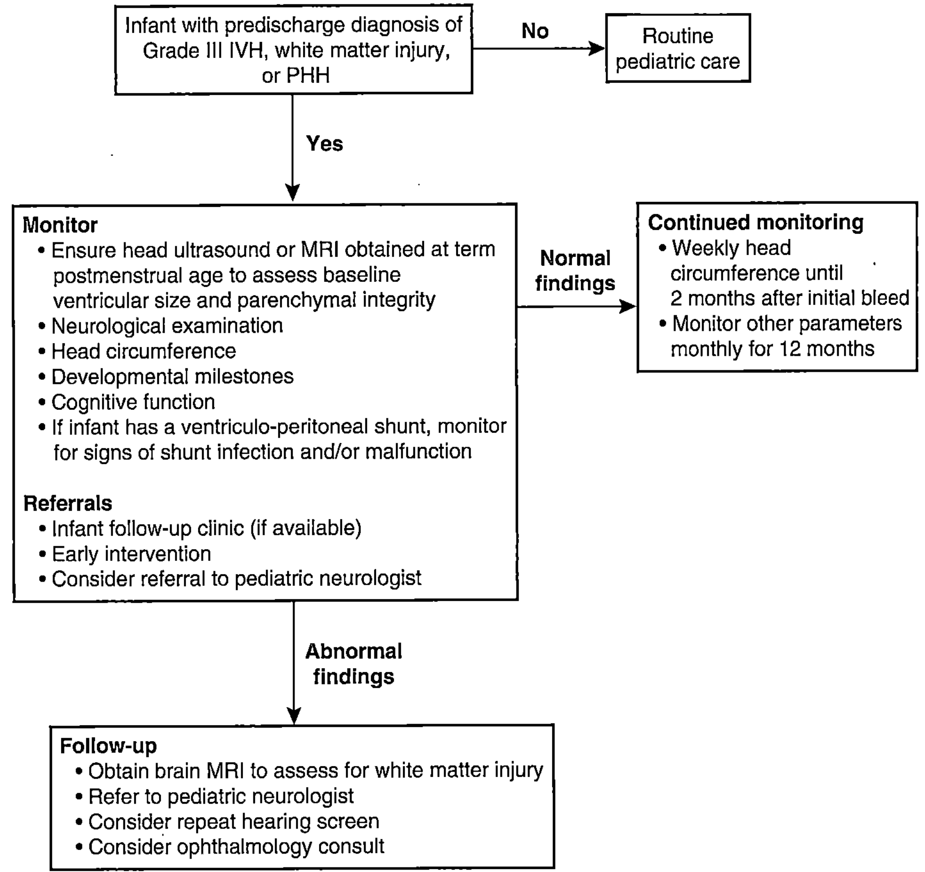

FIGURE 5A-2 Algorithm for outpatient management of an infant with grade III IVH, white matter injury, or PHH. *Refer to Chapter 5C. Please note that this is a recommended algorithm that does not represent a professional standard of care; care should be revised to meet individual patient needs.

Resources for Families and Clinicians

Hydrocephalus Association (HA)
870 Market Street, Suite 705, San Francisco, CA 94102
Phone: (415) 732-7040; (888) 598-3789 (provides personal one-on-one support)
www.hydroassoc.org

Hydrocephalus Foundation, Inc. (HyFI)
910 Rear Broadway, Saugus, MA 01906
Phone: (781) 942-1161
www.hydrocephalus.org

Provides support, educational resources, and networking opportunities to patients and families affected by hydrocephalus.

REFERENCES

1. Allan WC, Holt PJ, Sawyer LR, et al: Ventricular dilation after neonatal periventricular-intraventricular hemorrhage. Natural history and therapeutic implications. *Am J Dis Child* 136(7):589-593, 1982.
2. Hill A: Ventricular dilation following intraventricular hemorrhage in the premature infant. *Can J Neurol Sci* 10(2):81-85, 1983.
3. Hudgins RJ: Posthemorrhagic hydrocephalus of infancy. *Neurosurg Clin N Am* 12(4):743-751, ix, 2001.
4. Linder N, Haskin O, Levit O, et al: Risk factors for intraventricular hemorrhage in very low birth weight premature infants: a retrospective case-control study. *Pediatrics* 111 (5 pt 1):e590-595, 2003.
5. Roland EH, Hill A: Intraventricular hemorrhage and posthemorrhagic hydrocephalus. Current and potential future interventions. *Clin Perinatol* 24(3):589-605, 1997.
6. Allan WC: The IVH complex of lesions: cerebrovascular injury in the preterm infant. *Neurol Clin* 8(3):529-551, 1990.
7. Papile LA, Burstein J, Burstein R, et al: Incidence and evolution of subependymal and intraventricular hemorrhage: a study of infants with birth weights less than 1,500 gm. *J Pediatr* 92(4):529-534, 1978.
8. Hanigan WC, Powell FC, Miller TC, et al: Symptomatic intracranial hemorrhage in full-term infants. *Childs Nerv Syst* 11(12):698-707, 1995.
9. Mitchell W, O'Tuama L: Cerebral intraventricular hemorrhages in infants: a widening age spectrum. *Pediatrics* 65(1):35-39, 1980.
10. Whitelaw A: Intraventricular haemorrhage and posthaemorrhagic hydrocephalus: pathogenesis, prevention and future interventions. *Semin Neonatol* 6(2):135-146, 2001.
11. Hansen AR, Snyder EY: Medical management of neonatal posthemorrhagic hydrocephalus. *Neurosurg Clin N Am* 9(1):95-104, 1998.
12. Goddard-Finegold J, Armstrong D, Zeller RS: Intraventricular hemorrhage, following volume expansion after hypovolemic hypotension in the newborn beagle. *J Pediatr* 100(5):796-799, 1982.
13. Perlman J, Thach B: Respiratory origin of fluctuations in arterial blood pressure in premature infants with respiratory distress syndrome. *Pediatrics* 81(3):399-403, 1988.
14. Whitelaw A: Postnatal phenobarbitone for the prevention of intraventricular hemorrhage in preterm infants. *Cochrane Database Syst Rev* (1):CD001691, 2001.
15. Ment LR, Duncan CC, Ehrenkranz RA, et al: Intraventricular hemorrhage in the preterm neonate: timing and cerebral blood flow changes. *J Pediatr* 104(3):419-425, 1984.
16. Osborn DA, Evans N, Kluckow M: Hemodynamic and antecedent risk factors of early and late periventricular/intraventricular hemorrhage in premature infants. *Pediatrics* 112(1 pt 1):33-39, 2003.
17. Vasileiadis GT: Grading intraventricular hemorrhage with no grades. *Pediatrics* 113(4):930-931; author reply 930-931, 2004.
18. Ment LR, Vohr BR, Makuch RW, et al: Prevention of intraventricular hemorrhage by indomethacin in male preterm infants. *J Pediatr* 145(6):832-834, 2004.
19. Herrera C, Holberton J, Davis P: Prolonged versus short course of indomethacin for the treatment of patent ductus arteriosus in preterm infants. *Cochrane Database Syst Rev* (1):CD003480, 2004.
20. Yanowitz TD, Baker RW, Sobchak Brozanski B: Prophylactic indomethacin reduces grades III and IV intraventricular hemorrhages when compared to early indomethacin treatment of a patent ductus arteriosus. *J Perinatol* 23(4): 317-322, 2003.
21. Ment LR, Duncan CC, Ehrenkranz RA, et al: Randomized indomethacin trial for prevention of intraventricular hemorrhage in very low birth weight infants. *J Pediatr* 107(6):937-943, 1985.
22. Fowlie PW, Davis PG: Prophylactic indomethacin for preterm infants: a systematic review and meta-analysis. *Arch Dis Child Fetal Neonatal Ed* 88(6):F464-466, 2003.
23. Schmidt B, Davis P, Moddemann D, et al: Long-term effects of indomethacin prophylaxis in extremely-low-birth-weight infants. *N Engl J Med* 344(26):1966-1972, 2001.
24. Vohr BR, Allan WC, Westerveld M, et al: School-age outcomes of very low birth weight infants in the indomethacin intraventricular hemorrhage prevention trial. *Pediatrics* 111(4 pt 1):e340-e346, 2003.
25. Leviton A, Kuban KC, Pagano M, et al: Antenatal corticosteroids appear to reduce the risk of postnatal germinal matrix hemorrhage in intubated low birth weight newborns. *Pediatrics* 91(6):1083-1088, 1993.
26. Murphy BP, Inder TE, Rooks V, et al: Posthaemorrhagic ventricular dilatation in the premature infant: natural history and predictors of outcome. *Arch Dis Child Fetal Neonatal Ed* 87(1):F37-F41, 2002.
27. Hill A, Shackelford GD, Volpe JJ: A potential mechanism of pathogenesis for early posthemorrhagic hydrocephalus in the premature newborn. *Pediatrics* 73(1):19-21, 1984.
28. Hudgins RJ, Boydston WR, Gilreath CL: Treatment of posthemorrhagic hydrocephalus in the preterm infant with a ventricular access device. *Pediatr Neurosurg* 29(6):309-313, 1998.
29. Ment LR, Vohr B, Allan W, et al: The etiology and outcome of cerebral ventriculomegaly at term in very low birth weight preterm infants. *Pediatrics* 104(2 pt 1):243-248, 1999.
30. Whitelaw A: Repeated lumbar or ventricular punctures in newborns with intraventricular hemorrhage. *Cochrane Database Syst Rev* (1):CD000216, 2001.
31. Bergman I, Bauer RE, Barmada MA, et al: Intracerebral hemorrhage in the full-term neonatal infant. *Pediatrics* 75(3):488-496, 1985.
32. Whitelaw A, Kennedy CR, Brion LP: Diuretic therapy for newborn infants with posthemorrhagic ventricular dilatation. *Cochrane Database Syst Rev* (2):CD002270, 2001.
33. Tubbs RS, Banks JT, Soleau S, et al: Complications of ventriculosubgaleal shunts in infants and children. *Childs Nerv Syst* 21(1):48-51, 2005.
34. Tubbs RS, Smyth MD, Wellons JC 3rd, et al: Alternative uses for the subgaleal shunt in pediatric neurosurgery. *Pediatr Neurosurg* 39(1):22-24, 2003.
35. Tubbs RS, Smyth MD, Wellons JC, 3rd, et al: Life expectancy of ventriculosubgaleal shunt revisions. *Pediatr Neurosurg* 38(5):244-246, 2003.
36. Fulmer BB, Grabb PA, Oakes WJ, et al: Neonatal ventriculosubgaleal shunts. *Neurosurgery* 47(1):80-83; discussion 83-84, 2000.

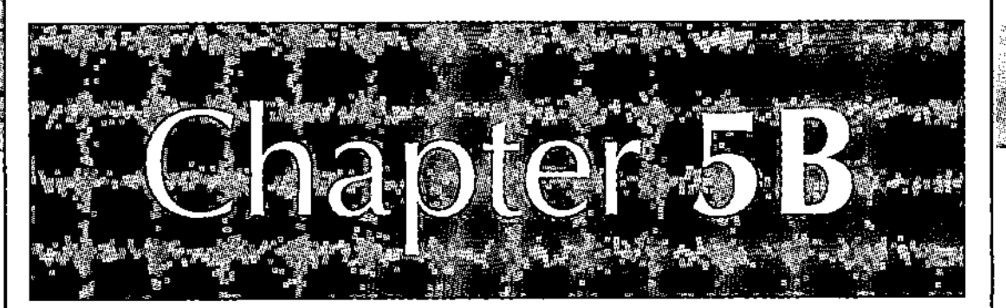

Surgical Management of Hydrocephalus and Postoperative Care of the Shunted Patient

Oguz Cataltepe, MD

Hydrocephalus arises from an imbalance between the production and absorption rates of cerebrospinal fluid (CSF) leading to excessive accumulation of CSF and enlarged ventricles. Enlarged ventricles, elevated intracranial pressure (ICP), and increased head circumference are frequently associated with hydrocephalus.[1,2]

Pathophysiology

The mechanism of hydrocephalus almost always is related to an obstruction along the CSF circulation pathways from the intraventricular level to arachnoid villi. Approximately 80% of CSF is produced by the choroid plexus in the lateral and third ventricles via an energy-dependent process. The CSF production rate is approximately 0.3 to 0.4 ml/min or 20 ml/hr. CSF circulates in the ventricular system through the foramen of Monro and aqueduct of Sylvius and reaches the fourth ventricle. CSF leaves the ventricular system through the foramens of Magendie and Luschka and enters the basal cisterns. It then circulates around the spinal cord and cerebral convexity. Finally, it is absorbed through the arachnoidal granulations around the sagittal sinus.

The major portion of CSF absorption is an ICP-dependent passive process and is determined by a pressure gradient between the cortical subarachnoid space and the sagittal sinus. However, infants do not have well-developed arachnoid villilike structures, and thus the exact mechanism of CSF absorption in newborns is unclear. Normal ICP values differ according to age. Although there is no consensus, normal ICP values typically are accepted as 10 to 16 cm Hg in adults and older children, 3 to 7 cm Hg in infants, and 2 to 4 cm Hg in newborns.[1-5]

Incidence

The overall incidence of hydrocephalus in infants is 3 to 4 per 1000 live births; congenital hydrocephalus is observed in 0.9 to 1.5 per 1000 live births. Approximately 30% of hydrocephalus cases occur in preterm infants secondary to intraventricular hemorrhage (IVH). The incidence of hydrocephalus associated with meningomyelocele is 1.3 to 2.9 per 1000 live births. It has been estimated that 45,000 to 50,000 shunts are placed in children and adults each year in the United States.[2,6]

Etiology

Numerous congenital and acquired disorders can cause hydrocephalus.[1,2] Table 5B-1 lists the most common causes of hydrocephalus.

Clinical Presentation

The most common finding of hydrocephalus in the newborn and infant is increased head circumference in association with a large and bulging fontanel, diastasis of the sutures, and distention of scalp veins. Other common presenting signs are

Table 5B-1 Common Causes of Hydrocephalus

Congenital malformations
Aqueduct stenosis
Dandy-Walker malformation
Meningomyelocele
Encephalocele
Posthemorrhagic
Intraventricular hemorrhage (11%)
Intraventricular hemorrhage of prematurity
Coagulation disorders
Postinfectious (7.6%)
Ventriculitis, meningitis
Intrauterine cytomegalovirus, toxoplasmosis, rubella, mumps, varicella
Neoplastic (11%)
Trauma/subarachnoidal hemorrhage (4.7%)

difficulty with head control, poor feeding, vomiting, lethargy and increased sleepiness, seizures, cranial nerve palsies, and papilledema. The Parinaud phenomenon, or "sunset sign," can be observed in severe cases of hydrocephalus.[1,2]

Radiologic Diagnosis

Ultrasonography (USG) and computed tomography (CT) are the most useful radiologic tools for diagnosing hydrocephalus. Magnetic resonance imaging (MRI) is another extremely valuable tool for assessing the etiology of hydrocephalus. The basic radiologic criteria for diagnosing hydrocephalus are enlarged ventricles and signs of increased ICP. Although enlarged ventricular size is a relative description, some radiologic criteria that are used to define enlargement include temporal horns greater than 2 mm in width in axial slices and ballooning of the frontal horns and third ventricle. Periventricular edema secondary to transependymal CSF flow, with obliteration of sylvian fissure, interhemispheric fissures, and cerebral sulci, are other signs of increased pressure. Another reliable sign of increased pressure is upward bowing of the corpus callosum and downward bowing of the third ventricle floor in midsagittal MRI sections.

Hydrocephalus can be classified into two radiologic groups: communicating and noncommunicating. Panventricular enlargement is the trademark of communicating hydrocephalus, characterized by rounded and dilated lateral, third, and fourth ventricles. In contrast, in noncommunicating hydrocephalus, ventricles become dilated proximal to the site of obstruction. For example, if there is an obstruction at the level of the aqueduct of Sylvius, the lateral and third ventricles become enlarged, while the fourth ventricle will have a normal appearance.[1,2]

Management

The treatment goal in a newborn with hydrocephalus is preventing and reversing neurologic damage secondary to raised ICP. An acceptable goal is to reach 3.5-cm thickness of the cerebral mantle by age 5 months.[2] Primarily, surgical management options for hydrocephalus are placement of a shunt or an endoscopic third ventriculostomy. Neonates with hydrocephalus secondary to a nonhemorrhagic cause can be shunted within the first few days of birth, depending on their clinical status. In contrast, premature infants with IVH can be shunted only after they reach a weight of more than 1500 g and CSF protein levels are <500 mg/dl. Although there is no well-defined cutoff weight for shunting infants, a birth weight less than 1500 to 1800 g can be problematic because of the small absorptive surface of the abdomen as well as an immature immune system. In general, neonates weighing more than 2000 g do not usually have any absorption problem and do not have a significantly increased risk for infection.[1,2,7,8]

Patients with hydrocephalus caused by IVH constitute a challenging group. Premature infants are at high risk for developing IVH because of the presence of fragile blood vessels in the germinal matrix. An unstable blood flow with high pressure to this vascular area can lead to IVH. Although the rate of IVH among very-low-birth-weight premature babies (<1500 g) decreased from 35% to 50% in the early 1980s to 15% by the late 1990s, it is still a significant problem among premature neonates. Despite this success in preventing IVH, no significant improvements have been made in the management of IVH-related hydrocephalus. Interventions such as early lumbar punctures (LP), diuretic drugs to reduce CSF production, and intraventricular fibrinolytic therapy to prevent the development of hydrocephalus have been tested but failed to prevent shunt dependency, disability, or mortality. Surgical interventions, such as placement of a subgaleal shunt, subcutaneous reservoir, or an external drain have been used for temporary management of hydrocephalus with very high ICP. However, the rate of shunt dependency in this group is still as high as 50% to 60%. In addition, the disability rate is approximately 60% and the mortality rate is approximately 20%.[2]

Hydrocephalus is observed in ≈25% of infants with a myelomeningocele. Most of the remaining 75% will develop symptomatic hydrocephalus after surgical repair of the myelomeningocele. Among this patient group, approximately 95% of infants with an Arnold-Chiari II malformation develop hydrocephalus, and 85% of them require shunting.[2,7]

Surgical Treatment

Surgical treatment of hydrocephalus includes shunting and use of neuroendoscopic techniques, such as third ventriculostomy. Currently, shunting is the main treatment option in newborns because of the relatively low success rate of endoscopic techniques during the first year of life. All shunt systems have three components: a proximal (ventricular) catheter, a shunt valve reservoir, and a distal (peritoneal or atrial) catheter. The shunt system is named on the basis of the location of the proximal and distal end, (e.g., ventriculoperitoneal, ventriculoatrial). The most commonly used shunt system is the ventriculoperitoneal shunt system, in which an intra-abdominally placed distal catheter allows for CSF absorption by the peritoneum.[7] The advantages of this abdominal placement include a more efficient absorption potential of the peritoneum and greater feasibility of placing a longer catheter into the abdomen.

The ventricular catheter is placed in the lateral ventricle (ideally into the frontal horn) through a frontal or parieto-occipital burr hole. The tip of the ventricular catheter has multiple tiny holes, and the other end of the catheter is connected to the reservoir and shunt valve. The shunt valve is placed under the galea. Numerous shunt valves can be classified on the basis of (1) the valve type, such as slit valve, ball-in-cone valve, or adjustable differential pressure valve; (2) the type of regulation, such as pressure or flow; or (3) the opening pressures, such as low pressure (<40 mm H_2O), medium pressure (40–80 mm H_2O), high pressure (>80 mm H_2O), or programmable valves. The shunt valve is connected to a distal catheter that most frequently is placed into the abdomen and, less frequently, into the atrium or pleural spaces.

Postoperative Care and Follow-up of a Shunted Patient

Ideal postoperative care and clinical follow-up of an infant with a shunt is the product of teamwork among the pediatric neurosurgeon, primary care provider, and family. This process begins in the hospital immediately after surgery and continues throughout the patient's life. A USG or CT scan and a shunt series should be obtained soon after surgery to determine whether the shunt tubing is in the correct position with no signs of disconnection or kinking. Other complications, such as IVH, also must be ruled out. Although the resultant decrease in ventricular size may take weeks in infants, the anterior fontanel should be soft before discharge.

Postoperative follow-up of a shunted infant can vary by center. We prefer to perform the first infant examination 1 week after surgery. The infant is assessed for any signs of infection or obstruction during this visit. One significant function of the first follow-up visit is to educate the family about the nature of the pathologic process, clinical signs of malfunction and/or infection, and how they should respond if any problem arises (Table 5B-2). Their concerns and questions should be clearly addressed. The family should have phone numbers to easily access the pediatric neurosurgeon's office if any problem arises. Families should maintain a well-documented shadow file that includes history; clinical and radiologic examination findings; surgical reports that include the dates of surgeries, types of surgeries, and shunt specifics.

Subsequent visits are recommended at 6 weeks, 3 months, and 6 months after the initial surgery. Depending on the pathology, an imaging study (USG or CT scan) can be obtained 6 weeks after surgery. Another follow-up CT scan usually is obtained at 6 months, and a copy of this study should be given to the family as a baseline imaging study. The most significant part of the assessment of a shunted patient is comparison of the current CT scan with a previous baseline study. Therefore, the family should bring this baseline study to all emergency department visits.

After 6 months postoperatively, the patient is seen once per year. Although routine imaging studies are not necessary every year, a CT scan should be obtained every 2 to 3 years, especially in patients with a myelomeningocele. The catheter length should be checked with a shunt series, especially during growth spurts.[2]

The primary care provider plays a significant role in the long-term care of a shunted infant. Routine follow-up examinations in the pediatrician's office should include questions about irritability, seizures, increased sleepiness, and decreased activity in infants. Questions about headaches, mental status changes, and visual changes should be geared to older children. The head circumference should be followed closely. The anterior fontanel should be assessed to

Table 5B-2 Family Responsibilities

- Have a basic understanding of the pathophysiology of hydrocephalus
- Maintenance of a file, which includes:
  - History
  - Clinical findings
  - Radiographic findings (including most recent computed tomographic scan)
  - Surgical reports (including dates of surgeries, types of surgeries, and shunt specifics)
- Phone numbers of neurosurgeon and primary care provider easily accessible
- Awareness of the clinical signs of shunt malfunction and infection

determine if it is sunken, soft, full, or tense. Primary care providers should note whether the sutures are separated or overriding. Any abnormality in the appearance and palpation of the shunt valve and tract can be significant. Persistent redness over the shunt tract can be a sign of shunt infection. Abdominal examination is important to rule out any distention or tenderness that may be signs of a pseudocyst or absorption problem.

Shunt-Related Problems

Shunt failure is most frequently seen within the first few months after surgery. The most common reasons for shunt failure are shunt malfunction and infection.[7,9] Other potential complications include skin problems, overdrainage, slit ventricle syndrome, and/or headaches. These specific complications and the management of these potential concerns are addressed in the following sections (Table 5B-3).

Shunt malfunction

Malfunction of the shunt system can be related to obstruction of any part of the shunt system. Ventricular catheter obstruction occurs because of improper placement of shunt catheters, migration of the catheter, or occlusion by the choroid plexus or cellular debris. The shunt valve can be occluded by cellular debris. The most common reasons for distal catheter obstruction are abdominal pseudocyst formation, indolent shunt infections, and occlusion by intra-abdominal tissues. Shunt obstruction is highest in the immediate postoperative period. Overall shunt malfunction rate is 25% to 40% in the first year and then 4% to 5% per year thereafter. Mean survival time for a shunt is approximately 5 years. Shunt migration, disconnection, or fracture can occur, especially at a later date.[6,7,10]

Shunt dysfunction causes increased ICP in a shunt-dependent patient. It is important to note that the signs of increased ICP change with a patient's age. These observations may be very subtle in an infant compared with an older child. An older child often will demonstrate increased sleepiness, drowsiness, headache, and vomiting. These signs may be of sudden onset and very severe or have a gradual, insidious onset. Children may have blurred or double vision, unstable balance, changes in personality, concentration problems, deterioration of school performance, lethargy, or unconsciousness. Seizures can occur in 5% to 48% of shunted children.

In contrast to children, infants have less obvious signs, such as irritability, downward eye deviation, delayed developmental milestones, and/or new or

Table 5B-3 Shunt Complications

Complication	Clinical Presentation	Evaluation
Shunt malfunction resulting from obstruction	Infant: Irritability Downward eye deviation Delayed developmental milestones New and/or increased seizure frequency Subcutaneous fluid collection Older child: Increased sleepiness Headache Vomiting Blurred or double vision Unstable balance Change in personality Concentration difficulty Lethargy Unconsciousness	Shunt series Head CT or USG Shunt tap Radioisotope shuntogram Shunt exploration if above tests inconclusive
Shunt infection	Fever Headache Irritability Skin changes Abdominal pain or tenderness	Blood tests WBC count Culture C-reactive protein CSF (post-CT scan) Gram stain Culture WBC/RBC counts Protein/glucose Abdominal ultrasound

CSF, Cerebrospinal fluid; *CT*, computed tomography; *RBC*, red blood cell; *USG*, ultrasonography; *WBC*, white blood cell.

increased seizure frequency. An infant with suspicious clinical findings should be assessed carefully for possible shunt failure. Clinical examination might reveal bulging fontanel, split sutures, increasing head circumference, papilledema, sixth nerve palsy, limited upward eye movements, bradycardia, and/or apnea. Another significant finding of shunt malfunction in infants is the development of a subcutaneous fluid collection. Any fluid collection around the shunt or catheter tract should be considered a shunt malfunction until proven otherwise.

Although pumping the shunt reservoir to assess for shunt malfunction is a common practice, even among parents, it is not a reliable test. If any signs and symptoms of shunt malfunction are seen, a shunt series should be obtained. A shunt series constitutes plain x-ray films of the head, neck, chest, and abdomen to assess the hardware of the shunt system. It is helpful to see whether there is any kink, disconnection, calcification, or broken piece of the shunt system. These images also can reveal the length of the abdominal or atrial catheter and displacement or migration of these catheters, as well as the type of the shunt system, if it is not known. Head CT or USG should be obtained to assess ventricular size and radiologic findings of increased ICP. Comparison with the previous CT scan is especially significant and often provides the simplest and clearest evidence of shunt malfunction. Although the sensitivity of a shunt tap to assess for a shunt malfunction is not high, tapping the shunt reservoir and removing CSF may be a lifesaving procedure in an unconscious patient with a distally obstructed shunt system. Finally, a radioisotope shuntogram can be performed to determine shunt function. Injection of a radioisotope (typically technetium 99m [^{99m}Tc]) into the reservoir can allow tracing of the flow of radioactive tracer along the shunt system and determine the degree of absorption through the peritoneum. Although this is a reliable technique, false-positive and false-negative results can be obtained. If all tests are inconclusive, then a shunt exploration can be performed as a last resort.

Infection

Infection rates range between 2% and 20% in large clinical studies. Following mechanical problems, infection is the second most common reason for shunt failure. Seventy percent of infections occur within the first 2 months after surgery. Young age is a significant risk factor for infection. This may be related to an immature immune system, thin skin, or wound healing difficulties. The infection might be related to direct inoculation of the microorganism during surgery (most common), hematogenous spread, or retrograde contamination from the peritoneal end. The most common etiologic agents are *Staphylococcus epidermidis* (40%) and *Staphylococcus aureus* (20%).[7,9,10]

Clinical symptoms of a shunt infection can vary. Fever, headache, and irritability are frequently associated with shunt infection. Color changes and erythematous skin over the shunt tract are significant signs of infection. Meningeal irritation signs are not frequently seen in infants or children. Patients infected with *S. epidermidis* may be quite well and have only intermittent fevers or irritability; leukocytosis may be the only sign in this patient group.[10] If untreated, a shunt infection can lead to meningitis, ventriculitis, peritonitis, pleural empyema, or bacteremia.

If a shunt infection is suspected, laboratory evaluation of the blood is necessary. In febrile patients, cultures should also be taken from other potential sources. Routine blood workup will frequently reveal an elevated white blood cell (WBC) count. However, a shunt infection with gram-positive organisms also may be associated with a low serum WBC count because of a mild inflammatory reaction.[9] Bacteremia can be seen in up to 25% of shunt infections. Sustained elevation of C-reactive protein levels in serum also correlates strongly with a shunt infection. An abdominal USG should be performed if the patient has abdominal pain or tenderness.

Obtaining CSF is critical to determining whether a shunt infection is present. Ideally, the fluid should be obtained by a shunt reservoir tap, which has a much higher yield (95%) compared with an LP (7%–50%) or ventricular tap (26%).[9] Before obtaining CSF fluid, a CT scan should be obtained to determine ventricular size and catheter location. If the CT scan shows slit, obliterated ventricles, CSF should be obtained using a slow aspiration to minimize the risk of a ventricular catheter obstruction. The shunt reservoir tap and CSF aspiration should be performed with a meticulous aseptic technique to prevent contamination of the system and CSF sample.

CSF should be tested by microbiologic analysis, including Gram stain, CSF culture, and cell counts as well as protein/glucose values. Because infections caused by indolent bacteria such as diphtheroids are difficult to diagnose, CSF cultures should be followed for 2 weeks to determine whether there are any anaerobic infections. CSF fluid with increased WBC counts, diminished glucose levels, and elevated protein levels are significant findings suggestive of an infection.

Management of an infected shunt is controversial and consists of two potential approaches. First, the entire shunt is removed, and an externalized ventricular drain is placed. The second approach involves externalizing the distal end of the shunt. In both strategies, antibiotics are administered until three consecutive negative CSF cultures are obtained.

A new shunt can then be placed. The first method has the greatest chance of curing the infection and the lowest mortality rate.[10]

Skin-related problems

Skin and wound complications usually are related to the surgical technique, the patient, the shunt, and/or the surgical material. Skin characteristics, such as thinness, loose subcutaneous tissue, prolonged skin compression secondary to a tight bandage, or lying down over the shunt valve, are the most common reasons for skin complications. Surgical precautions, such as making a small incision, creating a subgaleal dissection just large enough to place the shunt valve, using age-appropriate shunt valve sizes, avoiding hard plastic pieces, attaining good skin closure with appropriate material, and down-faced knots, are technical details that can help to prevent skin-related complications. After surgery, avoiding pressure over the shunt valve is especially important.

Overdrainage

Overdrainage of CSF is generally related to a low opening pressure of the valve system and/or siphon effect. Although daily activities, such as postural changes, rapid eye movement (REM) sleep, or straining may induce increased CSF drainage, most patients tolerate these changes. Overdrainage of the CSF can cause significant clinical problems, especially in neonates. Upgrading the opening pressure of the shunt, placing an antisiphon device, or using flow-regulating valves can solve this problem. However, in some cases these changes are ineffective and slit ventricle syndrome can develop (see following section).[9]

Slit ventricle syndrome

Slit ventricle syndrome is a very challenging complication of shunt placement. Although the actual incidence is not known, slit ventricle syndrome has been reported to occur in 0.9% to 33.3% of shunted children and more commonly in older children than in infants.[9] Radiographically, it appears as very small, slitlike ventricles. Clinically, it is associated with frequent headaches. The mechanism is controversial and probably related to multiple causes. Intermittent shunt malfunction, overdrainage of CSF, periventricular fibrosis, and decreased intracranial compliance all are suggested mechanisms. Thus it may be associated with increased or decreased ICP. Management is controversial and includes medical options such as furosemide, acetazolamide, and antimigraine medications, as well as surgical options such as revising the shunt, upgrading the pressure on the valve, changing the valve to a flow resistance valve, adding an antisiphon device, subtemporal decompression, and performing endoscopic third ventriculostomy.

Headache

Headache is a frequent complaint in shunted patients. Although most headaches are not clinically significant, a persistent headache must be evaluated. A headache may be due to a shunt obstruction associated with increased ICP. However, a headache also can be due to overdrainage that is frequently seen with slit ventricle syndrome. This type of headache typically is worse when the patient is in the upright position and improves when the patient is recumbent.

Care and Assessment of Shunted Neonates

Neonates constitute a special group of patients with hydrocephalus. Because of their postural flat-lying position and the anatomy of their open sutures and fontanels, infants have specific CSF flow dynamics within their shunts. These physiologic neonatal characteristics place them at increased risk for shunt complications. Noninfectious complications in newborns have been reported to be as high as 22%.[11] As expected, premature neonates with low birth weight have a higher risk for infection and other complications because of their immature immune system, thin skin, and subcutaneous tissue.[12]

Attentive perioperative care of shunted neonates can be helpful in attempting to minimize potential complications. Surgical technical details specific for neonates include placing the drill hole into the thicker part of the skull bone, making a minimal dural incision for ventricular catheter placement to prevent CSF leakage through the dural opening, choosing thicker cortical areas to place the catheter to minimize CSF leak, minimizing the subcutaneous dissection, and placing the shunt frontally to prevent skin necrosis related to positioning. Postoperatively, complications can be minimized by placing the infant in a semi-upright position for 1 to 2 weeks after shunt insertion to promote rapid drainage of CSF. If the fontanel becomes more depressed or sutures become overriding, the head position should be lowered. If CSF collects around the shunt, the infant's head should be raised.

Neonates must be closely observed for potential long-term complications. Overdrainage may lead to collapse of the thin cortex layer and development of a subdural effusion/hematoma after shunt implantation.[13] Infants may develop craniosynostosis, especially if significant loss of brain tissue occurs. Overdrainage-related problems are evidenced by a sunken fontanel and overlapping sutures. Patients who cannot be managed with positional precautions may require an upgrade or readjustment of the valve setting. A good strategy for preventing oscillation between overdrainage and underdrainage of CSF can be using a programmable valve and setting the opening pressure to 30 to 40 mm H_2O for the first 2 weeks and then increasing the pressure to a higher level after satisfactory wound healing is obtained.[13]

Wound breakdown can be a significant postoperative problem in premature infants because of loose subcutaneous tissue and thin skin with less resistance to CSF. For these reasons, CSF might easily migrate along the catheter, complicating wound healing and increasing the chance for infection.

Shunted infants with a myelomeningocele constitute a special subgroup. These infants have a high rate of Arnold-Chiari II malformation, which is associated with a 5% to 10% risk for brainstem dysfunction secondary to compression. These infants show severe retropulsion of the head, stridor, drooling, and increased tone in their extremities. Therefore, brainstem findings should be closely followed in this patient group and the patients referred to neurosurgery without delay.

Outcome

Outcome is closely correlated with etiologic factors. Patients with IVH-related hydrocephalus have a poorer outcome. In a large series of 299 preterm infants with IVH, 68 patients developed hydrocephalus and 23 died. In the long term, 15% were developmentally normal, 35% had mild neurologic symptoms and/or slight developmental delay, 28% had handicaps and/or moderate mental retardation, and 17.5% had severe handicaps and/or severe mental retardation. Patients with intraparenchymal IVH and hydrocephalus (i.e., grade IV IVH) and/or patients who required a VP shunt had significantly worse outcomes. Infants with shunt infection and a high number of revisions also have significantly worse neurodevelopmental outcome.[14] In general, the shunt failure rate is 40% in the first 2 years after surgery, with an overall 1% yearly mortality rate in this patient group. Thus the primary care provider must be attuned to recognizing a malfunctioning shunt.

Resources for Families and Physicians

Hydrocephalus Association (HA)
870 Market Street, Suite 705, San Francisco, California 94102
www.hydroassoc.org
Phone: (415) 732-7040; (888) 598-3789 (provides personal, one-on-one support)

Hydrocephalus Foundation, Inc. (HyFI)
910 Rear Broadway, Saugus, MA 01906
Phone: (781) 942-1161
www.hydrocephalus.org

Provides support, educational resources, and networking opportunities to patients and families affected by hydrocephalus.

REFERENCES

1. Carey CM, Tullous MW, Walker ML: Hydrocephalus, etiology, pathologic effects, diagnosis and natural history. In Cheek WR, editor: *Pediatric neurosurgery*. New York, 1994, WB Saunders.
2. Rekate HL: Treatment of hydrocephalus. In Albright AL, Pollack IF, Adelson PD, editors: *Principles and practice of pediatric neurosurgery*. Philadelphia, 1999, Thieme.
3. McComb JG, Zlokoviz BV: CSF and the bloodbrain interface. In Cheek WR, editor: *Pediatric neurosurgery*. New York, 1994, WB Saunders.
4. Bergsneider M: Evolving concepts of cerebrospinal fluid physiology. *Neurosurg Clin N Am* 36(4):661-684, 2001.
5. Tamburrini G, DiRocco C, Velardi F, et al: Prolonged intracranial pressure monitoring in non-traumatic pediatric neurosurgical diseases. *Med Sci Monit* 10(4):53-63, 2004.
6. McAllister JP, Chovan P: Neonatal hydrocephalus, mechanisms and consequences. *Neurosurg Clin N Am* 9(1):73-94, 1998.
7. Kestle JRW, Garton HJL, Drake JM: Treatment of hydrocephalus with shunts. In Albright AL, Pollack IF, Adelson PD, editors: *Principles and practice of pediatric neurosurgery*. Philadelphia, 1999, Thieme.
8. Frim DM, Scott RM, Madsen JR: Surgical management of neonatal hydrocephalus. *Neurosurg Clin N Am* 9(1): 105-110, 1998.
9. Marlin AE, Gaskill SJ: CSF shunts: complications and results. In Cheek WR, editor: *Pediatric neurosurgery*. New York, 1994, WB Saunders.
10. Drake JM, Sainte-Rose C: *Shunt book*. Cambridge, Mass, 1995, Blackwell Science.
11. Korinth MC, Gilsbach JM: What is the ideal initial valve pressure setting in neonates with ventriculoperitoneal shunts? *Pediatr Neurosurg* 36:169-174, 2002.
12. Benzel EC, Reeves JP, Nguyen PK, et al: The treatment of hydrocephalus in preterm infants with intraventricular hemorrhage. *Acta Neurochir (Wien)* 122:200-203, 1993.
13. Drake JM, Kestle JR, Milner R, et al: Randomized trial of CSF shunt valve design in pediatric hydrocephalus. *Acta Neurochir (Wien)* 43:294-303, 1999.
14. Resch B, Gedermann A, Maurer U, et al: Neurodevelopmental outcome of hydrocephalus following intra/periventricular hemorrhage in preterm infants: short- and long-term results. *Childs Nerv Syst* 12:27-33, 1996.

Chapter 5C

White Matter Injury

Xianhua Piao, MD, PhD

White matter injury in preterm infants is commonly referred to as *periventricular leukomalacia* (PVL). PVL typically results from insults to the developing brain between 23 and 32 weeks' gestation, when the developing white matter is particularly vulnerable. PVL rarely occurs in term infants. This lesion has a 5% to 15% prevalence rate among infants born before 32 weeks and is one of the best predictors of cerebral palsy (CP) in preterm infants.

Although ultrasound evidence of PVL is apparent at approximately 1 month of age, the actual insult usually occurs in the first week of postnatal life. Only a small percentage of PVL cases occur prenatally or after 2 weeks of age. Antenatal etiologies associated with PVL include intrauterine growth restriction, intrauterine infections, monozygous twin gestation, maternal use of cocaine during pregnancy, and oligohydramnios. Late-onset PVL can occur in extremely-low-birth-weight infants after 1 month postnatal age. These late-onset cases may be associated with intercurrent events associated with a systemic inflammatory response preceding the appearance of cysts.[1]

Ultrasonographically, PVL generally appears first as an echodensity in the periventricular white matter adjacent to the lateral ventricles; this subsequently undergoes cystic change. Magnetic resonance imaging (MRI) studies of preterm infants have revealed that cystic PVL is present in only a very small percentage of surviving premature infants. In fact, a greater proportion of infants have white matter abnormalities that are diffuse and not detected by ultrasonography.[2,3]

Pathogenesis

The pathogenesis of PVL is both complex and multifactorial. Extremely preterm birth is the principal risk factor. Other factors associated with PVL include birth trauma, asphyxia, respiratory failure, cardiopulmonary defects, neonatal surgery, and hypocarbia. In this chapter we describe the three major incitors of PVL: hypoxic–ischemic injury, intrinsically vulnerable oligodendroglia, and maternal/fetal infection and/or inflammation.

Hypoxic-ischemic injury

The developing brain is most vulnerable to white matter injury between 23 and 32 weeks' gestation. Impaired cerebrovascular autoregulation and anatomic watershed areas are two major factors underlying a propensity for focal cerebral ischemia affecting the white matter.

Impaired cerebrovascular autoregulation

The stage of cerebrovascular development is critical for regulating blood flow. In the preterm or growth-restricted newborn, a possible mechanism for development of PVL is the fact that immature vessels have a limited capacity for vasodilatation; therefore, a severe hypoxic insult cannot be adequately compensated. In addition, the cerebral circulation in the immature fetus or neonate depends upon an adequate systemic blood pressure because this population has poor intracranial vascular autoregulation. The causes of PVL might be mediated by excessive variations in the systemic blood pressure, resulting in secondary fluctuations in cerebral perfusion.[4,5] Poor cerebral perfusion can then lead to ischemic infarction. Approximately 20% of patients with infarctions can have secondary hemorrhage following reperfusion to these areas.

Watershed areas

The vascular supply to the cerebral white matter consists of the long and short penetrating arteries. The border zones of the cerebral blood supply, called *watershed areas*, are most susceptible to a fall in perfusion pressure and decreased cerebral blood flow.[4] After 32 weeks' gestation, the periventricular vascular supply increases substantially, and this mechanism of PVL is less common.

Intrinsic vulnerability of the oligodendroglia

The intrinsic vulnerability of oligodendrocyte precursors is central to the pathogenesis of PVL. The greatest risk period for PVL corresponds to the time when oligodendrocyte precursors dominate the cerebral white matter, at approximately 23 to 32 weeks' gestation in humans.[4,6] Although the specific mechanism responsible for oligodendrocyte injury is unknown, the major contributors include glutamate excitotoxicity, free radical and cytokine-mediated injury, and a developmental lack of antioxidant enzymes in oligodendrocytes that normally regulate oxidative stress.[4,7]

Maternal/fetal infection and/or inflammation

Ischemia-induced inflammation, intrauterine infection, and chorioamnionitis have been proposed as primary causes of white matter injury in the premature infants, all mediated by proinflammatory cytokines. Chorioamnionitis and postnatal infection have been shown to be associated with the development of PVL and subsequent CP.[8,9] Higher levels of proinflammatory cytokines, such as tumor necrosis factor-α (TNF-α), interleukin-1 (IL-1), and interleukin-6 (IL-6), have been detected more often among infants who later develop PVL than in those who do not, providing circumstantial evidence that proinflammatory mediators are involved in the development of PVL.[10,11] Antenatal maternal treatment with betamethasone is associated with a reduction in the incidence of PVL, potentially by blocking the release of proinflammatory cytokines, providing indirect evidence for the role of inflammation in the development of PVL.[12]

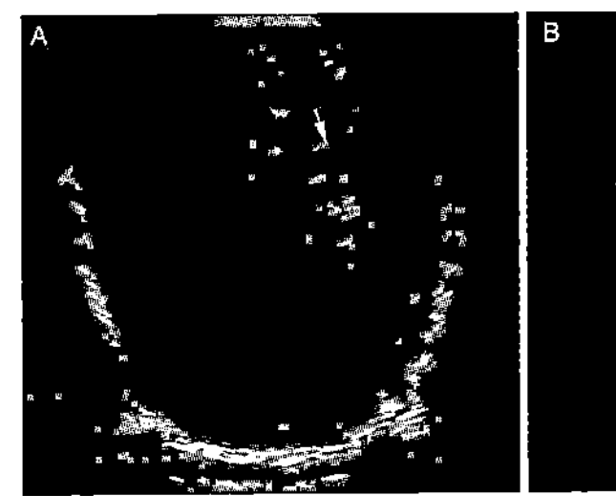

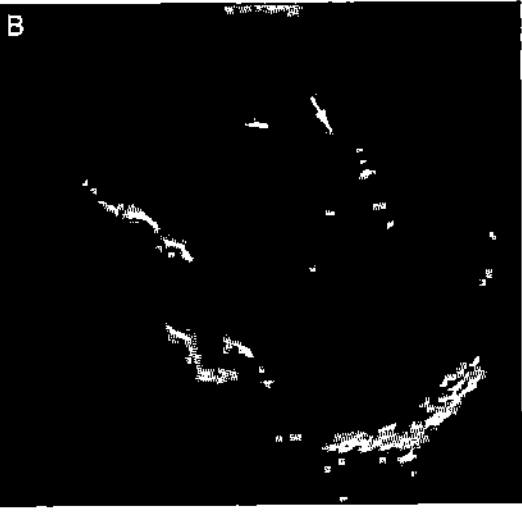

FIGURE 5C-1 Cystic periventricular leukomalacia on ultrasonographic images. Coronal (A) and left parasagittal (B) views at 39 days of age. Widespread multiple cystic changes were observed in the periventricular whiter matter *(white arrows)*. (Images courtesy of Dr. George Taylor, Department of Radiology, Children's Hospital, Harvard Medical School.)

Diagnosis

Cranial ultrasonography is useful in detecting severe lesions of the white matter in preterm infants. It is the standard method for initial evaluation. The ultrasonographic diagnosis of PVL is made when cystic changes and/or prolonged or severe periventricular echodensities are observed (Figure 5C-1). Pierrat et al.[13] described two types of cystic white matter disease: stage II, consisting of small periventricular cysts, which usually occur after 28 postnatal days and often are transient; and stage III, which is characterized by more diffuse and persistent cystic lesions and usually occurs within the first postnatal month.[13] Because the majority of cystic changes occur well after birth, serial ultrasonographic examinations are recommended for extremely preterm infants until they are at or near term gestation.

Neonatal cranial ultrasonography of the preterm infant demonstrates high reliability in the detection of cystic white matter injury but has significant limitations for the more common *noncystic* white matter injury. As a result, two more sensitive tests, MRI and electroencephalography (EEG), are emerging. MRI has been shown to be substantially more sensitive than ultrasonography in detecting PVL, especially diffuse white matter changes.[2,3] A study suggests that, in combination with cranial ultrasonography, EEG can detect more than 90% of infants with PVL, on the basis of the presence of acute and chronic EEG abnormalities.[14] Periventricular hyperintensity, which may be associated with enlarged lateral ventricles or irregularity of the lateral ventricular wall, observed in late infancy on T2-weighted MRI images (Figure 5C-2), is closely related to PVL.[15] From 20% to 50% of preterm infants at term-equivalent age appear to have areas of diffuse excessive high-signal intensity within the cerebral white matter,

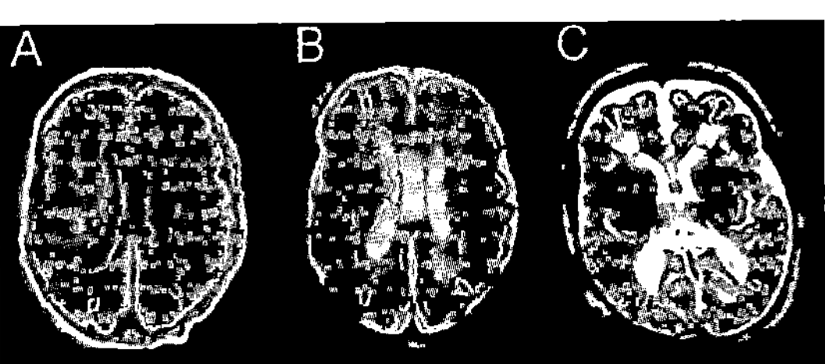

FIGURE 5C-2 Periventricular leukomalacia associated with enlarged lateral ventricles on magnetic resonance images. Transverse T1-weighted image (A) and T2-weighted image (B) at 28 weeks' gestational age. Cystic periventricular leukomalacia is evident within the cerebral white matter anterior and posterior to the lateral ventricles *(arrows)*. (C) T2-weighted image of the same infant at 40 weeks' postmenstrual age. These images demonstrate cystic lesions anterior to the anterior horns of the lateral ventricles *(arrowheads)*, squared off posterior horns of the lateral ventricles *(arrows)*, and diminished white matter posteriorly. (Modified from Counsell SJ, Rutherford MA, Cowan FM, et al: *Arch Dis Child Fetal Neonatal Ed* 88(4):F269-F274, 2003.)

indicating a high incidence of diffuse white matter injury[2,3] and possible impaired overall[16] and regional[17] brain growth.

Morbidity

PVL is the most common brain lesion associated with extreme prematurity and correlates strongly with subsequent neurodevelopmental disabilities. Spastic diplegia is the most common form of long-term deficit associated with white matter injury. In more severe cases, quadriplegia, cerebral visual impairment, and/or cognitive impairment can occur.

Cerebral palsy (CP). Approximately 60% to 100% of infants with PVL later develop signs of CP. Spastic diplegia is the most common form of CP following mild PVL. Severe PVL might lead to quadriplegia.

Intellectual impairment. Varying degrees of intellectual impairment, developmental delay, or both, have been reported in association with PVL.

Visual impairment. Fixation difficulties, nystagmus, strabismus, and severe visual impairment are associated with PVL.

Prevention

Preventing premature birth is the most important method of reducing the incidence of PVL. Other management strategies are speculative and unproven at this time.

Perinatal management has focused on reducing fetal effects of chorioamnionitis and minimizing fluctuations in fetal cerebral blood flow. Strategies have included administration of prenatal betamethasone, early treatment of chorioamnionitis, intervention to prevent placental insufficiency, and avoidance of maternal cocaine use.

Postnatal management strategies aim to minimize cerebral blood flow fluctuations by minimizing rapid fluctuations in blood pressure, treating a symptomatic patent ductus arteriosus, and avoiding hypocarbia in mechanically ventilated infants.

Long-term Follow-up

PVL usually is asymptomatic until the neurologic sequelae of white matter damage become apparent in later infancy, as evidenced by spastic motor deficits and, in some cases, visual and/or cognitive deficits. Infants in whom PVL is suspected should undergo close neurodevelopmental follow-up. Because cystic changes can develop several weeks to months after the initial insult, serial ultrasonography is recommended for extremely low gestational age infants at risk for developing PVL before discharge home. When feasible, cranial MRI should be considered at term gestation for extremely premature infants, in addition to neurologic examination and neurodevelopmental assessment. Cranial MRI should also be used to evaluate late infancy or early toddler developmental delay or neurologic abnormalities. Infants with evidence of PVL should be followed on an outpatient basis by a pediatric neurologist.

Acknowledgment

The author thanks Linda J. Van Marter, MD, MPH, for critical review of this chapter.

REFERENCES

1. Andre P, Thebaud B, Delavaucoupet J, et al: Late-onset cystic periventricular leukomalacia in premature infants: a threat until term. *Am J Perinatol* 18:79-86, 2001.
2. Inder TE, Anderson NJ, Spencer C, et al: White matter injury in the premature infant: a comparison between serial cranial sonographic and MR findings at term. *AJNR Am J Neuroradiol* 24:805-809, 2003.
3. Maalouf EF, Duggan PJ, Counsell SJ, et al: Comparison of findings on cranial ultrasound and magnetic resonance imaging in preterm infants. *Pediatrics* 107:719-727, 2001.
4. Volpe JJ. Neurobiology of periventricular leukomalacia in the premature infant. *Pediatr Res* 50:553-562, 2001.
5. Okumura A, Toyota N, Hayakawa F, et al: Cerebral hemodynamics during early neonatal period in preterm infants with periventricular leukomalacia. *Brain Dev* 24:693-697, 2002.
6. Back SA, Luo NL, Borenstein NS, et al: Late oligodendrocyte progenitors coincide with the developmental window of vulnerability for human perinatal white matter injury. *J Neurosci* 21:1302-1312, 2001.
7. Inder T, Mocatta T, Darlow B, et al: Markers of oxidative injury in the cerebrospinal fluid of a premature infant with meningitis and periventricular leukomalacia. *J Pediatr* 140: 617-621, 2002.
8. Wu YW, Colford JM Jr: Chorioamnionitis as a risk factor for cerebral palsy: a meta-analysis. *JAMA* 284:1417-1424, 2000.
9. De Felice C, Toti P, Laurini RN, et al: Early neonatal brain injury in histologic chorioamnionitis. *J Pediatr* 138:101-104, 2001.
10. Kadhim H, Tabarki B, Verellen G, et al: Inflammatory cytokines in the pathogenesis of periventricular leukomalacia. *Neurology* 56:1278-1284, 2001.
11. Kadhim H, Tabarki B, De Prez C, et al: Interleukin-2 in the pathogenesis of perinatal white matter damage. *Neurology* 58:1125-1128, 2002.
12. Baud O, Foix-L'Helias L, Kaminski M, et al: Antenatal glucocorticoid treatment and cystic periventricular leukomalacia in very premature infants. *N Engl J Med* 341:1190-1196, 1999.
13. Pierrat V, Duquennoy C, van Haastert IC, et al: Ultrasound diagnosis and neurodevelopmental outcome of localised and extensive cystic periventricular leucomalacia. *Arch Dis Child Fetal Neonatal Ed* 84:F151-156, 2001.
14. Kubota T, Okumura A, Hayakawa F, et al: Combination of neonatal electroencephalography and ultrasonography: sensitive means of early diagnosis of periventricular leukomalacia. *Brain Dev* 24:698-702, 2002.
15. Hashimoto K, Hasegawa H, Kida Y, et al: Correlation between neuroimaging and neurological outcome in periventricular leukomalacia: diagnostic criteria. *Pediatr Int* 43:240-245, 2001.
16. Inder TE, Huppi PS, Warfield S, et al: Periventricular white matter injury in the premature infant is followed by reduced cerebral cortical gray matter volume at term. *Ann Neurol* 46:755-760, 1999.
17. Peterson BS, Vohr B, Staib LH, et al: Regional brain volume abnormalities and long-term cognitive outcome in preterm infants. *JAMA* 284:1939-1947, 2000.

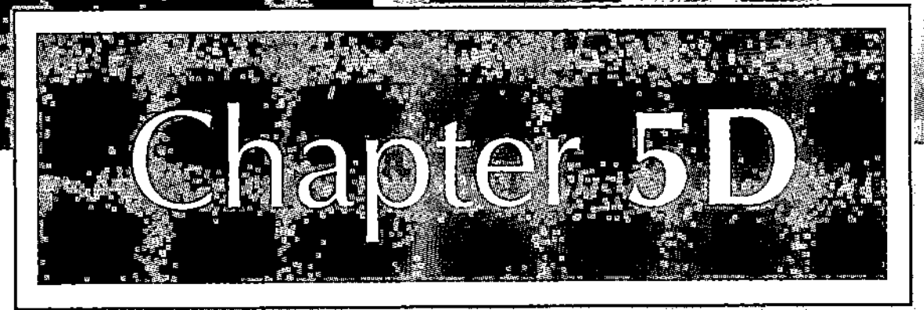

Cerebral Palsy

Emily Jean Davidson, MD, MPH

Cerebral palsy (CP) represents a spectrum of neurodevelopmental syndromes resulting from a nonprogressive insult to the developing brain that manifests as deficits in motor functioning and may be associated with additional deficits in cognitive, sensory, and other areas. Although the underlying insult is static, the presentation may change over time. The overall incidence of CP is 1.5 to 2.0 per 1000 live births.[1] Approximately half of children diagnosed with CP are born prematurely. The prevalence of CP is estimated at 100,000 patients younger than 18 years in the United States.[2] The United Cerebral Palsy Association estimates that 764,000 children and adults in the United States have CP (*http://www.ucp.org/ ucp_generaldoc.cfm/ 1/9/37/ 37-37/447*). Current estimates are $11.5 billion lifetime costs (in 2003 dollars) for persons with CP born in 2000.[3] Survival of people with CP is increasing because of improved supportive care so that currently 87% of individuals with CP live past age 30 years.[4]

Most cases (70%–80%) of CP result from a prenatal insult to the developing brain, with relatively few cases (6%–7%) arising from birth asphyxia.[5] Multiple factors may be responsible for the development of CP, and usually the exact cause cannot be determined.

Classification of CP

The four types of CP are spastic, dyskinetic, ataxic, and mixed (Figure 5D-1). Spastic diplegia is the most common type of CP found in premature infants. The proportion of different subtypes of CP varies in different studies.

1. *Spastic or "pyramidal"* CP (72%–93% of all CP)[6] is due to an upper motor neuron defect and thus presents with increased tone with a clasp knife quality, increased deep-tendon reflexes, pathologic reflexes, and spastic weakness. Spastic CP is further divided topologically according to the limbs that are most affected:
   - Diplegia (14%–55%):[6] lower extremities more involved than upper extremities
   - Hemiplegia (18%–35%):[6] one side of the body; arm generally affected more than leg
   - Quadriplegia (9%–43%):[6] all limbs affected; legs more affected than arms

   The following terms also can be used:

   - Double hemiplegia: all four extremities; upper extremities more involved than lower
   - Monoplegia: one extremity, usually upper
   - Triplegia: one upper, two lower extremities; either hemiplegia plus diplegia, or variant of quadriplegia
2. *Dyskinetic CP* (≈5% of all CP)[7] generally involves the basal ganglia and is characterized by involuntary movements and fluctuating muscle tone. Tone often is lower (even hypotonic) when the child is sleeping. Tone also varies while the patient is awake. Dyskinetic CP is further divided by movement difficulty:
   - Athetoid: characterized by chorea (random, jerky motions) and athetosis (slow, writhing movements often involving face and arms)
   - Dystonic: characterized by rigid posturing of trunk and head
3. *Ataxic CP (3.5%–3.7% of CP)*[7] involves injury to the cerebellum and is characterized by difficulty in balance and positioning the body in space.
4. *Mixed CP* is diagnosed when there is a combination of the three other types and one type does not predominate.

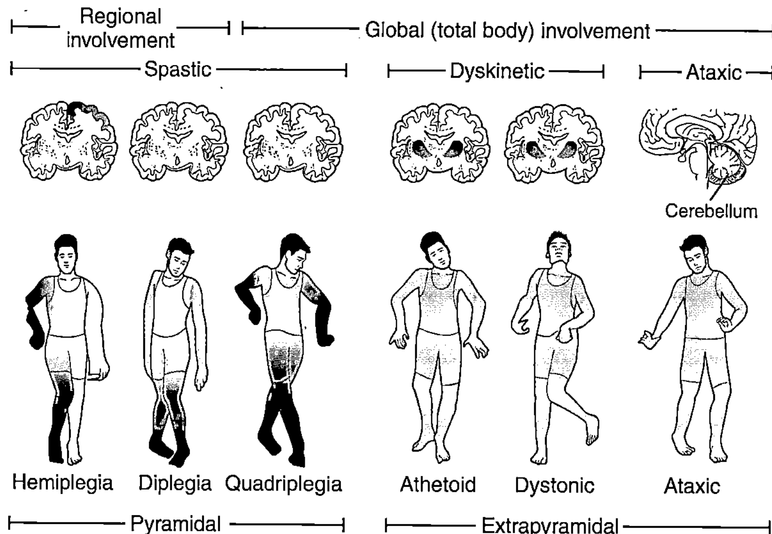

FIGURE 5D-1 This figure demonstrates the affected brain region in different types of pyramidal and extrapyramidal CP. From Pellegrino L: Cerebral palsy. *In* Batshaw ML (editor): *Children with Disabilities,* 4th ed. Brookes, Baltimore, 1997, p. 502.

Etiology

The clinician always should attempt to identify a cause of CP because other neurologic disorders (e.g., chromosomal abnormalities, spinal cord disorders, mitochondrial disorders, or metabolic disorders such as Smith-Lemli-Opitz syndrome) initially may be misdiagnosed as CP. It is particularly critical to find such causes when treatment could halt progression of the condition (e.g., in cases of ongoing child abuse leading to traumatic brain injury or a treatable metabolic disorder such as phenylketonuria) or could have implications for the family's future child-bearing plans (e.g., hereditary metabolic disorders such as Tay-Sachs disease). However, the etiology of CP often is difficult to determine. Historically, birth injury often was blamed, but birth injury causes only approximately 6% to 7% of CP, and much of CP is thought to result from prenatal causes. Current data show that preterm infants make up at least 25% of cases of CP.[8] The birth prevalence of CP increases with decreasing gestational age, from approximately 4% at 32 weeks and increasing to approximately 20% for infants born at or before 27 weeks' gestation.[8]

Common findings in preterm infants with CP

Cranial ultrasound scans performed on preterm infants often reveal findings associated with CP, including white matter abnormalities and cerebral hemorrhage. However, it is important to note that approximately 4% of infants less than 32 weeks' gestation present with CP despite the absence of ultrasonographic abnormalities. Conversely, 75% of infants with white matter abnormalities on ultrasound, and the majority of those with grade I to III intraventricular hemorrhage detected on ultrasound, do not go on to develop CP.[8]

The most common findings on ultrasound include the following:

1. *Periventricular Leukomalacia (PVL) or White Matter Injury:* The infant with PVL presents with a bilateral, symmetric, nonhemorrhagic lesion in the periventricular white matter. Clinically, PVL presents as spastic diplegia with weakening of all extremities but affecting lower more prominently than upper extremities. The intellectual deficits seen in 25% to 50% may be related to more diffuse white matter injury (see Chapter 5C for more details).
2. *Intraparenchymal Hemorrhage (IPH):* This usually is a large, primarily unilateral hemorrhage that is located in the periventricular white matter. Clinically common symptoms include hemiparesis, involvement of lower extremity greater than upper extremity, and intellectual deficits.
3. *Intraventricular Hemorrhage (IVH):* IVHs previously were described by a grading system, with grade I representing subependymal hemorrhage, grade II representing IVH without ventricular dilatation, and grade III representing IVH with ventricular dilatation. Although this grading system is still used in some institutions, it recently has been replaced by a descriptive method. Clinically, IVH is associated mainly with bilateral spastic CP (see Chapter 5A for more details).

Prenatal, perinatal, and postnatal risk factors have been associated with CP (see Table 5D-2). A variety of factors may be involved in each type of cerebral injury in CP, including particular vulnerabilities of the developing brain at different gestational ages and altered development of the blood supply to the white matter. There is evidence that infection can play an important role in the development of cystic PVL in preterm infants and CP in both term and preterm infants.[9] The literature suggests that, rather than a single discrete event or cause, many cases of CP result from the interaction of multiple causal factors.[10]

In contrast to preterm infants with CP who are most likely to present with spastic diplegia, infants born at term are more likely to present with hemiplegic CP, which most often is due to cerebral injury in the distribution of the middle cerebral artery.[11] Approximately 25% of cases of CP in term infants result from newborn encephalopathy, and these are most likely to result in spastic quadriplegia (although any type of CP may result from newborn encephalopathy).[12] Brain malformations also may be etiologic factors, and the risk factors (see Table 5D-2) should be considered in term infants as well.

Associated Problems

The injury to the brain that causes damage to the motor cortex and/or basal ganglia or cerebellum also may be responsible for injury to other areas of the brain and lead to problems that extend beyond the motor domain. There is an increased incidence of seizures in children with CP. Damage to the optic tracts and/or visual cortex may lead to visual impairment. Infants with CP may have a cortical hearing impairment and/or cognitive disabilities. Many other medical sequelae of CP result from the abnormalities in muscle tone, including increased respiratory difficulty (restrictive lung disease may be more severe if the child has significant scoliosis), recurrent aspirations, and reactive airway disease. Difficulty with muscle weakness and coordination may contribute to inadequate clearance of respiratory secretions and lead to respiratory distress. Orthopedic problems are especially common, including increased tone leading to joint problems (hip dislocation is particularly common) and scoliosis. Difficulty with oromotor function can lead to communication impairment and dysphagia. Swallowing difficulties can lead to poor nourishment, as well as aspiration pneumonia and reactive airway disease.

Although the type of CP often determines whether specific associated medical problems must be monitored, visual, hearing, and/or cognitive impairment and seizures are sufficiently common in all types of CP to merit screening for these conditions by history and, for vision and hearing, by formal screening. Table 5D-1 lists the percentage of specific impairments associated with different types of CP.

Monitoring for CP after Discharge from the Neonatal Intensive Care Unit

Signs of CP may not be evident during the infant's hospital stay. In other situations, infants who later develop CP may present with hypotonia in the newborn period. However, in these infants, it may be difficult to distinguish the normal hypotonia of the premature infant from hypotonia caused by a cerebral insult. Many centers have coordinated programs in which infants born prematurely receive routine neurology follow-up along with assessments by physical therapy, physiatry, orthopedics, and other specialties. If a child does not receive routine monitoring through such a center, it is particularly important for the primary care provider to monitor for signs of CP.

The prenatal and perinatal history is helpful in identifying children who are at risk for CP. Potential risk factors are listed in Table 5D-2. A thorough review of systems with questions about the child's current functioning directed at areas that may be affected in CP can be helpful as well. We recommend using the questions listed in Table 5D-3 as a starting point.

In addition to a general assessment, the physical examination should include careful attention to the

Table 5D-1 Percentage of Associated Impairments in Different Types of Cerebral Palsy

Impairment	Quadriplegia	Hemiplegia	Diplegia	Dyskinetic	Mixed
Visual impairment	55	23	38	50	64
Auditory impairment	22	8	17	17	21
Mental retardation	67	38	56	92	79
Seizure disorder	45	12	12	45	12

Modified from Robinson RO: *Dev Med Child Neurol* 15:305-312, 1973.

Table 5D-2 Risk Factors for Development of Cerebral Palsy

Prenatal Risk Factors	Perinatal/Postnatal Risk Factors
Intrauterine infection	Prematurity (greater risk with lower gestational age)
Teratogenic exposures	Low birth weight
Placental complications (e.g., abruption, insufficiency)	Perinatal depression
Multiple births	Intracranial hemorrhage
Maternal mental retardation	Infection
Maternal seizures	Seizures
Maternal hyperthyroidism	Hypoglycemia
Long menstrual cycles	Hyperbilirubinemia
History of fetal loss	Newborn encephalopathy
Low socioeconomic status	
Abnormal fetal presentation	
Congenital malformation	

Modified from: Cooley WC, American Academy of Pediatrics Committee on Children with Disabilities: *Pediatrics* 114(4):1107, 2004, and Kuban KC, Leviton A: *N Engl J Med* 330(3):188-195, 1994.

neurologic examination. The infant should be examined, looking for appropriate motor milestones; increased, decreased, variable, or asymmetric muscle tone; persistence of primitive reflexes; and delays in postural and protective reflexes (Table 5D-4).

Diagnosis

When the findings of physical examination and history obtained during the primary care visit suggest a diagnosis of CP, the primary care provider should discuss this possibility with the family and make a prompt referral to a pediatric neurology specialist to confirm the diagnosis or to continue monitoring. Although the diagnosis may be made on a clinical basis, current recommendations from the American Academy of Neurology suggest neuroimaging, preferably with magnetic resonance imaging, to delineate abnormalities that may be useful in both diagnosis and prognosis. Figure 5D-2 provides an algorithm of a child with suspected CP.

Management

Children with CP are at risk for associated difficulties in many areas. Well-child care should include a comprehensive review of systems, specifically asking about the issues listed in Table 5D-5. Any positive answers should prompt more in-depth evaluation and possible referral. In addition to the medical workup, it is important to look at all areas of the child's life (school, home, mobility, communication) with the goal of improving functional status.

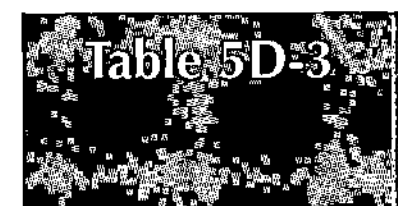

Table 5D-3 Questions for Families of Infants with Risk Factors for Cerebral Palsy

NEUROLOGIC

Have you noticed anything that made you concerned about seizures?
Have you seen any staring episodes?
Does the baby seem to show a preference for one side of his or her body over the other?
Does the baby seem stronger on one side than the other?
Does the baby's body seem to be stiffer or more floppy than other babies or his or her age?
Does the baby have a preference for one hand over the other?
Does the baby seem to startle very easily?

DEVELOPMENT

Do you have concerns about or have you noticed any delays in the baby/child's development?
Are any of the motor skills surprisingly early? (Early rolling or standing supported with stiff legs may be a sign of spasticity; early hand preference before 18 months can indicate hemiplegia.)

VISION

Does the baby follow things with his or her eyes?
Do you have any concerns about his or her vision?

HEARING

Does the baby react to loud noises?
Do you have any concerns about his or her hearing?

SPEECH AND COMMUNICATION

Is the baby babbling?

FEEDING

Is the baby feeding well from breast or bottle?
Does the baby choke, gag, or cough when she or he eats?
Is the baby gaining weight well?

Areas of concern and recommendations for referral follow.

Ophthalmology

Children diagnosed with CP should be seen by an ophthalmology specialist for an initial evaluation and have follow-up as directed by the specialist. Visual impairment is common in children with CP. The brain injury associated with CP often is coupled with amblyopia or cortical visual impairment. For former premature infants, retinopathy of prematurity is a major cause of visual abnormalities (see Chapter 8A).

Audiology/ear nose throat

Children with CP who did not have or did not pass the hearing screen at birth should have a hearing screen (see Chapter 8C). Children with CP are at risk for cortically based hearing impairment. In addition, children with other complications of CP,

Table 5D-4 Technique of Eliciting Primitive Reflexes and Expected Age of Disappearance

Reflex	Position	Method	Response	Age at Disappearance
Palmar grasp	Supine	Placing the index finger in the palm of the infant	Flexion of fingers, fist making	6 months
Plantar grasp	Supine	Pressing a thumb against the sole just behind the toes of the foot	Flexion of toes	15 months
Galant	Prone	Scratching the skin of the infant's back from the shoulder downward, 2–3 cm lateral to the spinous processes	Incurvation of the trunk, with the concavity on the stimulated side	4 months
Asymmetric tonic neck reflex	Supine	Rotation of the infant's head to one side for 15 seconds	Extension of the extremities on the chin side and flexion of those on the occipital side	3 months
Suprapubic extensor	Supine	Pressing the skin over the pubic bone with the fingers	Reflex extension of both lower extremities, with adduction and internal rotation into talipes equinus	4 weeks
Crossed extensor	Supine	Passive total flexion of one lower extremity	Extension of the other lower limb, with adduction and internal rotation into talipes equinus	6 weeks
Rossolimo	Supine	Light tapping of the second to fourth toes at their plantar surface	Tonic flexion of the toes at the first metacarpophalangeal joint	4 weeks
Heel	Supine	Tapping on the heel with a hammer, with the hip and knee joint flexed and the ankle in neutral position	Rapid reflex extension of the lower extremity in question	3 weeks
Moro	Supine	Sudden head extension produced by a light drop of the head	Abduction followed by adduction and flexion of upper extremities	6 months
Babinski	Supine	Striking along the lateral aspect of the sole extending from the heel to the head of the fifth metatarsal	Combined extensor response: simultaneous dorsiflexion of the great toe and fanning of the remaining toes	Presence always abnormal

From: Zafeiriou DI: *Pediatr Neurol* 31(1):1-8, 2004.

such as gastroesophageal reflux disease (GERD), may be at higher risk for otitis media.

Developmental/early intervention

The primary care provider should refer any child younger than 3 years who is diagnosed with CP to Early Intervention (EI). Many of the risk factors for CP also will meet criteria for EI eligibility (see Chapter 12E for further details). Children older than 3 years with CP should be evaluated by the public school system. If educational needs are identified, the Federal Individuals with Disabilities Education Act (IDEA) mandates that the school develop an Individualized Education Plan (IEP) that, when indicated, should include therapies such as physical therapy, occupational therapy, and speech therapy. If the child is on target cognitively but requires physical accommodation, the federal law known as Section 504 prohibits discrimination against students with disabilities and requires the school to provide accommodations for access to full participation in school, including the same academic curriculum and extracurricular activities.

Clinicians who are experienced with this patient population should perform regular developmental assessments. Testing must appropriately account for visual and hearing impairments, as well as motor limitations.

Communication

It is essential that children with CP have maximal ability to communicate, and this issue should be addressed as early as possible. Infants with CP or at risk for CP should be followed by EI as discussed earlier.

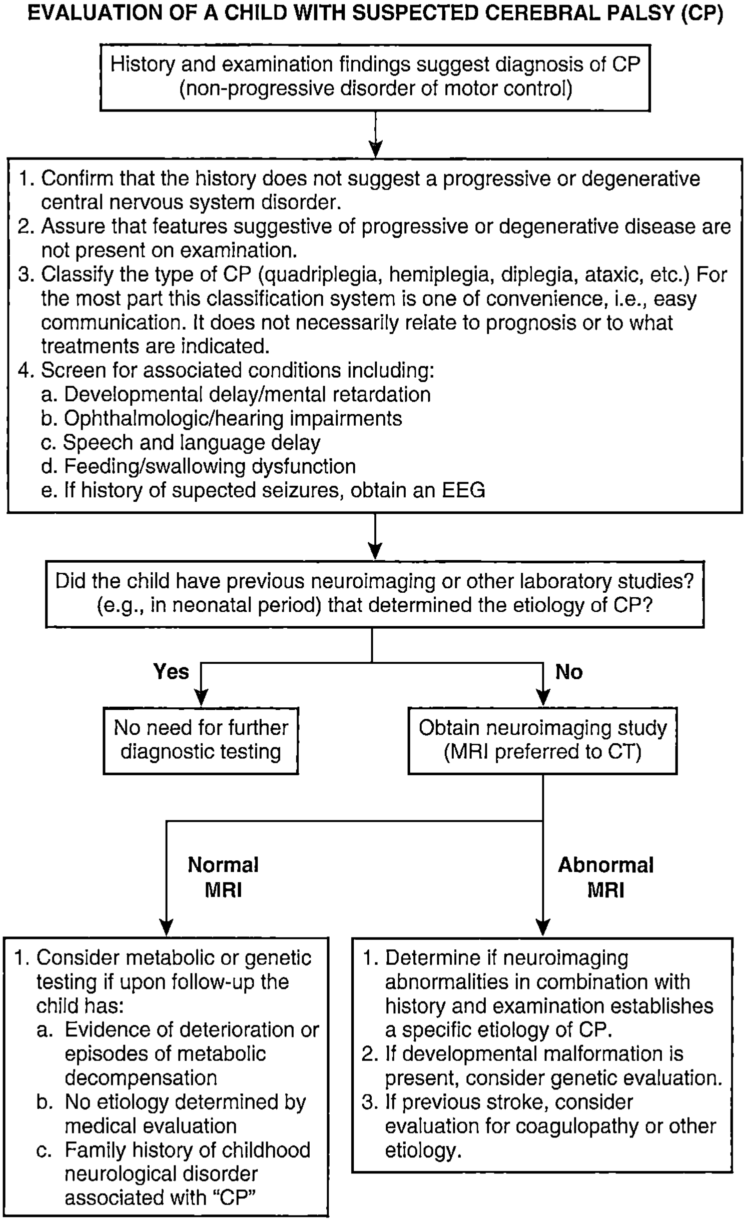

FIGURE 5D-2 Algorithm for the evaluation of the child with CP. Screening for associated conditions (mental retardation, vision/hearing inpairments, speech and language delays, oral motor dysfunction, and epilepsy is recommended. Neuroimaging (MRI preferred to CT) is recommended for further evaluation if the etiology of the child's CP has not been determined. In some children, additional metabolic or genetic testing may be indicated. From: Ashwal S, Russman BS, Blasco PA, et al: *Neurology* 62:851-63, 2004.

EVALUATION OF A CHILD WITH SUSPECTED CEREBRAL PALSY (CP)

History and examination findings suggest diagnosis of CP (non-progressive disorder of motor control)

↓

1. Confirm that the history does not suggest a progressive or degenerative central nervous system disorder.
2. Assure that features suggestive of progressive or degenerative disease are not present on examination.
3. Classify the type of CP (quadriplegia, hemiplegia, diplegia, ataxic, etc.) For the most part this classification system is one of convenience, i.e., easy communication. It does not necessarily relate to prognosis or to what treatments are indicated.
4. Screen for associated conditions including:
   a. Developmental delay/mental retardation
   b. Ophthalmologic/hearing impairments
   c. Speech and language delay
   d. Feeding/swallowing dysfunction
   e. If history of supected seizures, obtain an EEG

↓

Did the child have previous neuroimaging or other laboratory studies? (e.g., in neonatal period) that determined the etiology of CP?

Yes → No need for further diagnostic testing

No → Obtain neuroimaging study (MRI preferred to CT)

Normal MRI →

1. Consider metabolic or genetic testing if upon follow-up the child has:
   a. Evidence of deterioration or episodes of metabolic decompensation
   b. No etiology determined by medical evaluation
   c. Family history of childhood neurological disorder associated with "CP"

Abnormal MRI →

1. Determine if neuroimaging abnormalities in combination with history and examination establishes a specific etiology of CP.
2. If developmental malformation is present, consider genetic evaluation.
3. If previous stroke, consider evaluation for coagulopathy or other etiology.

Children with CP may have difficulty with communication because vision and hearing impairments may affect exposure to language. Cognitive impairment and dysarthria also may affect language (and speech) production. Communication specialists (who may be trained in occupational therapy or speech language pathology) can assess for the child's need for communication strategies or devices. Initially, simple switches that activate lights or voice recordings can help teach young children with CP the concept of cause and effect. Sophisticated computer systems can be set up with nested menus that can be operated by hand or head switches. Programming appropriate conversation starters into these devices (e.g., "Hi, I'm Joe, what's your name?" or a favorite joke) can help to promote peer interaction for children with CP.

Neurology

A neurology specialist should follow children with CP. The frequency of visits will be determined by the acuity and nature of the child's neurologic issues and will be directed by the neurology specialist. For example, if a child with CP has poorly controlled seizures or difficulty with spasticity, more frequent follow-up would be needed. For children who are stable, annual visits may be appropriate.

Table 5D-5 Monitoring for Potential Associated Problems in Children with Celebral Palsy

Potential Associated Problem	Primary Care Provider Role
Audiology: cortical hearing impairment, otitis media	Ensure one hearing screen has been done and passed Low threshold for repeat hearing screen
Communication	If problem with communication, refer to a communication specialist (occupational therapy specialist or speech language pathology specialist)
Developmental	Developmental assessments by clinician experienced with cerebral palsy Child <3 yr: EI referral Child >3 yr: Evaluation by public school system If educational needs are identified, develop an Individualized Education Plan (to include physical therapy, occupational therapy, speech therapy if needed) If child requires only physical accommodations, school should develop a 504 plan
Feeding and Growth: oromotor dysfunction, poor weight gain, gastroesophageal reflux disease, aspiration	Monitor weight/head circumference/length at each visit. Goal weight for height or body mass index is 25%–50%. Special growth charts for children with quadriplegic cerebral palsy are available (see text). Adjust calories as needed Referral to dietician/nutritional specialist if overweight or underweight If frequent coughing, choking, or gagging with feeds or diagnosis of pneumonia, obtain a modified barium swallow to assess for aspiration; if result is abnormal, refer to gastroenterology specialist for gastrostomy tube Monitor for gastroesophageal reflux disease; treat as indicated Monitor for constipation; treat as indicated
Neurologic: abnormalities of tone, strength, reflexes; seizures; cognitive impairment	All children with cerebral palsy should be followed by a neurology specialist Monitor for seizure activity Monitor for cognitive disabilities
Ophthalmologic: cortical visual impairment, amblyopia	All children with cerebral palsy should have consultation with an ophthalmology specialist with follow-up as needed
Orthopedic: increased tone, contractures, scoliosis, hip dislocation	If spasticity present, referral to specialist in physical medicine and rehabilitation for possible medication, physical therapy, and assessment for adaptive equipment (e.g., orthotics, splints, casting, positioning devices); referral to physical therapy for initial evaluation and ongoing therapy. (*Note:* this may be provided in the EI or school setting.) Monitor hip examination at each visit Referral to orthopedic specialist if decreased range of motion
Respiratory: aspiration pneumonia, reactive airway disease, restrictive lung disease, obstructive sleep apnea	Monitor for respiratory issues at primary care visits Consider referral to pulmonology specialist if recurrent aspiration pneumonia or suspected restrictive lung disease or poorly controlled reactive airway disease Consider referral for sleep study if evidence of obstructive sleep apnea Annual flu shot

EI, Early Intervention program.

Feeding and growth

Children with CP are at risk for feeding difficulties as a result of oromotor dysfunction. Often, children with CP present with poor feeding early in infancy but may be able to take adequate calories for growth. However, they may not be able to keep up with their caloric needs as demands increase. Any child with CP who presents with aspiration pneumonia or with coughing, choking, or gagging with feeds should undergo a videofluoroscopic swallow study (modified barium swallow) by an experienced radiology specialist and a speech pathology specialist to assess for aspiration risk. For children who aspirate only thin liquids, thickening feeds with cereal or yogurt may be sufficient to prevent aspiration. Children who aspirate all consistencies should be referred to a gastroenterology specialist for possible placement of a gastrostomy tube. It is important to emphasize that, although the injury leading to CP is static, the child's presentation may change over time, and feeding issues may arise at any point in childhood. Conversely, some children who have poor oromotor function as infants may develop improved functioning as they grow, and oral feedings may be reintroduced.

For children with CP, weight, height, and head circumference should be measured at each primary care visit. The goal weight for height or body mass index (BMI) for children with CP is between 25% and 50%. Excess weight gain accentuates mobility challenges, progression of scoliosis, and hip subluxation and makes care more difficult for caregivers. Special growth charts that can be used for children with quadriplegic CP are available from the Kennedy Krieger Institute (*http://www.kennedykrieger.org/kki_misc.jsp?pid=2694*). Children with CP are shorter than their typically developing peers (by 5% at 2 years and >10% at 8 years).[13] Children with CP who are overweight or underweight, as well as children with CP who are fed by gastrostomy tube, should be referred for evaluation by a registered dietitian.

Gastroenterology

In addition to their risk for poor nutrition, children with CP are at increased risk for GERD. Mild GERD may respond to antacids, but more severe GERD, especially in children who cannot protect their airways, can lead to aspiration and require more aggressive interventions, which may include a gastrostomy tube with fundoplication or a gastrojejunostomy tube (see Chapter 4A for more details).

Children with CP should be monitored and treated for constipation. Constipation is most notable in children with severe spastic quadriplegia (see Chapter 4D).

Orthopedic

The increased and often asymmetric muscle tone in children with CP can lead to significant orthopedic issues. Common problems include scoliosis, contractures, and hip dislocation. Whereas all infants should be monitored for developmental hip dislocation, children with CP must be monitored their entire lives. High tone in the adductor muscles can lead to posterior displacement of the femoral head and ultimately to hip dislocation. Hip dislocation can be quite painful and may be associated with new onset of agitation or crying. Children with CP should be referred to an orthopedic specialist for assessment if they are found to have a change in their range of motion.

Physiatry

Physicians specializing in physical medicine and rehabilitation can provide assessments of function and treatment for management of spasticity, including medication, botulinum toxin (Botox), and phenol injections. These specialists also can direct physical therapy and review adaptive equipment.

Spasticity management

A combination of approaches may be needed to help manage spasticity and prevent contractures. Orthotics may be used to maintain the joint in a neutral position. For example, ankle–foot orthoses commonly are used to keep the ankle at 90 degrees and prevent shortening of the Achilles tendon. These molded plastic braces may be hinged at the ankle or solid and are designed to fit inside the child's shoe. Hand splints may be used to help keep the hand open and the wrist in a neutral position. A body jacket or soft spinal orthosis may be used to help stabilize the trunk. Serial casting may be used alone or in conjunction with Botox to gradually lengthen spastic muscles. Positioning is important, and a variety of devices can be used to help keep the child in appropriate alignment. Figure 5D-3 provides some examples.

Physical therapy can be used to maintain range of motion and stretch spastic muscles. Children diagnosed with CP should be referred to the physical therapy department for assessment and ongoing treatment. Another device that may be recommended by the physical therapy or physiatry department is therapeutic electrical stimulation. This device contains electrodes that are applied at nighttime to weak and nonspastic antagonist muscles and deliver low-level electrical stimulation while the patient sleeps. Possible benefits include decreased hyperreflexia and tone, as well as growth in muscle bulk.

When spasticity interferes with functioning despite mechanical interventions, medical treatments may be needed. Medications are most commonly used in children with more significant spasticity, as in spastic quadriplegia. Most commonly used medications include diazepam (Valium), which works in the central nervous system to enhance inhibitory γ-aminobutyric acid (GABA) effects. Clonazepam (Klonopin) has similar effects but lasts longer. Baclofen (Lioresal), a GABA analogue that inhibits spinal monosynaptic and polysynaptic reflexes, also can be prescribed. Dantrium sodium (Dantrolene), which acts directly on skeletal muscle, is used less commonly, and tizanidine (Zanaflex) is approved for use only in adults.

Direct nerve and muscle blocks may be used to treat specific muscle groups and have the advantage of avoiding systemic side effects. Botox (botulinum type A toxin) inhibits acetylcholine release at the neuromuscular junction and leads to temporary muscle weakness (duration of effect ≈ 3–6 months). Botox is most useful for smaller muscle groups, such as the gastrocsoleus, and select muscles in the arms, neck, etc. These injections can be administered with local anesthetic in the office. For larger muscle groups such as the hamstrings, the larger quantity of Botox needed could cause systemic side effects, so phenol injections may be used instead. The phenol is injected where the nerve branch enters the muscle and causes demyelination lasting 4 to 12 months. These injections are uncomfortable and are administered in the operating

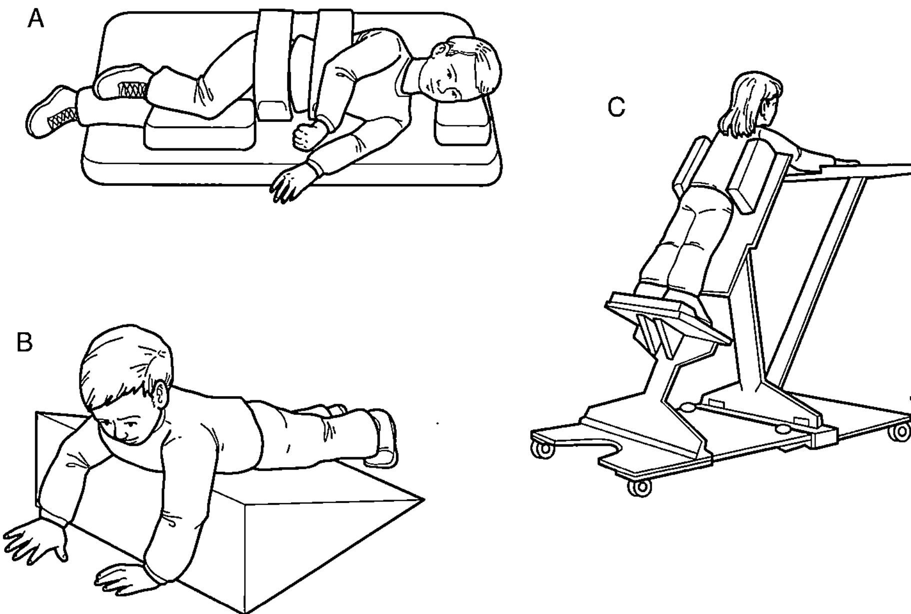

FIGURE 5D-3 This figure shows the various positioning devices for a child with CP. *A,* sidelyer, *B,* prone wedge; *C,* prone stander. From: Pellegrino L: Cerebral palsy. *In* Batshaw ML (editor): *Children with disabilities.* 4th ed. Brookes, Baltimore, 1997, p. 512.

room under general anesthesia. For patients who have had a good response to baclofen but have difficulty with systemic side effects, a baclofen pump can be implanted by a neurosurgeon. The pump delivers a continuous infusion of low-dose baclofen intrathecally and produces the desired effect without the same degree of systemic effects. Another surgical approach is the dorsal rhizotomy, in which the 1-α afferent input to the cord is selectively and permanently disrupted. Results may be variable and are best with a select subgroup of patients, most commonly those with spastic diplegia.

Conclusion: Comprehensive Care and the Medical Home

Premature infants are at increased risk for CP, and the primary care provider plays a key role in ongoing assessment to screen for risk factors and signs of CP. Once a child is diagnosed with CP, the primary care provider must assess and treat associated health and developmental problems.

The role of the primary care provider is particularly important for children with CP who have one or more of the complex associated medical problems described. Ideally, the primary care provider can work within the medical home framework to provide care that is "accessible, continuous, comprehensive, family centered, coordinated, compassionate, and culturally effective."[14] In practical terms, this requires regularly reviewing systems, making appropriate referrals, ensuring office practices that are welcoming to children with physical or cognitive impairments and their families, and helping families keep track of and prioritize medical evaluations and treatments. As the supportive care for children with CP continues to improve, pediatric providers should anticipate providing comprehensive care for children with CP from birth through young adulthood and assisting families with transition to adult care systems.

Resources for Families and Clinicians

American Academy for Cerebral Palsy and Developmental Medicine (AACPDM)
6300 North River Road, Suite 727
Rosemont, IL 60018-4226
Phone: (847) 698-1635
http://www.aacpdm.org/index?service=page/Home

This organization is a multidisciplinary scientific society devoted to the study of cerebral palsy and other childhood-onset disabilities, promoting professional education for the treatment and management of these conditions and improving the quality of life for people with these disabilities.

KidsHealth.Org
http://kidshealth.org/kid/health_problems/brain/cerebral_palsy.html

KidsHealth.Org is a website developed by The Nemours Foundation's Center for Children's Health Media. The website has separate sections for kids, teens, and parents and explains medical conditions in language that people at each level can understand. Physicians working in the field review each article for accuracy. The URL provided here is a link for the article on CP.

March of Dimes

http://www.marchofdimes.com/professionals/14332_1208.asp

Provides a brief overview of cerebral palsy for families.

National Institutes of Neurological Disorders and Stroke

http://www.ninds.nih.gov/disorders/cerebral_palsy/detail_cerebral_palsy.htm

This organization is the US government's leading supporter of biomedical research on brain and nervous system disorders, including cerebral palsy. Provides a lengthy overview of cerebral palsy for families.

NICHCY

http://www.nichcy.org/pubs/factshe/fs2txt.htm

NICHCY is the National Dissemination Center for Children with Disabilities. The Center serves as a centralized source of information on a wide variety of disabilities, special education law, and other information about related laws, such as No Child Left Behind and other information on educational research. The handouts (such as the one on cerebral palsy) on their website are without copyright, so families can freely copy and distribute them.

United Cerebral Palsy Foundation (UCP)

660 L Street, NW Suite 700
Washington, DC 20036-5602
Phone: (800) 872-5827
http://www.ucp.org

The organization's mission is to advance the independence, productivity, and full citizenship of people with cerebral palsy and other disabilities. They are a leading source about cerebral palsy and a strong advocate for the rights of persons with any disability. Their services include therapy; community living; assistive technology training; state and local referrals; early intervention programs; employment assistance; individual and family support; advocacy; social and recreation programs.

REFERENCES

1. Murphy CC, Yeargin-Allsopp M, Decoufle P, et al: Prevalence of cerebral palsy among 10-year old children in metropolitan Atlanta, 1985 through 1987. *J Pediatr* 123: S13-S20, 1993.
2. Boyle CA, Doucfle P, Yeargin-Allsopp M: Prevalence and health impact of developmental disabilities in US children. *Pediatrics* 93(3):399-403, 1994 (for percentage of US children with CP; US Bureau of the Census, population estimates available at *http://www.childstats.gov/americaschildren/index.asp* for estimate of number of children in the United States).
3. MMWR: Economic costs associated with mental retardation, cerebral palsy, hearing loss, and vision impairment—United States, 2003 *MMWR Morb Mortal Wkly Rep* 50(03):57-59, 2004.
4. Crichton JU, Mackinnon M, White CP: The life-expectancy of persons with cerebral palsy. *Dev Med Child Neurol* 37:567-576, 1995.
5. Nelson KB, Ellenberg JH: Antecedents of cerebral palsy: multivariate analysis of risk. *N Engl J Med* 315: 81-86, 1986.
6. Surveillance of Cerebral Palsy in Europe (SCPE): Surveillance of cerebral palsy in Europe: a collaboration of cerebral palsy registers. *Dev Med Child Neurol* 42: 816-824, 2000.
7. Surman G, Bonellie S, Chalmers J, et al: UKCP: a collaborative network of cerebral palsy registers in the United Kingdom. *J Public Health (Oxf)* Jun;28(2):148-156, 2006. Epub 2006 Mar 23.
8. Ancel PY, Livinec F, Larroque B, et al: EPIPAGE Study Group. Cerebral palsy among very preterm children in relation to gestational age and neonatal ultrasound abnormalities: the EPIPAGE cohort study. *Pediatrics* 117(3): 828-835, 2006.
9. Wu YW, Colford JM Jr: Chorioamnionitis as a risk factor for cerebral palsy: a meta-analysis. *JAMA* 284(11): 1417-1424, 2000.
10. Keogh JM, Badawi N: The origins of cerebral palsy. *Curr Opin Neurol* 19(2):129-134, 2006.
11. Kuban KC, Leviton A: Cerebral palsy. *N Engl J Med* 330(3):188-195, 1994.
12. Badawi N, Felix JF, Kurinczuk JJ, et al: Cerebral palsy following term newborn encephalopathy: a population-based study. *Dev Med Child Neurol* 47(5):293-298, 2005.
13. Krick J, Murphy-Miller P, Zeger S, et al: Pattern of growth in children with cerebral palsy. *J Am Diet Assoc* 96(7): 680-685, 1996.
14. Cooley WC, American Academy of Pediatrics Committee on Children with Disabilities: Providing a primary care medical home for children and youth with cerebral palsy. *Pediatrics* 114(4):1107, 2004.

GENERAL REFERENCES

Ashwal S, Russman BS, Blasco PA, et al: Practice parameter: diagnostic assessment of the child with cerebral palsy: report of the Quality Standards Subcommittee of the American Academy of Neurology and the Practice Committee of the Child Neurology Society. *Neurology* 62;851-863, 2004.

Morton RE, Hankinson J, Nicholson J: Botulinum toxin for cerebral palsy; where are we now? *Arch Dis Child* 89(12):1133-1137, 2004.

Pellegrino L: Cerebral palsy. In Batshaw ML, editor: *Children with disabilities*, ed 4. Baltimore, 1998, Brookes.

Ratanawongsa B: Cerebral palsy. In *eMedicine*. Available at: *http://www.emedicine.com/neuro/topic533.htm*. Last updated August 2005.

Reyes AL, Cash AT, Green SH, et al: Gastroesophageal reflux in children with cerebral palsy. *Child Care Hlth Dev* 19:109-118, 1993.

Sochaniwskyj AE, Koheil RM, Bablich K, et al: Oral motor functioning, frequency of swallowing and drooling in normal children and children with cerebral palsy. *Arch Phys Med Rehabil* 67: 861-874, 1986.

Wood NS, Marlow N, Costeloe K, et al: Neurologic and developmental disability after extremely preterm birth. EPICure Study Group. *N Engl J Med* 343(6):378-384, 2000.

Zafeiriou DI: Primitive reflexes and postural reactions in the neurodevelopmental examination. *Pediatr Neurol* 31(1):1-8, 2004.

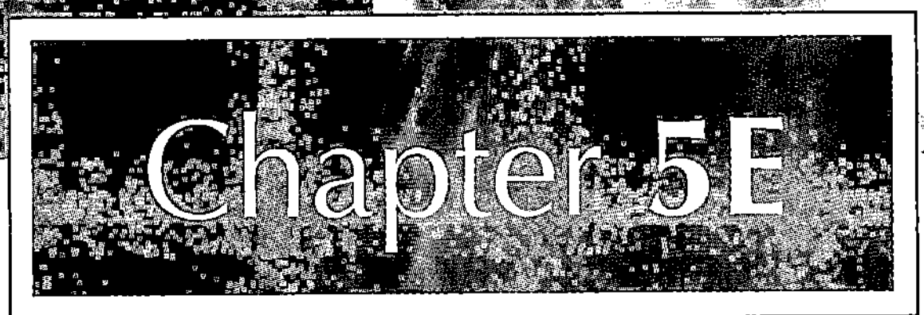

Neurodevelopmental Assessment and Care of Premature Infants in Primary Care: An Evidence-Based Approach

Jack Maypole, MD, and Steven Parker, MD

Neither consensus nor any accepted practice guidelines are available regarding the role of primary care providers in monitoring the health, growth, and development of preterm infants. Additionally, the neurodevelopmental and behavioral assessment of the premature infant is especially complex. In this chapter we provide an overview of the unique neurologic, developmental, and behavioral problems that many premature infants face and offer, when possible, evidence-based strategies for evaluating and managing these issues in the primary care setting.

The Medical Home

The American Academy of Pediatrics recommends that children born prematurely, especially those with potential developmental challenges, should be exposed to "a medical home."[1] In this model, the primary care provider provides the family of a premature infant with routine healthcare maintenance, anticipatory guidance, coordination of multiple specialty evaluations, family advocacy and support, and assessment of neurodevelopment or behavioral issues. The medical home provides a context and contract for healthcare providers and families to form therapeutic approaches consistent with standards of care, remaining respectful of a family's cultural and health beliefs.

The medical home movement espouses a philosophy that the healthcare of infants, children, and adolescents ideally should be accessible, continuous, comprehensive, family centered, coordinated, compassionate, and culturally effective. In this context, primary care should be delivered or directed by healthcare providers with continuous involvement of families in order to collaboratively manage and facilitate all the important aspects of the child's pediatric care. Ideally, clinicians and families develop a partnership of mutual responsibility and trust.

Neurodevelopmental and Behavioral Outcomes

Infants born before week 37 of gestation are at greater risk for short-term and long-term neurologic, developmental, and behavioral problems. Greater degrees of prematurity and/or lower birth weights have been found to correlate with risks and complications in these areas. Because of technologic and medical advances, a greater number of lower gestational age infants are surviving, causing the prevalence of issues such as neurologic impairment, mental retardation, and/or cerebral palsy (CP) to remain stable or increase over this time period. Table 5E-1 lists the risks associated with prematurity that are known to have adverse developmental and/or behavioral sequelae.

Table 5E-1 Risk Factors for Developmental and/or Behavioral Problems in the Preterm Infant[13]

PRENATAL

Lower birth weight (<1500 g)
Gestational age <28 weeks
Intrauterine growth restriction
Male gender

POSTNATAL

Neonatal seizures
Abnormal head imaging (including white matter injury/periventricular leukomalacia, grade 3–4 intraventricular hemorrhage)
Chronic lung disease
Prolonged mechanical ventilation
Infections (including necrotizing enterocolitis requiring surgery, sepsis, meningitis)
Feeding problems (beyond 34 weeks' postconceptual/postmenstrual age)
Extracorporeal membrane oxygenation
Low socioeconomic status
Maternal depression

Table 5E-2 Prevalence of Significant Disabilities in Children Born Weighing <1500 g

Mental retardation	10%–20%
Cerebral palsy	5%–21%
Blindness	2%–11%
Deafness	1%–3%
Motor delay	24%
Language problems	23%–42%
Attention deficit hyperactivity disorder	7%–10%
Need for special education	9%–28%
Psychological/behavioral problems	25%

From: Wolke D: *Arch Dis Child* 78:567-570, 1998; Hack M, Flanner DJ, Schluchter M, et al: *N Engl J Med* 346:149-157, 2002; and Msall ME: *J Pediatr* 137(5):600-602, 2000.

Data on neurodevelopmental outcomes of the prematurely born child may be difficult to interpret, partly because of the diverse population as a result of the numerous potential factors that can contribute to premature delivery. In addition, complications in the first months of life vary greatly from child to child. Furthermore, technology and management strategies have advanced over the past 3 decades, limiting our ability to compare recent literature with earlier data. Finally, evolving study designs confound research results. For example, most older studies describing the outcome of premature infants are based on birth weight. This technique confounds the outcomes of preterm infants with those who experienced intrauterine growth restriction.

A growing number of recent investigations have formally assessed the neurologic and behavioral outcomes of preterm infants. Consistently (and perhaps surprisingly), up to 40% to 50% of children born with extremely low birth weight (ELBW, <1000 g) have normal neurologic, developmental, and behavioral trajectories over the first 3 years of life.[2-4] However, primary care providers still should be vigilant in following the outcomes for the "other half" of children born prematurely. The recent prevalence of some of these morbidities is provided in Tables 5E-2 and 5E-3. Because preterm infants may present subtly or demonstrate signs later in childhood, the healthcare provider should integrate and adapt assessments of development, neurologic status, and behavior for each child at each encounter. Using tools and concepts described in this chapter, clinicians can ascertain whether children are performing at expected levels or require further evaluation or referral. Some useful recommendations are listed in Table 5E-4.

The long-term outcome of the premature infant arises from a complex interplay of biologic, genetic, social, and environmental factors. This interplay is most apparent as the child's motor skills develop. In the first 2 years, biologic factors serve as stronger predictors of long-term function and potential. Premature infants may demonstrate improving developmental performance during the first years of life as they recover from perinatal and prenatal insults and chronic health impairments. As children approach school age, analysis has shown that genetic and environmental factors account for more variation in cognitive development than do perinatal factors. In a transactional model of development, most preterm children demonstrate a "normalizing" tendency whereby eventually positive environmental influences can ameliorate many biologic risk factors.

Prematurely born children may demonstrate additional or shifting developmental dysfunction over time, as more subtle disabilities become increasingly apparent and testable, designated as "new morbidities." These children are at increased risk for having neurocognitive challenges in areas of learning and academic achievement, visual/motor integration, language skills, minor developmental abnormalities, motor delays, and behavioral problems. Some studies even have suggested that some children born prematurely show deteriorations in academic performance in specific areas over time. For example, a survey of British children born prematurely revealed that this group required more assistance in school and/or had a decrease in their intelligence quotient (IQ) when measured at school age and later during adolescence.[5]

Table 5E-3 Prevalence of Motor Abnormalities, Speech Development, and Ophthalmic Assessment in Premature Infants*

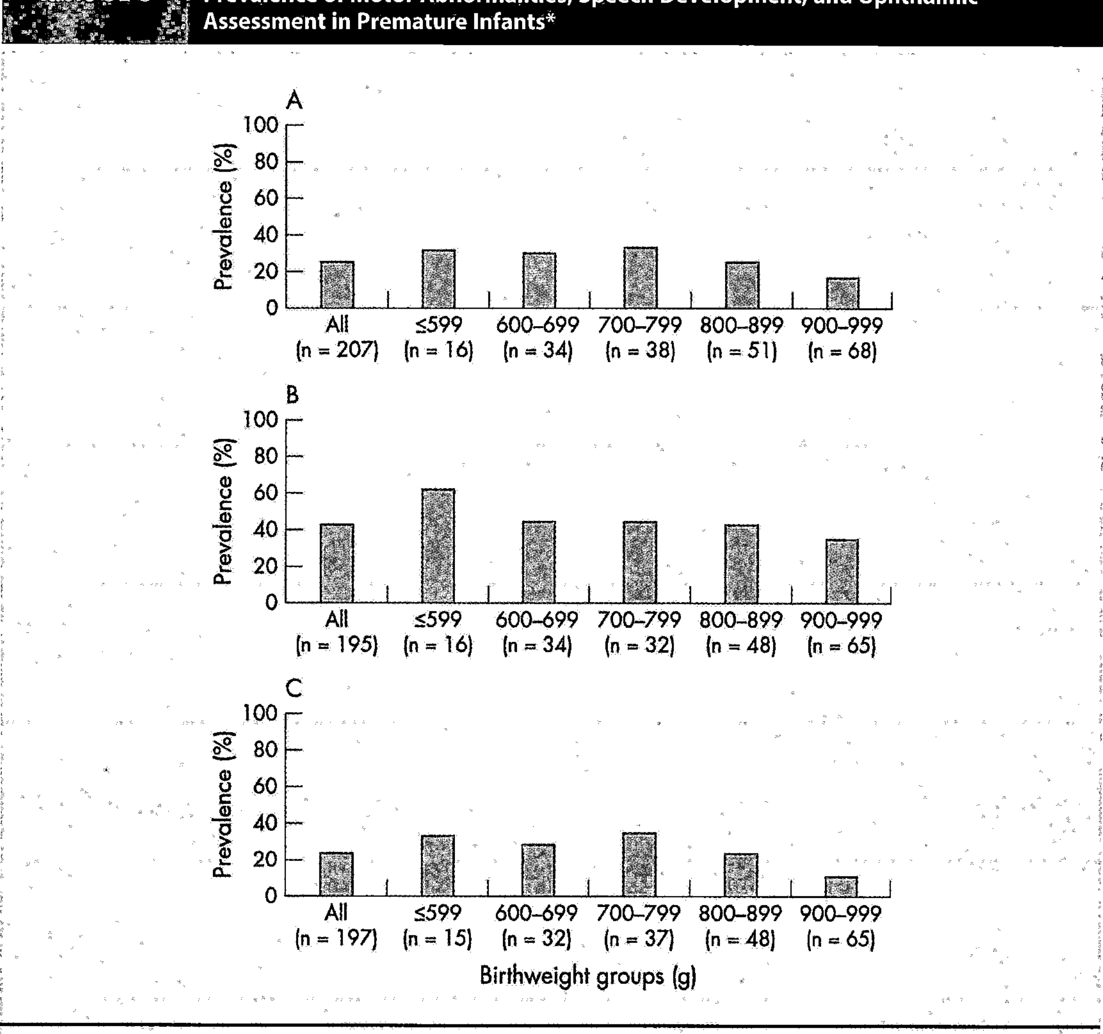

*Outcomes were assessed at 18 months' corrected age in surviving extremely-low-birth-weight infants born at 22–26 weeks' gestation. **A:** Motor impairment (including cerebral palsy). **B:** Delay in speech development. **C:** Abnormalities in ophthalmic assessment.

From: Tommiska V, Heinonen K, Kero P, et al: *Arch Dis Child Fetal Neonatal Ed* 88:F29-F35, 2003.

Correction for prematurity

Controversy exists about the age that one should stop correcting for gestational age. Most authorities recommend that the correction for developmental milestones be continued until age 2 years. At this age, for example, correcting for a 28-week gestation produces up to a 12% difference in developmental age.[6] For more premature children, this correction should be continued longer, as the measurable difference in expected performance will be significant up to 3 years. For simplicity, we recommend correction for prematurity up to 3 years of age when considering neurologic, developmental, or behavioral issues, unless otherwise indicated by a standardized evaluation.

Specific Medical Issues Complicating Outcomes

Numerous chronic and complex medical issues experienced by many children born prematurely have a global impact on neurodevelopment and behavior. Awareness and optimal management of these medical problems will maximize the potential for better outcomes (Table 5E-5). Investigation of low-birth-weight preterm infants at 36 months of age revealed they had lower IQ scores and were much smaller than matched infants with failure to thrive.[7] Those with ongoing respiratory and cardiovascular issues (e.g., poor cerebral perfusion, cardiovascular instability, or persistent hypoxia) are at

Table 5E-4 Pearls for the Primary Care Provider on Outcomes of Preterm Infants

- More frequent and significant disabilities are associated with decreasing birth weight and lower gestational age.
- Cognitive deficits are more common than motor deficits.
- Disabilities or delays in neurodevelopmental areas may be subtle or appear latently. Deficits in cognitive, verbal, perceptual, motor, and visual-motor measures may not manifest until school age, even in prematurely born children classified as "nondisabled" in early childhood[25] (Castro et al., 2004).
- Up to 50% of infants born at extreme prematurity (≤25 weeks' gestation) may be found without disability at follow-up over the first 3 years of life.[4,24]
- Nearly all infants with normal findings on neurodevelopmental examination at the infant's expected due date continue to develop normally. If a child shows no developmental delays during infancy, the risk of mental retardation or cerebral palsy is low.[3]

From references 3, 4, 24, and 25, and Castro L, Yolton K, Haberman B, et al: *Pediatrics* 114:404-410, 2004.

greater risk for having long-term developmental and cognitive dysfunction. Ischemia and meningitis are associated with a moderate risk of developmental problems. Although hypocalcemia and intraventricular hemorrhage are risk factors for neurodevelopmental problems, comparably they pose less risk.[8]

Ophthalmologic

Retinopathy of prematurity (ROP), strabismus, and myopia occur more frequently in children born prematurely. Studies have found a higher incidence (45%–59%) of overall visual impairment in this population. There are two possible explanations for associations between visual and neurodevelopmental impairments. Both areas of disability may have a common etiology (i.e., a consequence of neurologic damage). Alternatively, poor visual function may directly affect the development of motor and cognitive skills. Generally, visual screening detects most visual deficits, but more subtle visual deficits may require specialized ophthalmologic testing and routine follow-up by a pediatric ophthalmology specialist.[9-13] Please see Chapters 8A and 8B for further details.

Table 5E-5 Specific Medical Issues Complicating Outcomes of Premature Infants

Issue	Potential Problems	Therapy	Potential Impact of Therapy	Role for Primary Care Physician
Growth and nutrition	Oromotor issues Gastroesophageal reflux disease, malabsorption, short gut, constipation Metabolic disorder	Optimize calories and feeding Minimize symptoms	Enhance brain growth and development	Consult with nutrition specialist, gastroenterology specialist, occupational therapist (OT), and physical therapist (PT) as indicated
Cardiac/respiratory	Hypoxia, hypotension, hypertension Congenital heart disease; bronchopulmonary dysplasia/chronic lung disease; infection	Optimize perfusion and oxygenation	Avoid acute or chronic hypoxic insult to developing central nervous system	Cardiac and pulmonary consultations as indicated
Neurologic	Seizures Hypertonia Hypotonia Intraventricular hemorrhage Ventriculoperitoneal shunts Periventricular leukomalacia Developmental delay	Seizure control Prevention of contractures Preserving strength and mobility	Optimize interactions and awareness Promote mobility and ability to obtain independence	Consult with neurology specialist, orthopedic specialist, OT, PT, or speech therapist or neurosurgeon regarding optimized anticonvulsant and musculoskeletal therapy
Vision	Retinopathy of prematurity, strabismus, myopia	Surgery, patches, corrective lenses	Interaction with environment and/or others	Ophthalmology evaluations at 6 months and as indicated
Auditory surveillance	Progressive or late-onset hearing problems	Assistive devices	Interaction with environment and/or others	Re-evaluate at 6 months

Audiologic

Premature infants with a family history of permanent childhood hearing loss, stigmata of a syndrome or neurodegenerative disorder associated with hearing loss, history of bacterial meningitis, congenital infection, history of exchange transfusion, need for extracorporeal membrane oxygenation, severe hyperbilirubinemia (bilirubin level ≥20 mg/dl), recurrent or persistent otitis media with effusion for at least 3 months, and/or prolonged use of ototoxic medications are at greater risk for progressive or later-onset hearing problems. In these infants, auditory re-evaluation should occur every 6 months until age 3 years.[14] Premature infants born at 32 weeks' gestation or less without any additional risk for hearing loss should have a hearing screen repeated at age 12 months (see Chapter 8C for further details).

Intraventricular hemorrhage

This complication occurs in approximately 35% to 50% of infants born at less than 35 weeks' gestation. Blood in the subependymal or germinal matrix (similar to previously described grade I hemorrhage) and blood in the ventricles without dilatation (i.e., grade II hemorrhage) are associated with only a 1% to 2% risk of CP or mental retardation. More severe hemorrhages, however, carry significant risks. Lesions with blood in the ventricle with ventricular dilatation (i.e., grade III hemorrhage) are associated with a 30% risk of CP or mental retardation and a 50% risk of some type of developmental disability. Intraparenchymal hemorrhage with potential cystic formations in the brain parenchyma (i.e., grade IV hemorrhage) can carry up to a 70% risk of CP or mental retardation and a 90% risk of developmental disability.[15] Please see Chapter 5A for further details.

White matter injury/periventricular leukomalacia

White matter injury adjacent to the lateral ventricles is associated with significant neurologic morbidities. Mental retardation or CP invariably occurs in infants with large bilateral cysts. Even small, focal, unilateral cysts are associated with a 50% to 80% risk of mental retardation or CP. Children also may have developmental delay or visual impairments, depending on the degree and location of the injury. Please see Chapter 5C for further details.

Neurologic Surveillance

Healthcare providers need to perform periodic neurologic examinations of the infant/child born prematurely. The four aspects of this examination that must be regularly surveyed are (1) tone (passive resistance); (2) strength (active resistance); (3) deep tendon reflexes; and (4) coordination, station and gait. This section focuses on tone and reflexes.

Evaluation of tone is especially important because it frequently is abnormal in the prematurely born child (Table 5E-6), and abnormalities of tone may provide a dynamic, evolving manifestation of the child's neurologic status. As discussed later, the primary care provider and the specialist must use their assessments of prematurely born children *over time* to establish a prognosis; single encounters provide a mere snapshot of ongoing developmental trajectories. Even then, the ability of clinicians to forecast neurodevelopmental outcomes has proven to be problematic during the first year of life.

Abnormal tone can be suggestive of CP, a permanent disorder of movement and posture, which is characterized by persistent motor delay and an abnormal motor examination (see Chapter 5D). The resultant abnormal voluntary muscular control and coordination arises from a nonprogressive defect in the brain. CP also may be associated with a variety of nonmotor disabilities (in cognitive, neurosensory, neurobehavioral domains) and/or with musculoskeletal issues. If a child's motor quotient severity (motor development age/corrected age) is ≤0.7, further evaluation is warranted (Table 5E-7).[16] If the child has no motor delay, CP is unlikely.[17]

Abnormal tone (especially in the lower extremities) in infants born prematurely may resolve in the first year of life without apparent sequelae. In contrast to CP, these "transient dystonias" resolve

Table 5E-6 Findings of Abnormal Tone on Physical Examination

Hypotonia	Hypertonia
Exaggerated head lag Excessive "slip through" when held at the shoulders Poor head control Poor truncal tone, leading to exaggerated curve in ventral suspension Persistent hypotonia with diminished deep tendon reflexes	Spastic form may be elicited by rapid movement of extremity by examiner Dyskinetic form, with rigid extension, may be "shaken out" by examiner Other manifestations: early rolling over, appearance of hypertonia with leg extension, absent weight bearing, and persistent/early feeding problems

Table 5E-7 Motor Quotient*

MQ	Interpretation
>.70	Normal
.50–.70	Suspicious—merits evaluation
<.50	Abnormal—prompt referral

*Motor quotient (MQ) = Motor age/Corrected gestational age.

by 15 to 18 months of age.[18] Other abnormalities of tone in the infant born prematurely may also be identified. These phenomena may have many manifestations in the first year of life, even evolving from one form into another. For example, an infant born with a "floppy" or hypotonic appearance may develop hypertonicity over the first year of life.

If any abnormalities are noted, input and evaluations by specialists in neurology or in programs such as early intervention are warranted. In addition, referrals to specialists in occupational, physical, or speech therapy may be indicated. The provider also should consider a referral to orthopedic, neurosurgery, developmental, or pharmacotherapeutic specialists or to a rehabilitative facility. Coordination of recommended therapies should occur among the primary care provider, specialty provider, and community-based services (e.g., early intervention program or via the educational system). More extensive evaluations may require magnetic resonance imaging or cytogenetic studies. Atypical findings, such as choreoathetosis, may suggest an undetermined metabolic disorder, and other studies (e.g., plasma lactate, amino acids, and urine organic acids and/or other assays) may be indicated as determined by the subspecialty consultation.

Assessing for the persistence or delay of reflexes is another important component of the neurologic examination in a child born prematurely. The primitive reflexes include the Moro, tonic labyrinthe, asymmetric tonic neck, and positive support reactions. Typically, these reflexes appear and are readily elicitable in the first 3 months of life. These reflexes should be symmetric but not obligatory." Obligatory primitive reflexes cause persistent eliciting of a reflex with ongoing application of a stimulus and cessation of the reflex only if the stimulus is removed.[16] Primitive reflexes should not be elicited beyond 6 to 8 months of age. In contrast, postural reflexes are complex, self-protective responses that involve righting, protection, and equilibrium movements. The onset of these reflexes may evolve slowly in children with central nervous system injury. If primitive reflexes persist or evolution of postural reflexes is delayed, further evaluation by a subspecialist is needed.

Developmental Surveillance

The primary care clinician may be unable to detect a multitude of developmental problems unless formal tools are used for developmental surveillance. In the general population, large numbers of children with disabilities are not identified before school entrance.[19] Children born prematurely are at increased risk for developmental delays, and a variety of strategies can be used by a busy practice to recognize these delays in a timely manner.

After discharge from the hospital, primary care providers can use the Newborn Behavioral Observations (NBO) system, which enables clinicians to make observations of newborn behavior and assists families to begin to understand their infants' development.[20] Please see Chapter 11 for further details. When the infant gets older, data can be obtained from neurodevelopmental screening tools, including the Denver Developmental Screening Test, Parent's Evaluation of Developmental Status (PEDS), Early Language Milestone Test, and others (Table 5E-8). (For further information on the use of developmental and behavioral screening tools, see Glasgoe and Shapiro's overview at *http://www.dbpeds.org/articles/detail.cfm?id=5*). The instruments identified on this site are practical, easy to use, efficient, and age appropriate for the premature infant in the first years of life. The American Academy of Pediatrics' recent policy statement (accessible at: *http://pediatrics.aappublications.org/cgi/content/full/118/1/405*) reviews algorithms of developmental surveillance. Other instruments and approaches may be appropriate when prematurely born children reach school age. In addition, the clinician may draw from the responses obtained from parent questionnaires, the history, and/or the discussion during the clinical encounter. It is essential that the primary care provider actively assess the child's neurodevelopmental and behavioral status by asking specific questions of family members (Table 5E-9).

To ensure that the clinician avoids the common pitfalls of screening for developmental issues in the primary care setting, we recommend the following steps:

- Use developmental tools consistently and as designed. Screening tools may be highly sensitive and may detect even a subtle delay in a developmental domain. Identifying areas for increased vigilance or having lower thresholds of referring premature infants for further evaluation by subspecialists should be a high priority.
- Be systematic, and use measures appropriate for the primary care setting. Clinicians should use screening tools that are both cost effective

Table 5E-8 Tools for Developmental and Behavioral Assessment*†

Screening Tests for Primary Care Providers	Reference	Appropriate Age Range
Newborn Behavioral Observations (NBO) System	*www.brazelton-institute.com*	Day of life 1 to 3 months' corrected gestational age
Parent's Evaluation of Developmental Status (PEDS)	*http://www.pedstest.com* and *www.forepath.org*	Birth–9 years
Infant Development Inventory	*http://www.childdevrev.com/idi_new.html*	3–18 months
Ages and Stages Infant Monitoring Questionnaire	*www.pbrookes.com*	4–60 months
Cognitive Adaptive Test/Clinical Linguistic and Auditory Milestone Scale (CAT/CLAMS)	*www.elsevier.com*	0–2 years
Early Language Milestone Test (ELMS)	Coplan J. *The early language milestone scale*, ed 2. Austin, Tex, 1993, PRO-ED.	0–4 years
Denver Developmental Screening Test (DDST-2)	Denver Developmental Materials, Inc., PO Box 6919, Denver, CO 80206	0–6 years
Vineland Adaptive Behavior Scales (VABS)	*http://www.agsnet.com/group.asp?n GroupInfoID=a3000*	3–18 years

*When using the developmental screening tests, we recommend full correction for prematurity until age 24–36 months, depending on the tool used.
†For further information regarding the use of developmental and behavioral screening tools, see Glasgoe and Shapiro's overview at *http://www.dbpeds.org/articles/detail.cfm?id=5*.

and practical. As Table 5E-8 notes, different assessments are appropriate for varying ages.

- Engage in network building and system savvy. To enhance utilization of services and one's sophistication of available resources, clinicians should identify key players at the local and state levels (including schools, departments of social services, and public health).
- Gain an understanding of community resources. Providers should use local coordinators responsible for implementing child-find and intervention programs under the Individuals with

Table 5E-9 Summary of Key Clinical Questions for the Family of a Child Born Prematurely

Specific Area of Assessment	Some Initial Questions to Ask the Family
General question	What are your concerns or questions about your child's progress, or overall development today?
Surveillance of abnormal tone	Do you think your child is either stiff or floppy? Does your child have any unusual movement patterns? Does your child move both sides of his or her body equally?
Surveillance of language delays	Are you worried about how your child communicates? Does your child respond to you and your voice?
Behavioral and socioemotional issues	Are you worried at all about your child's behavior? Does your child have trouble finishing tasks? Do you think your child is more active than other children? Are you concerned about your child being unusually shy, sad, or fearful? Is your child's behavior getting in the way of doing well in child care and/or school, with friends, or at home?
Sensory integration	Is your child easily overstimulated? Does your child have trouble "multitasking" or performing complicated tasks compared with his or her peers?
Temperament	How are you and your child getting along? Are there any problems that you are worried about?
Attachment disorders	Do you have any concerns regarding how your child relates to family, friends, or new contacts?
Sleep	Do you have any concerns about your child's sleeping?
Crying	How many hours per day does your baby cry?
Vulnerable child syndrome	Do you see your child as especially fragile or sick compared with other children? Are you worried your child might die?

Disabilities with Education Act (IDEA). For information on programs, the National Early Childhood Technical Assistance Center has a website *(www.nectac.org)* with contact information for every state and usually region for children 0 to 3 or 3 to 5 years of age. For children older than 5 years, a school psychologist or the local school board may offer services for identified children.

In the child born prematurely, developmental issues may be subtle and may elude casual or superficial observation in the primary care setting. Furthermore, some developmental deficits may exist in isolation from other physical or focal neurologic findings in the first years of life. For example, in a study of infants born at less than 29 weeks' gestation, 23% of children with no diagnosed physical impairment required additional special school services at ages 4 to 10 years.[21] In addition to neurologic and motor delays, sensory processing deficits or hypersensitivity to sensory stimuli (e.g., touch, sound, and movement) frequently occur in children born prematurely and may have long-term impacts on the performance and level of function in later childhood, adolescence, and adulthood of these individuals.

As discussed earlier, healthy premature infants usually "catch up" to their peers in developmental functioning by 2 years of age. As the child's chronologic age increases, the proportion of prematurity (and thus the impact of a correction for gestational age) correspondingly diminishes. When using the developmental screening tests, we recommend full correction for prematurity until age 24 to 36 months, depending on the tool used.

Delays in speech and language are among the most common developmental challenges observed in children born prematurely. These delays may arise from a premature infant's inability to (1) perceive or process auditory and visual information, (2) learn and conceptualize verbal language, and/or (3) produce spoken words. Evaluation of speech and language skills of the child born prematurely requires placing current skills in the context of the child's developmental and medical history. This includes the child's neurologic and oromotor function, current level of cognitive function, and overall impression following a physical examination. The primary care provider can refer to Table 5E-10 to recognize red flags that correlate with a delay in language as well as other developmental areas. Specifically, a language delay describes a child with fewer than 20 meaningful words at 18 months' corrected age, a child who is unable to follow one-step commands, and a child with abnormal hearing, vision, or speech and language assessment. If the primary care provider is concerned about the child's language development, the clinician should administer a language-focused screening test, such as the Early Language Milestone Test (ELMS) or the Cognitive Adaptive Test/Clinical Linguistic and Auditory Milestone Scale (CAT/CLAMS), as described in Table 5E-8.

For the busy clinician, it is most practical to master some (not all) of the testing instruments outlined in Table 5E-8. The primary care provider should integrate the use of these test instruments into a well-child visit and when a specific neurodevelopmental concern arises. It is important to emphasize that these tools are used as a screening tool for neurodevelopmental issues and not for diagnostic purposes. When results of concern are found, the clinician should consult an appropriate and accessible specialist, such as a developmental pediatric specialist, pediatric neurology specialist, child psychiatrist, or child psychologist.

Behavioral and Socioemotional Surveillance

Outcomes for social and behavioral issues among children born prematurely differ from those of children born at term gestation. Anticipatory guidance with continued surveillance and assessments in the primary care setting is essential to identify children with behavioral and/or socioemotional concerns. This surveillance should continue during middle childhood and into adolescence.

Prematurely born children can demonstrate specific "externalizing behaviors." Some research suggests that by school age and into adulthood, children born prematurely may be more likely to demonstrate symptoms of attention deficit hyperactivity disorder (ADHD). Interestingly, a survey of former very-low-birth-weight (VLBW) infants at age 20 years found the odds ratios for parent-reported rates for attention problems was 2.4 (compared with adults born at term), whereas no differences in young adult self-reports of ADHD were found.[22] In particular, studies have found that children born prematurely manifest a greater deficit in attention over time but with less of a hyperactive component.[6] Interestingly, the attentional issues found in premature infants do not appear to be linked to the development of antisocial behaviors, such as conduct disorder or oppositional/defiant behavior evident later in childhood, adolescence, or adulthood.[6]

During the school-age and adolescence periods, children born prematurely are more likely to experience so-called *internalized behaviors*, such as social shyness, depression, and anxiety.[6,23] These issues appear to be more pronounced in girls than in boys. A survey of former VLBW women at age 20 years

Table 5E-10 Red Flags for Delays in Developmental Milestones of Premature Infants between 2 and 36 Months' Corrected Gestational Age

Age	Social	Self-help	Gross Motor	Fine Motor	Language
2 months		Not alert to mother, with special interest			
3 months	No social smile				
4 months			Does not pull up to sit Unable to lift head up to 45 degrees in prone position	Persistence of grasp Hands fisted most of time	No responsive vocalization
5 months			Does not roll over	Unable to hold rattle	
6 months		No effort to reach at objects	Persistence of primitive reflexes past 6 months Poor head control		Does not attempt to make sounds
7 months		Not searching for dropped object		Unable to hold an object in each hand	
8 months	No laugh in playful situations	No interest in peek-a-boo	Does not sit without support		
9 months				Lack of hand-to-hand transfer of objects	Not saying "da" or "ba"
10 months			Does not stand while holding on	Absence of pincer grasp	Not saying "dada" or "baba"
12 months	Stiffens when approached Hard to console	Does not search for hidden object			
15 months			Not walking	Unable to put in or take out objects	
18 months		No interest in cause-and-effect games			Has fewer than three words
21 months				Unable to remove socks or gloves by self	
24 months	Rocks back and forth in crib Kicks, bites, screams easily and w/o provocation Poor eye contact	Does not categorize similarities	Not climbing down stairs	Unable to stack 5 blocks; not scribbling	No two-word phrases or repetition of phrases
30 months			Not jumping with both feet	Unable to turn single page of a book	Not using at least one personal pronoun
36 months	Does not play with other children In constant motion Resists discipline	Does not know own full name	Unable to stand on one foot	Unable to stack eight blocks; cannot draw straight line	Speech only half-understandable

From: Blasco PA: Motor delays. In Parker S, Zuckerman B, Augustyn M, editors: *Developmental and behavioral pediatrics: a handbook for primary care.* New York, 2005, Lippincott, Williams & Wilkins; and First LR, Palfrey JS: *N Engl J Med* 330(7):478-783, 1994.

reported significantly more withdrawn behaviors and fewer delinquent behavioral problems than in control subjects. Their rates of internalizing behaviors (which included anxious, depressed, and withdrawn behaviors) were above the borderline clinical cutoff.[22] A New Zealand survey of VLBW infants had similar findings.[23]

The increased risk for children who were born prematurely to have behavioral and socioemotional issues probably plays a role in their higher incidence of developing significant school problems. Prematurely born children without major handicaps and with IQs in the lower range of normal who attend regular school are still at higher risk for school achievement problems compared with same-age peers (Table 5E-11). Hack et al.[24] found that fewer VLBW young adults (74%) compared with young adults with normal birth weights (83%) had graduated from high school. VLBW participants also had a lower mean IQ (87 vs. 92) and lower academic achievement scores. However, these young adults also reported less alcohol and drug use and had lower rates of pregnancy than did normal-birth-weight controls. The authors speculate that, because of the early history of medical risk in VLBW children, their parents may have provided the children with more attention and supervision compared with their less vulnerable, full-term peers. Data on adult outcomes continue to emerge as increasing numbers of children born prematurely survive to adulthood and are analyzed against a background of improving medical and technical interventions.

Specific Behavioral Issues

(Table 5E-9)

Sensory integration

Children born prematurely are more likely to experience challenges processing a variety of stimuli at the same time. Such difficulty may make them more prone to sensory (e.g., taste, touch, sound) hypersensitivity. In particular, educators or families may report that school-aged children born prematurely are more challenged in visual motor integration or logical reasoning tasks.[6,25] If there is any concern about the premature infant's ability to process stimuli and/or tolerate textures or handling of food during his or her first year of life, the primary care provider should obtain a targeted evaluation and/or therapy from a pediatric occupational therapy specialist.

Table 5E-11 Educational Outcomes of Children Born Prematurely

Specific Issue	Incidence
Attending age-appropriate classes in regular primary school	40%–45%
General school problems	12%–52%
Educated below age level	22%–26%
School failure	19%–22%

From: O'Brien F, Roth S, Stewart A, et al: *Arch Dis Child* 89:207-211, 2004; and Indredavik MS, Vik T, Heyerdahl S, et al: *Arch Dis Child Fetal Neonatal Ed* 89:F445-F450, 2004.

Temperament

Based on observations, infants born prematurely may be perceived as "more difficult" to their caregivers. In particular, these infants are more likely to be described as having diminished spontaneous activity and vigor; having a decreased ability to maintain and modulate their emotional responses; and being less alert and attentive, less responsive, less interested in game playing, less contingent, less prone to smile, and less content. The primary care provider must work with the family to distinguish whether these behaviors are manifestations of an underlying medical condition (e.g., gastroesophageal reflux, encephalopathy) or are a characteristic of an infant's temperament. Some parents may experience their preterm infant to have a more negative affect and greater irritability than matched full-term infants.[26] These issues may exacerbate a poor fit of temperaments between caregiver and child, increasing stress and presenting challenges to bonding.

Primary care providers should obtain further evaluation when an infant's temperamental style is causing significant emotional distress for the parents; parents view the child as "bad" or behaviorally damaged; and/or if the parental response to difficult temperamental traits is maladaptive and appears to exacerbate the situation.

A study from France suggests that later temperamental distinctions between children born prematurely (before 29 weeks' gestation) and full-term counterparts disappear at 9 months of age.[27] The analysis included 266 singleton infants born at less than 29 weeks' gestation and 546 full-term singleton infants from the same regions. Further studies in this field are warranted.

Attachment disorders

Research has demonstrated higher rates of insecure or problematic attachment of prematurely born children to their mothers in early life. As noted earlier, children born prematurely also have higher rates of some emotional problems (e.g., anxiety) that may inhibit their ability to communicate or to form new relationships. Again, the primary care provider must work with the family to distinguish whether these behaviors are manifestations of an underlying medical condition (e.g., neurosensory deficit, gastroesophageal reflux, encephalopathy) or are a characteristic of an infant's temperament or cognitive function. Further evaluation is warranted if the parent–child relationship lacks nurturing and caring interactions.

Sleep

By 4 months of age most full-term infants can sleep for up to 6 to 8 hours per night. Infants born prematurely tend to wake more frequently during the first 3 to 4 months of life. Extended sleep for infants born prematurely does not often occur until 6 months' corrected gestational age.[28,29]

To attempt to prevent sleeping problems, consistent sleep hygiene (e.g., regular nighttime rituals, reducing noise and lights, swaddling, adding white noise) should be emphasized. Overstimulation of these children also may occur with routine play/cuddling. Thus, calm and established routines around bedtime may enhance sleep onset. Fortunately, contrary to anecdotal reports, children born prematurely have not been found to have more sleeping problems in the preschool years compared with their peers.

As with healthy infants, the premature infant should sleep on his or her back to lower the risk of sudden infant death syndrome (SIDS). Soft mattresses and other surfaces that could trap exhaled air are also associated with SIDS and should be avoided.

Crying and colic

In full-term infants, crying peaks at approximately 6 weeks of age, lasting approximately 2 to 4 hours per day. The escalation in crying may be difficult to interpret in a term child but may be experienced as even more worrisome by a parent who still views his or her infant as more vulnerable to new medical and other problems. Surveys have found that children of premature birth are fussier, cry longer, and are less consolable than their full-term counterparts. Furthermore, children born prematurely tended to be more labile, changing their behavioral state more frequently. In turn, this might precipitate an unsuccessful cycle of crying and soothing between parent and child.[29] Premature infants appear to have the same peak amount of crying (6 weeks' corrected gestational age) as full-term infants.[30] Please refer to Chapter 4B for further details.

Adapting elements from practices in neonatal intensive care units, such as the Newborn Individualized Developmental Care and Assessment Program, may offer some approaches that are developmentally supportive of a premature infant's needs. These principles include consistent caregiving styles, providing a predictable structure in a day, providing care based on the infant's behavioral cues, building in help/lead time for transitions, and maintaining an individualized environment and stimulation for the infant.[28]

Vulnerable child syndrome

The vulnerable child syndrome (VCS), also known as *compensatory parenting*, was originally defined in 1964 by Green and Solnit.[31] It refers to any instance in which parents, because of earlier events, perceive their children to be abnormally susceptible to illness or death. This creates a continuing, overprotective, anxiety-ridden relationship that may adversely affect the child's development.[32] This syndrome is more common in specific circumstances, such as prematurity, death of a previous child, abnormal screening results in pregnancy, pregnancy or delivery complications, false-positive screening results, or self-limited illness early in life (particularly one that required hospital admissions).

It is extremely important for healthcare providers to reinforce the idea of normal interactions with other children, family members, and extended communities, limited only by the child's tolerance. A frequent mistake made by some practitioners is to inadvertently reinforce overprotective behaviors. Consequently, it is always useful to promote, explore, or recommend activities that promote self-esteem, independence, and mastery of the prematurely born child, such as classes, summer camp, or after-school activities with "well children."

The primary care provider should consider a diagnosis of VCS in the following scenarios: if a parent is excessively worried; if a child frequently is brought to the provider with minor complaints; if there are recurring symptoms that might be psychosomatic; if the child has behavioral problems; if the parents have difficulty separating from their child; and if a school-age child is not participating in activities or social events. Persistent concerns may merit referral of a family and child to psychological or emotional counseling, peer or family support groups, or community-based services.[33]

Communication with Families

Optimal communication between the primary care provider and the parents of a prematurely born child requires a number of interpersonal and communication tools. These interactions involve activated reflective listening, facilitating dialogue with open-ended questions as appropriate. The primary care provider should allow the parent to enumerate concerns and clearly identify the parental agenda at the outset of clinical encounters and conversations. Thereafter, the clinician must acknowledge concerns and establish a follow-up plan of identified issues before ending the visit.[34] Health visits with complex children may require flexibility in planning and sometimes a departure from anticipated tasks and management. Hence, a clinician working to provide counseling or interpretation of complicated issues may need to allow time for discussions of psychosocial issues, support systems, stressors, or problem-solving strategies.

The primary care provider should communicate specifically with families about their adjustment to having a premature infant. After discharge from the hospital, the arrival of a formerly premature, potentially sick infant into the home raises a number of issues for parents and the rest of the family unit. Procedures or periods of critical illness may be traumatic[35] and may contribute to long-term concerns about the infant's survival and neurodevelopmental potential. The complexity of caring for a complicated or chronically ill premature infant may pose a persistent degree of stress upon a household. Tommiska et al.[35] studied parents of ELBW infants born in the late 1990s and found that mothers demonstrated significantly more distress than did fathers with respect to role restriction, incompetence, and spouse relationship problems. Male parents reported a greater degree of social isolation. However, most parents seemed to have recovered by the time the child reached the age of 2 years. To provide continued support and ensure appropriate family adjustment, the primary care provider should perform the following:

- Schedule a "decompression visit" for the first session, to allow for venting of stress, brainstorming, and problem solving;
- Identify family stressors and support systems; start each visit by inquiring about the family members' concerns and ascertain that questions or concerns have been discussed during each encounter; and
- Consider referral to a family support group and/or counseling for overwhelmed, grieving, or depressed parents.

In some instances, primary care providers must communicate bad news or an uncertain or negative prognosis to the family of a prematurely born child. To optimize the therapeutic alliance, the primary care provider may need to invest time, energy, and advance planning to this process—all of which are scarce resources in primary care settings. Hopefully, the strategies listed in Table 5E-12 will improve the communication of difficult issues for providers working with families of children born prematurely.[36]

Table 5E-12 Strategies for Primary Care Providers to Communicate Difficult Information to Families

Planning the discussion	Tell the family as soon as possible
	Communicate in a private, undistracted setting
	Assemble "key people" for important communications
Specific focus during discussion	Personalize the discussion
	Get to the point "Stop, look, listen"
	Answer/pause for questions
	Invite affect
Format of discussion	Titrate the message
	Verify that key points are understood
	Discuss "next steps"

Conclusion

It is essential that primary care providers actively assess the child's neurodevelopmental and behavioral status by asking specific questions to the family (Table 5E-9). Regardless of the type of neurodevelopmental or behavioral issue, once a clinician has identified a problem, similar therapeutic strategies must be undertaken. These include (1) assisting in the coordination of input and management strategies from multiple subspecialty and paramedical providers (i.e., orthopedic specialists, occupational, physical, and speech therapy specialists); (2) facilitating the parental role as caretaker and advocate; (3) including and empowering families to assist in the administration and oversight of therapies and progress; and (4) promoting long-term function of the child as effectively and normally as possible. It is hoped that this chapter has provided clinicians with important tools to ensure adequate recognition and referral of neurologic, developmental, and behavioral issues of children born prematurely.

Resources for Families and Clinicians

American Academy of Pediatrics
www.medicalhomeinfo.org
Scroll to Screening Initiatives, then Developmental Screening, and then For Providers or To Families.
http://www.aap.org/healthtopics/stages.cfm
Provides extensive information about developmental stages and screening and provides an overview and resources for integrating a medical home approach into a primary care setting.
http://pediatrics.aappublications.org/cgi/content/full/118/1/405
Provides an AAP policy statement about identifying infants and young children with developmental disorders in the medical home: an algorithm for developmental surveillance and screening. Included within this statement is an easy-to-use algorithm that serves as a decision-making tool for conducting developmental surveillance and screening.
Centers for Disease Control and Prevention
http://www.cdc.gov/ncbddd/child/screen_provider.htm
This website discusses the role of the primary care provider in a child's developmental health.
Developmental Screening Tools
www.dbpeds.org/
This website provides information about the specific use of developmental and behavioral

screening tools *(http://www.dbpeds.org/articles/detail.cfm?TextID=539).*

Exceptional Parent Magazine

www.eparent.com

Provides information, support, ideas, encouragement, and outreach for families and service providers of children with disabilities.

Federation for Children with Special Needs

95 Berkley Street, Suite 104, Boston MA 02116

www.fcsn.org

The mission of this organization is to provide information, support, and assistance to parents of children with disabilities, the professionals serving them, and their communities. This website primarily services Massachusetts but has a link to the Family Resource database, a national database of agencies across the country, which provides information/services to families of children with special needs.

Internet Resource for Special Children

www.irsc.org

This site is dedicated to children with disabilities and other health-related disorders. It provides a directory for links for families, educators, and medical professionals caring for these children.

National Early Childhood Technical Assistance System

www.nectac.org

This site provides contact information about intervention programs for every state and usually region for children 0 to 3 or 3 to 5 years of age.

Other websites

www.brightfutures.org

Information on this website is based on published guidelines for health supervision of infants, children, and adolescents. It is funded by the U.S. Department of Health and Human Services, under the direction of the Maternal and Child Health Bureau.

www.generalpediatrics.com

Clearinghouse of information, handouts, and problem-based information for clinicians and parents.

REFERENCES

1. The American Academy of Pediatrics Statement: medical home. *Pediatrics* 110(1):184-186, 2002.
2. Tommiska V, Heinonen K, Kero P, et al: A national two year follow up study of extremely low birthweight infants born in 1996–1997. *Arch Dis Child Fetal Neonatal Ed* 88:F29-F35, 2003. Available at: *http://fn.bmjjournals.com/cgi/content/full/88/1/F29#SEC3.*
3. Hoekstra RE, Ferrara TB, Couser RJ, et al: Survival and long-term neurodevelopmental outcomes of extremely premature infants born at 23-26 weeks' gestational age at a tertiary center. *Pediatrics* 113:e1-e6, 2004.
4. Wood NS, Marlow N, Costeloe K, et al: Neurologic and developmental disability after extremely preterm birth. *N Engl J Med* 343:378-384, 2000.
5. O'Brien F, Roth S, Stewart A, et al: The neurodevelopmental progress of infants less than 33 weeks into adolescence. *Arch Dis Child* 89:207-211, 2004.
6. Wolke D: Psychological development of prematurely born children. *Arch Dis Child* 78:567-570, 1998.
7. Kelleher KJ, Casey PH, Bradley RH, et al: Risk factors and outcomes for failure to thrive in low birth weight preterm infants. *Pediatrics* 91(5):941-948, 1993.
8. Trachtenbarg DE, Golemon TB: Care of the premature infant: part I. Monitoring growth and development. *Am Fam Physician* 57(9):2123-2130, 1998.
9. Burgess P, Johnson A: Ocular defects in infants of extremely low birth weight and low gestational age. *Br J Ophthalmol* 75:84-87, 1991.
10. Cooke RW: Factors affecting survival and outcome at 3 years in extremely preterm infants. *Arch Dis Child Fetal Neonatal Ed* 71:F28-F31, 1994.
11. Dowdeswell HJ, Slater AM, Broomhall J, et al: Visual deficits in children born at less than 32 weeks' gestation with and without major ocular pathology and cerebral damage. *Br J Ophthalmol* 79:447-452, 1995.
12. Powls A, Botting N, Cooke RW, et al: Visual impairment in very low birthweight children. *Arch Dis Child Fetal Neonatal Ed* 76:F82-F87, 1997.
13. Vohr BR, Wright LL, Dusick AM, et al: Neurodevelopmental and functional outcomes of extremely low birth weight infants in the National Institute of Child Heath and Human Development Neonatal Research Network, 1993–1994. *Pediatrics* 105:1216-1226, 2000.
14. Blackman JA, Boyle RJ: Prematurity: primary care follow-up. In Parker S, Zuckerman B, Augustyn M, editors: *Developmental and behavioral pediatrics: a handbook for primary care.* New York, 2005, Lippincott, Williams & Wilkins.
15. Graziani LJ, Pasto M, Stanley C, et al: Neonatal neurosonographic correlates of cerebral palsy in preterm infants. *Pediatrics* 78:88-95, 1986.
16. Blasco PA: Motor delays. In Parker S, Zuckerman B, Augustyn M, editors: *Developmental and behavioral pediatrics: a handbook for primary care.* New York, 2005, Lippincott, Williams & Wilkins.
17. Palmer FB, Hoon AH: Cerebral palsy. In Parker S, Zuckerman B, Augustyn M, editors: *Developmental and behavioral pediatrics: a handbook for primary care.* New York, 2005, Lippincott, Williams & Wilkins.
18. Hack M: Follow-up for high risk neonates. In Fanaroff AA, Martin RJ, editors: *Neonatal-perinatal medicine,* ed 6. St. Louis, 1997, Mosby.
19. Glasgoe FP, Shapiro HL. Introduction to developmental and behavioral screening. Available at: ***http://www.dbpeds.org/articles/detail.cfm?id=5.*** Last accessed March 15, 2005.
20. Nugent JK, Keefer CH, Minear S, et al: *Understanding newborn behavior and early relationships: the newborn behavoral observations (NBO) system handbook.* Baltimore, 2007, Paul H. Brookes.
21. D'Angio CT, Sinkin RA, Stevens TP, et al: Longitudinal, 15-year follow-up of children born at less than 29 weeks' gestation after introduction of surfactant therapy into a region: neurologic, cognitive, and educational outcomes. *Pediatrics* 110:1094-1102, 2002.
22. Hack M, Youngstrom EA, Cartar L, et al: Behavioral outcomes and evidence of psychopathology among very low birth weight infants at age 20 years. *Pediatrics* 114:932-940, 2004.
23. Horwood J, Mogridge N, Darlow B: Cognitive, educational, and behavioural outcomes at 7 to 8 years in a national low birthweight cohort. *Arch Dis Child Fetal Neonatal Ed* 79:F12-F20, 1998.
24. Hack M, Flanner DJ, Schluchter M, et al: Outcomes in young adulthood for very-low-birth-weight infants. *N Engl J Med* 346:149-157, 2002.
25. Saigal S: Follow-up of very low birthweight babies to adolescence. *Semin Neonatol* 5:107-118, 2000.

26. Field TM: High risk infants "have less fun" during early interactions. *Top Early Child Spec Educ* 3(1):77-87,1983.
27. Larroque B, N'guyen The Tich S, Guedeney A, et al: Temperament at 9 months of very preterm infants born at less than 29 weeks' gestation: the Epipage study. *J Dev Behav Pediatr* 26(1):48-55, 2005.
28. Berger SP, Holt-Turner I, Cupoli JM, et al: Caring for the graduate from the neonatal intensive care unit. *Pediatr Clin North Am* 45:701-712, 1998.
29. Bennett FC: Developmental outcome. In Avery GB, Fletcher MA, MacDonald MG, editors: *Neonatology: pathophysiology and management of the newborn*, ed 5. Philadelphia, 1997, Lippincott, Williams & Wilkins.
30. Barr RG, Chen S, Hopkins B, et al: Crying patterns in preterm infants. *Dev Med Child Neurol* 38:345-355, 1996.
31. Green M, Solnit AJ: Reactions to the threatened loss of a child; a vulnerable child syndrome. Pediatric management of the dying child, part III. *Pediatrics* 34:58-66,1964.
32. Forsyth B: Vulnerable children. In Parker S, Zuckerman B, Augustyn M, editors: *Developmental and behavioral pediatrics: a handbook for primary care.* New York, 2005, Lippincott, Williams & Wilkins.
33. Sherman MP, Steinfeld MP, Phillipps AF, et al. Follow-up of the NICU patient. Available at: *http://www.emedicine.com/ped/topic2600.htm.* Last accessed January 15, 2007.
34. Korsch B. Talking with parents. In Parker S, Zuckerman B, Augustyn M, editors: *Developmental and behavioral pediatrics: a handbook for primary care.* New York, 2005, Lippincott, Williams & Wilkins.
35. Tommiska V, Ostberg M, Fellman V: Parental stress in families of 2 year old extremely low birthweight infants. *Arch Dis Child Fetal Neonatal Ed* 86(3):F161-F164, 2002.
36. Shonkoff JP, Yatchmink YE: Helping families deal with bad news. In Parker S, Zuckerman B, Augustyn M, editors: *Developmental and behavioral pediatrics: a handbook for primary care.* New York, 2005, Lippincott, Williams & Wilkins.

Chapter 6A

Anemia of Prematurity

Jennifer Hyde, MD

Anemia is a common condition in premature infants. Primarily, anemia occurs in this population because premature infants lack a critical intrauterine period of hematologic development. These infants are not exposed to the extremely high rate of red blood cell (RBC) production and iron storage that occurs during the last trimester of pregnancy, particularly after 32 weeks' gestation.[1] Figure 6A-1 shows the increasing RBC mass in relation to gestational age.[1] After delivery, the newborn premature infant has limited RBC production, decreased RBC survival, and rapid weight gain, all of which contribute to the development of a pathologic anemia whereby the hemoglobin (Hgb) concentration can fall to less than 10 g/dl.[2,3] Frequent blood sampling in sick premature infants exacerbates this anemia.

Development of Anemia: Three Phases

Three phases of anemia of prematurity have been described.[2] Primary care providers should be aware of these phases because monitoring and treatment strategies vary among the stages.

Phase I

The first phase occurs during the first 2 months of life and is attributed to multiple factors. In utero, the fetus is relatively hypoxemic, inducing erythropoietin (EPO) production. After birth, the rise in PaO_2 suppresses EPO production.[3] Indeed, plasma EPO is essentially undetectable in the first weeks after birth.[1] As a result, the production of RBCs decreases by a factor of approximately 10 during the first week of life. EPO production, and therefore Hgb synthesis, is lowest at 2 weeks of life (Figure 6A-2).[1]

In addition to low EPO levels, the RBC lifespan in premature infants is shorter than that of term infants or adults. Whereas the RBC lifespan in premature infants is estimated to be 35 to 50 days, the RBC lifespan in term infants is 60 to 70 days and in adults is 120 days.[1,3]

An Hgb nadir is attained when the initial RBCs have surpassed their lifespan without being

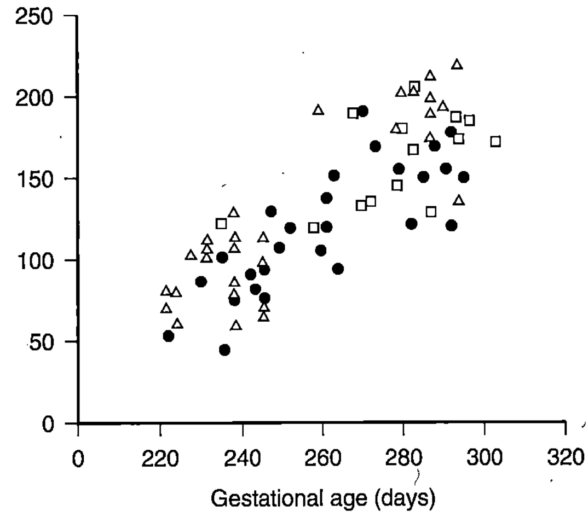

FIGURE 6A-1 The circulating red blood cell mass in newborn infants in relation to the gestational age. Circles represent values obtained by ^{51}Cr dilution method; triangles represent values obtained from plasma volume measurements. From: Brugnara CP, Orah S: The neonatal erythrocyte and its disorders. In Nathan DG, Orkin SH, Ginsburg D, Look AT, and Oski FA, editors: *Hematology of infancy and childhood*. Philadelphia, WB Saunders, 2003, p 24. Originally from: Bratteby L-E: *Acta Pediatr Scand* 57:132, 1968.

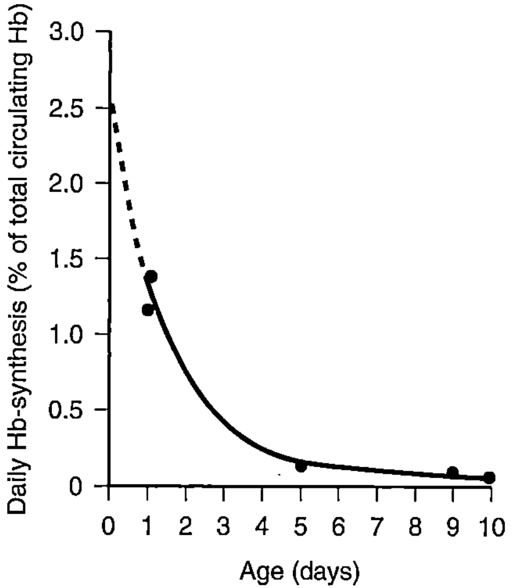

FIGURE 6A-2 The relative rate of hemoglobin synthesis at birth and during the first 10 days of life. From: Brugnara CP, Orah S: The neonatal erythrocyte and its disorders. In Nathan DG, Orkin SH, Ginsburg D, Look AT, Oski FA, editors: *Hematology of infancy and childhood*. Philadelphia, 2003, WB Saunders, p 23. Originally from: Garby L, Sjoelin S, Vuille JC: *Acta Paediatr* 52:537-53, 1963.

adequately replaced because of the abrupt termination of EPO production. The nadir for a premature infant occurs at approximately 5 to 8 weeks of life (mean Hgb 8 g/dl). A term infant has a later nadir, occurring at 8 to 12 weeks of life (mean Hgb 11 g/dl).[1,3] Premature infants have an Hgb nadir that is broader and deeper than in normal term infants. For example, the average Hgb is 8 g/dl for infants born weighing 1000 to 1500 g, 8.5 g/dl for infants born weighing 1500 to 2000 g, and 9 g/dl for those born weighing 2000 to 2500 g.[2]

During this first phase of anemia, iron is not excreted from the body. As red cells are lost as a consequence of their shorter life spans, iron accumulates. Therefore, iron availability is normal, and iron supplementation in the first few weeks of life does not prevent the inevitable nadir.[2] Thus, this first stage of anemia is a normochromic, non–iron-deficient anemia.

Phase II

Following this first phase, EPO production, and therefore erythropoiesis, resumes, and the second phase of anemia begins. During this intermediate phase, the Hgb mass begins to increase. Because of the infants' rapid weight gain and concomitant volume expansion, the hematocrit rises only slightly. Although the fall and subsequent rise in hematocrit are dependent on initial Hgb concentrations, generally by 3 months of age the same level of anemia is obtained in most infants (Figure 6A-3).[2] The source of iron for this early rise in Hgb is the iron that had been freed and stored during the early phase. The length of this second phase depends directly on the initial Hgb mass, which contains all the iron stored from birth. In general, this stage lasts approximately 6 to 8 weeks and ends with the exhaustion of available iron stores.[2]

Phase III

If exogenous iron is not provided, the late phase of anemia develops (at approximately 3–4 months of age). This is a hypochromic, microcytic anemia associated with a further drop in Hgb concentration.[2] Significant iron deficiency can persist into the second year of life. To limit and/or prevent this phase of anemia, iron therapy is recommended in all premature infants. Iron therapy results in a swift increase in Hgb concentration and correction of the anemia (Figure 6A-4).

Prevention of Anemia

Iron supplementation

To minimize the risk for significant anemia, infants should receive an appropriate dietary intake of iron. Earlier studies have found that when iron was

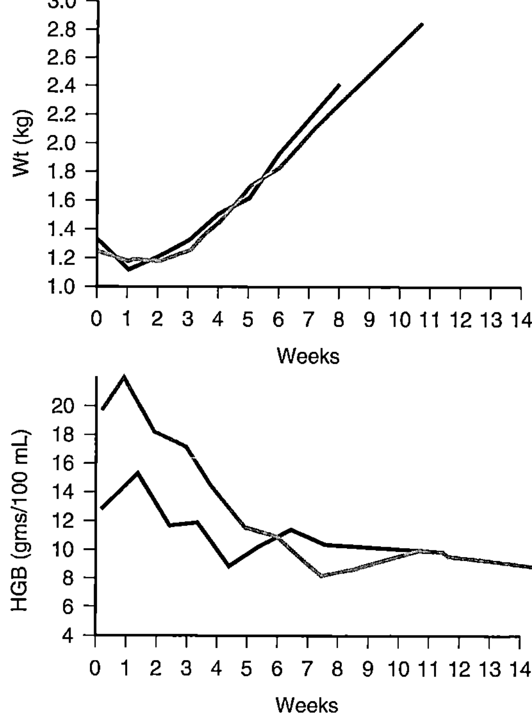

FIGURE 6A-3 The course of hemoglobin concentration in two infants with similar weight curves but with different initial hemoglobin concentrations. From: Schulman I: *J Pediatr* 54:665, 1959.

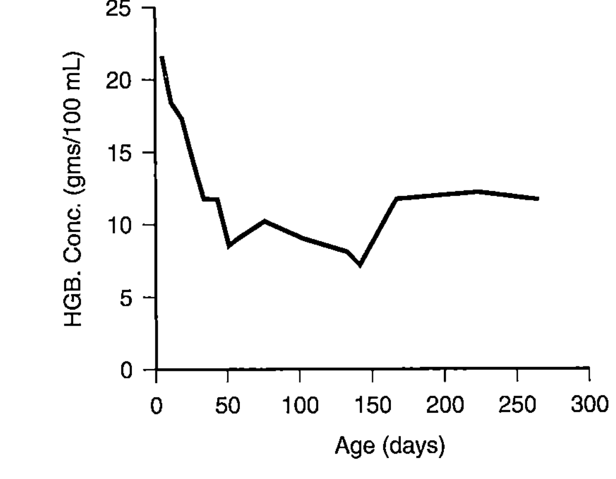

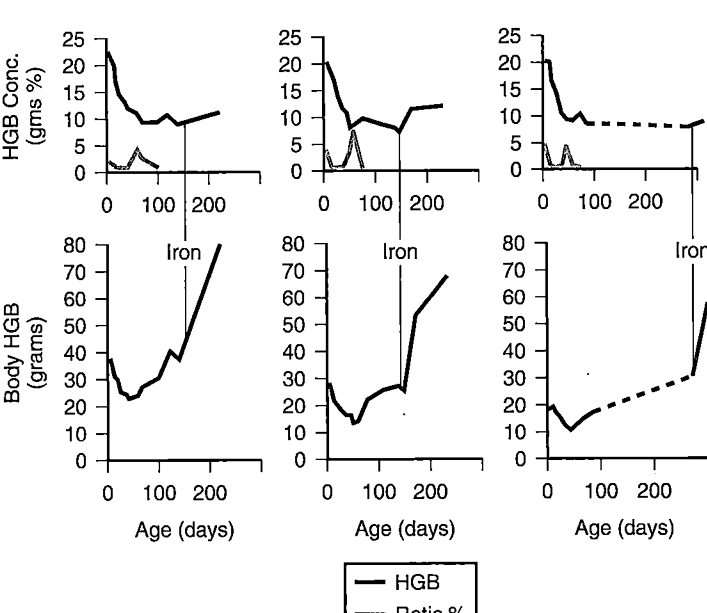

FIGURE 6A-4 Top graph: Typical course of the hemoglobin concentration in a premature infant. Bottom two graph sets: Changes in hemoglobin concentration, circulating hemoglobin mass, and reticulocyte percentage in premature infants of different birth weights. From: Schulman I: *J Pediatr* 54:667, 1959.

initiated at 4 months of age, Hgb levels rose quickly (Figure 6A-4).[2] Another study found that 2 mg/kg/day of iron supplementation in 2-week-old infants born weighing 1000 to 2000 g prevented iron deficiency at 3 months of age compared with nonsupplemented control infants (Figure 6A-5).[4] Some families worry that supplemental iron will contribute to constipation or fussiness in their infants, but therapeutic iron up to 6 mg/kg/day has been shown to be well tolerated without evidence of these concerns.[5]

Generally, it is thought that if iron supplementation is started early (beginning in the neonatal intensive care unit [NICU]) and continued for several months beyond, iron stores should be sufficient to support the infant through the necessary rebuilding of RBC mass and overall growth that occurs post nadir. Today, most premature infants are discharged from the NICU with iron therapy. The primary care provider then is faced with the challenge of determining the continued iron dose and the length of therapy required. The total enteral dose for the preterm infant who is not receiving EPO ranges from 2 to 4 mg/kg/day, depending on the degree of prematurity.[6] The American Academy of Pediatrics (AAP) recommends that the breastfed preterm infant receive at least 2 mg/kg/day of elemental iron supplementation beginning at 1 month of age until 12 months of age.[3] Because preterm or postdischarge formulas supply approximately 1.8 mg/kg/day to the average preterm infant taking 150 ml/kg/day of formula,[7] these infants may benefit from an additional 1 mg/kg/day of elemental iron.[6] Recommended doses for iron supplementation are listed in Table 6A-1.

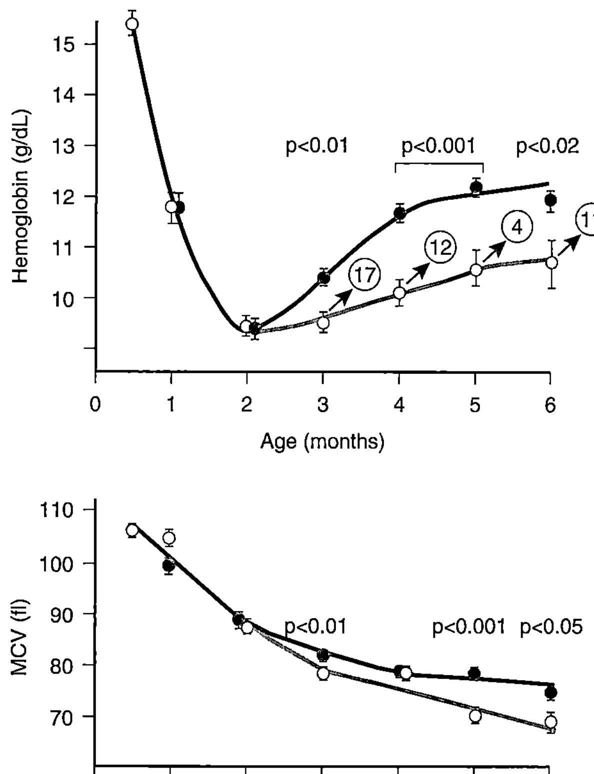

FIGURE 6A-5 Concentration of hemoglobin and mean corpuscular volume in low-birth-weight infants who received no iron supplementation (open circles) or 2 mg iron/kg/day starting at two weeks (closed circles). Means +/– SEM are indicated. Differences between the groups became significant at 3 months of age. The number of unsupplemented infants at each age started on iron supplementation on the basis of anemia is showing within circles. From: Lundstrom U, Siimes MA, Dallman PR: *J Pediatr* 91:879, 1977.

Screening

In addition to adequate dietary iron intake, screening for anemia will help to identify those infants who require more aggressive therapy. Whereas most full-term infants regain their birth Hgb level by 6 months postnatal age,[2,4] iron stores in preterm infants are sufficient for 2 to 3 months postnatally.[7] The infants at greatest risk for significant anemia are those born less than 32 weeks' gestation who were treated with recombinant EPO or never required a transfusion and who did not receive adequate iron supplementation.[7]

There are no official guidelines about screening for anemia in premature infants. If Hgb levels are measured too early (i.e., at the 2-month office visit), the measurement will correspond to the infant's nadir, independent of iron supplementation. Measuring an Hgb level at 4 or 6 months of age should correspond to the rebuilding phase of the infant. Thus, the AAP recommends screening preterm infants for anemia at approximately 4 months of age.[7] To obtain accurate results, screening should be performed by venipuncture and when the infant is healthy. A normal Hgb level at this time indicates that the infant probably can maintain his or her RBC mass on the infant's current diet and iron supplementation. For infants without anemia, the primary care provider should repeat the screening by 9 to 12 months of age (see the management section for recommendations about treating infants with anemia).

Management

Blood transfusions

Because the decline of Hgb level is directly related to the birth weight of the infant as a result of iatrogenic causes, many very-low-birth-weight premature infants will require blood transfusions during their time in the NICU. Usually a combination of clinical signs and symptoms determines the timing of transfusions. Signs of hypoxemia include tachycardia, tachypnea, poor feeding, and apnea and bradycardia spells. Although there are no clear guidelines, some common indications for transfusion include the following:

1. Replacing blood after >10% of the infant's blood volume has been removed,

Table 6A-1 Iron Supplementation Guidelines in the Preterm Infant

Nutrient	Breastfed	Formula-fed
Elemental iron*	2 mg/kg/day iron supplementation starting at 1 month until 12 months† Iron supplementation should be provided as elemental iron drops; a vitamin preparation with iron is less likely to provide sufficient iron for the preterm breastfed infant	Only iron-fortified formulas are recommended Because iron-fortified formulas (including postdischarge formulas) supply ≈1.8 mg/kg/day at an intake of 150 ml/kg/day, some infants may benefit from an additional 1 mg/kg/day until 12 months of age (this can be administered as either iron drops or in a vitamin preparation with iron)

Data from: Rao R, Georgieff: Microminerals. In Tsang RC, Uauy R, Koletzko B, et al., editors: *Nutrition of the preterm infant: scientific basis and practical guidelines*, ed 3. Cincinnati, Ohio, 2005, Digital Educational Publishing; and American Academy of Pediatrics (AAP) Committee on Nutrition: Iron deficiency. In Kleinman RE, editor: *Pediatric nutrition handbook*, ed 5. Elk Grove Village, Ill, 2004, American Academy of Pediatrics.

Note: This is a recommended guideline that does not represent a professional standard of care; care should be revised to meet individual patient needs.

*Infants who are receiving erythropoietin should be given 6 mg/kg/day iron supplementation.

†This is the current American Academy of Pediatrics recommendation, which does not stipulate chronological vs corrected age. Tsang et al.[10] continue to recommend 2–4/mg/kg/day for ELBW and VLBW infants.

2. Maintaining a hematocrit >35% to 40% in patients with severe respiratory distress or symptomatic heart disease,
3. Maintaining hematocrit >30% in neonates with mild-to-moderate cardiopulmonary problems, growth failure, or significant apnea, and/or
4. Transfusing any asymptomatic infant with a hematocrit <21% and reticulocytes <3%.[1,3]

There is a high variability of transfusion guidelines among different centers. Because of the high cost of transfusions and the small risk of bloodborne infections, minimizing the need for transfusions is an area of active investigation.

Erythropoietin

EPO levels decrease in the first several weeks of life, precipitating anemia of prematurity.[1,8] Recombinant human erythropoietin (rhEPO) has been given to premature infants to stimulate RBC production in an attempt to minimize the need for transfusions. Treatment with rhEPO has been shown to reduce, but not eliminate, the need for blood transfusions. Unfortunately, therapy is extremely expensive. Furthermore, results have not been consistent enough to recommend rhEPO therapy as a standard of care.[1,8,9] To assist the stimulated bone marrow, iron (6 mg/kg/day) and vitamin E should be given to infants treated with rhEPO.[1]

Iron supplementation

If an infant has evidence of anemia, the presumptive iron deficiency anemia can be treated with a higher oral elemental iron dose (3–6 mg/kg/day of elemental iron) for 4 weeks.[7] If the Hgb level increases by more than 1 g/dl or if the hematocrit increases by more than 3%, the diagnosis of iron deficiency anemia can be confirmed, and the iron regimen should be continued for 2 months before rechecking values.[7] It is important to monitor Hgb and hematocrit values after 6 months of successful therapy.

If the repeat Hgb or hematocrit values have not improved after 4 weeks of a higher supplemental iron dose, further laboratory evaluation is indicated.[7] A serum ferritin value and RBC indexes (i.e., mean corpuscular value and RBC distribution width) may be helpful. If possible, a reticulocyte cellular Hgb (CHr) level should be obtained; if this value is low, there is a high probability of iron deficiency.

Conclusion

This chapter highlights the major components of iron physiology in the newborn. Because premature infants are at high risk for developing anemia, the primary care provider should ensure that these infants receive the current recommended iron supplementation. In addition, screening for anemia at approximately 4 months of age will identify those infants at greatest risk and determine whether additional iron supplementation is necessary. Further evaluation is required for infants who remain anemic.

Acknowledgment

The author thanks Ellis Neufeld, MD, PhD, for critical review of this chapter.

REFERENCES

1. Brugnara CP, Orah S: The neonatal erythrocyte and its disorders. In Nathan DG, Orkin SH, Ginsburg D, et al., editors: *Hematology of infancy and childhood.* Philadelphia, 2003, WB Saunders.
2. Schulman I: The anemia of prematurity. *J Pediatr* 54:663-672, 1959.
3. Salsbury DC: Anemia of prematurity. *Neonatal Netw* 20:13-20, 2001.
4. Lundstrom U, Siimes MA, Dallman PR: At what age does iron supplementation become necessary in low-birth-weight infants? *J Pediatr* 91:878-883, 1977.
5. Iron fortification of infant formulas. American Academy of Pediatrics. Committee on Nutrition. *Pediatrics* 104:119-123, 1999.
6. Rao R, Georgieff: Microminerals. In Tsang RC, Uauy R, Koletzko B, et al., editors: *Nutrition of the preterm infant: scientific basis and practical guidelines,* ed 3. Cincinnati, Ohio, 2005, Digital Educational Publishing.
7. American Academy of Pediatrics (AAP) Committee on Nutrition: Iron deficiency. In Kleinman RE, editor: *Pediatric nutrition handbook,* ed 5. Elk Grove Village, Ill, 2004, American Academy of Pediatrics.
8. Juul SE: Erythropoietin in the neonate. *Curr Probl Pediatr* 29:129-149, 1999.
9. Kling PJ, Winzerling JJ: Iron status and the treatment of the anemia of prematurity. *Clin Perinatol* 29:283-294, 2002.
10. Gracey M, Tsang R, Abrams S, editors: *Nutrition of the preterm infant,* ed 2. Cincinnati, Ohio, 2005, Digital Educational Publishing.

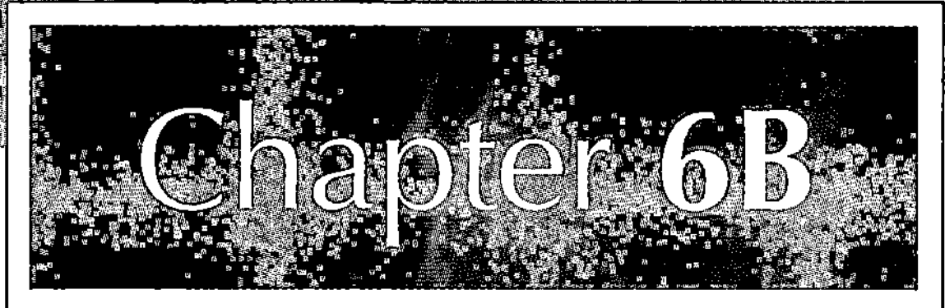

Indirect Hyperbilirubinemia

Steven A. Ringer, MD, PhD

Indirect or unconjugated hyperbilirubinemia is one of the most common and important issues for all newborns. It is of even greater significance for premature newborns, among whom both the incidence and potential risks are increased. The serum level of bilirubin in all newborns is elevated by adult standards, but as many as 60% of term infants will have levels that rise above 5 to 7 mg/dl,[1] and the percentage is higher in preterm infants. In a subset of babies the level gets high enough to be associated with a risk of bilirubin toxicity, but effective therapy to reduce the level is available if started in a timely fashion. Therefore, the global management of hyperbilirubinemia is geared toward early identification of the subset of babies at risk for elevated levels, the rapid institution of appropriate therapy, and avoidance of toxicity. The key to identification must be based on the recognition of the factors commonly associated with a greater elevation in serum bilirubin and a system of screening and follow-up. Screening based on the appearance of symptoms is of little help because most affected babies are otherwise well, with no other signs or symptoms.

Except in unusual cases, the most critical period for the development of significant hyperbilirubinemia is in the days immediately following birth. For premature infants born at gestational ages less than 34 weeks, significant hyperbilirubinemia is extremely common, with as many as 80% of babies requiring therapy, including nearly 100% of those born before 30 weeks' gestation. In part, this is because levels that might be considered moderate or normal in term infants are of greater concern in small premature infants, so therapy is instituted earlier. This normal physiologic hyperbilirubinemia is compounded by several factors. Bilirubin production may be increased as a result of infection, altered metabolic status, skin bruising, or intraventricular hemorrhage, all of which are more common in immature infants. Bilirubin excretion is diminished as a result of limited or absent enteral feedings. Finally, the multiple care needs and the changing characteristics of the skin make it more difficult to maintain adequate hydration, and even a relatively minor degree of dehydration may contribute to increased bilirubin levels.

In very immature infants, hyperbilirubinemia will have resolved or will be substantially diminished by the time of discharge from the hospital, so evaluation and treatment of these patients is not of direct clinical concern to the practicing pediatrician. In contrast, premature infants born at late preterm gestational ages (34–37 weeks' gestation) may be discharged while still in the early stages of hyperbilirubinemia. As many as one fourth of this group may develop hyperbilirubinemia requiring therapy, and they are at increased risk for sequelae.[2] These infants require close monitoring in the first several days of life.

The care for premature infants after discharge is enhanced by an understanding of the normal physiology of bilirubin production and metabolism, the pathologic conditions that result in significant hyperbilirubinemia, and the diagnosis and treatment of the possible sequelae. It is particularly important to understand the important differences between the full-term infant and the late preterm infant, and how this affects evaluation and treatment of hyperbilirubinemia.

Pathophysiology of Neonatal Hyperbilirubinemia

Bilirubin is the breakdown product of heme from red blood cells and some other proteins (Figure 6B-1). Heme is converted to biliverdin, a greenish compound, and carbon monoxide. Heme oxygenase catalyzes this rate-limiting step in which the biliverdin and carbon monoxide are produced in amounts equimolar to the amount of degraded hemoglobin. Biliverdin then is converted to

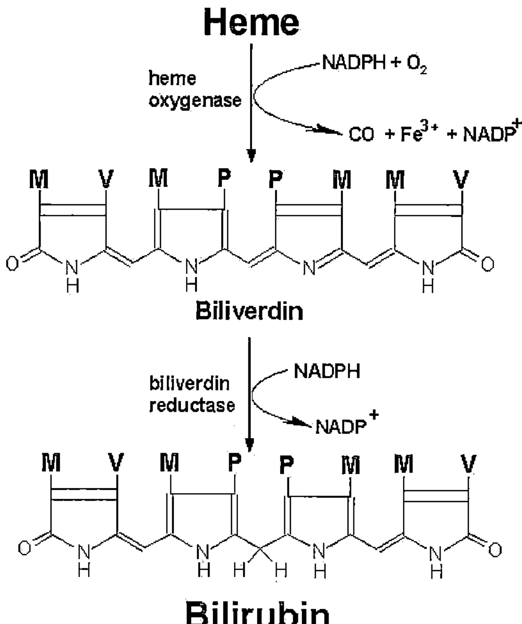

FIGURE 6B-1 Heme is broken down to biliverdin, carbon monoxide, and iron by heme oxygenase. Biliverdin is then converted to bilirubin by biliverdin reductase. Bilirubin can then be conjugated by glucuronyl transferase to form bilirubin diglucuronide. From: *http://isu.indstate.edu/mwking/heme-porphyrin.html*

bilirubin, a reaction that is catalyzed by biliverdin reductase. Bilirubin normally is bound to albumin in the serum, transported to the liver, taken up by hepatocytes, and converted to monoglucuronyl-bilirubin and diglucuronyl-bilirubin by uridine diphosphate glucuronosyltransferase (UDPGT). The conjugated species are excreted via the bile into the intestinal tract.

Some hyperbilirubinemia develops in all newborns because of physiologic processes that increase bilirubin production and decrease excretion. The normal hematocrit of a term infant is between 45% and 60% and that of a premature infant is 40% to 50%, depending on gestational age, so a greater load of hemoglobin per unit of body weight is available for degradation than is the case in older patients. Newborn red cells also turn over faster because they contain fetal hemoglobin (hemoglobin F), and their lifespan is only approximately 90 days, much shorter than the 120-day lifespan of cells, which contain adult hemoglobin.[3]

Newborns also are deficient in UDPGT activity, so they are less able to conjugate and excrete bilirubin.[4] Immediately after birth, almost no conjugation occurs, and, at most, monoglucuronides are formed on the first day of life. Bilirubin itself induces enzymatic activity, so by day 2 to 3 a significant percentage of the bilirubin is fully conjugated and excretion increased. In patients of East Asian ethnicity and within some families, and in some pathologic cases,[5] newborn jaundice is worse because UDPGT activity is diminished as a result of expansion of thymine-adenine repeats in the promoter region of the primary coding gene (Figure 6B-2). Bilirubin levels also are normally higher in males and in infants born to mothers with diabetes.[6]

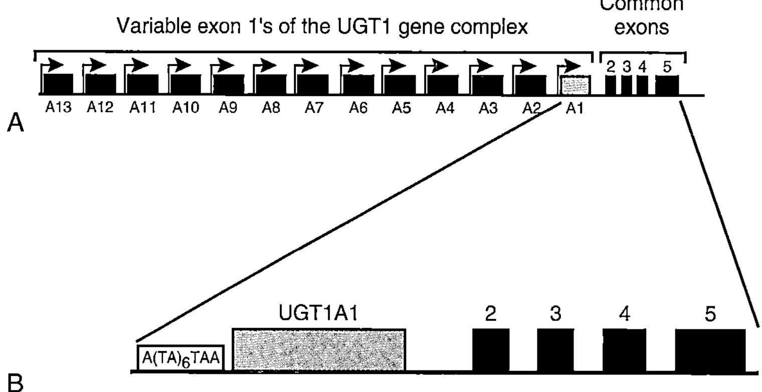

FIGURE 6B-2 The upper panel shows a schematic representation of the genomic structure of the UDPGT gene complex. The exploded area in the lower panel shows the exons 1A1 and 2-5 that have been identified as the sites for mutations leading to absent or decreased activity. From: Clarke DJ, Mogharbi N, Monaghan G, et al: *Clin Chim Acta* 266:63-74, 1997.

Excretion is diminished because newborns, especially those who are premature or breastfed,[6] have a much slower rate of intestinal transit. This magnifies the effect of enterohepatic circulation on decreasing net excretion. Conjugated bilirubin, especially the monoglucuronide form commonly found in newborns, is unconjugated by β-glucuronidase in the intestinal wall, and the bilirubin is reabsorbed and returned to the serum. The bacterial flora, which would prevent this action by reducing conjugated bilirubin to nonresorbable urobilinogen, are lacking in newborns.

Prematurity exacerbates hyperbilirubinemia because slower intestinal motility and immature or discoordinated feeding result in decreased intake, diminished bilirubin excretion, and increased enterohepatic circulation, especially among breastfed babies. Among well, late preterm infants, the bilirubin levels are similar to those of term babies in the first 3 to 4 days, when the levels usually peak and begin to decline in term infants. Levels in premature infants continue to rise slightly thereafter, reach peak levels on days 5 to 7,[7] and decline more slowly thereafter.

Distinguishing normal from abnormal

The challenges posed by hyperbilirubinemia in the newborn include determining which babies have "normal" or physiologic jaundice and which have a pathologic reason for the jaundice. Equally important, the practitioner must determine what degree of elevation in bilirubin level is concerning in each baby and what therapy might be required. This task is difficult even in term infants because, although serum concentrations usually peak at 5 to 6 mg/dl (86–103 μmol/L), they may rise as high as 7 to 17 mg/dl (104–291 μmol/L) and still be normal.

The assessment is even more complex in premature babies in whom the usual level of bilirubin is somewhat higher than in term infants of equivalent weight and postnatal age, but the risk of a particular level may be increased by additional factors common in these babies. The best approach is to consider the bilirubin level at a known postnatal age in hours and to determine whether this fits into the normal pattern of bilirubin rise after birth or predicts the development of an abnormally high or risky level. The abnormal patterns that strongly suggest a pathologic cause include a rapid increase on the first day, a rise above 15 to 17 mg/dl, or hyperbilirubinemia that is unresponsive to phototherapy.

Contribution of breastfeeding to hyperbilirubinemia

Breastfeeding is a normal phenomenon that should be actively encouraged and supported because the benefits in terms of newborn health and maternal–infant interaction are enormous. Breastfeeding influences the course of hyperbilirubinemia in healthy babies more than any other factor, especially in premature infants. The adequacy of feeding in the first few days tends to influence the maximum level of bilirubin, whereas factors related to the properties of human milk itself tend to influence the duration of hyperbilirubinemia.

When breastfeeding is optimized, the serum levels of bilirubin in the first 5 days of life are similar to those in infants fed artificial formula (Figures 6B-3 and 6B-4), with the same maximum levels. In otherwise healthy breastfed babies, bilirubin levels in the first several days may significantly exceed those in formula-fed infants. This phenomenon is well known, often considered part of the normal pattern of hyperbilirubinemia in these babies, and thus is dismissed as being without consequence. However, excessively high levels should *not* be expected in a breastfeeding baby, and dismissing them increases the likelihood of missing a more serious condition. The common confusion

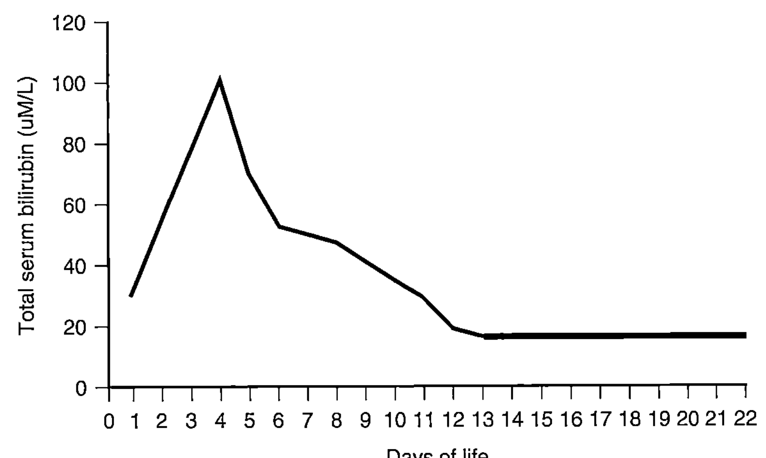

FIGURE 6B-3 In artificially fed infants the bilirubin level peaks about 3-4 days and declines thereafter. Premature infants may have a later and/or higher peak with a slower decline. From: Gartner L: *Journal Perinatol* 21:2001, p S29.

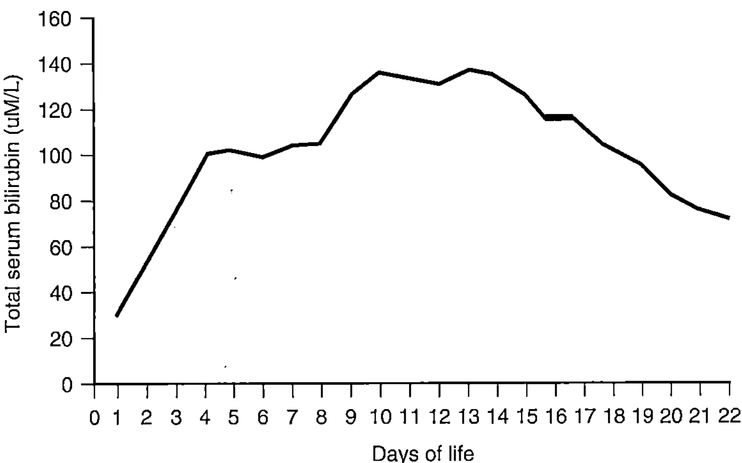

FIGURE 6B-4 In optimally fed infants the peak bilirubin level is similar to that in artificially fed infants, but it occurs several days later and declines more slowly thereafter. In premature infants the peak may be higher and the rate of decline is often very slow. To convert umol/L to ~mg/dL divide by 17. From: Gartner L: *Journal Perinatol* 21:2001, p S29.

is due to inaccurate terminology, as this early hyperbilirubinemia has often been termed *breastfeeding jaundice*, implying that it is a *normal* process. Gartner[8] has urged that the more precise term *breast-nonfeeding jaundice* be used. This term makes it clear that the early hyperbilirubinemia is the result of decreased or inadequate intake of milk, which is abnormal and potentially dangerous to the baby. Successful breastfeeding depends on the production of adequate quantities of milk, which is best achieved by the initiation of breastfeeding within the first hour after birth and then giving 10 to 12 feedings per day of breast milk alone for the first 1 to 2 weeks. Considerable support of mother and baby is required, including help with proper positioning of the infant to support his or her ability to suckle. The effectiveness of feeding can be assessed by monitoring overall weight loss; weight loss that is less than 8% to 10% from birth weight is a very reassuring sign.[8]

The addition of water or formula feedings is not recommended because this will diminish maternal confidence and disrupt maternal–infant interaction, effects that will result in decreased milk production and thereby worsen the underlying problem. The rise in bilirubin levels under conditions of decreased feeding volume almost certainly occurs as a result of diminished caloric intake and not simply from dehydration. In human adults and newborn monkeys,[9] a state of partial starvation results in increased intestinal reabsorption of bilirubin, and this enhanced enterohepatic circulation most likely is the cause of elevated bilirubin in human newborns as well.

Prematurity, especially late preterm infants, increases the likelihood of significant breast nonfeeding jaundice. Babies born at even lower gestational ages are closely monitored as inpatients, and their feedings are closely measured, but babies born at 35 to 36 weeks' gestation usually are cared for in newborn nurseries, where estimates of intake are only approximate. Because of their immaturity, these babies may feed sluggishly or in a poorly coordinated manner, making it more likely that their intake will be diminished. They may be discharged from the hospital at approximately 2 days of age, often before their mother's milk letdown has occurred or adequate intake has been established. To reduce the possibility of significant jaundice, routine screening of the bilirubin level should be performed before discharge (see later), and these babies should be evaluated within 1 to 2 days of discharge. Thereafter, they should be seen at an interval dictated by their individual progress and not according to a standard protocol. In this way, a significant increase in bilirubin level among breastfed premature babies can be prevented or minimized; the importance of this benefit cannot be overestimated. Pathologic causes of hyperbilirubinemia are relatively uncommon, but the incidence of feeding difficulties in late preterm infants is high and, within this population, is the cause of the greatest potential risk for both hyperbilirubinemia and bilirubin toxicity.

Although peak bilirubin levels in adequately breastfed infants do not exceed those in infants fed artificial formula, the overall course of hyperbilirubinemia in these infants is different and more prolonged, especially in premature babies. After day 5, the levels typically rise somewhat or remain stable over the following 10 days. Thereafter, they begin to decline slowly but may remain elevated for several weeks. Originally, this "breast milk jaundice" was thought to result from pregnanediol, an inhibitor of hepatic glucuronyl transferase,[10] in the milk. It now seems more likely that some unidentified factor in mature human milk increases the intestinal reabsorption of bilirubin, resulting in a persistence of increased serum levels. This normal process may result in levels of 10 to 12 mg/dl that persist in a breastfed premature infant for 3 to 4 weeks. It is a diagnosis of exclusion; if levels reach 18 to 20 mg/dl, a pathologic cause must be ruled out.

Pathologic Causes of Hyperbilirubinemia

A bilirubin level higher than 17 mg/dl in a full or preterm newborn in the first several days of life is unusual enough that it should be evaluated because it is much more likely to have an underlying pathologic cause.[11] The causes of elevated indirect hyperbilirubinemia in the newborn are listed in Table 6B-1. The diagnosis of pathologic hyperbilirubinemia is very important because neurologic injury is more likely in these instances. The two major exceptions, as stressed earlier, are late preterm birth and/or inadequate breastfeeding, which often occur together. Even in these clinical settings, an additional cause for an excessive level of bilirubin should always be ruled out, once treatment is initiated.

The serum level of bilirubin reflects the balance between production and elimination, so the level peaks as conjugation and excretion begin to increase, and production either slows or remains constant. Pathologic causes of jaundice include an abnormally increased rate of bilirubin production, an abnormally diminished uptake or conjugation by the liver or increased enterohepatic circulation,[12] or a combination of factors.

Hemolytic diseases

Increased production of bilirubin occurs as a result of increased or accelerated red cell (erythrocyte) destruction. The most common cause is immune-mediated hemolysis caused by blood group

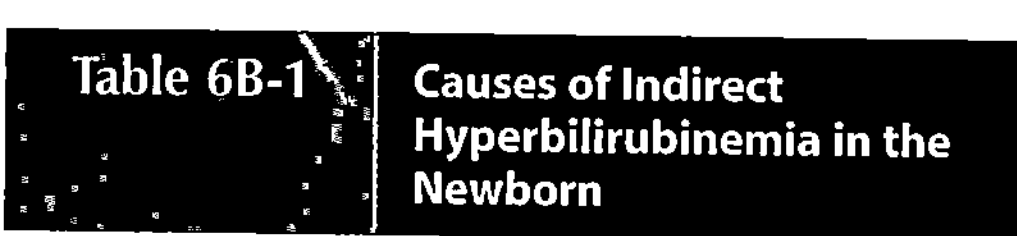
Table 6B-1 Causes of Indirect Hyperbilirubinemia in the Newborn

INCREASED BILIRUBIN PRODUCTION

Hemolytic disease resulting from fetal–maternal blood group incompatibilities
  Rh, AB-O, Kell, Duffy, c, E
Structural defects of red cell membrane
  Spherocytosis, elliptocytosis
Red cell enzyme deficiencies
  Glucose-6-phosphate dehydrogenase, pyruvate kinase, hexokinase
Significant extravascular blood
Polycythemia
Sepsis

DECREASED EXCRETION

Prematurity
Breast *non*feeding
Increased enterohepatic circulation
Gilbert disease
Crigler-Najjar syndrome
Congenital hypothyroidism
Sepsis

incompatibilities between baby and mother. In these disorders, an antigen present on the surface of the fetal erythrocytes is foreign to the mother, and maternal antibodies are formed against this antigen when fetal erythrocytes enter the maternal circulation via small fetomaternal hemorrhages or transplacental exchange. These immunoglobulin G (IgG) antibodies then cross the placenta into the fetal circulation and bind to fetal cells, which are then hemolyzed. The released hemoglobin is metabolized to bilirubin.

The most severe immune reactions are those caused by incompatibilities in the Rh factor or D antigen. However, Rh disease is rarely seen now because of vigilant monitoring of Rh-negative women during gestation and prophylactic treatment with concentrated anti-D immunoglobulin G (RhoGAM). Hyperbilirubinemia resulting from incompatibility between A or B type blood in the fetus and type O in the mother is now the most common immune-mediated cause. ABO disease tends to be much less severe than Rh disease but occasionally can result in severe hemolysis and hyperbilirubinemia, especially among cases of B-O incompatibility. Other blood group incompatibilities, such as those attributable to antigens Kell, Duffy, c, or E, occasionally cause severe hemolytic disease and severe hyperbilirubinemia of the newborn. These cases can be identified by routine testing of all pregnant women for blood type and screening for serum antibodies.

Nonimmune hemolysis can occur when structural defects in the red cell membrane result in increased cell destruction, as in spherocytosis and elliptocytosis.[13,14] Spherocytosis presents with hemolytic anemia, reticulocytosis, and spherocytes observed on the peripheral blood smear. The red cells in this disorder are susceptible to hemolysis because of osmotic stress as they age, but the osmotic fragility test for this characteristic is unreliable in the newborn because most of the red cells are relatively young. Many cases of this autosomal dominant disorder are the result of new mutations, so a family history may be absent.

Deficiencies of several red cell enzymes, including glucose-6-phosphate dehydrogenase (G6PD), pyruvate kinase, or hexokinase, make red cells susceptible to oxidative injury and rapid destruction and lead to excessive bilirubin production. The most common is G6PD deficiency, which also is associated with a significant decrease in bilirubin conjugation[15,16] as a result of a gene interaction between the G6PD deficiency and the promoter polymorphism for the variant gene of UDPGT. The combination leads to extremely high bilirubin levels in affected infants after the first few days of life. This disorder is more common among those of African descent, but it occurs in virtually all ethnic groups.

Hemolytic diseases appear to increase the risk of bilirubin toxicity for reasons that are not yet clear. The level at which bilirubin poses a risk of acute or permanent injury is lower in these patients, so therapy should begin at levels lower than in infants with nonhemolytic hyperbilirubinemia. Hemolysis should be suspected if the hematocrit is low or is dropping, and if the reticulocyte count is elevated at birth. Abnormal red cell forms, such as spherocytes or microspherocytes, may be identified on the blood smear. A Coombs test may be positive in the presence of immune-mediated hemolysis, although the reliability of this test is limited in the newborn.

Nonhemolytic causes of production

Hyperbilirubinemia can result from polycythemia (hematocrit >70), a high–normal hematocrit, and any significant amount of extravascular blood collection, such as hematoma or bruises. Severe bacterial infection may cause elevated bilirubin levels both by hemolysis and by impairing hepatic conjugation and excretion.

Disorders of excretion

Elevated levels of bilirubin can result from deficient hepatic uptake or excretion. Gilbert syndrome[17] is a benign disorder occurring in 3% to 7% of the population and is characterized by chronic unconjugated jaundice. The male/female ratio is approximately 4:1, and both homozygous and heterozygous forms exist. The clinical manifestations are not usually significant until the second decade of life, but patients with the disorder will have an accelerated increase in bilirubin level in the newborn period.[17] The disorder appears to be partially caused by abnormalities in either the function or the amount of hepatic membrane uptake proteins, which limits hepatic uptake.[18] However, the primary defect appears to be a diminution in the activity of the conjugating enzyme UDPGT resulting from an expansion of thymine-adenine (TA) repeats in the promoter region of the primary coding gene.[19] Other variations in this gene may also result in hyperbilirubinemia, and combined abnormalities may occur in a single patient, including such variable presentations as G6PD deficiency and Gilbert syndrome occurring together.[17,20]

Crigler-Najjar syndrome type I is a severe autosomal recessive deficiency of the conjugating enzyme, which presents with a rapid rise in serum bilirubin to a concentration of 30 to 40 mg/dl and frank encephalopathy.[21,22] Therapy may extend beyond exchange transfusion and aggressive phototherapy to include both liver transplantation and auxiliary orthotopic transplantation in order to prevent injury.[23] Crigler-Najjar syndrome type II is a milder disorder in which serum levels of bilirubin rarely rise above 20 mg/dl.[24]

Congenital hypothyroidism results in hyperbilirubinemia because of diminished excretion and should be considered in patients with prolonged jaundice and diminished stool output. Other rare causes of diminished excretion are Lucey-Driscoll syndrome and transient familial neonatal hyperbilirubinemia. In this familial disorder, severe early hyperbilirubinemia develops because of an uncharacterized inhibitor of UDPGT in the serum and then gradually resolves over 2 weeks. The bilirubin concentration may initially rise to dangerous levels, so close monitoring of infants from affected families is necessary.[21,25]

Especially in premature infants in whom feeding is inadequate, bacterial flora are decreased, and intestinal motility is diminished,[26] exaggerated enterohepatic circulation may be viewed as a pathologic state.

Toxicity of hyperbilirubinemia

Indirect or unconjugated bilirubin is a neurotoxin. Injury occurs when serum levels are markedly elevated and/or certain predisposing factors are present, allowing enough bilirubin to reach the central nervous system. The first clinical descriptions of bilirubin encephalopathy, or kernicterus, were reported in the United States between 50 and 100 years ago. Most cases at that time occurred as a result of Rh isoimmunization and the resultant hemolysis, leading to extremely high serum levels of bilirubin. The availability of immune anti-D globulin and intrauterine transfusion resulted in a marked reduction in the incidence and severity of this disorder. Phototherapy has provided a noninvasive therapy that can be easily used to prevent most cases of excessive elevations in bilirubin levels from any cause. Consequently, toxicity from hyperbilirubinemia became an extremely rare condition in the United States, unfamiliar to most practitioners.

Over the past 15 years the incidence of bilirubin encephalopathy apparently has increased, in part because of a more relaxed approach to therapy as the disease disappeared and earlier hospital discharge after birth. The relatively recent inclusion of otherwise healthy late preterm infants in the group discharged in 2 days has added a population at increased risk for the problem. This is compounded by the fact that the large increase in breastfeeding has outstripped the availability of adequate support measures in many places, making inadequate feeding more likely (discussed earlier).

The term *kernicterus* refers to the pathologic changes that occur in the brain correlating with bilirubin toxicity, including staining and necrosis of the basal ganglia, hippocampal cortex, subthalamic nuclei, and cerebellum. If the patient survives the acute phase of injury, gliosis will develop in the affected areas of the brain, but the cerebral cortex generally is not involved.[27,28] The mechanism of cytotoxicity appears to be mitochondrial injury to astrocytes and neurons. MRP1/Mrp1 protein levels in central nervous system endothelia and cells mediate active export of bilirubin. Genetic differences in the upregulation of these proteins in response to bilirubin may explain differential sensitivity to injury between patients[29] and the reason that associated risk factors are important.

Normally, bilirubin is carried bound to albumin in the bloodstream, and the capacity for binding is very high. In the healthy infant, each gram of albumin can bind 8.2 to 8.5 mg of bilirubin. Thus, an infant with a normal serum albumin of 3.0 g/dl should be able to fully bind all serum bilirubin up to a level of approximately 25 mg/dl. Only levels in excess of this value might then pose a danger to the infant, and an albumin/bilirubin ratio can be used to estimate risk in a healthy term infant. The binding capacity of albumin is altered by changes in serum pH, hypercarbia, hypoxemia, or the presence of certain drugs or clinical conditions, making it especially difficult to estimate a "danger level" of bilirubin in ill or premature infants.

Direct measurement of bilirubin binding capacity is not clinically available, so rough rules are used to determine the level that might pose a danger in a particular infant. In general, a maximum level of 20 to 25 mg/dl is considered safe for healthy term infants in the absence of hemolysis. For premature infants, the estimates are based in part on older autopsy data demonstrating pathologic changes in premature infants at levels well below 20 to 25 mg/dl. Conventionally, a bilirubin level (in milligrams per deciliter) that is less than 1% of the birth weight (e.g., a level of 14 mg/dl for a baby with a birth weight of 1350–1400 g) is reasonably considered to be safe for a particular infant. Such an estimate must be lowered when factors are present that can diminish bilirubin binding or alter the permeability of the blood-brain barrier. Binding is reduced by decreased pH, elevated pCO_2, drugs, and preservatives, most notably the strongly contraindicated sulfa drugs and benzoates.[30] Illness, particularly infection, can affect the integrity of the blood-brain barrier. These factors increase the risk of bilirubin toxicity at lower serum levels, and clinical practice must be adjusted accordingly.[31]

The duration of excessive hyperbilirubinemia appears to determine the degree and chronicity of toxicity. No information on how long the level must be elevated in order to result in permanent and severe damage is available, but it is clear that prompt treatment of elevated levels, by whatever mechanism is likely to decrease the levels the fastest, can correct early neurologic symptoms and prevent sequelae.[32-35] Shapiro and Nakamura[35] make this point very directly: "the faster and more aggressive the treatment, the more reversible and better the outcome."

Kernicterus also refers to the clinical presentation of bilirubin-induced neurologic injury. Clinical features vary considerably among patients[12]; as many as 15% have no acute neurologic symptoms at all. The disease course consists of an acute phase, which consists of three overlapping periods, and a later chronic phase if the baby survives. The earliest signs begin soon after birth (days 1–2) and include poor suck, hypotonia, depressed sensorium, and seizures in a jaundiced infant, problems which may progress to death. The second phase begins at about the middle of the first week of life and presents as fever and a high-pitched cry. Overall tone typically alternates between hypertonia and hypotonia, and a paralysis of upward gaze occurs. During this phase, spasm of extensor muscles becomes a prominent sign, resulting in the arching of the back and neck, the hallmark opisthotonus and retrocollis of kernicterus. The third phase of the acute disease occurs after 7 days of age. The initial hypertonia, a prominent sign, gradually diminishes over time. During the entire acute phase, brainstem auditory evoked potentials will be either absent or distinctly abnormal, and magnetic resonance imaging demonstrates hyperintense lesions in the globus pallidus.[35,36]

Over the first year, an affected infant will manifest hypotonia and motor delay, with preserved or even active deep tendon reflexes. Later in childhood, dysplasia of the dental enamel is noted, along with paralysis of upward gaze and sensorineural hearing loss. The most prominent findings include movement disorders, such as choreoathetosis, ballismus and tremor, and moderate-to-severe developmental delay.[36]

The initial presentation in premature infants is more subtle and often much more difficult to diagnose accurately. The early mortality approaches 100%, whereas the rate is approximately 50% in term infants. In both groups, most deaths occur in the first few days.[3,37]

Individual differences in susceptibility and the effectiveness of early treatment in reversing toxicity in some infants make it difficult to predict either the severity or long-term outcome in a particular infant. In addition, although peak serum levels lower than those predicted to be dangerous are unlikely to lead to injury, this question has not been answered conclusively. Almost 30 years ago, The Collaborative Perinatal Project studied 27,000 infants and demonstrated a relationship between overall neurodevelopment in the first year of life and maximum serum bilirubin. Similar correlations have been reported elsewhere, but only among infants whose birth weights exceeded 1500 g, and the differences disappeared by 5 years of age.[38,39]

A 17-year follow-up of a large study of infants with neonatal hyperbilirubinemia in excess of 20 mg/dl demonstrated an association between high levels and slightly reduced IQ in males alone.[40]

Although the primary cause of neurologic damage is an elevated bilirubin level, other factors definitely can increase the risk of any particular level in any particular baby. Prematurity or the presence of hemolysis are important, but sex, genetic factors, and overall clinical status, including asphyxia, acidosis, or sepsis, also have been identified as contributing to risk.[12] The contribution of these factors appears to be particularly important for the premature infant with underlying acute or chronic morbidity, and these factors need to be considered when the physician is evaluating a specific patient and making decisions about treatment and follow-up.

Diagnosis and Management

Diagnosis and management of hyperbilirubinemia that is of concern are complicated by the variability in course, vulnerability, and cause among different patients, and by the fact that some hyperbilirubinemia is normal. Patients who develop clinical jaundice soon after birth are most obviously at risk, making early identification important. The traditional diagnostic tool has been direct clinical assessment, with increased vigilance in the presence of the factors associated with increased risk. If an infant is viewed under good lighting conditions with a white light source or natural daylight, the serum bilirubin level generally has been estimated on the basis of how much of the baby appears visibly jaundiced, progressing in a cephalocaudal manner.[41] This method may be somewhat helpful once the baby already appears jaundiced, but studies show that this method is variably reliable and may miss infants with significant hyperbilirubinemia, including those with darker skin or those in whom significant jaundice develops after the first 1 to 2 days of life.[42,43] There now is no doubt that a better approach to early diagnosis is to complement the clinical examination with a system of universal screening and risk assessment, based on the development of nomograms to predict the probable course of hyperbilirubinemia in newborns.

Clinical practice guidelines

Prompted by an increase in reported cases of kernicterus, the American Academy of Pediatrics (AAP) Subcommittee on Hyperbilirubinemia developed a set of Clinical Practice Guidelines to aid practitioners in the management of hyperbilirubinemia.[44] These guidelines reflect the additional difficulties of assessing patients who are discharged from the hospital within 48 hours, and they recognize the new challenges of an expanding population of babies who are sent home at less than 37 weeks' gestation. They are not intended to establish a specific standard of care, because variation based on individual circumstances often is appropriate, but they are an excellent framework for clinical decision making.

The 10 key elements of the recommendations are as follows: (1) promoting and supporting successful breastfeeding by encouraging early frequent feedings and avoidance of supplementation; (2) establishing protocols to identify patients at risk for hyperbilirubinemia, including screening of pregnant women for blood type and frequent assessment of all infants for jaundice; (3) measuring bilirubin level in any infant who appears jaundiced at less than 24 hours of age; (4) avoiding the use of visual assessment alone; (5) interpreting all bilirubin levels as a function of the infant's age in hours rather than days; (6) highlighting the increased risk of hyperbilirubinemia in infants born at less than 38 weeks' gestation, especially those who are breastfed; (7) systematically screening all infants before discharge, including an assessment of the risk of high levels based on developed nomograms; (8) providing complete information to parents about the risks of hyperbilirubinemia; (9) ensuring appropriate follow-up based on risk assessment and time of discharge; and (10) appropriately treating with phototherapy or exchange transfusion. Figure 6B-5 shows the algorithm for management.

Universal screening

For full-term and late preterm infants, the most widely accepted nomograms (Figure 6B-6) were derived by Bhutani et al.[45] Similar nomograms have been constructed for populations limited to late preterm infants alone, but the variations from the population as a whole are minimal.[45] The percentile-based nomograms of the hour-specific values for bilirubin were constructed using serum bilirubin levels measured at known times during the first 2 days of life in a diverse population of newborns. Measurements also were made later in the first week of life in a subset of babies, and these values were used to classify the risk of significantly elevated levels of hyperbilirubinemia at any time in the early neonatal period. In a system of universal early screening, levels usually are obtained at 36 hours of age, or earlier if the baby appears jaundiced. Based on these levels, infants can be stratified into three risk groups. Infants in the high-risk stratum have a 40% risk of subsequently developing moderate or severe jaundice. For those in the lowest risk category, the risk of subsequent severe hyperbilirubinemia is essentially zero, and those in the intermediate group are at intermediate risk.

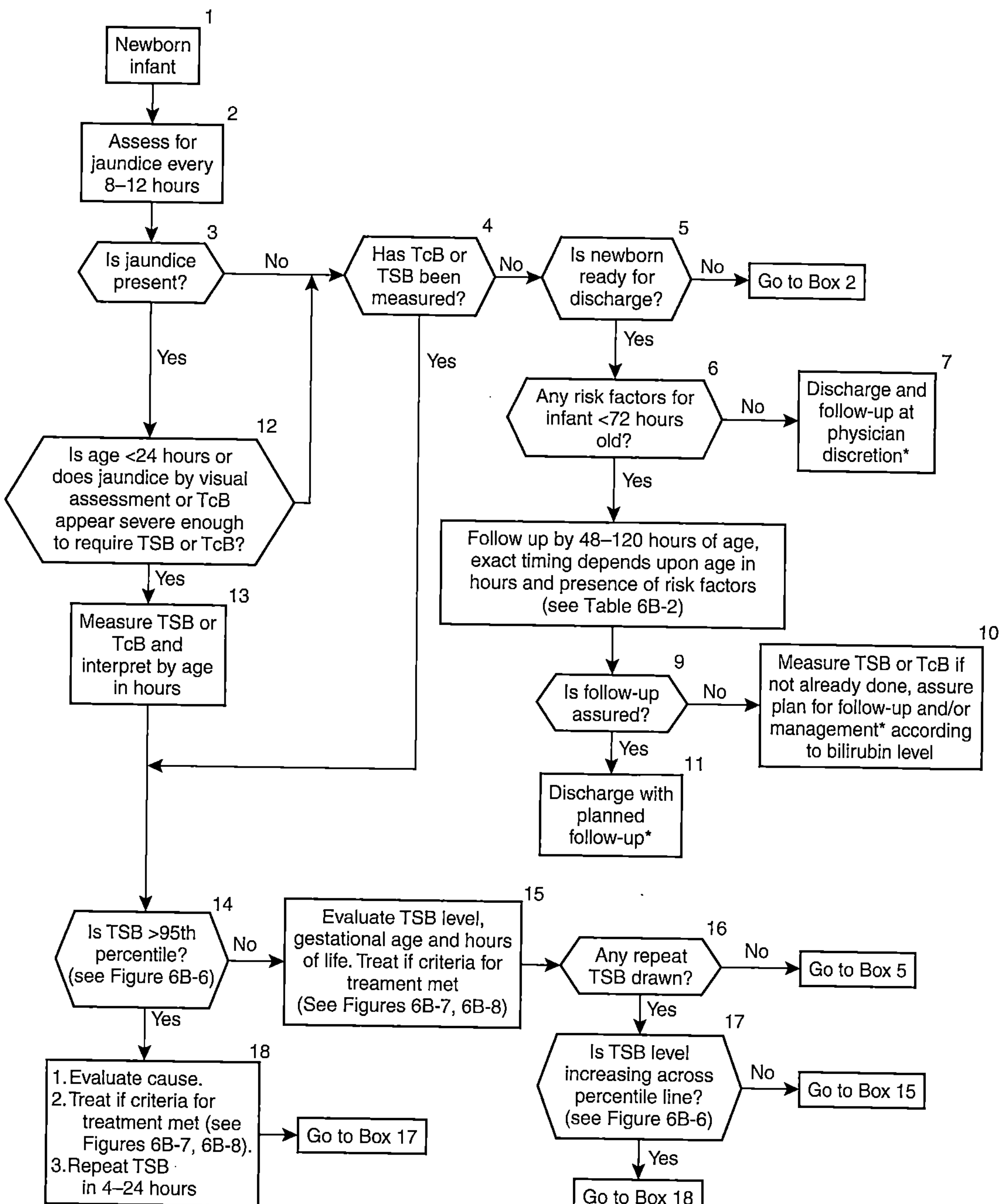

FIGURE 6B-5 This algorithm outlines the management of jaundice in the newborn nursery. From: American Academy of Pediatrics Clinical Practice Guideline, *Pediatrics* 114: 2004, p 299. *TcB*, transcutaneous bilirubin; *TSB*, total serum bilirubin.

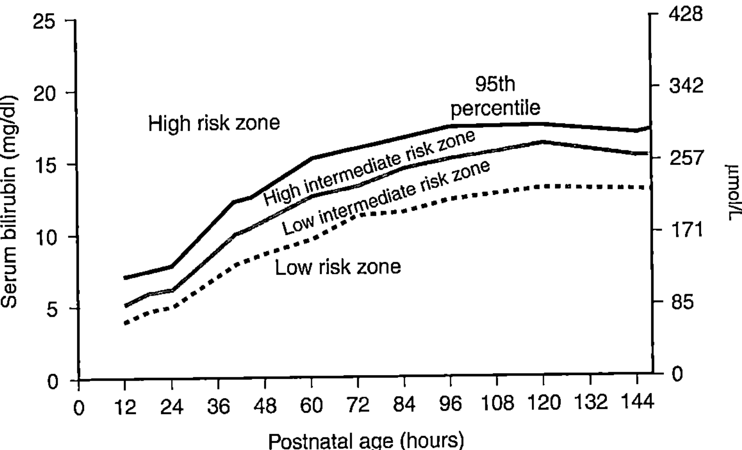

FIGURE 6B-6 The risk is of developing levels in the highest percentiles and is not the risk of developing bilirubin induced neurologic damage. From: Bhutani VK, Johnson L, Sivieri EM: *Pediatrics* 103: 1999, p 9.

Treatment should be started in high-risk patients in whom the level already exceeds the threshold (discussed later), but the majority of patients identified as being at high risk of developing severe jaundice can be scheduled for follow-up visits and determination of bilirubin levels in the days immediately following discharge. The number and timing of these evaluations can be individually tailored on the basis of bilirubin levels and the presence of risk factors.

Universal screening can require a large increase in laboratory testing, but the cost and patient discomfort can be minimized without decreasing effectiveness. Screening bilirubin levels can be obtained coincident with metabolic screening, eliminating an additional heel stick and economizing personnel costs for phlebotomy. Transcutaneous measurements also can be substituted for some serum determinations. Older devices designed for this purpose were not reliable and were difficult to use,[46] but these concerns have been addressed in currently available devices.[47] The BiliChek bilirubinometer (BiliChek Noninvasive Bilirubin System, Respironics, Inc., Carlsbad, CA) uses the entire spectrum of visible light (380–760 nm) reflected from the skin, and the Jaundice Meter JM-102 (Minolta/Hill-Rom Air-Shields, Hatboro, PA) uses two wavelengths for measurement. Both systems compare the incident and reflected light at each wavelength, from which the concentration in the skin is derived and the serum level of bilirubin is calculated by using the known absorbance pattern of bilirubin. Bilirubin levels derived in this manner are more accurate (compared with gas chromatographic analysis) than levels obtained in many hospital-based laboratories, and their use in a screening program has been validated.

Measurement of exhaled carbon monoxide (CO) can be used to determine elevated bilirubin production and increased risk of a high level[48,49] because equimolar amounts of CO and bilirubin are produced by metabolism of hemoglobin. This measurement may be the best way to assess the severity of hemolysis but has not yet been shown to be generally useful in clinical care.

Timing of follow-up visit

Early follow-up is important for infants discharged before 72 hours of age, and the timing should be based on stratification of the predischarge screening bilirubin and modified as needed if the risk factors listed in Table 6B-2 are present. Earlier and/or more frequent visits should be arranged when risk factors are present and when discharge occurs before 36 hours of age.

Full-term infants discharged before 24 hours of age should be seen by 72 hours of age, those discharged between 24 and 48 hours should be seen by 96 hours, and those discharged between 48 and 72 hours should be seen by 120 hours of age. Prematurity is such an important risk factor that it usually is prudent to schedule the first visit within 1 day of discharge. The nomogram still should be used at these subsequent visits, so high-risk babies can be monitored more and treated when necessary.

Treatment

The first line of therapy is ensuring adequate hydration and food intake. For breastfeeding babies, this requires frequent feedings and adequate maternal support; it almost never requires abandonment of breastfeeding. If the bilirubin level is elevated despite these actions, phototherapy should be instituted. The threshold level for phototherapy may vary among individual infants, depending on gestational age and other risk factors.

Table 6B-2 Risk Factors for Development of Severe Indirect Hyperbilirubinemia in the Late Preterm Newborn

MAJOR RISK FACTORS
Predischarge bilirubin level in the high-risk zone on nomogram
Jaundice observed in the first 24 hours of life
Blood group incompatibility with positive direct antiglobulin test or other hemolytic disease
Gestational age 35–36 weeks
Previous sibling with significant hyperbilirubinemia
Significant extravascular blood
Breastfeeding not well established
East Asian race
MINOR RISK FACTORS
Screening bilirubin level in the intermediate nomogram zone
Clinical jaundice or family history of jaundice
Infant of diabetic mother

Modified from: American Academy of Pediatrics Subcommittee on Hyperbilirubinemia: *Pediatrics* 114:297-316, 2004.

If the bilirubin level is high enough to require therapy and/or the direct-reacting bilirubin level is significantly elevated, further testing should be performed to discern the underlying cause of the hyperbilirubinemia. Measurement of the G6PD level also is recommended if the jaundice requires therapy and if the family history or ethnicity suggests the likelihood of this disorder. This is more important in African Americans, in whom the incidence of G6PD deficiency is high and is a major cause of kernicterus.

Phototherapy

The effectiveness of phototherapy is well established.[50,51] The practice involves illuminating the infant's skin surface with visible light, preferably with peak intensity at a wavelength of 460 to 470 nm, which includes the absorption maximum of both unbound and albumin-bound bilirubin. This blue-green light causes photoisomerization and photooxidation of bilirubin, but the major reaction is a structural isomerization. This irreversibly converts bilirubin to lumirubin, a water-soluble compound that is excreted in bile and urine. The therapy depends on good hydration because visible light increases insensible water losses from the skin. Three major factors determine the effectiveness of therapy: the wavelength of the light, the surface area of the exposed skin, and the intensity of the light.

Commercial phototherapy units are designed to produce maximum illumination at wavelengths close to the absorption maximum of bilirubin while minimizing exposure to either infrared or ultraviolet radiation. Older units typically used special fluorescent bulbs designed to emit higher intensities of blue light, and these units usually incorporated a plastic shield to minimize ultraviolet light. Newer units use spotlights or fiberoptic blankets with enhancement of irradiation at the most effective wavelengths.

The use of regulated phototherapy units provides an assurance of both effectiveness and safety. Encouraging parents to place a jaundiced infant in a sunny window to treat jaundice usually is not advisable for several reasons. Exposure to the ultraviolet radiation in sunlight is associated with both short- and long-term dangers, and unfiltered sunlight includes infrared wavelengths that could result in dangerous overheating in a small infant. This type of recommendation could trivialize the importance of therapy and the potential dangers of hyperbilirubinemia in the parent's minds and thus may lead them away from adequate surveillance of both the baby and the bilirubin levels.

Overhead, spotlight, and blanket units all are roughly equivalent. Less intense therapy with a single phototherapy unit often is all that is required, and it should reduce the bilirubin level by 6% to 20% in the first 24 hours.[52-54] If the initial level already is significantly high or if the level continues to increase despite phototherapy, additional units should be added to deliver intensive phototherapy (defined as irradiance of 30 $\mu W/cm^2$ to the maximum surface area). This usually will result in a decrease in serum bilirubin of 30% to 40% in the first 24 hours. If the bilirubin level continues to rise or does not significantly decrease with intensive phototherapy, underlying hemolysis is likely to be the cause.

The exposed surface area should be maximized while ensuring adequate temperature control, including reducing the diaper coverage to a minimum and/or using a bed with incorporated phototherapy. Although maximizing the time of exposure should increase the efficacy of phototherapy, comparisons of intermittent versus continuous exposure have not provided definitive proof in the clinical setting.[55] Continuous phototherapy should be used, but it usually can be safely interrupted for brief periods to permit feeding or parent–infant interaction. If the bilirubin level is close to that at which an exchange transfusion might be performed, uninterrupted phototherapy is the best course.

Figure 6B-7 is a guide for instituting phototherapy in premature infants on the basis of bilirubin levels obtained at a known postnatal age in hours. The graphs are based on the AAP practice guidelines, recognizing that prematurity alone increases

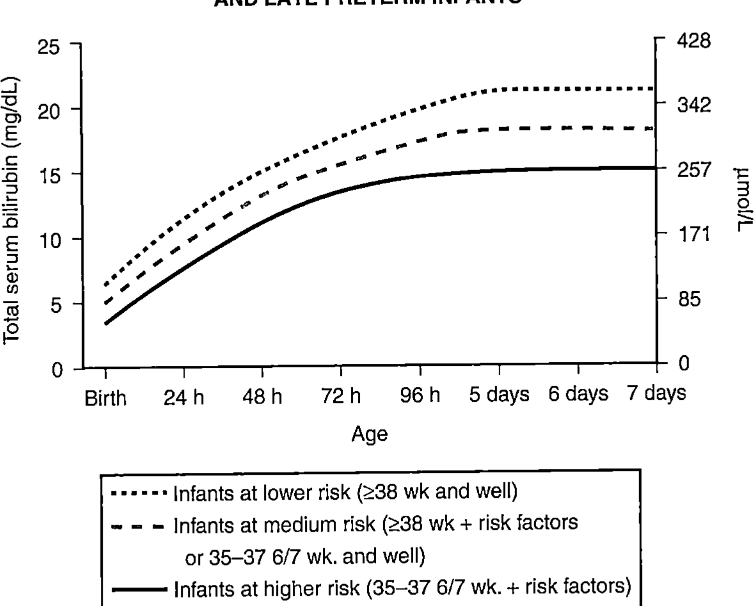

FIGURE 6B-7 All premature infants should be considered to be at medium risk or high risk if factors in Table 6B-2 are present (dashed or dotted line). From: American Academy of Pediatrics Clinical Practice Guideline. *Pediatrics* 114: 2004, p 304.

the risk of more severe hyperbilirubinemia and potential sequelae. When other risk factors are present, therapy should be started at the lower levels indicated. Table 6B-3 can be used in a nursery program that performs screening bilirubin levels at a single postnatal age, but a bilirubin level obtained at any hour of age should prompt the use of phototherapy if the level exceeds the limits given in Figure 6B-7. A late preterm infant who requires phototherapy should be evaluated for a hemolytic cause of the hyperbilirubinemia.

Treatment decisions should be guided by the use of total bilirubin level without subtracting the direct-reacting fraction unless this fraction is 50% or more. In such rare cases, additional evaluation should be performed, and decisions about phototherapy should be individualized.

Phototherapy should be stopped when the hyperbilirubinemia is resolving. The stopping level depends on the initial level that was used as the starting point, the postnatal age, and the underlying cause. A follow-up level should be measured after therapy has been stopped to ensure the adequacy of therapy. A normal rebound of 0.5 to 1.0 mg/dl may occur in the first 12 hours, but this small rise should not prompt restarting therapy. If the infant is doing well with a clear downward trend in the level and breastfeeding is well established, phototherapy usually can be safely stopped, often without the need for a rebound level. Phototherapy for hemolytic disease should be continued longer until a clear downward trend is established, and a follow-up level should be measured within 1 day of discharge.

Home versus hospital phototherapy

For infants who already have been discharged and for those in whom control of hyperbilirubinemia seems likely, administering phototherapy at home is an attractive idea. It allows optimal parent–infant interaction, ensures greater ease in feeding, and should decrease the need for readmission. However, most home phototherapy units provide lower irradiance, and the ease of exposing maximal surface area while ensuring good temperature control is more difficult at home. Therefore home phototherapy should be used only for infants in whom the therapy is considered "optional" or marginally necessary. It must include regular monitoring of bilirubin levels.

Additional therapy for immune-mediated hemolysis

Immune-mediated hemolytic disorders may result in a rapid early rise in bilirubin levels, and the risk of injury is greater than for nonhemolytic causes, particularly when coupled with prematurity. Early and aggressive therapy may be indicated. In addition to intensive phototherapy, treatment with intravenous immune globulin (IVIG) can be effective for these disorders. The most common treatment regimens include 0.5 to 1.0 g/kg/day, given for 2 days; this will reduce the need for exchange transfusions in Rh and ABO disease[56-58] and blunt the rise in bilirubin levels. This therapy is likely to be effective for other immune hemolytic diseases, as well.

Following this therapy, bilirubin levels tend to plateau at moderately high levels and then slowly decline. The length of phototherapy can be

Table 6B-3 Guidelines for Instituting Phototherapy in Premature Infants* Based on Total Bilirubin Level at Postnatal Age

	Postnatal Age			
Risk Factors†	**12 Hours**	**24 Hours**	**36 Hours**	**48 Hours**
Medium risk (well)	7.5	9.6	11.6	13
High risk (additional risk factors)	6	7.9	9.4	11.2

All bilirubin levels are given in milligrams per deciliter.
*For infants of gestational age 35–37 6/7 weeks' gestation.
†See Table 6B-2 for list of risk factors. Note that bilirubin levels can be obtained at any hour of age.

shortened, but some low-grade hemolysis continues, and moderate levels of bilirubin often persist for several weeks. The normal postnatal nadir of the hematocrit that occurs at 4 to 6 weeks of age often is even lower in these patients, especially if they are premature. This late anemia may require treatment by transfusion if symptoms occur. In infants who have received IVIG, primary care providers should monitor hematocrit levels every 1 to 2 weeks until the nadir is reached.

Exchange transfusion

If the bilirubin level continues to rise significantly or if any symptoms of bilirubin encephalopathy are present despite aggressive phototherapy, an exchange transfusion should be performed, unless circumstances are such that that the bilirubin level is more likely to decrease at the same rate or faster without the intervention. The threshold levels for term and late preterm infants are shown in Figure 6B-8, based on the AAP Clinical Practice Guidelines. Before the availability of screening and treatment for Rh incompatibility, this procedure was commonly performed.[59] Today it is performed infrequently and should be undertaken only in centers with adequate experience, equipment, and personnel to ensure maximum safety.

The exchange transfusion most often is performed through a single large umbilical venous line, but it can be performed using a venous and arterial line simultaneously. The details of the procedure are available elsewhere.[60] The total volume of blood exchanged should be twice the calculated circulating blood volume of 80 ml/kg, and the procedure should be completed over approximately 90 to 120 minutes. In most instances, a bilirubin level drawn immediately after the procedure will be approximately 50% of the pre-procedural level but will increase over 2 to 3 hours to approximately two thirds of the pre-exchange level, as equilibration occurs.

A measured serum albumin level and a calculated bilirubin/albumin ratio can be used to more accurately assess the risk of bilirubin encephalopathy,

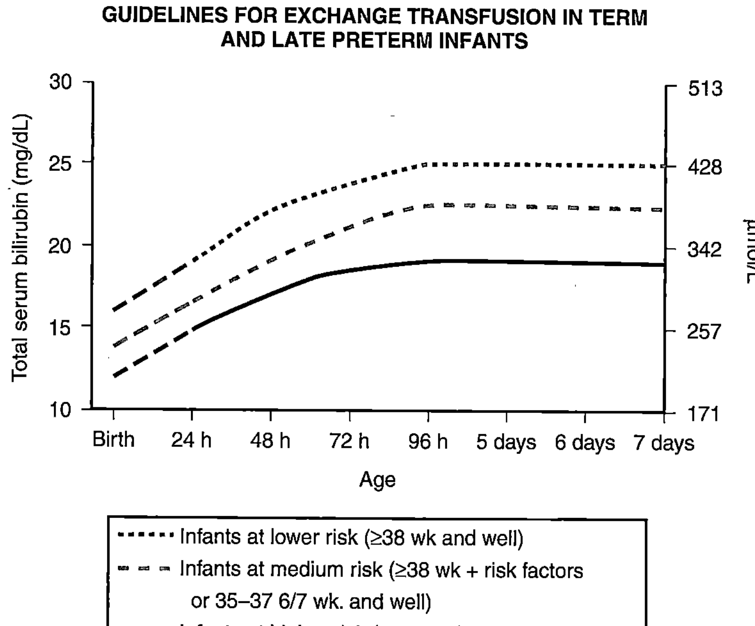

FIGURE 6B-8 All premature infants should be considered to be at medium risk or high risk if factors in Table 6B-2 are present (dashed or dotted line). These are suggested levels, and the utility at less than 24 hours of age may be limited. From: American Academy of Pediatrics Clinical Practice Guideline. *Pediatrics* 114: 2004, p 305.

especially when an exchange transfusion is being considered. For premature infants a ratio >7.2, or >6.8 when other risk factors are present, should prompt consideration of exchange transfusion. Any serum bilirubin level high enough to require exchange transfusion, including any level >25 mg/dl, is a medical emergency, and direct admission to an appropriate hospital should occur as quickly as possible. If an infant already has signs of bilirubin encephalopathy, immediate exchange transfusion is recommended, even if the serum level is already falling.

Future Directions

To date, the approach to the late preterm infant generally has followed that for a full-term baby, with the added vigilance that comes from recognition of the greater potential risk in this population. The current management described here enables prevention of almost all cases of kernicterus. As the mechanism of bilirubin-induced neurologic injury is more completely elucidated and the genetic factors that create risk are defined, management will become less dependent on generalized estimates about risk in whole populations of infants and instead will be determined individually with greater reliability. The current cost of testing, as well as worry and concern for the families and caregivers of the babies who never develop a problem, will be eliminated. Focus then can shift to a more complete exploration of the risks of possible subtle injury caused by bilirubin so that even this potential problem can be understood and eliminated.

Resources for Families and Clinicians

American Academy of Pediatrics
http://www.aap.org/family/jaundicefeature.htm
This website provides clinical practice guidelines for managing hyperbilirubinemia in infants ≥35 weeks' gestation.

March of Dimes
http://www.marchofdimes.com/professionals/14332_9268.asp
This website provides information about jaundice to families.

Mayo Clinic
http://www.mayoclinic.com/invoke.cfm?objectid=EDFE58D5-87F3-4231-91E36178255A37D9&dsection=1
This website provides information about jaundice to families.

Tool for Bilirubin Management
http://www.bilitool.org/
The clinical provider can enter the infant's age and bilirubin level, and the website will use the Bhutani normogram to determine the infant's level of risk.

REFERENCES

1. Maisels MJ: The clinical approach to the jaundiced newborn. In Maisels MJ, Watchko JF, editors: *Neonatal jaundice.* Amsterdam, 2000, Harwood Academic Publishers.
2. Sarici SU, Serdar MA, Korkmaz A, et al: Incidence, course and prediction of hyperbilirubinemia in near-term and term newborns. *Pediatrics* 113:775-780, 2004.
3. Broulliard R: Measurement of red cell life span. *JAMA* 230:1304, 1974.
4. Green RM, Gollan JL: Crigler-Najjar disease type I: therapeutic approaches to genetic liver diseases into the next century. *Gastroenterology* 112:649, 1997.
5. Clarke DJ, Mogharbi N, Monaghan G, et al: Genetic defects of the UDP-glucuronosyl transferase gene that cause familial non-haemolytic unconjugated hyperbilirubinaemias. *Clin Chim Acta* 266:63-74, 1997.
6. Maisels MJ, Gifford K, Antle CE, et al: Normal serum bilirubin levels in the newborn and the effect of breast-feeding. *Pediatrics* 78:837-843, 1986.
7. Ulrich D, Fevery J, Sieg A, et al: The influence of gestational age on bilirubin conjugation in newborns. *Eur J Clin Invest* 21:83-89, 1991.
8. Gartner L: Breastfeeding and jaundice. *J Perinatol* 21:S25-S29, 2001.
9. Gartner U, Goeser T, Wolkoff AW: Effect of fasting on the uptake of bilirubin and sulfobromophthalein by the isolated perfused rat liver. *Gastroenterology* 113:1707-1713, 1997.
10. Arias IM, Gartner LM: Production of unconjugated hyperbilirubinemia in full-term newborn infants following administration of pregnane-3(alpha)20(beta)-diol. *Nature* 203:1292-1293, 1964.
11. Halamek LP, Stevenson DK: Neonatal jaundice and liver disease. In Fanaroff AA, Martin RJ, editors: *Neonatal-perinatal medicine: diseases of the fetus and infant, vol. 2,* ed 6. St. Louis, 1997, Mosby Yearbook.
12. Dennery PA, Seidman DS, Stevenson DK: Neonatal hyperbilirubinemia. *N Engl J Med* 344:581, 2001.
13. Fischer AF, Nakamura H, Uetani Y, et al: Comparison of bilirubin production in Japanese and Caucasian infants. *J Pediatr Gastroenterol Nutr* 7:27, 1988.
14. Johnson JD, Angelus P, Aldrich M, et al: Exaggerated jaundice in Navajo neonates: the role of bilirubin production. *Am J Dis Child* 140:889, 1986.
15. Kaplan M, Rubatelli FF, Hammerman C, et al: Bilirubin conjugation, reflected by serum conjugated bilirubin fractions, in glucose-6-phosphate dehydrogenase deficient neonates: a determining factor in the pathogenesis of hyperbilirubinemia. *Pediatrics* 102(3):E37, 1998. Available at: *http://www.pediatrics.org/cgi/content/full/102/3/e37.*
16. Kaplan M, Renbaum P, Levi-Lahad E, et al: Gilbert syndrome and glucose-6-phosphate dehydrogenase deficiency: a dose-dependent genetic interaction crucial to neonatal hyperbilirubinemia. *Proc Natl Acad Sci U S A* 94:12128, 1997.
17. Bancroft JD, Kreamer B, Gourley GR: Gilbert syndrome accelerates development of neonatal jaundice. *J Pediatr* 132:656, 1998.
18. Wolkoff, AW, Chowdhury JR, Arias IM: Hereditary jaundice and disorders of bilirubin metabolism. In Scriver CR, Sly WS, Childs B et al., editors: *The metabolic basis of inherited disease,* ed 6. New York, 1989, McGraw-Hill.
19. Bosma PJ, Chowdhury JR, Bakker C, et al: The genetic basis of the reduced expression of bilirubin UDP-glucuronosyl transferase 1 in Gilbert's syndrome. *N Engl J Med* 333:1171, 1995.
20. Yusoff, S, Van Rostenberghe H, Yusoff NM, et al: Frequencies of A(TA)7TAA, G71R, and G493R mutations of the UGT1A1 gene in the Malaysian population. *Biol Neonate* 2006;89(3):171-6.

21. Green RM, Gollan JL: Crigler-Najjar disease type I: therapeutic approaches to genetic liver diseases into the next century. *Gastoenterology* 112:649, 1997.
22. Kadakol A, Ghosh SS, Sappal BS, et al: Genetic lesions of bilirubin uridine-diphosphoglucuronate glucuronosyltransferase (UGT1A1) causing Crigler-Najjar and Gilbert syndromes: correlation of genotype to phenotype. *Hum Nutr* 16:297, 2000.
23. Rela M, Muiesan P, Vilca-Melendez H, et al: Auxiliary partial orthotopic liver transplantation for Crigler-Najjar syndrome type 1. *Ann Surg* 229:565, 1999.
24. Rubaltelli FF, Novello A, Zancan L, et al: Serum and bile bilirubin pigments in the differential diagnosis of Crigler-Najjar disease. *Pediatrics* 94:553, 1994.
25. Gartner U, Goeser T, Wolkoff AW: Effect of fasting on the uptake of bilirubin and sulfobromophthalein by the isolated perfused rat liver. *Gastroenterology* 113:1707, 1997.
26. Kotal P, Vitek L, Fevery J: Fasting-related hyperbilirubinemia in rats: the effect of decreased intestinal motility. *Gastroenterology* 111:217, 1996.
27. Claireaux AE, Cole PG, Lathe GH: Icterus of the brain in the newborn. *Lancet* 2:1226, 1953.
28. Turkel SB: Autopsy findings associated with neonatal hyperbilirubinemia. *Clin Perinatol* 17:381, 1990.
29. Ostrow JD, Pascolo L, Brites D, et al: Molecular basis of bilirubin-induced neurotoxicity. *Trends Mol Med* 10(2):65-70, 2004.
30. Robertson A, Karp W, Brodersen R: Bilirubin displacing effect of drugs used in neonatology. *Acta Paediatr Scand* 80:1119, 1991.
31. Newman TB, Xiong B, Gonzales VN, et al: Prediction and prevention of extreme neonatal hyperbilirubinemia in a mature health maintenance organization. *Arch Pediatr Adolesc Med* 154:1140-1147, 2000.
32. Harris MC, Bernbaum JC, Polin JR, et al: Developmental follow-up of breastfed term and near-term infants with marked hyperbilirubinemia. *Pediatrics* 107:1075-1080, 2001.
33. Gupta AK, Mann SB: Is auditory brainstem response a bilirubin neurotoxicity marker? *Am J Otolaryngol* 19:232-236, 1998.
34. Agrawal VK, Shukla R, Misra PK, et al: Brainstem auditory evoked response in newborns with hyperbilirubinemia. *Indian Pediatr* 35:513-518, 1998.
35. Shapiro SM, Nakamura H: Bilirubin toxicity in the developing nervous system. *Pediatr Neurol* 29:410-421, 2003.
36. Scheidt PC, Mellits ED, Hardy JB, et al: Toxicity to bilirubin in neonates: infant development during the first year of life in relation to maximal neonatal serum bilirubin concentrations. *J Pediatr* 91:292, 1997.
37. Govaert P, Lequin M, Swarte R, et al: Changes in globus pallidus with (pre)term kernicterus. *Pediatrics* 112(6):1256-1263, 2003.
38. Van de Bor M, van Zeben-van der Aa TM, Verloove-Vanhorick SP, et al: Hyperbilirubinemia in preterm infants and neurodevelopmental outcome at 2 years of age: results of a national collaborative survey. *Pediatrics* 83:915, 1989.
39. Van de Bor M, Ens-Dolkkum M, Schreuder AM, et al: Hyperbilirubinemia in low birth weight infants and outcome at 5 years of age. *Pediatrics* 89:359, 1992.
40. Seidman DS, Paz I, Stevenson DK, et al: Neonatal hyperbilirubinemia and physical and cognitive performance at 17 years of age. *Pediatrics* 88:828, 1991.
41. Kramer LI: Advancement of dermal icterus in the jaundiced newborn. *Am J Dis Child* 118:454, 1969.
42. Penn AA, Enzmann DR, Hahn JS, et al: Kernicterus in a full term infant. *Pediatrics* 93:17, 1993.
43. Maisels MJ, Newman TB: Kernicterus in otherwise healthy, breastfed term newborns. *Pediatrics* 96:730, 1995.
44. American Academy of Pediatrics Subcommittee on Hyperbilirubinemia: Management of hyperbilirubinemia in the newborn infant 35 or more weeks of gestation. *Pediatrics* 114:297-316, 2004.
45. Bhutani VK, Johnson L, Sivieri EM: Predictive ability of a predischarge hour-specific serum bilirubin for subsequent significant hyperbilirubinemia in healthy term and near-term infants. *Pediatrics* 103:6-14, 1999.
46. Stevenson DK, Fanaroff AA, Maisels MJJ, et al: Prediction of hyperbilirubinemia in near-term and term infants. *Pediatrics* 108(1):31-39, 2001.
47. Yamanouchi I, Yamuchi Y, Igarishi I: Transcutaneous bilirubinometry: preliminary studies of noninvasive transcutaneous bilirubin meter in the Okayama National Hospital. *Pediatrics* 65:195, 1980.
48. Ruabtelli FF, Gourley GR, Loskamp N, et al: Transcutaneous bilirubin measurement: a multicenter evaluation of a new device. *Pediatrics* 107:1264, 2001.
49. Vreman HJ, Stevenson DK, Oh W, et al: Semiportable electrochemical instrument for determining carbon monoxide in breath. *Clin Chem* 40:1927, 1994.
50. Vreman HJ, Baxter LM, Stone RT, et al: Evaluation of a fully automated end-tidal carbon monoxide instrument for breath analyses. *Clin Chem* 42:50, 1996.
51. Cremer RJ, Perryman PW, Richards DH: Influence of light on the hyperbilirubinemia of infants. *Lancet* 1:1094-1097, 1958.
52. Lucey J, Ferreiro M, Hewitt J: Prevention of hyperbilirubinemia of prematurity by phototherapy. *Pediatrics* 41(6):1947-1954, 1986.
53. Maisels MJ, Kring E: Bilirubin rebound following intensive phototherapy. *Arch Pediatr Adolesc Med* 56:669-672, 2002.
54. Garg AK, Prasad RS, Hifzi IA: Controlled trial of high-intensity double-surface phototherapy on a fluid bed versus conventional phototherapy in neonatal jaundice. *Pediatrics* 95:914-916, 995.
55. Tan K: Comparison of the efficacy of fiberoptic and conventional phototherapy for neonatal hyperbilirubinemia. *J Pediatr* 125:607-612, 1994.
56. Lau SP, Fung KP: Serum bilirubin kinetics in intermittent phototherapy of physiologic jaundice. *Arch Dis Child* 59:892-894, 1984.
57. Gottstein R, Cooke RW: Systematic review of intravenous immunoglobulin in haemolytic disease of the newborn. *Arch Did Child Fetal Neonatal Ed* 88:F6-F10, 2003.
58. Miqdad A, Abdelbasit O, Shaheed M, et al: Intravenous immunoglobulin G (IVIG) therapy for significant hyperbilirubinemia in ABO hemolytic disease of the newborn. *J Matern Fetal Neonatal Med* 16(3):163-166, 2004.
59. Mukhopadhyay K, Murki S, Narang A, et al: Intravenous immunoglobulins in rhesus hemolytic disease. *Indian J Pediatr* 70(9):697-699, 2003.
60. Diamond LK, Allen FH, Thomas WO: Erythroblastosis fetalis VII. Treatment with exchange transfusion. *N Engl J Med* 244:39-49, 1951.

Chapter 7A

Hypothyroidism in the Preterm Infant

Mandy Brown Belfort, MD, MPH, and Rosalind S. Brown, MD

Thyroxine (T_4) is critical for fetal and infant brain development and plays an important role in normal growth. Abnormalities of thyroid function are common in preterm infants and must be managed properly to prevent adverse sequelae, including neurodevelopmental impairment. A basic appreciation of fetal and neonatal thyroid physiology is necessary to understand the thyroid hormone abnormalities that can occur in preterm infants, the effect these abnormalities may have on the infant, and the rationale for diagnosis and therapy.

Fetal and Neonatal Thyroid Physiology

T_4 is first detected in the fetus at 10 to 12 weeks when organogenesis is complete. Early in gestation, T_4 is provided to the fetus from the mother via the placenta. T_4 begins to rise at 18 to 20 weeks' gestation, coincident with maturation of the hypothalamus and pituitary gland as well as increasing thyroid-stimulating hormone (TSH) levels in the circulation. Both T_4 and TSH levels continue to rise with advancing gestational age (Figure 7A-1).[1,2] At birth in full-term infants, a rapid surge in TSH level is followed by an increase in T_4 to values much higher than at any other time of life. Over the subsequent 1 to 2 weeks, T_4 and TSH levels drop slowly (Figure 7A-2).[2,3]

Fetal thyroid-binding globulin (TBG) follows a similar pattern to T_4 and TSH both in utero and after birth (Figures 7A-1 and 7A-2)[1,2,4] TBG levels rise progressively after 20 weeks' gestation, correlating with increasing liver maturity. Unlike the levels of T_4, TSH, and TBG, levels of triiodothyronine (T_3) remain low in the fetal circulation through most of gestation as a result of immaturity of the type 1 deiodinase enzyme that converts T_4 to T_3. Despite low serum levels of T_3, brain and pituitary T_3 levels are considerably higher. This adaptation may explain the relatively normal cognitive outcome in infants with congenital hypothyroidism who have received early and adequate postnatal therapy.[5]

Thyroid function in the preterm infant reflects the relative immaturity of the hypothalamic–pituitary–thyroid axis of the fetus at a comparable gestational age. In the premature infant, both the TSH and T_4 postnatal surges are blunted and the subsequent T_4 drop is exaggerated, particularly in the very-low-birth-weight (VLBW) infant (<1500 g), in whom transient thyroid disorders are common (Figure 7A-3).[4] Loss of maternal T_4 contribution and thyroid suppression from acute illness both contribute to the drop in T_4 concentration after birth. Premature infants are particularly sensitive to iodine exposure because the ability of the thyroid to reduce iodide trapping in response to excess iodide (Wolff-Chaikoff effect) does not mature until 36 to 40 weeks' gestation. For these reasons, the T_4 concentration in the extrauterine preterm infant may actually be lower than in the fetus of a comparable gestational age.

Maternal thyroid disease and treatment can affect the term and preterm infant alike. Maternal antithyroid medications used for Graves' disease (propylthiouracil or methimazole), maternal iodine excess or deficiency, and transplacental passage of maternal TSH receptor-blocking antibodies all can lead to transient neonatal hypothyroidism. TSH receptor-blocking antibodies can persist for many years in the maternal circulation, so the recurrence rate in subsequent offspring is high.

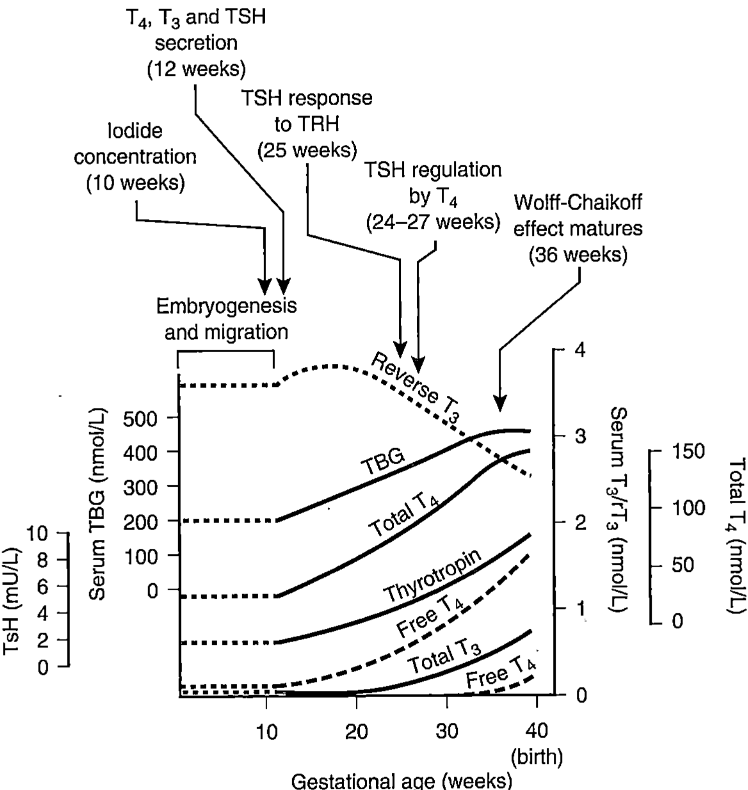

FIGURE 7A-1 Maturation of thyroid gland function during gestation. From: Brown RS, Larsen PR: Thyroid gland development and disease in: *http://www.thyroidmanager.org*. Version Nov 2006, Leslie J DeGroot, MD, editor.

Diagnosis and Management

Newborn screening

Abnormalities of thyroid function in the premature infant usually are first detected on the newborn screen. Screening programs in many regions of the United States measure T_4 as the primary screen and use TSH as a backup when T_4 is low. Other programs measure TSH levels and then test T_4 if the TSH level is abnormal. Both approaches are equivalent in detecting permanent cases of congenital hypothyroidism. Some programs measure both T_4 and TSH in high-risk infants. Reference ranges appropriate for gestational age must be used for proper interpretation of test results (Table 7A-1)[6] because thyroid function varies with the degree of prematurity as well as chronological age.[7,8] Abnormal screening tests occur disproportionately in preterm infants, reflecting their physiologic immaturity and the relatively high incidence of transient disorders of thyroid function in this population. Abnormalities can be physiologic or represent either transient or permanent disorders and require close follow-up (Figure 7A-4).

Newborn screening is highly effective in identifying thyroid hormone abnormalities. Occasionally, cases of congenital hypothyroidism are missed because of failure to collect a specimen, incorrect timing of specimen collection, hospital transfer, critical illness, and laboratory error. The newborn screen should be sent between 36 and 72 hours of life, and nurseries should establish and maintain a system to ensure that specimens are collected promptly and sent for all infants, including those who are acutely ill. If the newborn screen is sent before 48 hours of life, appropriate normal values should be used. Although nonspecific in premature infants, signs and symptoms of hypothyroidism are important to recognize and include prolonged jaundice, a large posterior fontanel, dry and mottled skin, hypothermia, bradycardia, poor weight gain, constipation, and goiter (Table 7A-2). The presence of one or more of these findings should prompt the clinician to verify that appropriate newborn screening has occurred and to consider further evaluation, including measurement of free T_4 and TSH levels in the hospital laboratory.

Thyroid function abnormalities in preterm infants

Low T_4 with normal TSH

Low T_4 with a normal TSH is the most common abnormality of thyroid function in premature infants and occurs in up to 50% of infants at less than 30 weeks' gestation. This abnormality usually

POSTNATAL THYROID HORMONE LEVELS

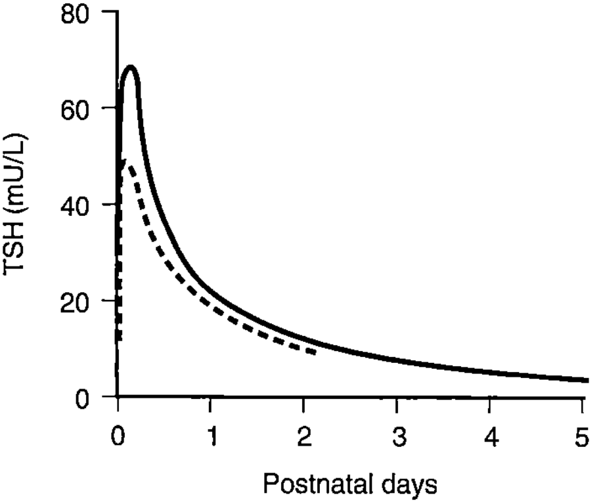

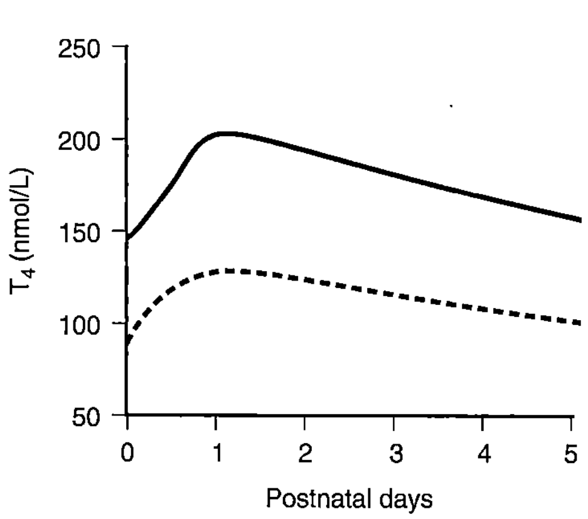

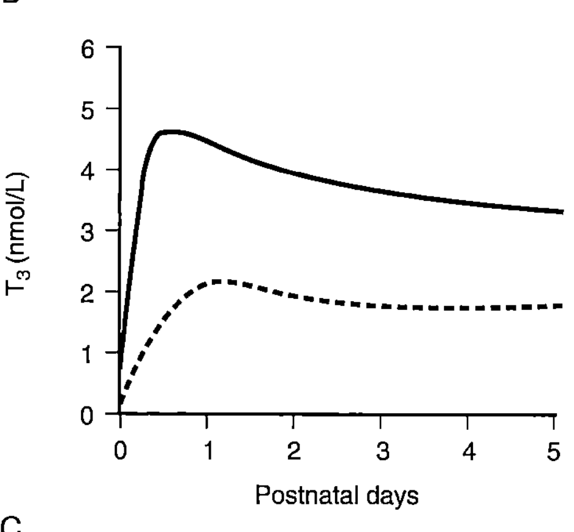

FIGURE 7A-2 Postnatal changes in the serum concentration of thyroid-stimulating hormone (TSH), thyroxine (T_4), and triiodothyronine (T_3) in term infants *(continuous line)* compared with premature infants (*broken line*) in the first week of life. Note that the postnatal surge in TSH is followed by an increase in T_4 and T_3 concentrations in the first few days of life. T_4, T_3, and TSH concentrations all subsequently decline. Changes in TSH, T_4, and T_3 in premature infants are similar to those in term infants, but in preterm infants the postnatal surge is blunted and the subsequent decline is more pronounced. Modified from: Fisher DA, Klein AH: *N Engl J Med* 304:702-712, 1981.

is transient and likely multifactorial in origin (Table 7A-3).[9] Immaturity of the hypothalamic–pituitary–thyroid axis, loss of the maternal thyroxine contribution, and thyroid suppression from acute illness, such as hyaline membrane disease, all can lead to hypothyroxinemia. Premature infants frequently are deficient in TBG as a result of liver immaturity, malnutrition, and illness, in which case the total T_4 is affected more than the free T_4. Rarely, permanent congenital hypothyroidism is the cause of low T_4 with an initially normal TSH in the premature infant.

Infants with primary hypothyroidism may present initially with a normal TSH, but because of immaturity of the hypothalamic–pituitary–thyroid axis they can have a delayed rise in TSH up to 8 weeks later. In these infants, thyroid function tests (TFTs), initially normal on newborn screening, subsequently become abnormal. These infants have evidence for primary hypothyroidism and require treatment (see following). This phenomenon of delayed rise in TSH is observed most frequently in premature infants in the neonatal intensive care unit (NICU) but also may occur in older infants.[10] Although the etiology is not usually determined, excess postnatal iodine exposure should always be considered in this setting. Monozygotic twins and infants with congenital heart disease or trisomy 21 also are at increased risk for a delayed rise in TSH.

The finding of a low T_4 for age and normal TSH on newborn screening should prompt submission of a repeat specimen and confirmation of these results in the serum, measured by the hospital laboratory. Free T_4 and TBG also should be measured to assess for TBG deficiency. Many infants with a normal free T_4, a normal TSH, and a low TBG have isolated TBG deficiency and do not require treatment. If the free T_4 is low, congenital hypopituitarism should be considered, particularly if prolonged hypoglycemia, microphallus, or a midline facial defect is present. Many infants with a low free T_4 and normal TSH can be followed for a short time without initiation of therapy. To monitor the T_4 concentration and to assess for a delayed rise in TSH, the newborn screen should be repeated every 2 weeks until the results normalize.[11] Initiation of therapy in premature infants with persistently low T_4 and normal TSH is controversial but should be considered in infants born at less than 27 weeks' gestation (see following).

Low T_4 with elevated TSH

Infants with low T_4 and elevated TSH, including those with a delayed rise in TSH, have evidence of primary hypothyroidism, which may be transient or permanent. This abnormality may be an appropriate but delayed response to hypothyroxinemia caused by loss of maternal thyroxine contribution,

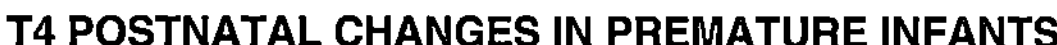

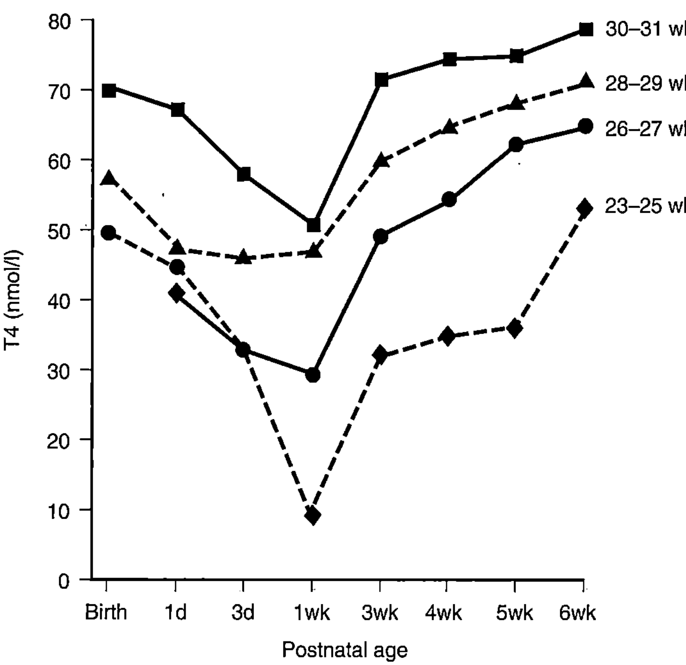

FIGURE 7A-3 Serum thyroxine (T_4) in the first 6 weeks of life according to gestational age. From: Mercado M, Yu VY, Francis I, et al: *Early Hum Dev* 16(2-3):131-141, 1988.

during recovery from the sick euthyroid syndrome, or as a result of inadequate endogenous iodine or excessive iodine exposure. Low T_4 and elevated TSH also may represent permanent congenital hypothyroidism, in which case the TSH frequently is > 40 mU/L. Presence of a thyroid gland of normal size and in a normal location on ultrasound is consistent with transient disease, as 85% of patients with permanent congenital hypothyroidism have dysgenesis or agenesis of the thyroid gland.

Compared with term infants, VLBW infants have eight times the incidence of having TSH >40 mU/L and low-birth-weight (LBW) infants (<2500 g) have twice the incidence.[12] However, the incidence of permanent congenital hypothyroidism is approximately one in 3500 to 4000 newborns, regardless of birth weight. Infants with low T_4 and elevated TSH should have repeat testing immediately and usually require treatment with thyroxine replacement therapy. Assessment of whether the disorder is transient or permanent is made at a later time.

Normal T_4 with elevated TSH

Normal T_4 and elevated TSH may be caused by mild transient or permanent compensated primary hypothyroidism (Table 7A-3). Controversy exists over whether infants with this abnormality require treatment, and data are lacking regarding the long-term neurodevelopmental effects of this disorder. Repeat testing should be performed every 2 weeks to assess for normalization of the TSH level. Reasonable guidelines for therapy include treating infants with persistent TSH elevation >10 mU/L

Table 7A-1 Reference Ranges for Thyroxine (T_4) and Thyrotropin in Premature and Term Infants in the First Week of Life

Age Group	Age (wk)	Weight (g)	Free T_4 (ng/dL)	Thyrotropin (mU/L)
Premature infants*	25–27	772 (233)	0.6–2.2 (1.4)	0.2–30.3
	28–30	1260 (238)	0.6–3.4 (2.0)	0.2–20.6
	31–33	1786 (255)	1.0–3.8 (2/4)	0.7–27.9
	34–36	2125 (376)	1.2–4.4 (2.8)	1.2–21.6
Term infants†	37–42	>2500	2.0–5.3 (3.8)	1.0–39

From: Fisher DA. *Clin Perinatol* 23:999-1014, 1998; as modified by Martin CR: Thyroid disorders. In Cloherty JP, Eichenwald EC, Stark AR, editors: *Manual of neonatal care*, ed 5. Philadelphia, 2004, Lippincott Williams & Wilkins. Values in parentheses are standard deviation for weight and mean for free T_4.
*Adams LM, Emery JR, Clarks SJ: *J Pediatr* 126:122, 1995.
†Nelson JC, Clark SJ, Borut DJ, et al: *J Pediatr* 123:899-905, 1993.

ALGORITHM FOR ABNORMAL THYROID SCREENING RESULTS IN THE PREMATURE INFANT

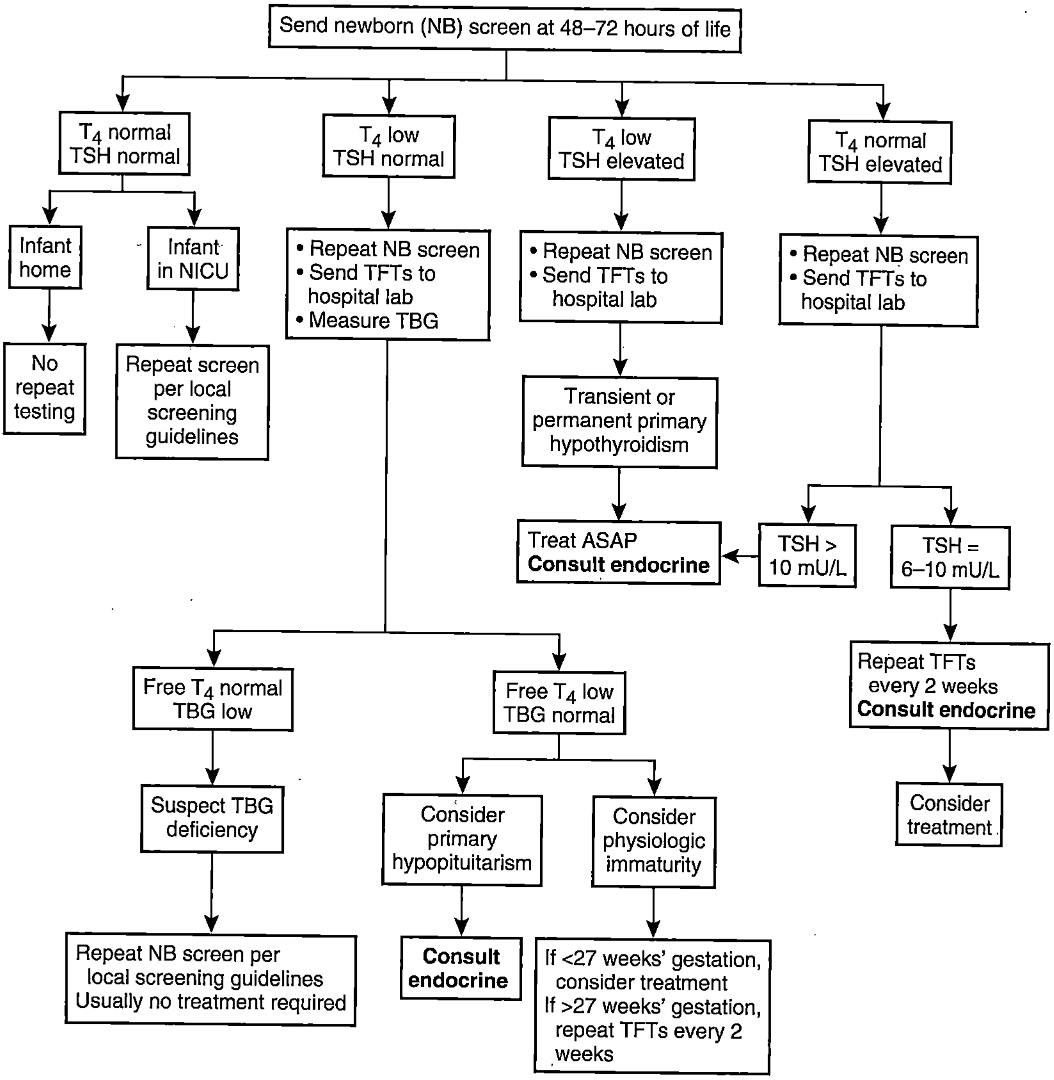

Send newborn (NB) screen at 48–72 hours of life

- T_4 normal / TSH normal
  - Infant home → No repeat testing
  - Infant in NICU → Repeat screen per local screening guidelines
- T_4 low / TSH normal → • Repeat NB screen • Send TFTs to hospital lab • Measure TBG
  - Free T_4 normal / TBG low → Suspect TBG deficiency → Repeat NB screen per local screening guidelines / Usually no treatment required
  - Free T_4 low / TBG normal
    - Consider primary hypopituitarism → **Consult endocrine**
    - Consider physiologic immaturity → If <27 weeks' gestation, consider treatment / If >27 weeks' gestation, repeat TFTs every 2 weeks
- T_4 low / TSH elevated → • Repeat NB screen • Send TFTs to hospital lab → Transient or permanent primary hypothyroidism → Treat ASAP / **Consult endocrine**
- T_4 normal / TSH elevated → • Repeat NB screen • Send TFTs to hospital lab
  - TSH > 10 mU/L → Treat ASAP / **Consult endocrine**
  - TSH = 6–10 mU/L → Repeat TFTs every 2 weeks / **Consult endocrine** → Consider treatment

FIGURE 7A-4 Suggested approach to the investigation of a premature infant with abnormal state thyroid screening test. Please note that this is a recommended algorithm that does not represent a professional standard of care; care should be revised to meet individual patient needs. *NICU*, neonatal intensive care unit; *TBG*, thyroid-binding globulin; T_4, thyroxine; *TFTs*, thyroid function tests; *TSH*, thyroid-stimulating hormone.

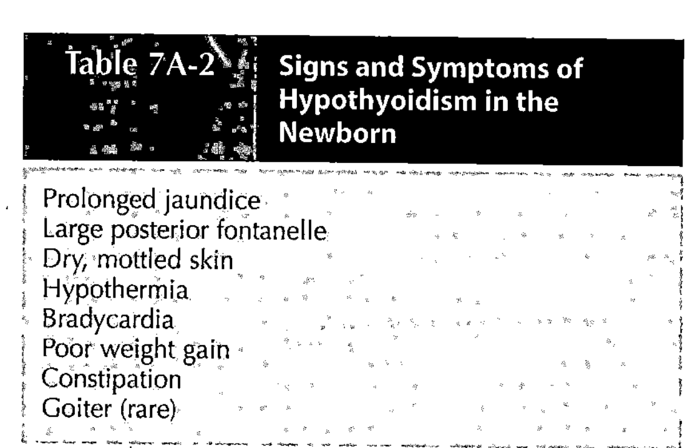

Table 7A-2 Signs and Symptoms of Hypothyroidism in the Newborn
Prolonged jaundice
Large posterior fontanelle
Dry, mottled skin
Hypothermia
Bradycardia
Poor weight gain
Constipation
Goiter (rare)

beyond 2 to 4 weeks of age, particularly if the TSH level is not decreasing or if the T_4 level is in the low–normal range or decreasing. Controversy exists over treatment of infants with persistent TSH in the 6 to 10 mU/L range, and decisions regarding treatment should be made in consultation with a pediatric endocrinology specialist.

Treatment (Table 7A-4)

Rationale for therapy

The decision to initiate thyroid hormone replacement is based on the known adverse neurodevelopmental

Table 7A-3 Thyroid Function Abnormalities in the Preterm Infant

Abnormality: Thyroxine (T_4)	Abnormality: Thyroid-Stimulating Hormone (TSH)	Causes
Low	Normal	**Transient** Immature hypothalamic–pituitary–thyroid axis Loss of maternal thyroxine contribution Thyroid suppression from acute illness (i.e., hyaline membrane disease) Thyroid-binding globulin deficiency (liver immaturity, malnutrition) **Permanent** Congenital hypothyroidism with delayed rise in TSH*
Low	High	**Transient** Recovery from loss of maternal T_4 contribution Recovery from sick euthyroid syndrome Decreased endogenous iodine stores Excessive exogenous iodine exposure **Permanent** Congenital hypothyroidism (TSH usually >40 mU/L)
Normal	High	Immature hypothalamic–pituitary–thyroid axis Compensated primary hypothyroidism (transient or permanent)

*Premature infants, monozygotic twins, and infants with trisomy 21 and/or congenital heart disease are at increased risk for delayed rise in TSH.

effects of hypothyroidism. Clearly, any infant with permanent congenital hypothyroidism requires prompt initiation of therapy to optimize outcome. However, decisions regarding therapy in premature infants are complicated by incomplete knowledge about the long-term neurocognitive sequelae of an isolated low T_4 caused by physiologic immaturity, the sick euthyroid syndrome, or mild transient hypothyroidism, all of which are relatively common in premature infants.

Retrospective studies have shown that severe hypothyroxinemia is associated with adverse motor and cognitive outcomes in infants born at 33 weeks' gestation or less, even after adjusting for severity of illness and other confounding factors.[13,14] However, whether this association is truly causal or simply

Table 7A-4 Treatment of Hypothyroidism in the Preterm Infant

Indications	**Clear** Primary hypothyroidism (low T_4 and TSH >20 mU/L). Compensated primary hypothyroidism that does not normalize in 2–3 weeks (normal T_4, TSH >10 mU/L). **Controversial** Persistently low T_4, normal TSH in infants <27 weeks' gestation. Normal T_4, persistently elevated TSH (6–10 mU/L).
Dose	Starting dose of thyroxine 8 µg/kg/day. Adjust dose based on thyroid function tests. No need to increase dose automatically to account for weight gain.
Administration	Crush tablet and administer with juice or formula/breast milk. Do not administer with soy-based formula, iron, or fiber, which inhibit absorption. Liquid preparations relatively unstable.
Monitoring	Measure: total and free T_4, TSH*, TBG. Frequency: After starting therapy or changing dose: every 2 weeks While in the NICU: every 2 weeks Year 1 of life: every 2 months Year 2 of life: every 3 months
Therapeutic goal	T_4 > median for age, TSH <6 mU/L (optimally 1–2 mU/L).
Duration of therapy	Continue until 3 years of age, then consider trial without medication to assess for resolution of transient hypothyroidism vs permanent hypothyroidism.

NICU, Neonatal intensive care unit; *T_4*, thyroxine; *TBG*, thyroid-binding globulin; *TSH*, thyroid-stimulating hormone.
*TSH is the most sensitive guide for determining therapy in primary hypothyroidism.

coincidental is unclear. A prospective, randomized, controlled trial of thyroxine supplementation in infants born at less than 30 weeks' gestation showed no overall improvement in either motor or cognitive outcomes in thyroxine-treated infants. Infants born at less than 27 weeks' gestation who received thyroxine had improved cognitive outcomes at school age; however, treated infants born after 29 weeks' gestation had slightly worse cognitive function than did infants who received placebo.[15,16]

The initial dose of levothyroxine in premature infants is 8 μg/kg/day, which is lower than the usual starting dose of 10 to 15 μg/kg/day used for term infants with congenital hypothyroidism. Thyroid hormone can be crushed and administered with juice or formula, and care should be taken that all of the medicine has been swallowed. Thyroid hormone should not be given with substances that interfere with its absorption, such as iron, soy, or fiber. Liquid preparations are relatively unstable and should not be used unless a pharmacist with special expertise is available.

TFTs including T_4, TSH, TBG, and free T_4 should be repeated 1 to 2 weeks after initiation of therapy and every 2 weeks thereafter while the infant remains in the NICU. The target T_4 is greater than the median for age, and the desired TSH is <6 mU/L and optimally 1 to 3 mU/L. In primary hypothyroidism, the serum TSH concentration is the most sensitive long-term guide to adequacy of therapy. Normalization of the TSH usually lags behind the T_4, so initially the T_4 level is used to assess adequacy of therapy. The dose of levothyroxine does not need to be adjusted for weight gain as long as the TFTs remain in the target range.

Postdischarge Follow-Up

Follow-up of infants discharged from the NICU on thyroid hormone replacement should be coordinated closely with a pediatric endocrinology specialist. Once an infant is established on a regimen of thyroxine, a reasonable strategy for follow-up is to repeat TFTs every 2 months in the first year of life and every 3 months in the second year of life. The goal is to normalize the T_4 and TSH for age, and the dose should be adjusted upward or downward as needed. If the dose is adjusted, repeat T_4 and TSH should be measured 2 weeks after the change. As noted earlier, the serum TSH concentration is the most sensitive long-term guide to adequacy of therapy in primary hypothyroidism, and the thyroxine dose does not need to be increased to account for weight gain as long as the TFTs remain in the target range. Because it is usually unknown whether the hypothyroidism is transient or permanent at the start of therapy, thyroid hormone replacement generally is continued until 2 to 3 years of age, when brain development is no longer dependent on thyroid hormone. At that time, a trial without medication can be attempted safely, particularly in children whose TSH values have remained normal without a need to increase the dosage of replacement.

Occasionally, infants with mild thyroid hormone abnormalities or persistent physiologic immaturity require follow-up testing after discharge from the NICU, even though they were not started on thyroxine replacement. TFTs should be repeated every 2 weeks until results normalize, as is done with hospitalized infants. A low threshold for treatment usually is adopted.

Resources for Families and Clinicians

The MAGIC Foundation
http://www.magicfoundation.org

The MAGIC Foundation is a national nonprofit organization created to provide support services for families of children with specific diseases that affect a child's growth. This site provides detailed information about congenital hypothyroidism for families.

National Newborn Screening & Genetic Resource Center (NNSGRC)
http://genes-r-us.uthscsa.edu/

This website provides information and resources about newborn screening to healthcare professionals and families. In addition, those interested should contact their own state screening program.

REFERENCES

1. Thorpe-Beeston JG, Nicolaides KH, Felton CV, et al: Maturation of the secretion of thyroid hormone and thyroid-stimulating hormone in the fetus. *N Engl J Med* 324(8):532-536, 1991.
2. Brown RS: The thyroid gland. In Brook CGD, Hindmarsh PC, editors: *Clinical pediatric endocrinology*, ed 4. Oxford, 2001, Blackwell Publishing.
3. Fisher DA, Klein AH: Thyroid development and disorders of thyroid function in the newborn. *N Engl J Med* 304(12): 702-712, 1981.
4. Mercado M, Yu VY, Francis I, et al: Thyroid function in very preterm infants. *Early Hum Dev* 16(2-3):131-141, 1988.
5. Burrow GN, Fisher DA, Larsen PR: Maternal and fetal thyroid function. *N Engl J Med* 331(16):1072-1078, 1994.
6. Martin CR: Thyroid disorders. In Cloherty JP, Eichenwald EC, Stark AR, editors: *Manual of neonatal care*, ed 5. Philadelphia, 2004, Lippincott Williams & Wilkins.
7. Adams LM, Emery JR, Clark SJ, et al: Reference ranges for newer thyroid function tests in premature infants. *J Pediatr* 126(1):122-127, 1995.
8. Frank JE, Faix JE, Hermos RJ, et al: Thyroid function in very low birth weight infants: effects on neonatal hypothyroidism screening. *J Pediatr* 128(4):548-554, 1996.
9. LaFranchi SH: Thyroid function in the preterm infant. *Thyroid* 9:71-78, 1999.
10. Larson C, Hermos R, Delaney A, et al: Risk factors associated with delayed thyrotropin elevations in congenital hypothyroidism. *J Pediatr* 143(5):587-591, 2003.

11. Hunter MK, Mandel SH, Sesser DE, et al: Follow-up of newborns with low thyroxine and nonelevated thyroid-stimulating hormone-screening concentrations: results of the 20-year experience in the Northwest Regional Newborn Screening Program. *J Pediatr* 132(1):70-74, 1998.
12. Delange F, Dalhem A, Bourdoux P, et al: Increased risk of primary hypothyroidism in preterm infants. *J Pediatr* 105(3):462-469, 1984.
13. Den Ouden AL, Kok JH, Verkerk PH: The relation between neonatal thyroxine levels and neurodevelopmental outcome at age 5 and 9 years in a national cohort of very preterm and/or very low birth weight infants. *Pediatr Res* 39(1): 142-145, 1996.
14. Reuss ML, Paneth N, Pinto-Martin JA, et al: The relation of transient hypothyroxinemia in preterm infants to neurologic development at two years of age. *N Engl J Med* 334(13):821-827, 1996.
15. van Wassenaer AG, Kok JH, de Vijlder JJ, et al: Effects of thyroxine supplementation on neurologic development in infants born at less than 30 weeks' gestation. *N Engl J Med* 336(1):21-26, 1997.
16. Briet JM, van Wassenaer AG, Dekker FW, et al: Neonatal thyroxine supplementation in very preterm children: developmental outcome evaluated at early school age. *Pediatrics* 107(4):712-718, 2001.

Chapter 7B

Osteopenia of Prematurity

Ruben Diaz, MD, PhD

The skeleton has important structural and metabolic functions in human physiology. In addition to shielding soft tissue organs and providing levers against which muscles contract, bones are the largest reservoir of calcium and a repository for blood cell precursors in the marrow cavity. One of the skeleton's unique characteristics is its ability to undergo mineralization, which increases the bone's strength and capacity to endure stress. Premature infants, especially those of very low birth weight (<1500 g) and young gestational age (<32 weeks), transition to extrauterine life before a period in fetal development when significant mineral deposition in bone occurs. Thus the skeleton of premature infants can be significantly hypomineralized compared with the skeleton of term infants.[1,2] In addition, bones of premature infants must adapt to postnatal changes much earlier than expected while experiencing significant physiologic stressors and medical interventions that can have direct adverse effects on bone physiology. Challenges in maintaining a good nutritional state during the first weeks of life of premature infants further affect bone growth. Consequently, it is important to identify, evaluate, and treat premature infants at high risk for having compromised bone development to prevent impaired linear growth and a high predisposition to fractures.

Bone development starts in utero. Under the influence of various hormonal, nutritional, and mechanical factors, bone growth and remodeling occur throughout infancy, childhood, and adolescence. Cartilaginous bone growth ceases in adulthood, but bone remodeling remains a tightly regulated process in response to changing metabolic needs and mechanical stressors. Bone formation requires the initial activity of osteoblasts to lay down osteoid, the organic bone matrix, followed by the physiologic process of mineralization, which represents the incorporation of calcium, phosphate, and other minerals into osteoid. Bone remodeling, on the other hand, requires the coordinated action of osteoclasts to break down mineralized bone, followed by osteoblast-mediated bone formation. Bone remodeling appears to be regulated by osteocytes that sense changes in mechanical stress and by various metabolic, hormonal, and nutritional factors.[3]

The combination of size, organic matrix composition, and mineralization density confers to bones the strength and flexibility to sustain weight and strain without fracturing. When deposition of extracellular matrix is impaired, as seen with mutations of the collagen I gene in osteogenesis imperfecta, bone becomes brittle and fractures easily. Likewise, decreased mineralization of the bony matrix is associated with long bone deformities because of strain, as described in various forms of rickets. An evaluation of bone quality in growing children must take into account how the metabolic environment, the availability of nutrients and minerals, and the mechanical demands affect the size and mineralized content of different bones. From a functional perspective, it probably is the degree of stability rather than the extent of mineralization that provides a better measure of good bone health.[2]

Abnormal Bone Mineralization

Current noninvasive methods to study bone structure in children rely on measurements of a real mineralized content. Plain x-ray radiographs provide a subjective measure of mineralized content, whereas dual-energy x-ray absorptiometry (DEXA) is used to obtain a more quantitative measurement.[4] Measures of bone mineralization are affected by changes in bone size in growing children. Accordingly, smaller and younger infants of similar age generally will have smaller bones, and a lower measure of mineral content may not necessarily represent a sign of pathology. Because standards that account for variables of size and age often are lacking, especially at very young ages, any comparative quantitative evaluation of mineral content is extremely difficult. A temporal rise in mineralized content in a given subject could represent an increase in bone mineral content per unit bone length, an increase in bone size, or both. Decreased bone mineralization, in turn, can be a reflection of decreased formation of osteoid by osteoblasts or a decrease in mineral incorporation into osteoid. These two possibilities correspond to the two most common pathologic conditions observed in the premature skeleton: osteomalacia and osteopenia. Osteomalacia occurs when incorporation of mineral content into osteoid is decreased. Because osteoblasts still are able to make organic matrix, the average mineral content in bone is decreased; the bones become soft and more radiolucent, and they bend easily when exposed to force. In growing children, this defect in mineralization also is present in calcified cartilaginous growth plates, and the appearance of growth plate widening and fraying describes the radiologic changes seen in rickets. Osteopenia, on the other hand, is diagnosed when bone trabeculae or thickness is decreased. It is caused by either decreased deposition or increased resorption of organic bone matrix without a defect in mineral incorporation. Because mineralization is not affected, the growth plate changes seen in osteomalacia/rickets are absent even though decreases in mineral density are easily detected. It is not uncommon to see the terms *decreased bone size, osteopenia,* and *osteomalacia* lumped together when describing pathologic bone disease in premature infants; however, efforts should be made to distinguish among them because the strategies for prevention and treatment of each condition can be different.

Mineral Homeostasis

Bone mineralization requires a continuous soluble source of calcium, phosphate, and other minerals. In the fetal period, active transplacental transport of calcium from the maternal side maintains the fetal serum calcium concentration higher than the concentration present in extrauterine life, presumably to sustain an active rate of bone mineralization.[5] In the postnatal period, the serum calcium concentration is regulated primarily by an endocrine feedback mechanism. A decrease in serum ionized calcium is sensed by the parathyroid glands, which secrete parathyroid hormone (PTH) in response to hypocalcemia. In the kidney, PTH promotes retention of calcium and 1α–hydroxylation of hydroxyvitamin D [25(OH)D] to produce $1,25(OH)_2D$, the bioactive form of vitamin D, which promotes the absorption of both calcium and phosphate in the small intestine. PTH also activates osteoclasts to release calcium from bone. The combined effect of PTH secretion is restoration of serum calcium levels to the normal range.[6] In the absence of an adequate enteral source of mineral or when stores of vitamin D are low, serum calcium levels will be maintained in the normal range at the expense of mineral mobilization from bone. Accordingly, in states of no adequate access to exogenous calcium, bone mineralization is decreased and bone matrix resorption is increased.

Phosphate is the anion required for formation of mineral hydroxyapatite in bone. The serum phosphate concentration is more variable than that of calcium, but phosphate is regulated by mechanisms that appear to rely primarily on the effects of PTH and other factors that affect glomerular filtration and tubular phosphate transport. Phosphate concentrations in the newborn period are higher than in adults. Low serum phosphate levels directly promote the production of $1,25(OH)_2D$ in the proximal tubule, enhancing intestinal absorption of phosphate. Hypophosphatemia also increases mobilization of calcium and phosphate from bone.

In the postnatal period, adequate stores of vitamin D are important to sustain the intestinal absorption of both calcium and phosphate. The neonate's vitamin D stores at birth correlate well with maternal status; thus, infants born to mothers with low vitamin D stores are at higher risk for developing vitamin D deficiency, especially when breastfed. Breast milk is a poor source of vitamin D, and infants' exposure to sun, a source of ultraviolet radiation to promote vitamin D synthesis in the skin, often is limited. Most commercially available infant formulas are supplemented with vitamin D. The American Academy of Pediatrics recommends that all term and preterm infants receive a total (from enteral feedings and supplements) of at least 200 IU/day and 400 IU/day of vitamin D, respectively.[7] Recently there is concern that higher doses of vitamin D supplementation may be more beneficial.[8] Thus, adequate stores of vitamin D and an abundant source of minerals are essential to ensure that the higher rates of mineralization are sustained throughout childhood.

Skeletal Changes in the Postnatal Period

Normal changes during the postnatal period include an approximately 30% decrease in the density of long bones in the first 6 months of life even though bone mineral content increases overall because of bone size growth.[9] This loss in density is due partly to an increase in the size of the marrow cavity that normally occurs after birth. It has been postulated that the mechanical stimulation in utero is greater as the fetus experiences continuous "resistance training" by kicking against the uterine wall. The decreased resistance outside the womb may reduce the bone mineralization rate. In addition, the substantial exposure to maternal estrogen and other placental hormones that may have an anabolic effect in bone is lost after birth. However, it is important to note that this decrease in bone density, often referred to as "physiologic osteoporosis of infancy," is not associated with increased bone fragility or fracture rate. In fact, bone strength increases threefold because of changes in geometry during the same period. Furthermore, the comparison of mineral content between term and premature infants at expected term may be inappropriate, because the postnatal adaptations expected to occur in preterm infants may be erroneously interpreted as pathologic.

Causes of Deficient Bone Mineralization in Premature Infants

During fetal development, approximately 20 to 30 g of calcium is accumulated in bone and 80% of mineral deposition occurs in the third trimester.[1] Intrauterine accretion of calcium has been estimated to be as high as 150 mg/kg at 36 weeks' gestation. Preterm infants, especially those less than 30 weeks' gestation, are born before experiencing this significant period of intrauterine calcium accretion, a situation often aggravated by compromised mineral reserves secondary to prolonged fetal stress. Parenteral sources of nutrition cannot provide sufficient amounts of calcium and phosphate to match intrauterine levels, and the supply of calcium and phosphorus in breast milk (25–35 mg/dl of calcium and 10–15 mg/dl of phosphate) and regular infant formulas is relatively low. This decrease in supply of both minerals, but especially of phosphate, predisposes premature infants to develop osteomalacia/rickets (Table 7B-1). Radiographic imaging is likely to show changes in the growth plates of long bones consistent with rickets. Prolonged parenteral nutrition aggravates this mineral deficit, as the mineral content of parenteral formulations is limited because of solubility concerns. Fluid restriction therapy, often implemented to preserve cardiac and respiratory function, also limits mineral intake. The special preterm formulas currently used provide much higher mineral content and help to overcome this deficit in supply when enteral feeds are initiated; however, the mineral supply through this route can be compromised by decreased intestinal

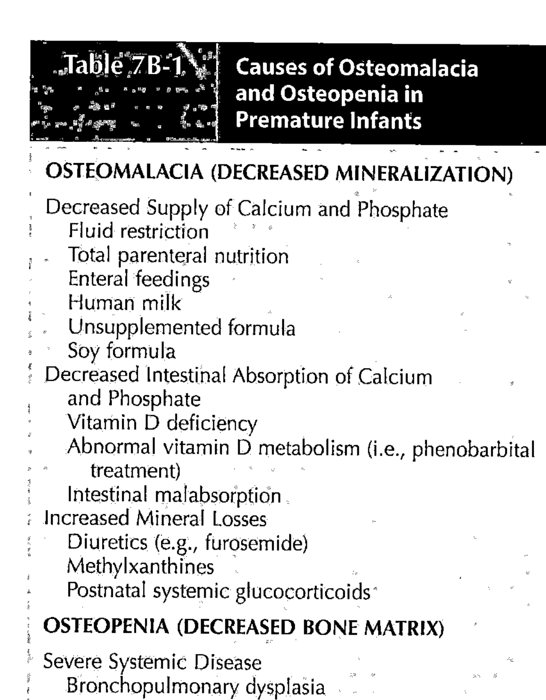

Table 7B-1 Causes of Osteomalacia and Osteopenia in Premature Infants

OSTEOMALACIA (DECREASED MINERALIZATION)

Decreased Supply of Calcium and Phosphate
- Fluid restriction
- Total parenteral nutrition
- Enteral feedings
- Human milk
- Unsupplemented formula
- Soy formula

Decreased Intestinal Absorption of Calcium and Phosphate
- Vitamin D deficiency
- Abnormal vitamin D metabolism (i.e., phenobarbital treatment)
- Intestinal malabsorption

Increased Mineral Losses
- Diuretics (e.g., furosemide)
- Methylxanthines
- Postnatal systemic glucocorticoids

OSTEOPENIA (DECREASED BONE MATRIX)

Severe Systemic Disease
- Bronchopulmonary dysplasia
- Sepsis
- Necrotizing enterocolitis

Drugs
- Diuretics
- Postnatal systemic glucocorticoids

Lack of Mechanical Stimulation
- Prolonged immobilization

bioavailability of minerals when present in high concentrations or in the presence of phytates (soy).[1] In addition, gastrointestinal complications, such as severe necrotizing enterocolitis, can compromise the intestinal capacity to absorb nutrients and minerals.

Calcium availability is compromised by increased urinary mineral losses normally seen in premature infants when compared with term babies. These losses are aggravated when methylxanthines, glucocorticoids, or diuretics are used as part of the medical management. Furosemide is known for its hypercalciuric effects, and even the thiazides, despite their hypocalciuric effects, have been shown to increase urinary mineral losses when used in conjunction with aldactone.

Vitamin D levels usually are not compromised in preterm infants unless the mother had poor vitamin D stores during pregnancy. In case of liver disease or when the infant is treated with an antiepileptic drug such as phenobarbital, inadequate hydroxylation limits the production of bioactive forms of vitamin D, decreasing the intestinal absorption of calcium and phosphate. Monitoring vitamin D levels and providing adequate supplementation in this group of patients is particularly important.

Causes of Osteopenia in Premature Infants

The skeleton, much like other organs, is highly sensitive to prolonged systemic illnesses, and the high rate of organic matrix deposition required during the postnatal period probably is very susceptible to metabolic stress. The hypoxia and acidosis associated with conditions such as bronchopulmonary dysplasia and necrotizing enterocolitis, for example, are likely to predispose premature infants to osteopenia (Table 7B-1). Recurrent sepsis may have similar consequences and compound the deleterious effect of limited supply of calcium and phosphate in supporting mineralization. Some of the drugs used to treat complications of prematurity have been associated with osteopenia in older patients and probably have similar consequences in premature infants. Glucocorticoids inhibit osteoblast function and increase urinary calcium losses. Besides their negative impact on mineral availability, diuretics often alter the physiologic acid-base balance when used chronically and affect bone growth.

More recently, the impact of prolonged immobilization of premature infants has received attention. The effects of gravity and muscle contraction place distinct functional requirements on bone strength and size to maintain mechanical stability. Prolonged immobilization as a result of severe sickness or prolonged intubation is likely to decrease the mechanical challenge to the skeleton. The absence of active mechanical activity results in a lack of drive to accrue mineral bone because stability can be maintained without an increase in bone thickness and length, even in the presence of a plentiful source of mineral. This may explain why osteopenia is still reported in premature infants who have not experienced many systemic postnatal complications or nutritional deficits. A rapid transition to a physical state with increased mechanical requirements on the skeleton will stress the stability of bones and predispose them to fractures.

Evaluation of Bone Disease in Premature Infants

Most premature infants, especially those born with low birth weight (<1500 g) and young gestational age (<32 weeks' gestation), are at risk for developing osteopenia and/or osteomalacia and should be evaluated periodically. Infants who have experienced severe respiratory or other systemic complications, who have undergone delayed initiation and advancement of enteral feeds, or who require chronic treatment with glucocorticoids or diuretics are at high risk for developing clinically significant bone disease even beyond the period of intensive neonatal care. Reliance on physical examination is not helpful in the diagnosis of osteopenia unless the disease has progressed to an advanced stage. In the neonatal intensive care unit (NICU), affected infants may experience tenderness at sites of fractures. In older patients, craniotabes or costochondral swelling in a characteristic distribution of a rachitic rosary may be observed. Upon discharge and with advancing age, long bone deformities and widening of joints should alert the primary care provider to the presence of osteomalacia.

Plain radiographs of long bones probably are the best imaging tool for diagnosing rickets and providing a subjective measure of bone mineralization.[10] However, a 30% to 40% loss of mineral content is necessary in order to be detected radiologically. More quantitative measurements with DEXA or other methods have proven useful as investigational tools, but in the absence of well-established standards, the use of these techniques remains of questionable clinical value in the primary care setting.

Biochemical screening should be directed primarily to the evaluation of metabolic bone disease (Table 7B-2). Calcium levels usually are within the normal range even in the presence of osteomalacia but can be elevated in states of significant phosphate depletion and hypophosphatemia. Phosphate levels usually are low or in the low–normal range, especially when the infant is not receiving phosphate-supplemented formula. In osteomalacia, osteoid production is relatively spared and osteoblast activity is markedly increased, so an elevated osteoblast-derived alkaline phosphatase level provides a biochemical measure of osteoblast activity and, indirectly, of the severity of osteomalacia. Alkaline phosphatase levels in the postnatal period normally can be quite elevated, and only relatively high values (>800 IU/ml or levels five times the adult normal range) have been correlated with radiologic evidence of osteomalacia. It is common to detect elevations of alkaline phosphatase level before osteomalacia is detected visually, not surprisingly because advanced progression of hypomineralization is required for detection by radiologic examination. Although serum alkaline phosphatase levels are derived from bone, liver, and other tissues, serum measurements correlate well with bone formation because the largest fraction in serum is derived from bone. The measurement of 25(OH)D, the product of liver-mediated hydroxylation of vitamin D, is the best measure of body vitamin D stores. Levels of 25(OH)D usually are normal at birth unless maternal stores were low. Without supplementation, premature infants are at risk for developing vitamin D deficiency, as are term infants, unless they receive substantial sun exposure. Because premature infants have a tendency for phosphate depletion, $1,25(OH)_2D$ levels

Table 7B-2 Outpatient Monitoring for Bone Disease in Premature Infants

Test	Expected Result
Serum	
Ca	Levels may be elevated in hypophosphatemia or low in severe vitamin D deficiency
PO_4	Normal or low in inadequately supplemented infants
Alkaline phosphatase	Elevated if osteomalacia is present
25(OH)D	Normal but may be low in unsupplemented infants, infants born to mothers with low stores, or infants treated with anticonvulsants
$1,25(OH)_2D$	Usually elevated at baseline
Parathyroid hormone	Usually normal but may be elevated in vitamin D deficiency
Urine	
Ca/Creatinine ratio	Broad range of variability during the first weeks of life, but ratios >1.5 when approaching postmenstrual term gestational age would be considered very elevated; ratio for infants >1 year usually is lower (<0.25)
Imaging	
Standard radiographs	Rickets, hypomineralization, or fractures
Dual-energy x-ray absorptiometry (DEXA)	Remains an investigational tool and may be recommended under the guidance of a pediatric endocrinology specialist

usually are mildly elevated, even in the absence of osteomalacia. PTH levels usually are within the normal range but can be elevated when there are significant urinary calcium losses and/or vitamin D deficiency, likely a response to mild hypocalcemia. Urinary studies typically are difficult to obtain outside the hospital in small infants, and, although a measure of both phosphate and calcium handling by the kidney generally is useful, spot urine calcium/creatinine ratios may be easier to include as part of the workup in the primary care setting. High urine calcium/creatinine ratios commonly are seen in premature infants, and this ratio decreases with age.[11] Normal term infants can have high ratios throughout the first year of life, up to 0.8 or even higher. The use of methylxanthines, furosemide, or dexamethasone is associated with even higher ratios, as is the degree of prematurity. Particularly high ratios (>1.5) may raise concern of significant hypercalciuria. Although various serum and urine markers of bone turnover currently are available (e.g., collagen-derived peptides), their clinical value in assessing bone health has not been established, especially in neonates.

Primary care providers should continue to monitor for bone disease in premature infants at high risk (Figure 7B-1). Discharged premature infants who remain on fluid restriction therapy or who are medicated with drugs known to affect bone or vitamin D metabolism (e.g., glucocorticoids, phenobarbital) should be monitored periodically every 4 to 8 weeks to ensure that they have no clinical or biochemical evidence of metabolic bone disease. During this interval, these infants should be examined for any physical evidence of bone fractures or visible ricketic changes. The initial biochemical screen should include at least a measurement of serum mineral (i.e., calcium and phosphate), alkaline phosphatase, and 25(OH)D levels. Urine measurements of calcium and creatinine may be appropriate for infants receiving diuretic therapy. If the physical examination or laboratory screen tests suggest the presence of bone disease, a plain radiograph of the long bones may help to confirm the presence of rickets or osteopenia. More stable patients also should be monitored periodically, especially if they have a history of prolonged parenteral nutrition or severe complications of prematurity. Although defining the period of time when vigilance is most important in the assessment of bone health in premature infants is difficult, a recommendation of close monitoring until at least 6 months' corrected gestational age appears reasonable. A significant catch-up in bone mass occurs during the first year of life, suggesting that aggressive monitoring beyond this period is not necessary.[12] Infants with significant active morbidity and poor nutritional state should be monitored longer.

Medical Intervention

Preventive steps starting as early as when infants are in the NICU can significantly improve the morbidity associated with poor bone mineralization. Advancements in neonatal care have allowed a decrease in immobilization periods, and improved nutritional management with the use of calcium- and phosphate-supplemented formulas has improved mineral availability to support bone mineralization. Most NICUs recommend the use of special transitional formulas enriched in minerals or fortified breast milk to ensure a high enteral content of minerals (e.g., Neosure, EnfaCare). These formulations often are recommended for use in very-low-birth-weight infants until they reach 6 to 12 months' corrected gestational age.[13] These formulas provide

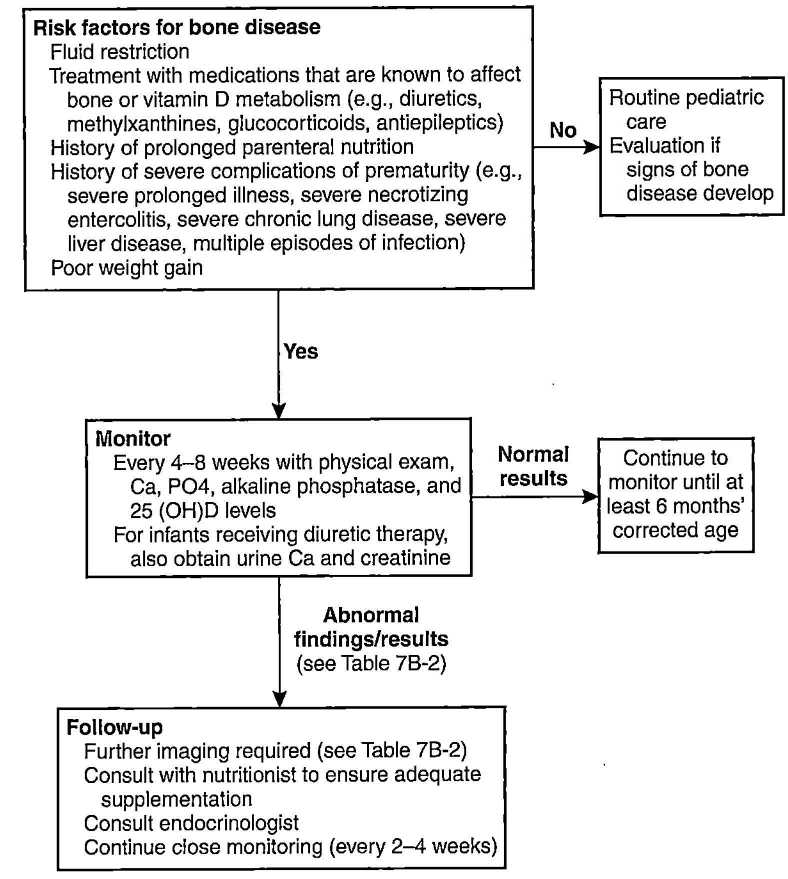

FIGURE 7B-1 Premature infants with risk factors for bone disease should be monitored closely and evaluated, as shown in this figure. Please note that this is a recommended algorithm that does not represent a professional standard of care; care should be revised to meet individual patient needs.

an adequate amount of vitamin D (400 IU/day) to minimize the chance of the infant's developing bone disease. Some studies have failed to show a measurable benefit from mineral-enriched formulas or breast milk, but differences in mineral bioavailability in these preparations may explain some of the variability reported.[14] Because no significant adverse effects have been noted from use of fortified breast milk or transitional formulas, they are commonly recommended by most nurseries. Because of the variability in mineral bioavailability and differences in infant's metabolic needs, clinical monitoring becomes essential to identifying infants at high risk. In cases of poor overall nutrition or clinical evidence of a deficit in mineral intake, efforts to increase both phosphate and calcium intake should be made with the aid of a nutrition specialist. For infants who show low or low–normal vitamin D stores (25OHD levels <20 ng/ml), vitamin D supplementation should be adjusted upward to normalize levels. Studies have not shown a benefit from increasing vitamin D supplementation above currently recommended levels (i.e, 400 IU/day) in vitamin D–sufficient infants, but infants who have fat malabsorption or who are treated with antiepileptics may require an increased dose to maintain normal levels. Although there are no clear guidelines about vitamin D dosing under those circumstances in young infants, a threefold increase in vitamin D requirements is often noted. Periodic monitoring of vitamin D levels (e.g., every 1–2 months) should ensure adequate supplementation. More recently, the role of physical therapy in promoting bone strength has been advocated, at least during periods of immobilization in the nursery,[15] but clinical studies showing a long-term benefit are not available. Discharged infants probably are no longer enduring prolonged periods of inactivity and will not require a regimented schedule of physical activity.

Conclusion

Premature infants are born at a time when bone mineral accretion is highest in utero. The metabolic complications often seen in the first few days of extrauterine life, together with the decreased mineral intake and mobility, can cause a decrease in bone mineral accretion. Both osteopenia and rickets have been observed in this setting, as well as a much higher predisposition to bone fractures. We have made significant progress in preventing metabolic bone disease in premature infants. The short-term impact of increased mineral supplementation has been to reduce the incidence of rickets in early life. The impact of these nutritional interventions on long-term bone health is unclear, but ensuring an adequate supply of minerals and an adequate source of vitamin D for efficient enteral absorption of these minerals has become acceptable practice. Some of the osteopenic changes noted in prematurity likely are the consequence of physiologic adaptation of bone to prolonged immobility associated with the early nursery course. Although various forms of physical activity have been shown to increase bone mass, much research is needed to optimize our interventions to ensure an adequate transition to the toddler years.

REFERENCES

1. Greer FR: Osteopenia of prematurity. *Annu Rev Nutr* 14:169, 1994.
2. Rauch F, Schoenau E: Skeletal development in premature infants: a review of bone physiology beyond nutritional aspects. *Arch Dis Child Fetal Neonatal Ed* 86:F82, 2002.
3. Rauch F, Schoenau E: The developing bone: slave or master of its cells and molecules? *Pediatr Res* 50:309, 2001.
4. Nelson DA, Koo WW: Interpretation of absorptiometric bone mass measurements in the growing skeleton: issues and limitations. *Calcif Tissue Int* 65:1, 1999.
5. Kovacs CS, Kronenberg HM: Maternal-fetal calcium and bone metabolism during pregnancy, puerperium, and lactation. *Endocr Rev* 18:832, 1997.
6. Broadus AE: Mineral balance and homeostasis. In Favus HJ, editor: *Primer on the metabolic bone diseases and disorders of mineral metabolism.* Washington DC, 2003, American Society for Bone and Mineral research.
7. Gartner LM, Greer FR: Prevention of rickets and vitamin D deficiency: new guidelines for vitamin D intake. *Pediatrics* 111:908, 2003.
8. Greer FR: Issues in establishing vitamin D recommendations for infants and children. *Am J Clin Nutr* 80:1759S, 2004.
9. Rauch F, Schoenau E: Changes in bone density during childhood and adolescence: an approach based on bone's biological organization. *J Bone Miner Res* 16:597, 2001.
10. Leonard MB, Shore, RM: Radiologic evaluation of bone mineral in children. In Favus HJ, editor: *Primer on the metabolic bone diseases and disorders of mineral metabolism.* Washington, DC, 2003, American Society for Bone and Mineral Research.
11. Aladangady N, Coen PG, White MP, et al: Urinary excretion of calcium and phosphate in preterm infants. *Pediatr Nephrol* 19:1225, 2004.
12. Fewtrell MS, Prentice A, Jones SC, et al: Bone mineralization and turnover in preterm infants at 8-12 years of age: the effect of early diet. *J Bone Miner Res* 14:810, 1999.
13. Carver JD, Wu PY, Hall RT, et al: Growth of preterm infants fed nutrient-enriched or term formula after hospital discharge. *Pediatrics* 107:683, 2001.
14. Faerk J, Petersen S, Peitersen B, et al: Diet and bone mineral content at term in premature infants. *Pediatr Res* 47:148, 2000.
15. Moyer-Mileur LJ, Brunstetter V, McNaught TP, et al: Daily physical activity program increases bone mineralization and growth in preterm very low birth weight infants *Pediatrics* 106:1088, 2000.

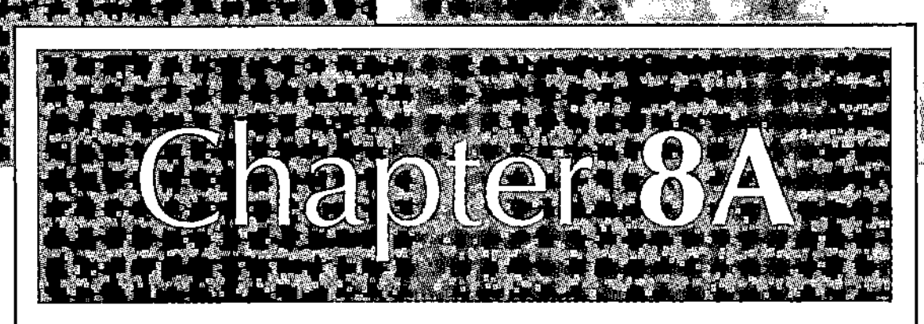

Retinopathy of Prematurity

John A.F. Zupancic, MD, ScD

Retinopathy of prematurity (ROP) is a disorder of abnormal vascular proliferation of the infant retina. It is the second most common cause of childhood blindness. The incidence of this condition is strongly correlated with gestation. It is rare in infants born after 32 weeks' gestation but increases in incidence to 51% of infants born between 28 and 31 weeks' gestation and 89% of infants born at or before 27 weeks' gestation.[1,2] In addition to prematurity and low birth weight, potential or confirmed risk factors include oxygen exposure and markers of neonatal illness severity, such as mechanical ventilation, systemic infection, blood transfusion, and intraventricular hemorrhage.[3]

Pathogenesis

The retina initially is avascular and receives its oxygen by diffusion from the hyaloid artery, which supplies the anterior eye and is resorbed in the third trimester. At 12 to 15 weeks' gestation, the retinal vessels appear at the optic disc and begin to migrate outward, reaching the nasal periphery by 36 weeks' postmenstrual age and the temporal periphery by 40 weeks.[4]

The pathogenesis of ROP appears to interrupt this normal progression in two phases.[5,6] In the first phase, a physiologic insult, such as hyperoxia, causes vasoconstriction of the developing vessels, resulting in hypoxia and ischemia. In the second phase, angiogenic factors associated with this ischemic state lead to neovascularization. The new vessels grow into the vitreous and are relatively permeable, resulting in hemorrhage and edema. In severe cases, fibrovascular proliferation in the vitreous may exert traction on the retina and lead to retinal detachment.

Vascular growth factors and their receptors, including insulinlike growth factor-I (IGF-I) and vascular endothelial growth factor (VEGF), are involved in the pathogenesis of ROP, although the mechanism is complex and incompletely understood.[5]

Classification

Classification of the severity of ROP is closely related to its pathogenesis and drives both prognosis and therapy. The International Classification of Retinopathy of Prematurity is a set of expert consensus definitions along four axes[7,8]:

1. The *location* of disease relates to the distance that normal and abnormal retinal vessels have progressed from the optic disc. As shown in Figure 8A-1, location is described as one of three zones, corresponding to three concentric circles. Zone 1 is centered on the optic disc and extends to a radius twice the distance from the disc to the macula. Zone 2 also is centered on the optic disc and extends from the perimeter of zone 1 to the nasal periphery and approximately halfway to the temporal periphery. Zone 3 extends from the perimeter of zone 2 to the temporal periphery.
2. The *stage* of disease describes the degree of vascular abnormality (Figures 8A-2 and 8A-3). In stage 1, there is a white demarcation line separating normal from avascular retina. In stage 2, a ridge of fibrous tissue between normal and avascular retina extends anteriorly into the vitreous. In stage 3, fibrous tissue and blood vessels appear along this ridge. In stage 4, scar tissue exerts traction and results in partial retinal detachment, either excluding (stage 4a) or including (stage 4b) the macula. Finally, in stage 5, the retina detaches completely, resulting in "cicatricial ROP."
3. The *extent* of disease refers to how much of the circumference of the retinal surface is involved.

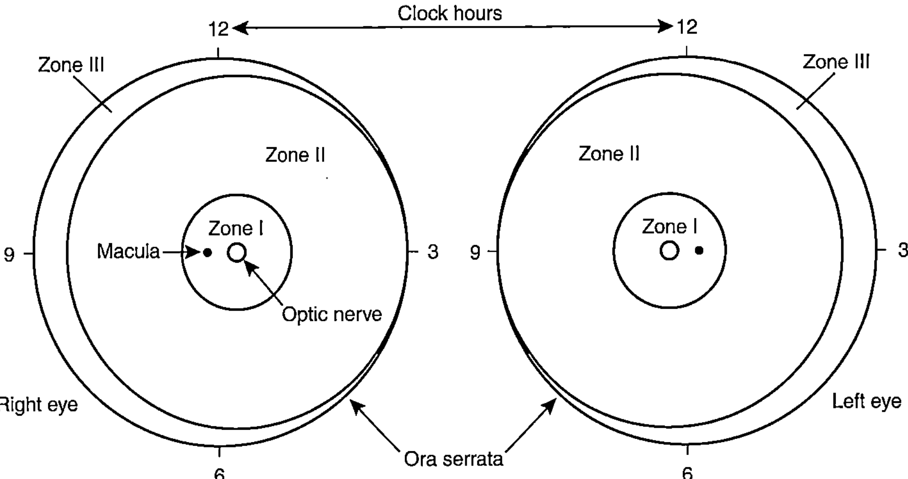

FIGURE 8A-1 This is a schematic demonstrating the 3 zones and clock hours of the retina. From: Screening examination of premature infants for retinopathy of prematurity. Section on Ophthalmology, American Academy of Ophthalmology and American Association for Pediatric Ophthalmology and Strabismus: *Pediatrics* 2006 117: p 574.

It is measured in contiguous or noncontiguous clock hours, with each hour covering a 30-degree segment.

4. *Plus disease* refers to dilatation and tortuosity of retinal vessels. This is a direct hemodynamic effect of extraretinal vascular proliferation and indicates a more severe form of the disease. It may be associated with anterior effects such as pupillary rigidity, iris vascular engorgement, or vitreous haze. The term *rush disease* refers to plus disease in zone 1, which tends to progress rapidly. An update of the consensus definitions describes an intermediate form of plus disease, referred to as *pre-plus disease.*[7]

Diagnosis

ROP is diagnosed by observation of the described findings on indirect ophthalmoscopy. Because these retinal abnormalities rarely are present before 30 weeks and because the presence of normal vitreous blood vessels ("primary vitreous haze") interferes with retinal visualization, examinations usually begin at 4 to 6 weeks' postnatal age or at 31 to 32 weeks' postmenstrual age, whichever is later. Given the therapeutic importance of accurate diagnosis and the variability in accuracy with level of experience, examinations should be performed by a pediatric ophthalmology specialist.

The American Academy of Pediatrics recommends screening of infants born at 30 weeks' gestational age or less or with a birth weight less than 1500 g.[9] In addition, selected infants with a birth weight between 1500 and 2000 g or gestational age of more than 30 weeks with severe cardiorespiratory instability should have retinal screening examinations.[9] Examinations continue every 2 weeks as long as retinal development is proceeding normally. Once ROP of any stage is noted, the examinations become more frequent, occurring weekly or even daily when therapeutic intervention appears imminent. Examinations can be discontinued once the retinal vessels have reached the perimeter of zone 3, at which point the retina is declared "mature."

Treatment

Because treatment of established ROP is invasive and of somewhat limited efficacy,[10] prevention is desirable. Severe physiologic instability or high levels of inspired oxygen are associated with development of ROP. Unfortunately, cardiorespiratory lability is an inherent feature of extreme prematurity, and oxygen saturation targets that safely balance the risk of ROP with the risk of hypoxia have not been established. Antioxidant therapies such as vitamin E and penicillamine have shown some promise in randomized trials, but the former may increase the risk of necrotizing enterocolitis or sepsis in the short term, and long-term outcomes have not been established for either.[11,12]

Once ROP has developed, the decision to intervene depends on the severity of disease. "Threshold" ROP involves stage 3 disease in five or more contiguous or eight cumulative clock hours, with plus disease, in either zone 1 or zone 2.[7] Threshold disease is associated with a risk of poor visual outcome of 50% and is thought universally to warrant treatment. "Prethreshold" ROP involves any of the following: (1) zone 1 ROP of any stage less than threshold; (2) zone 2 ROP with stage 2

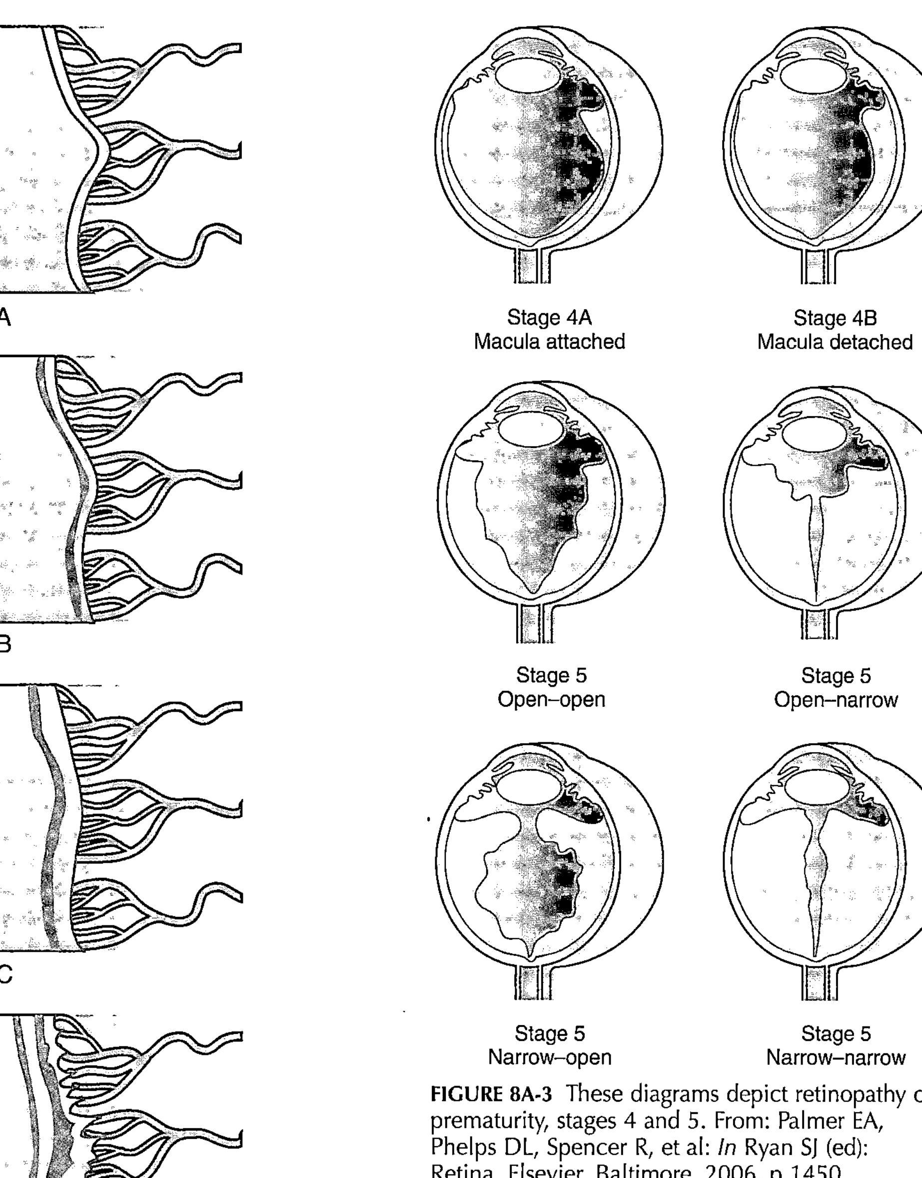

FIGURE 8A-3 These diagrams depict retinopathy of prematurity, stages 4 and 5. From: Palmer EA, Phelps DL, Spencer R, et al: *In* Ryan SJ (ed): Retina. Elsevier, Baltimore, 2006, p 1450. Courtesy Rand Spencer, MD.

FIGURE 8A-2 These diagrams show the 3 stages of retinopathy of prematurity. The vascularized, more mature retina is seen to the right and the avascular retina is to the left in the diagrams. **A**, The demarcation line of stage 1. **B**, The characterstic ridge of stage 2 is noted. **C**, Extraretinal fibrovascular proliferative tissue of "mild" stage 3. **D**, "Moderate" proliferation of extraretinal fibrovascular tissue from the ridge in more advanced stage 3. Modified from: Committee for the Classification of Retinopathy of Prematurity. An international classification of retinopathy of prematurity: *Arch Ophthalmol* 102:1130-1134, 1984.

and plus disease; (3) zone 2 ROP with stage 3 without plus disease; and (4) zone 2 ROP with stage 3 and plus disease, but without the required extent to qualify as threshold ROP. Approximately 30% of infants with prethreshold ROP will progress to threshold ROP.

Administration of supplemental oxygen to infants with prethreshold ROP may, theoretically, overcome retinal hypoxia, which leads to neovascularization. However, a large clinical trial showed reduction in progression of ROP only in infants with prethreshold ROP without plus disease.[13]

Definitive therapy for ROP involves ablation of the retina anterior to the abnormality in order to prevent neovascularization and the potential for retinal detachment. This ablation is performed using cryotherapy through the posterior sclera or, more recently, laser photocoagulation through the lens. Because both techniques involve destruction of retinal tissue, they previously were reserved for infants with threshold ROP. However, a large randomized trial later showed that laser therapy in "high-risk prethreshold ROP," as defined by a set of demographic and clinical risk factors,[3] also resulted in improved outcomes.[14] Therefore, current recommendations for retinal ablation include the following: (1) threshold disease; (2) prethreshold disease with zone 1 ROP, any stage with plus disease; (3) prethreshold disease with zone 1, stage 3 without plus disease; or (4) zone 2, stage 2 or 3 with plus disease.[14]

Once retinal detachment has occurred, retinal ablation is no longer effective. At this stage, surgical procedures are used to encourage reattachment of the retina. These include the scleral buckle, in which the globe is banded to bring the retina into contact with the wall of the eye, and vitrectomy, in which the vitreous is removed along with the pathologic fibrous tissue in order to reduce retinal traction. These procedures are of limited utility.[4]

Prognosis

Stage 1 or 2 ROP usually resolves, as does ROP in zone 3. Approximately 18% of infants weighing less than 1250 g will develop prethreshold ROP, and one third of these infants will progress to threshold ROP.[15] Infants with untreated threshold disease have a 45% risk of structural abnormality (e.g., detachment) and a 62% risk of poor visual acuity (Snellen 20/200 or worse).[16]

Treatment at threshold reduces poor structural outcome by half, to approximately 27%; poor visual acuity is reduced to 45%. Early treatment of infants with high-risk prethreshold disease, as described earlier, reduces the risk of poor visual acuity outcome from 20% to approximately 15%, but at the cost of more invasive treatments.[14]

Among infants who undergo vitrectomy and scleral buckle, normal visual acuity is attained in only 20%.[17]

It should be noted that premature infants with all severities of ROP remain at risk for other ophthalmologic problems.[18] Strabismus (ocular misalignment) may develop in 13% to 25% of premature infants. Myopia occurs in approximately 15% and high myopia in 4% of premature infants. Both strabismus and myopia may result in amblyopia (reduced visual acuity because of nonuse of one eye during a critical window of development, before age 7 years). Uncorrected differences in refractive error between the eyes (anisometropia) also may contribute to the risk of amblyopia.

Considerations for Primary Care

Although the peak intensity of ROP and the need for therapy occur before discharge of most extremely-low-birth-weight infants, there are several important considerations for clinicians providing primary care to this population.

First, infants sometimes are discharged home or transferred to convalescent nurseries away from ophthalmologic referral services before retinal maturation is completed. It is essential that infants closely adhere to the timetable of examinations. Prethreshold disease may progress rapidly to threshold, and a delay even of days may have catastrophic consequences.

Given the risk for strabismus, refractive error, amblyopia in premature infants, and cataract or late retinal detachment in infants who undergo ablation therapy, all premature infants born at less than 32 weeks' gestation should undergo ophthalmologic screening at 6 to 9 months' chronologic age, whether or not they were screened for ROP, developed ROP, or received treatment for ROP. The frequency of further examinations will depend on risk factors for visual problems, but formal acuity screening should be performed at least once in the preschool years.

Finally, in infants who have adverse consequences of retinopathy, global developmental outcomes will depend critically on the intensity of supportive interventions for blindness. In addition to the secondary effects of blindness, many of these infants will have other primary neurodevelopmental impairments that will interact with visual problems to create therapeutic challenges. The primary care clinician will be essential in coordinating a medical home and guiding families to appropriate community resources (Table 8A-1).

Resources for Families and Clinicians

American Academy of Pediatrics
http://www.aap.org/policy/060023.html

Provides a policy statement for screening examinations of premature infants for retinopathy of prematurity.

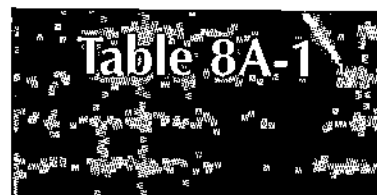

Table 8A-1 Outpatient Monitoring for Infants at Risk for Retinopathy of Prematurity

Confirm that retinal maturation is complete on recent ophthalmologic examination.
- If retina is mature, arrange for ophthalmologic follow-up at 6–9 months to monitor for amblyopia, strabismus, and/or refractive errors.
- If retina is immature, arrange for ophthalmologic follow-up per guidelines recommended in text. Emphasize to the family the extreme importance of a critical time window that must be met if treatment is to be successful and that timely follow-up examination is essential to successful treatment.[9]

All premature infants should have formal visual acuity screening that is performed once during the preschool years.

If evidence of visual difficulties is seen, refer to appropriate community resources (some federal resources highlighted in Resources for Families and Clinicians).

American Council of the Blind
1155 15th Street NW, Suite 1004, Washington, DC 20005
Phone: (800) 467-5081; Fax: (202) 467-5085
www.acb.org

This council strives to improve the well-being of all blind and visually impaired people by improving educational and rehabilitation facilities/opportunities, assisting and encouraging institutions and organizations servicing this population, and educating the public. The website provides an extensive list of links to resources and an online store.

American Foundation for the Blind
11 Penn Plaza, Suite 300, New York, NY 10001
Phone: (800) AFB-LINE (232-5463)
www.afb.org

Addresses issues of literacy, independent living, employment, and access through technology for the blind and visually impaired.

Association for Retinopathy of Prematurity and Related Diseases
PO Box 250425, Franklin, MI 48025
http://ropard.org/

The purpose of this organization is to fund clinically relevant basic science and clinical research to eliminate retinopathy of prematurity and associated retinal diseases. This organization funds innovative work leading directly to the development of new low-vision devices and teaching techniques and services for children who are visually impaired and their families.

National Association for Parents of Children with Visual Impairment (NAPVI)
http://www.spedex.com/napvi/

APVI is a national organization that enables parents to find information and resources for their children who are blind or visually impaired.

National Federation of the Blind (NFB)
http://www.nfb.org

The purpose of the National Federation of the Blind is twofold: to help blind persons achieve self-confidence and self-respect and to act as a vehicle for collective self-expression by the blind. By providing public education about blindness, information and referral services, *scholarships, literature* and publications about blindness, *aids and appliances* and other adaptive equipment for the blind, advocacy services and protection of civil rights, development and evaluation of *technology*, and support for blind persons and their families, members of the NFB strive to educate the public that the blind are normal individuals who can compete on terms of equality.

National Information Clearinghouse on Children Who Are Deaf-Blind
Western Oregon State College, 35 North Monmouth Avenue, Monmouth, OR 97361
Phone: (800) 438-9376; TTY: (800) 854-7013
www.dblink.org

The goal of this organization is to help parents, teachers, and others by providing information to foster the skills, strategies, and confidence necessary to nurture and empower deaf-blind children. DB-LINK is a federally funded service that identifies, coordinates, and disseminates, at no cost, information related to children and youth from birth through 21 years of age.

REFERENCES

1. Good WV, Hardy RJ, Dobson V, et al: The incidence and course of retinopathy of prematurity: findings from the early treatment for retinopathy of prematurity study. *Pediatrics* 116(1):15-23, 2005.
2. Palmer EA, Flynn JT, Hardy RJ, et al: Incidence and early course of retinopathy of prematurity. The Cryotherapy for Retinopathy of Prematurity Cooperative Group. *Ophthalmology* 98(11):1628-1640, 1991.
3. Hardy RJ, Palmer EA, Dobson V, et al: Risk analysis of prethreshold retinopathy of prematurity. *Arch Ophthalmol* 121(12):1697-1701, 2003.
4. Good WV, Gendron RL: Retinopathy of prematurity. *Ophthalmol Clin North Am* 14(3):513-519, 2001.
5. Smith LE: IGF-1 and retinopathy of prematurity in the preterm infant. *Biol Neonate* 88(3):237-244, 2005.
6. Smith L: Pathogenesis of retinopathy of prematurity. *Semin Neonatol* 8(6):469-473, 2003.
7. International Committee for the Classification of Retinopathy of Prematurity: The international classification of retinopathy of prematurity revisited. *Arch Ophthalmol* 123:991-999, 2005.
8. Committee for the Classification of Retinopathy of Prematurity. An international classification of retinopathy of prematurity. *Arch Ophthalmol* 102: 1130-1134, 1984.
9. Section on Ophthalmology American Academy of Pediatrics; American Academy of Ophthalmology; American Association for Pediatric Ophthalmology and

Strabismus: Screening examination of premature infants for retinopathy of prematurity. *Pediatrics* 117(2):572-576, 2006. Erratum in: *Pediatrics.* 118(3):1324, 2006.

10. Andersen CC, Phelps DL: Peripheral retinal ablation for threshold retinopathy of prematurity in preterm infants. 1999. Available at: *http://www.mrw.interscience.wiley.com/cochrane/clsysrev/articles/CD001693/frame.html.*
11. Brion LP, Bell EF, Raghuveer TS: Vitamin E supplementation for prevention of morbidity and mortality in preterm infants. 2003. Available at: *http://www.mrw.interscience.wiley.com/cochrane/clsysrev/articles/CD003665/frame.html.*
12. Phelps DL, Lakatos L, Watts JL: D-Penicillamine for preventing retinopathy of prematurity in preterm infants. *Cochrane Database Syst Rev* (1);CD001073, 2001.
13. Supplemental Therapeutic Oxygen for Prethreshold Retinopathy Of Prematurity (STOP-ROP), a randomized, controlled trial. I: primary outcomes: *Pediatrics* 105(2): 295-310, 2000.
14. Early Treatment for Retinopathy of Prematurity Cooperative Group: Revised indications for the treatment of retinopathy of prematurity: results of the early treatment for retinopathy of prematurity randomized trial: *Arch Ophthalmol* 121(12):1684-1694, 2003.
15. Schaffer DB, Palmer EA, Plotsky DF, et al: Prognostic factors in the natural course of retinopathy of prematurity. The Cryotherapy for Retinopathy of Prematurity Cooperative Group: *Ophthalmology* 100(2):230-237, 1993.
16. Cryotherapy for Retinopathy of Prematurity Cooperative Group: The natural ocular outcome of premature birth and retinopathy. Status at 1 year. *Arch Ophthalmol* 112(7): 903-912, 1994.
17. Repka MX, Tung B, Good WV, et al: Outcome of eyes developing retinal detachment during the Early Treatment for Retinopathy of Prematurity Study (ETROP). *Arch Ophthalmol.* 124(1):24-30, 2006.
18. O'Connor AR, Stephenson T, Johnson A, et al: Long-term ophthalmic outcome of low birth weight children with and without retinopathy of prematurity. *Pediatrics* 109(1):12-18, 2002.

Chapter 8B

Ophthalmologic Follow-up of the Premature Infant

Munish Gupta, MD

The premature infant is at risk for numerous complications and morbidities related to visual development that can arise during infancy and childhood. Retinopathy of prematurity (ROP) is the most important of these, but even in its absence, other significant ophthalmologic conditions can occur that can affect long-term vision. This chapter reviews ophthalmologic considerations other than ROP that are important in the outpatient management of the premature infant.

Background

Independent of prematurity, ophthalmologic abnormalities are common in the general pediatric population. Periodic vision screening is an important element of routine pediatric care because early identification of abnormalities can prevent long-term disabilities. Normal vision requires continued development of visual pathways from birth to approximately 10 years of age, and factors that impair vision during this time period can lead to permanent central visual loss if left uncorrected.

The most common pediatric ophthalmologic problems include strabismus, refractive errors, and amblyopia. *Strabismus* is an abnormality in ocular alignment and can be unilateral or bilateral. It includes vertical and horizontal deviations and occurs in approximately 4% of children.[1] *Refractive errors* refer to an inability of the eye to focus images precisely on the retina. They include *myopia*, in which images are focused anterior to the retina, *hyperopia*, in which images are focused posterior to the retina, and *astigmatism*, in which irregularities of the cornea or lens produce more than one focal point in the eye. *Anisometropia* refers to a significant difference in refractive state of one eye compared with the other. Refractive errors increase with age, occurring in 5% to 7% of preschool children and up to 20% of teenage children.[1,2] *Amblyopia* is a reduction in visual acuity of an eye that is not associated with structural or organic damage or abnormalities. It is caused by factors that cause disuse of an eye, and in childhood most commonly results from strabismus or anisometropia. If uncorrected, it can lead to permanent visual loss. Amblyopia is estimated to occur in 2% to 4% of preschool children.[1,2]

Visual impairment can result from structural abnormalities of the eye or other parts of the visual system, including damage to the visual cortex. However, this is very uncommon in otherwise healthy children.

Outcomes in Premature Infants

Children born prematurely appear to be at increased risk for numerous ophthalmologic conditions compared with children born full term. These conditions include common problems such as alignment and refractive errors, as well as long-term impairment of visual acuity. Much of our recent knowledge on the visual outcomes of premature infants comes from observational and interventional studies examining ROP performed 15 to 20 years ago. The largest series is reported by the Multicenter Trial of Cryotherapy for Retinopathy of Prematurity (CRYO-ROP). This study enrolled more than 4000 infants with birth weight less than 1251 g at multiple sites across the United States from 1986 to 1987 and followed more than 1200 of these infants at selected centers up to 5 years of age.[3-6] Numerous other prospective studies also have been reported, primarily from Europe and New Zealand. In general, these studies enrolled premature infants born in the late

1980s to early 1990s and followed them to 5 to 10 years of age, with sample sizes of several hundred infants. As with CRYO-ROP, these studies focused on very premature infants, with entry criteria of birth weight less than 1500 to 1700 g or gestational age less than 32 weeks. Several also examined matched controls of children born at full term.[7-16] The results of these various studies are summarized here according to ophthalmologic outcome.

Strabismus

Most cases of strabismus associated with prematurity are detected within the first year of life, although a significant number also develop later in childhood.[17] In CRYO-ROP, strabismus was noted in more than 14% of the infants within the first year of life and in a similar percentage of infants seen at 2 years of age.[3,4] The risk of strabismus was highly correlated with ROP, but it also was identified in more than 5% of infants without a history of ROP.[4] Other studies supported these findings, reporting overall childhood rates of strabismus of 12.5% to 22% among premature infants and 10% to 19% among premature infants without a history of ROP.[7,12,13,15,16] In comparison, rates of strabismus among full-term controls were 1.4% to 3%.[12,13]

Refractive errors

Infants and young children normally have mild physiologic hyperopia that is self resolving and does not require treatment. Myopia typically appears in childhood and increases in incidence through adolescence. Preterm infants appear to be at particular risk for both more severe hyperopia and myopia. CRYO-ROP found that, among its preterm cohort at age 5 to 6 years, 13.6% had significant hyperopia and 7.7% had significant myopia; 5.3% were classified as severe myopia.[6] Development of myopia was strongly associated with a history of ROP, but it also was seen in 10% of those without a history of ROP.[5] Other series examining preterm infants at 7 to 10 years of age used varying definitions but reported overall similar results: hyperopia in 4% to 18%, myopia in 14% to 22%, and severe myopia in 5% to 7%.[8,13,15] Among full-term controls, myopia was found in approximately 9% and severe myopia in approximately 2%.[8,13] Of note, although severe ROP did increase the risk of refractive errors, mild ROP was not associated with an increased risk compared with prematurity alone.[10,13,15]

Visual acuity

In most cases, strabismus and refractive errors can be managed with medical or surgical therapy. Severe cases, however, can lead to amblyopia and long-term visual impairment. Furthermore, it appears that premature infants are at increased risk for decreased visual acuity even after correction of refractive errors. Among the CRYO-ROP cohort at 5 to 6 years of age, 12.2% had best-corrected visual acuity worse than 20/60, with 5.1% worse than 20/200. This risk was strongly associated with ROP; among those without a history of ROP, 5.2% had visual acuity worse than 20/60 and none worse than 20/200. Of note, 92% of the children without a history of ROP had good visual outcomes, with an acuity of 20/40 or better.[6] Other studies reported similar results, with impaired visual acuity seen in approximately 4% to 8% of former preterm infants compared with 0% to 1% of term controls.[9,12,13,15] Visual acuity of 20/20 or better was seen in 76% to 86% of the preterm group.[9,13] As a group, these studies were consistent in showing generally favorable visual acuity outcomes in preterm infants, but with a small but significantly increased risk of impairment. Because these impairments were observed despite optimal correction of refractive errors and strabismus, they presumably were the result of structural abnormalities of the visual cortex or other elements of the visual pathway.

Other

In addition to the outcomes discussed, premature infants may be at risk for other ophthalmologic complications, including optic nerve atrophy, cataracts, glaucoma, and retinal detachment. However, these complications are rare, and their incidence has not been well studied.[17]

Recommendations

Vision screening during infancy and childhood should be a standard element of pediatric primary care for all children. The severity of potential long-term vision complications in preterm infants suggests that routine examination by an ophthalmology specialist in addition to screening by the primary care provider may be warranted for high-risk infants. Specific guidelines defining which infants require evaluation and at what age are not well defined, but recommendations for screening based on current knowledge are outlined here.

Identification of high-risk infants

It appears that, among premature infants, the highest risk for subsequent ophthalmologic complications is found in those born at less than 32 weeks' gestation or with birth weight less than 1500 g. These are the same infants who are at highest risk for ROP, and the majority of the studies discussed focused on these groups. Moderately premature infants born at greater than 32 weeks' gestation do not appear to be at increased risk for long-term visual morbidities compared with full-term infants.[11] In addition, although the risk of ophthalmologic complications is highest in extremely premature infants, it still is significant in those born between 28 and 32 weeks' gestation or birth weight 1000 to 1500 g.[11,13,16,18] Finally, in addition to ROP, other neurologic complications during the neonatal period, particularly intraventricular hemorrhage (IVH) and hydrocephalus, increase the risk for subsequent ophthalmologic morbidities.[17,19,20]

Timing of examination

Early detection of significant alignment or refractive errors is essential to allow for optimal intervention and management. External examination and retinoscopy can measure alignment and refraction even in very young infants.[1] However, many abnormalities detected in early infancy are transient. Furthermore, in premature infants, although strabismus and refractive errors can be detected as early as 3 months of age, later examination appears to be a more reliable predictor of significant changes requiring monitoring or intervention.[4,5,10] Most current recommendations suggest initial outpatient evaluation at 6 to 9 months' chronological age, with repeated examinations as indicated.[17,21]

Recommendations for outpatient monitoring

High-risk premature infants should receive routine evaluation by an ophthalmology specialist after discharge in addition to monitoring by their primary care provider (Table 8B-1). These include preterm infants born at less than 32 weeks' gestation, infants with birth weight less than 1500 g, and infants with significant neurologic complications, including IVH and hydrocephalus. The initial examination by the ophthalmology specialist should be performed at approximately 6 to 9 months' chronologic age, and repeated examination may be indicated later in childhood. All other premature infants should have their vision monitored through routine eye examinations and vision assessments by their primary care provider, as recommended for all children by groups including the American Academy of Pediatrics and the American Academy of Ophthalmology. These screening examinations should include external inspection, beginning in infancy, to assess for light reflexes, ocular alignment, and visual tracking, and age-appropriate visual acuity testing beginning at approximately 3 years of age.[1,22]

Table 8B-1 Outpatient Ophthalmologic Monitoring of Premature Infants

Characteristics	Recommendation(s)
Premature infants with: Gestational age <32 weeks, Birth weight <1500 g, or Intraventricular hemorrhage, hydrocephalus, or other neurologic injury	Routine vision screening by primary care provider; Examination by ophthalmology specialist at 6 to 9 months' chronologic age
All other premature infants	Routine vision screening by primary care provider

Conclusion

Premature infants are at increased risk for various ophthalmologic morbidities during childhood compared with full-term infants. These include treatable conditions such as strabismus and refractive errors, as well as less common but more serious conditions such as amblyopia and impaired visual acuity. Infants with a history of moderate or severe ROP are at highest risk, but premature infants without a history of ROP remain at increased risk for subsequent ophthalmologic complications. Although overall visual outcomes in premature infants generally are favorable, careful monitoring and follow-up can minimize the risk of long-term visual impairment.

REFERENCES

1. American Academy of Ophthalmology: Pediatric eye evaluations. San Francisco, CA, 2002.
2. U.S. Preventive Services Task Force: Screening for visual impairment in children younger than age 5 years: recommendation statement. *Ann Fam Med* 2(3):263-266, 2004.
3. Summers G, Phelps DL, Tung B, et al., for the Cryotherapy for Retinopathy of Prematurity Cooperative Group: Ocular cosmesis in retinopathy of prematurity. *Arch Ophthalmol* 110(8):1092-1097, 1992.
4. Bremer DL, Palmer EA, Fellows RR, et al: Strabismus in premature infants in the first year of life. Cryotherapy for Retinopathy of Prematurity Cooperative Group. *Arch Ophthalmol* 116(3): 329-333, 1998.
5. Quinn GE, Dobson V, Kivlin J, et al: Prevalence of myopia between 3 months and 5 1/2 years in preterm infants with and without retinopathy of prematurity. Cryotherapy for Retinopathy of Prematurity Cooperative Group. *Ophthalmology* 105(7):1292-1300, 1998.
6. Editorial Committee for the Cryotherapy for Retinopathy of Prematurity Cooperative Group: Multicenter trial of cryotherapy for retinopathy of prematurity: natural history ROP: ocular outcome at 5(1/2) years in premature infants with birth weights less than 1251 g. *Arch Ophthalmol* 120(5): 595-599, 2002.
7. Holmstrom G, el Azazi M, Kugelberg U: Ophthalmological follow up of preterm infants: a population based, prospective study of visual acuity and strabismus. *Br J Ophthalmol* 83(2):143-150, 1999.
8. Larsson EK, Rydberg AC, Holmstrom GE: A population-based study of the refractive outcome in 10-year-old preterm and full-term children. *Arch Ophthalmol* 121(10):1430-1436, 2003.
9. Larsson EK, Rydberg AC, Holmstrom GE: A population-based study on the visual outcome in 10-year-old preterm and full-term children. *Arch Ophthalmol* 123(6):825-832, 2005.

10. Holmstrom GE, Larsson EK: Development of spherical equivalent refraction in prematurely born children during the first 10 years of life: a population-based study. *Arch Ophthalmol* 123(10):1404-1411, 2005.
11. Schalij-Delfos NE, de Graaf ME, Treffers WF, et al: Long term follow up of premature infants: detection of strabismus, amblyopia, and refractive errors. *Br J Ophthalmol* 84(9):963-967, 2000.
12. Cooke RW, Foulder-Hughes L, Newsham D, et al: Ophthalmic impairment at 7 years of age in children born very preterm. *Arch Dis Child Fetal Neonatal Ed* 89(3):F249-F253, 2004.
13. O'Connor AR, Stephenson T, Johnson A, et al: Long-term ophthalmic outcome of low birth weight children with and without retinopathy of prematurity. *Pediatrics* 109(1):12-18, 2002.
14. O'Connor AR, Stephenson TJ, Johnson A, et al: Visual function in low birthweight children. *Br J Ophthalmol* 88(9): 1149-1153, 2004.
15. Darlow BA, Clemett RS, Horwood LJ, et al: Prospective study of New Zealand infants with birth weight less than 1500 g and screened for retinopathy of prematurity: visual outcome at age 7-8 years. *Br J Ophthalmol* 81(11):935-940, 1997.
16. Pennefather PM, Clarke MP, Strong NP, et al: Risk factors for strabismus in children born before 32 weeks' gestation. *Br J Ophthalmol* 83(5):514-518, 1999.
17. Repka MX: Ophthalmological problems of the premature infant. *Ment Retard Dev Disabil Res Rev* 8(4):249-257, 2002.
18. O'Connor AR, Stewart CE, Singh J, et al: Do infants of birth weight less than 1500 g require additional long term ophthalmic follow up? *Br J Ophthalmol* 90(4):451-455, 2006.
19. O'Keefe M, Kafil-Hussain N, Flitcroft I, et al: Ocular significance of intraventricular haemorrhage in premature infants. *Br J Ophthalmol* 85(3):357-359, 2001.
20. Christiansen SP, Fray KJ, Spencer T: Ocular outcomes in low birth weight premature infants with intraventricular hemorrhage. *J Pediatr Ophthalmol Strabismus* 39(3): 157-165, 2002.
21. Clarke MP: The Boer War and fuzzy logic in screening. *Br J Ophthalmol* 90(4):400-401, 2006.
22. American Academy of Pediatrics: Eye examination in infants, children, and young adults by pediatricians. *Pediatrics* 111(4 Pt 1):902-907, 2003.

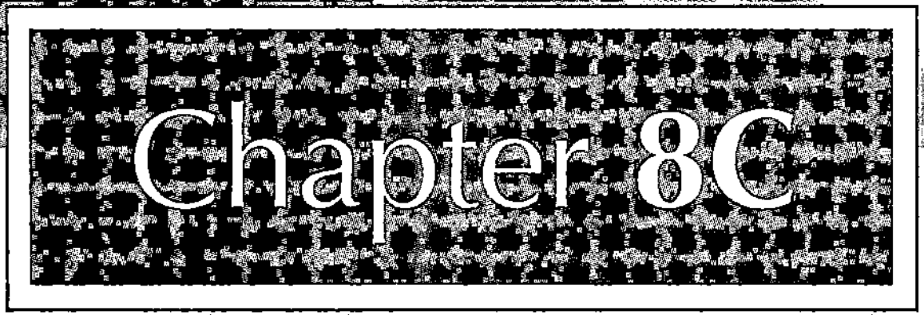

Hearing Loss in Premature Infants

Jane E. Stewart, MD, and Marcy Chant, AuD

Premature infants are at increased risk for hearing loss. Although the overall incidence of severe congenital hearing loss is 1 to 3 per 1000 live births, 2 to 4 per 100 infants who are born at less than 32 weeks' gestation will develop some degree of hearing loss.[1,2] The decibel ranges of hearing losses are defined in Table 8C-1. This chapter provides an introduction to hearing loss in premature infants, highlighting the types of hearing loss, etiologies, risk factors, detection, screening tests, follow-up testing and medical evaluation, prognosis, and management.

Types of Hearing Loss

There are four types of hearing loss in premature infants. *Conductive* hearing loss results from interference in the transmission of sound from the external auditory canal to a normal inner ear. The most common cause of conductive hearing loss is fluid in the middle ear or middle ear effusion. Less common causes include microtia, canal stenosis, or stapes fixation, conditions found in infants with craniofacial malformations. Another type of hearing loss is *sensorineural* hearing loss, which results from abnormal development or damage to the cochlear hair cells (sensory end organ) or auditory nerve. The third type of hearing loss—*auditory dyssynchrony or auditory neuropathy*—is less common. In this type, the inner ear or cochlea appears to receive sounds normally; however, processing of the signal from the cochlea to the auditory nerve is abnormal or disorganized, or the auditory nerve itself does not process the signal normally. The sound and speech perception of children with this disorder appears to be worse than predicted by their degree of hearing loss. The cause of this disorder is not known but is associated with neonatal risk factors such as hyperbilirubinemia, prematurity, hypoxia, and immune disorders, as well as a genetic predisposition in some families. The last type of hearing loss is *central* hearing loss. In this type, the auditory canal and inner ear are intact and sensory and neural pathways are normal, but auditory processing at higher levels of the central nervous system is abnormal.

Etiology

Current thinking is that hearing loss is of unknown etiology in 25% of cases, genetic in 50%, and nongenetic in 25%.

Of the genetic causes, 70% are estimated to be recessive, approximately 15% are autosomal dominant, and the remaining 15% are the result of other types of genetic transmission. The most common genetic cause of hearing loss is a mutation in the connexin 26 (Cx26)gene, located on chromosome 13q11-12. The carrier rate for this mutation is 3%,

Table 8C-1 Definitions of Degree of Hearing Loss

Degree of Hearing Loss	Decibel Range (dB)
Normal range or no hearing loss	−10–15
Slight loss/minimal loss	16–25
Mild loss	26–40
Moderate loss	41–55
Moderate/severe loss	56–70
Severe loss	71–90
Profound loss	≥91

Modified from: Yantis PA: Puretone air-conduction threshold testing. In Katz J, editor: *Handbook of clinical audiology,* Baltimore, 1994, Williams & Wilkins.

and it causes approximately 20% to 30% of congenital hearing loss. Approximately 30% of infants with a hearing loss have other associated medical problems included within a syndrome. More than 200 syndromes are known to include hearing loss (e.g., Alport syndrome, Pierre Robin sequence, Usher syndrome, Waardenburg syndrome, and trisomy 21).[3]

A nongenetic cause of childhood hearing loss is identified in 25% of cases. Hearing loss develops secondary to injury to the developing auditory system in the intrapartum or perinatal period. This injury may be secondary to infection, hypoxia, ischemia, metabolic disease, ototoxic medication, and/or hyperbilirubinemia. Premature infants are more commonly exposed to this type of injury and are particularly vulnerable to it.

Cytomegalovirus (CMV) congenital infection is the most common cause of nonhereditary sensorineural hearing loss. Approximately 1% of all infants are born with CMV infection. Of these infants (approximately 40,000 per year), 10% (4000) are born with clinical signs of infection (small for gestational age, hepatosplenomegaly, jaundice, thrombocytopenia, neutropenia, intracranial calcifications, skin rash). About half of all infants with these signs of infection at birth develop a hearing loss. Although the majority (90%) of infants born with CMV infection have no clinical signs of infection, hearing loss still develops in 10% to 15% of these infants. Because there is no established treatment of CMV in the newborn, prevention of hearing loss is not possible. Treatment with the antiviral agent ganciclovir is being studied, and preliminary data indicate that it may prevent the development and/or progression of hearing loss.[4]

Risk Factors

The Joint Committee on Infant Hearing has listed the following as risk indicators that place an infant at risk for progressive or delayed-onset sensorineural and or conductive hearing loss[5,6]:

1. Parental or caregiver concern regarding hearing, speech, language, or developmental delay;
2. Family history of permanent childhood hearing loss;
3. Stigmata or other findings associated with a syndrome known to include a sensorineural or conductive hearing loss or eustachian tube dysfunction;
4. Postnatal infections associated with sensorineural hearing loss, including bacterial meningitis;
5. In utero infections, such as CMV, herpes, rubella, syphilis, human immunodeficiency virus, and toxoplasmosis;
6. Neonatal indicators, specifically hyperbilirubinemia at a serum level requiring exchange transfusion (some centers use a level ≥20 mg/dl as a general guideline, regardless of the need for exchange transfusion; audiologic assessment with auditory brainstem responses within 2 months of age), persistent pulmonary hypertension of the newborn associated with mechanical ventilation, and conditions requiring use of extracorporeal membrane oxygenation (ECMO);
7. Syndromes associated with progressive hearing loss, such as neurofibromatosis, osteopetrosis, and Usher syndrome;
8. Neurodegenerative disorders, such as Hunter syndrome, or sensorimotor neuropathies, such as Friedreich ataxia and Charcot-Marie-Tooth syndrome;
9. Head trauma;
10. Recurrent or persistent otitis media with effusion for at least 3 months; and
11. Prolonged use of potentially ototoxic medications.

Detection

Universal newborn hearing screening is now recommended for all newborns. The Joint Committee on Infant Hearing and the American Academy of Pediatrics endorse a goal that 100% of infants need to be tested during their hospital birth admission. Implementation of this recommendation is under way. Most states are striving toward this goal, and many states have passed legislation to ensure that this goal is achieved promptly.

Screening Tests

Currently acceptable methodologies for physiologic screening of hearing in newborns include auditory brainstem response (ABR) and evoked otoacoustic emissions (EOAE). A threshold of ≥35 dB has been established as a cutoff for an abnormal screen, which prompts further testing.

The *ABR* measures the electroencephalographic waves generated by the auditory system in response to clicks via three electrodes on the infant's scalp. The characteristic waveform recorded from the electrodes becomes more well defined with increasing postconceptional age. The technique is reliable after 34 weeks' postmenstrual age. The automated version of ABR allows this test to be performed quickly and easily by trained hospital staff. At present, because of the increased risk of injury to the auditory pathway beyond the cochlea (auditory nerve), including auditory dyssynchrony, ABR is the preferred initial screening method in the neonatal period for evaluation of hearing loss in the neonatal intensive care unit graduate.[7]

Following a click stimulus, the *EOAE* test records acoustic "feedback" from the cochlea through the ossicles to the tympanic membrane and ear canal. EOAE is quicker to perform than ABR but is more likely to be affected by debris or fluid in the external and middle ear, resulting in higher referral rates. EOAE is unable to detect some forms of sensorineural hearing loss. EOAE often is combined with automated ABR in a two-step screening system. If an infant has not passed the initial EOAE, the ABR is performed ideally while the infant is still in the hospital.

Follow-up Testing and Medical Evaluation

All infants with abnormal screening ABRs should have follow-up testing with a pediatric audiology specialist. Figures 8C-1 and 8C-2 provide general guidelines for screening for a hearing loss in infants. Infants who refer in both ears should undergo diagnostic ABR within 2 weeks after their original test. Infants with unilateral abnormal results should have follow-up testing within 3 months. Follow-up testing should include a full diagnostic frequency-specific ABR to measure threshold. Evaluation of middle ear function, observation of the infant's

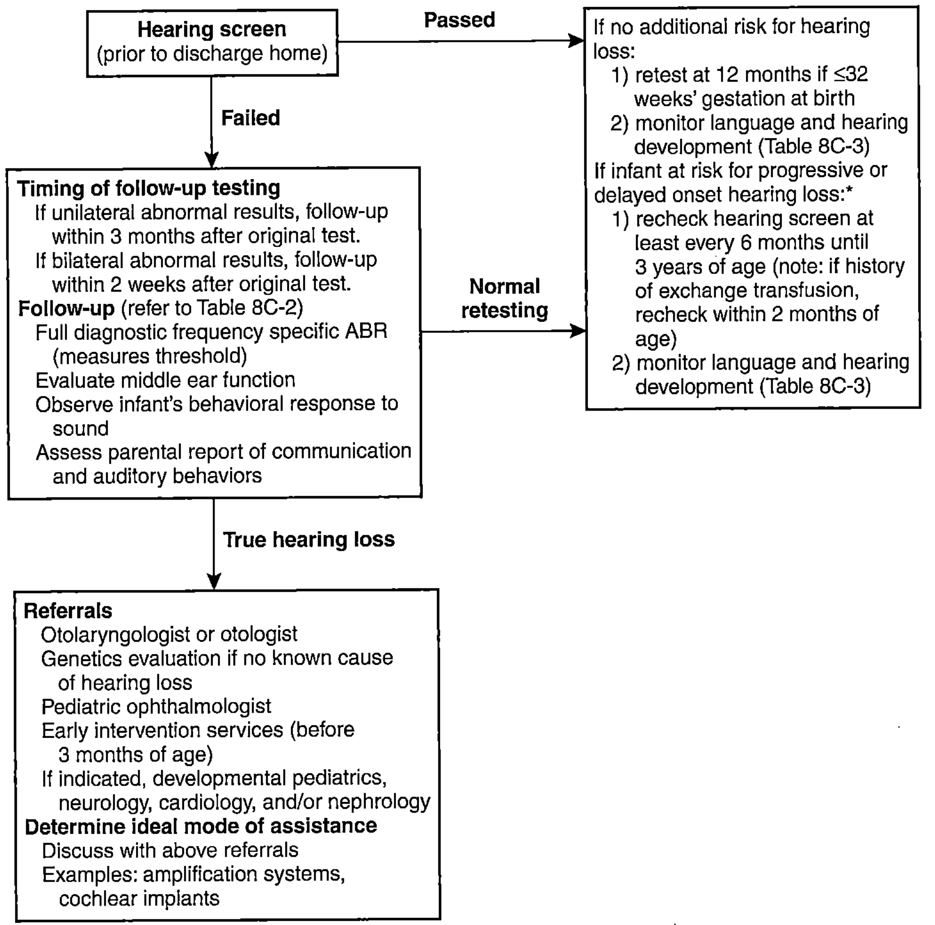

FIGURE 8C-1 *Risk factors: caregiver concern about hearing, speech, language, or developmental delay; family history of permanent childhood hearing loss; stigmata of a syndrome or neurodegenerative disorder associated with hearing loss; history of bacterial meningitis; in utero infection; exchange transfusion; hyperbilirubinemia ≥20 mg/dL; head trauma; recurrent or persistent otitis media with effusion for at least 3 months; and prolonged use of ototoxic medications.
Please note that this a recommended algorithm that does not represent a professional standard of care; care should be revised to meet individual patient needs.

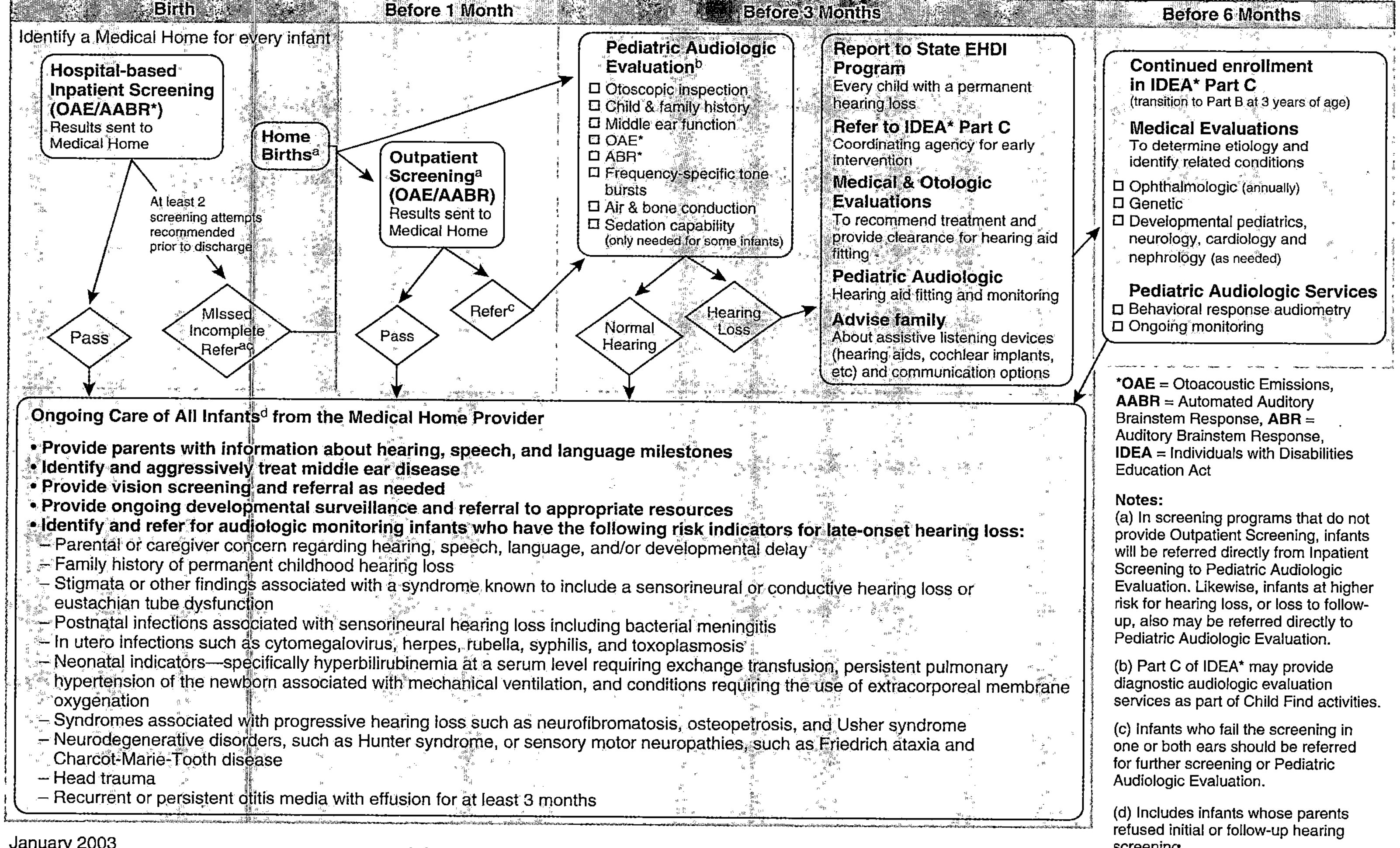

FIGURE 8C-2 Guidelines for pediatric medical home providers. From: the American Academy of Pediatrics. Available at: *http://www.medicalhomeinfo.org/screening/screen%20materials/algorithm.pdf.*

behavioral response to sound, and parental report of emerging communication and auditory behaviors also should be included. Table 8C-2 summarizes guidelines for appropriate follow-up audiologic testing.

Any infant at risk for progressive or delayed-onset sensorineural and/or conductive hearing loss (see Risk Factors) should warrant close audiologic monitoring (at least every 6 months for the first 3 years of life), even if the infant passes the original hearing screen in the newborn period. It is our practice to recommend follow-up hearing assessments at 1 year of age in all infants born at 32 weeks' gestation or less. In addition, primary care providers

Table 8C-2 Guidelines for Follow-up of Abnormal Audiologic Testing

Age	Testing	Description of Testing
Birth–4 months	**Case History**	
	Otoscopy	
	Physiologic Assessment	
	ABR testing for threshold estimation	Measures electrical activity of the auditory nerve and brainstem
	Evoked otoacoustic emissions	Measurement of sounds in the external ear canal that are a reflection of the working of the cochlea
	Acoustic immittance assessment	Objective means of assessing the integrity and function of the peripheral auditory mechanism
	Behavioral Assessment of Hearing Function	
	Behavioral observational assessment is not used for threshold estimation in infants < 4 months	
5–24 months	**Case History**	
	Otoscopy	
	Physiologic Assessment	
	Tympanometry	Objective measure of the compliance of the tympanic membrane
	Acoustic reflex thresholds	Determines the signal threshold at which the stapedial muscle contracts
	EOAE and ABR when behavioral testing is unreliable or inconclusive, or if ear-specific thresholds are not obtained	
	Behavioral Assessment of Hearing Function	
	Visual reinforcement audiometry (VRA) • Speech- and frequency-specific intervals using insert earphones • Sound field testing may be necessary if insert earphones are not tolerated	Head turn response following auditory stimulus is rewarded with an interesting visual event or reinforcer
25–60 months	**Case History**	
	Otoscopy	
	Physiologic Assessment	
	Threshold for speech: speech awareness threshold (SAT), speech recognition threshold (SRT)	
	Word recognition testing	
	Tympanometry	
	Acoustic reflex thresholds	
	EOAE and ABR when validity or adequacy of behavioral tests are limited or neural integrity of the auditory pathway up to the brainstem is in question	
	EOAE when ear-specific testing cannot be obtained	
	Behavioral Assessment of Hearing Function	
	Method depending on developmental level of child (e.g., VRA, CPA, conventional testing)	CPA: Children learn to engage in an activity each time they hear the test signal

Modified from: American Speech-Language-Hearing Association. *Guidelines for the Audiologic Assessment of Children From Birth to 5 years of Age, 2004*. Available at *http://www.asha.org/members/deskref-journals/deskref/default*
ABR, Auditory brainstem response; *CPA,* conditioned play audiometry; *EOAE,* evoked otoacoustic emissions; *VRA,* visual reinforcement audiometry.

Table 8C-3 Guidelines for Normal Development of Hearing and Early Language

Age	Hearing and Understanding	Talking
Birth–3 months	Startles to loud sounds Quiets around everyday voices Increases or decreases sucking in response to sound	Makes gurgling sounds Cries differently for different needs
4–6 months	Moves eyes in direction of sounds Responds to changes in tone of your voice Pays attention to music	Makes babbling sounds that are more speechlike and include the sounds "p", "b", and "m" Vocalizes excitement and displeasure Makes gurgling sounds when left alone and playing with you
7–9 months	Turns and looks in direction of sounds Recognizes words for common items such as "cup," "shoe," "juice" Listens when spoken to	Imitates different speech sounds Uses speech or noncrying sounds to get and keep attention
10–12 months	Begins to respond to requests: "Come here," "Want more?" Points to favorite toys	Has one or two words (bye-bye, dada, mama) although they might not be clear
1–2 years	Points to a few body parts when asked Follows simple commands and understands simple questions, such as "Roll the ball" and "Kiss the baby" Listens to simple stories, sounds, and rhymes Points to pictures in a book when named	Says more words every month Uses some one- to two-word questions, such as "Go bye-bye?" and "What's that?" Uses many different consonant sounds at the beginning of words Puts two words together, such as "more cookie" and "no juice"

Modified from: American Speech-Language Hearing Association: *How does your child hear and talk?* Available at: *www.asha.org.*

should monitor all infants for normal hearing and language development and refer any infant with delays for a hearing assessment (Table 8C-3).

Once an infant is diagnosed with a true hearing loss, the following referrals should be made (Figures 8C-3 and 8C-4):

1. Complete evaluation by an otolaryngology specialist or otology specialist who has experience with infants;
2. All infants diagnosed with hearing loss for whom there is not a definite etiology should be referred for genetic evaluation and counseling;
3. Evaluation by a pediatric ophthalmology specialist to evaluate for additional sensory loss;
4. Referral to developmental pediatric, neurology, cardiology, and/or nephrology specialist as indicated by other clinical findings and known associated problems with syndromes.

Prognosis

The prognosis depends largely on the degree of loss, as well as the time of diagnosis and treatment. For optimal auditory brain development, normal maturation of the central auditory pathways is dependent on early maximizing of auditory input. There is a critical window of neuroplasticity during the first 3 years of childhood. Thus, the earlier habilitation starts, the better the child's chance of achieving age-appropriate language and communication skills.[8,9]

Fitting of hearing aids in the neonatal period has been associated with improved speech outcome. Thus, current practice is to fit infants with amplification as soon as possible after diagnosis. Initiation of early intervention services before 3 months of age also has been associated with improved cognitive developmental outcome. Families should receive information to make decisions regarding communication choices as promptly as possible. Children with severe to profound bilateral hearing loss may be candidates for cochlear implants by the end of the first year of life. Language and communication outcomes for children receiving early cochlear implants and the accompanying intensive multidisciplinary team therapy are extremely promising.

Habilitation/Management

Once a diagnosis of true hearing loss is made, infants and families should be referred for early intervention services to enhance the child's acquisition of developmentally appropriate language skills. Each child is unique. It is important to understand

Appropriate Referrals

1. Audiologist knowledgeable in pediatric screening and amplification

Name:
Telephone number:
Fax:
Date of referral:

2. Otolaryngologist knowledgeable in pediatric hearing loss

Name:
Telephone number:
Fax:
Date of referral:

3. Local early intervention system

Name:
Telephone number:
Fax:
Date of referral:

4. Family support resources, financial resources

Name:
Telephone number:
Fax:
Date of referral:

5. Speech/language therapy and/or aural rehabilitation therapy

Name:
Telephone number:
Fax:
Date of referral:

6. Sign language classes if parents choose manual approach

Name:
Telephone number:
Fax:
Date of referral:

7. Ophthalmologist knowledgeable in co-morbid conditions in children with hearing loss

Name:
Telephone number:
Fax:
Date of referral:

8. Clinical geneticist knowledgeable in hearing impairment

Name:
Telephone number:
Fax:
Date of referral:

9. Equipment vendor(s)

Name:
Telephone number:
Fax:
Date of referral:

10. State EHDI coordinator
http://www.infanthearing.org/status/cnhs.html

Name:
Telephone number:
Fax:
Date of referral:

11. AAP Chapter champion
http://www.medicalhomeinfo.org/screening/Champions%20Roster.pdf

Name:
Telephone number:
Fax:
Date of referral:

12. Family physician(s)

Name:
Telephone number:
Fax:
Date of referral:

National Resources

Alexander Graham Bell Association for the Deaf and Hard of Hearing (AG Bell)
202/337-5220
www.agbell.org

American Academy of Audiology (AAA)
800/AAA-2336
www.audiology.org

American Academy of Pediatrics
www.aap.org

American Society for Deaf Children
717/334-7922
www.deafchildren.org

American Speech-Language-Hearing Association (ASHA)
800/498-2071
www.asha.org

Boys Town Center for Childhood Deafness
www.babyhearing.org

Centers for Disease Control and Prevention
www.cdc.gov/ncbddd/ehdi

Cochlear Implant Association, Inc.
202/895-2781
www.cici.org

Families for Hands and Voices
303/300-9763
www.handsandvoices.org

Laurent Clerc National Deaf Education Center and Clearinghouse at Gallaudet University
www.clerccenter.gallaudet.edu/InfoToGo

National Association of the Deaf (NAD)
301/587-1788
www.nad.org

National Center on Hearing Assessment and Management (NCHAM)
www.infanthearing.org

National Institute on Deafness and Other Communication Disorders
www.nidcd.nih.gov

Oberkotter Foundation
www.oraldeafed.org

The recommendations in this document do not indicate an exclusive course of treatment or serve as a standard of medical care. Variations, taking into account individual circumstances, may be appropriate.

This project is funded by an educational grant from the Maternal and Child Health Bureau, Health Resources and Services Administration, US Department of Health and Human Services.

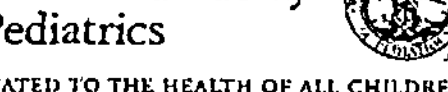

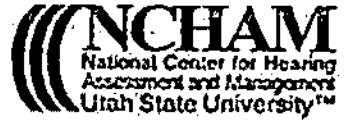

FIGURE 8C-3 Appropriate referrals. From: the American Academy of Pediatrics. Available at: *http://www.medicalhomeinfo.org/screening/Screen%20Materials/Template.pdf.*

Universal Newborn Hearing Screening, Diagnosis, and Intervention

Patient Checklist for Pediatric Medical Home Providers

Patient Name: ____________________

Date of Birth: ___/___/___

Birth

Hospital-based Inpatient Screening Results (OAE/AABR) DATE: ___/___/___
(also Home Births)

Left ear:	☐ Missed	☐ Incomplete	☐ Refer[a, c]	☐ Pass
Right ear:	☐ Missed	☐ Incomplete	☐ Refer[a, c]	☐ Pass

Before 1 month

Outpatient Screening Results (OAE/AABR) ___/___/___

Left ear:	☐ Incomplete	☐ Refer[a, c]	☐ Pass
Right ear:	☐ Incomplete	☐ Refer[a, c]	☐ Pass

Before 3 months

☐ **Pediatric Audiologic Evaluation**[b] ___/___/___

☐ Hearing Loss ☐ Normal Hearing

Documented child and family auditory history ___/___/___

- ☐ **Report to State EHDI Program** results of diagnostic evaluation ___/___/___
- ☐ **Refer to Early Intervention** (IDEA, Part C) ___/___/___
- ☐ **Medical & Otologic Evaluations** to recommend treatment and provide clearance for hearing aid fitting ___/___/___
- ☐ **Pediatric Audiologic** hearing aid fitting and monitoring ___/___/___
- ☐ **Advise family** about assistive listening devices (hearing aids, cochlear implants, etc.) and communication options ___/___/___

Before 6 months

☐ **Enrollment in Early Intervention (IDEA, Part C)** ___/___/___
(transition to Part B at 3 years of age)

Medical Evaluations to determine etiology and identify related conditions

- ☐ Ophthalmologic (annually) ___/___/___
- ☐ Genetic ___/___/___
- ☐ Developmental pediatrics, neurology, cardiology, and nephrology (as needed) ___/___/___

☐ **Ongoing Pediatric Audiologic Services**

Ongoing Care of All Infants[d]

- ☐ Provide parents with information about hearing, speech, and language milestones
- ☐ Identify and aggressively treat middle ear disease
- ☐ Vision screening and referral as needed
- ☐ Ongoing developmental surveillance/referral
- ☐ Referrals to otolaryngology and genetics, as needed
- ☐ Risk indicators for late onset hearing loss: ____________________

(refer for audiologic monitoring)

Service Provider Contact Information

Pediatric Audiologist:

Early Intervention Provider:

Other:

Other:

Other:

(a) In screening programs that do not provide Outpatient Screening, infants will be referred directly from Inpatient Screening to Pediatric Audiologic Evaluation. Likewise, infants at higher risk for hearing loss, or loss to follow-up, also may be referred directly to Pediatric Audiologic Evaluation.

(b) Early Intervention (IDEA, Part C) may provide diagnostic audiologic evaluation services as part of Child Find activities.

(c) Infants who fail the screening in one or both ears should be referred for further screening or Pediatric Audiologic Evaluation.

(d) Includes infants whose parents refused initial or follow-up hearing screening.

OAE = Otoacoustic Emissions
AABR = Automated Auditory Brainstem Response
ABR = Auditory Brainstem Response
IDEA = Individuals with Disabilities Education Act
EHDI = Early Hearing Detection & Intervention

This project is funded by an educational grant from the Maternal and Child Health Bureau, Health Resources and Services Administration, US Department of Health and Human Services.

American Academy of Pediatrics
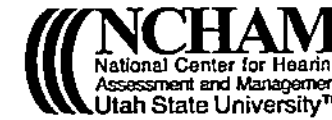
DEDICATED TO THE HEALTH OF ALL CHILDREN™

NCHAM National Center for Hearing Assessment and Management Utah State University™

March 2004

FIGURE 8C-4 Patient checklist for pediatric medical providers. From: American Academy of Pediatrics. Available at: *http://www.medicalhomeinfo.org/screening/EHDI/EHDIinfoproviders/checklistbw.pdf.*

the full nature and extent of a child's hearing loss or deafness. It also is important to understand how each family member and caregiver will communicate with the child. Primary care providers need to know the services available in the community for children in preschool and elementary school.

The most common forms of communication include auditory/verbal communication, auditory oral communication, cued speech, simultaneous communication, and American Sign Language. This section discusses the specific amplification methods.

Infants who are appropriate candidates and whose parents have chosen to use personal *amplification* systems should be fitted with hearing aids as soon as possible. Advances in technology have provided children with hearing loss an exciting array of amplification options. As increasingly more universal newborn hearing screening programs are being implemented across the United States, newborns are being identified earlier and fitted with amplification systems as young as the first few weeks of life. Hearing aid manufacturers are producing options specifically for this population, such as visible controls that can be adjusted easily by parents, childproof battery compartments, and volume controls. The price of digital hearing aids has been reduced so that many children can be fit with this technology, which provides flexible electroacoustic parameters. Newborns most commonly are fitted with behind-the-ear (BTE) hearing aids and direct audio input (DAI), often linked with FM systems.

Use of an FM system coupled with personal hearing aids is designed to provide better signal-to-noise ratio (SNR) in difficult listening situations. The signal from a remote microphone can be sent directly into the ear of a listener via the hearing aid or a variety of receivers. Young children depend on good speech perception abilities for speech and language acquisition, and it has been demonstrated that children with all degrees of hearing loss require an SNR advantage to preserve optimal speech perception in noise. FM technology is especially helpful in certain situations, such as traveling in the car, listening to a teacher at school, and listening to music.

The *cochlear implant* is one of the most significant technology advances in hearing and deafness since the development of the hearing aid. A cochlear implant is a surgically inserted device designed to take over the function of an inner ear that does not work properly by providing direct electrical stimulation to the auditory nerve. The cochlear implant is made up of external and internal components. The external component consists of a microphone worn at ear level (similar to a BTE hearing aid), a speech processor, which can be cased with the microphone or worn on the body, and the transmitter attached to the skin just behind the ear. The internal components consist of the receiver located just under the skin and the array of electrodes surgically placed in the cochlea.

Children as young as 12 months may be candidates for cochlear implants. To meet the criteria, a child must have severe to profound, bilateral, sensorineural hearing loss, receive little to no benefit from appropriately fitted hearing aids, realistic expectations from family with high motivation, and no medical conditions that will interfere with the cochlear implant procedure. Six weeks after the cochlear implant is placed, the child has a "stimulation" or "mapping" session. The internal and external components are hooked up, and the audiology specialist will program the speech processor for the child's individual needs. Following the initial programming, each child will have several mapping sessions to fine tune the cochlear implant. Benefits from cochlear implant are not always immediate and require a multidisciplinary team of audiology specialists, speech language pathology specialists, and educators to teach the child to hear.

Conclusion

Premature infants are at increased risk for hearing loss. Early diagnosis and initiation of therapeutic options have dramatically improved the outcome for infants with hearing loss. New recommendations for identifying infants at risk for late-onset hearing loss and progressive hearing loss are expected from the Joint Committee on Newborn Hearing Screening in the near future.

Resources for Families and Clinicians

American Academy of Audiology
http://www.audiology.org
American Academy of Pediatrics (AAP)
www.aap.org/policy/re9846.html and *www.medicalhomeinfo.org/screening/hearing.html*

These websites provide the recent AAP policy statement on screening for hearing loss.

American Society for Deaf Children
PO Box 3355, Gettysburg, PA 17325
Phone/TTY: (717) 334-7922; Fax: (717) 334-8808; Parent Hotline: (800) 942-ASDC
www.deafchildren.org

This is a national organization for families and professionals whose mission is to educate, empower, and support parents and families of the deaf and hard of hearing.

American Speech-Language-Hearing Association (ASHA)
10801 Rockville Pike, Rockville, MD 20852

Phone and TTY: (800) 638-8255 (public); (800) 498-2071 (professionals)
www.asha.org

This organization's mission is to ensure that all people with speech, language, and hearing disorders have access to quality services to help them communicate more effectively.

Better Hearing Institute (BHI)
http://www.betterhearing.org/

The BHI is a not-for-profit corporation that educates the public about the neglected problem of hearing loss and what can be done about it.

Boys Town National Research Center*
http://www.babyhearing.org

This team from Boys Town National Research Hospital provides parents with information about newborn screening and hearing loss. The team consists of audiology specialists, speech language pathology specialists, teachers of the deaf, genetic specialists, and parents of deaf and hard of hearing children.

Center for Disease Control and Prevention
http://www.cdc.gov/ncbddd/ehdi/default.htm

Provides information about the Early Hearing Detection and Intervention Program.

Hands & Voices
http://www.handsandvoices.org/

Hands & Voices is a nonprofit, parent-driven national organization dedicated to supporting families of children who are deaf or hard of hearing.

Harvard Medical School Center for Hereditary Deafness*
http://hearing.harvard.edu

Excellent booklets for families are available from this website.

Marion Downs National Center for Infant Hearing
http://www.colorado.edu/slhs/mdnc/

This website provides information from the Marion Downs National Center for Infant Hearing, which coordinates statewide systems for screening, diagnosis, and intervention for newborns and infants with hearing loss.

Massachusetts Universal Newborn Hearing Screening
http://www.mass.gov/dph/fch/unhsp/index.htm

This organization oversees statewide implementation of universal hearing screening initiative, ensures access to follow-up services, provides information about newborn hearing screening, provides parent-to-parent support, and helps families pay for audiologic diagnostic tests in Massachusetts.

National Association for the Deaf
814 Thayer Avenue, Silver Spring, MD 20910-4500
Phone and TTY: (301) 587-1788
www.nad.org

This organization was established in 1880 and is the oldest and largest constituency organization safeguarding the accessibility and civil rights of deaf and hard of hearing Americans in education, employment, healthcare, and telecommunications.

*Excellent first resources for families.

National Center for Hearing Assessment and Management (NCHAM)*
http://www.infanthearing.org/

The goal of NCHAM is to ensure that all infants and toddlers with hearing loss are identified as early as possible and provided with timely and appropriate audiologic, educational, and medical intervention.

National Cued Speech Association
www.cuedspeech.org

National Deaf Education Center Gallaudet University
800 Florida Avenue NE, Washington, DC 20002
Phone: (202) 651-5051; TTY (202) 651-5052
http://clerccenter.gallaudet.edu

This website provides a centralized source of information on topics dealing with deafness and hearing loss in children and individuals younger than 21 years.

National Institute on Deafness and Other Communication Disorders (NIDCD)
One Communication Avenue, Bethesda, MD 20892
Phone: (800) 241-1044l TTY (800) 241-1055
www.nidcd.nih.gov

The NIDCD is part of the National Institutes of Health (NIH) and is mandated to conduct and support biomedical and behavioral research and research training in the normal and disordered processes of hearing, balance, smell, taste, voice, speech, and language. It addresses special biomedical and behavioral problems associated with people who have communication impairments and supports efforts to create devices that substitute for lost and impaired communication function.

Oberkotter Foundation
Phone: (877) 672-5442; TTY: (877) 672-5889
www.oraldeafed.org

Comprehensive website for parents and professionals providing numerous links. It offers many materials for parents and professionals, including:

- Parent Information Kit, a resource guide for parents of newly diagnosed deaf and hard of hearing children.
- The ABCs of Early Intervention.

REFERENCES

1. Marlow ES, Hunt LP, Marlow N: Sensorineural hearing loss and prematurity. *Arch Dis Child Fetal Neonatal* 82:F141-144, 2000.
2. Van Naarden K, Decouflye P: Relative and attributable risk for moderate to profound bilateral sensorineural hearing impairment associated with lower birth weight in children 3 to 10 years old *Pediatrics* 104:905-910, 1999.

*Excellent first resources for families.

3. Kimberlin DW, Lin C-Y, Sanchez PJ, et al: Effect of ganciclovir therapy on hearing in symptomatic congenital cytomegalovirus disease involving the central nervous system: a randomized controlled trial. *J Pediatr* 143:16-25, 2003.
4. Rehm HL, Williamson RE, Kenna, et al: *Understanding the genetics of deafness: a guide for patients and families.* Harvard Medical School Center for Hereditary Deafness, Cambridge, Massachusetts. Available at: *http://hearing.harvard.edu.*
5. NIH Joint Committee on Infant Hearing. Year 2000 position statement: principles and guidelines for early hearing detection and intervention programs. *Pediatrics* 106:798-817, 2000.
6. Cunningham M, Cox DO: Hearing assessment in infants and children: recommendations beyond neonatal screening. *Pediatrics* 111:436-440, 2003.
7. Valkama Am, Laitakari KT, Tolonen EU, et al: Prediction of permanent hearing loss in high-risk preterm infants at term age. *Eur J Pediatr* 159:459-464, 2000.
8. Yoshinaga-Itano C: Efficacy of early identification and intervention. *Semin Hear* 16:115-120, 1995.
9. Yoshinaga-Itano C, Sedey Al, Coulter DK, et al: Language of early and later-identified children with hearing loss. *Pediatrics* 102:1161-1171, 1998.

GENERAL REFERENCES

AAP Task Force on Newborn Hearing and Infant Screening: Newborn and infant hearing loss: detection and intervention. *Pediatrics* 103:527-530, 1999.

Hone SW, Smith RJ: Genetics of hearing impairment. *Semin Neonatol* 6:531-541, 2001.

Institute of Better Hearing: *A guide to your child's hearing.* Alexandria, VA, 2005, Better Hearing Institute. Available at: *www.betterhearing.org.*

Moeller MP: Early intervention and language development in children you are deaf and hard of hearing. *Pediatrics* 106:E43, 2000.

Northern JL, Downs MP: *Hearing in children*, ed 4. Baltimore, 1991, Williams & Wilkins.

Schwartz Sue, editor: *Choices in deafness: a parents' guide to communication options*, ed 2. Bethesda, 1996, Woodbine House.

Serving the family from birth to the medical home. Newborn screening: a blueprint for the future—a call for a national agenda on state newborn screening programs. *Pediatrics* 106:389-422, 2000.

Chapter 9A

Cryptorchidism

Pankaj B. Agrawal, MD, MMSc

Cryptorchidism is failure of one or both testes to descend completely into the scrotum. In term neonates, the incidence ranges from 3.4% to 5.8%, whereas the incidence is as high as 30% in premature neonates.[1] By 9 months of age, approximately 75% of full-term and 90% of preterm infants have complete testicular descent without any therapeutic intervention.[2] The incidence of cryptorchidism decreases to 0.8% at 1 year of age. One third of the cryptorchidism cases are bilateral. The etiologies of cryptorchidism are diverse and listed in Table 9A-1. Cryptorchidism can be isolated or associated with other anomalies, including inguinal hernias, epididymal malformations, hypospadias, and upper urinary tract defects. There is an association of cryptorchidism with maternal history of exposure to exogenous hormones (e.g., diethylstilbestrol). In addition, there may be a family history of cryptorchidism, other congenital anomalies, neonatal deaths, precocious puberty, infertility, and consanguinity.

Evaluation

Determination of unilateral or bilateral cryptorchidism should be made. The testis should be located to assess whether it is palpable in the upper scrotum, superficial inguinal pouch, or inguinal canal, or not palpable at all. If the testis is palpable, assess whether it is retractile by determining whether it remains in the scrotum after it is pulled down and maintained in the scrotum for a minute. The nonretractile testis will immediately return back to the ascended location.

If the testis is not palpable, it may be absent, atrophied, in the inguinal canal, or located intra-abdominally. Infants with bilateral nonpalpable testes and those with unilateral nonpalpable testis and severe hypospadias may have ambiguous genitalia. If an infant has bilateral nonpalpable testes with virilization of external genitalia, the infant should be evaluated for congenital adrenal hyperplasia presenting as female pseudohermaphroditism.

An extensive *laboratory evaluation* is necessary in infants with *bilateral* nonpalpable testes. The evaluation includes the following:

1. Chromosomal analysis to assess for genetic sex and chromosomal anomalies;
2. Tests such as 17-hydroxyprogesterone (17-OHP) to rule out congenital adrenal hyperplasia or other virilizing disorders; and
3. Serum luteinizing hormone (LH), follicle-stimulating hormone (FSH), and testosterone

Table 9A-1. Causative Factors for Cryptorchidism[1-3]

Hypothalamic–pituitary–testicular axis	Hypopituitarism Prader-Willi syndrome Leydig cell failure Testosterone biosynthesis defects Androgen insensitivity 5α-Reductase deficiency Testicular dysgenesis Congenital anorchia Persistent Müllerian duct syndrome
Low intra-abdominal pressure	Umbilical hernia Gastroschisis Omphalocele Prune-belly syndrome
Neurologic	Meningomyelocele Cerebral palsy
Chromosomal/syndromic	Trisomy 13, 18 Sex chromosome mosaicism, chimerism, Y-chromosome translocation Noonan, Robinow, Smith-Lemli-Opitz, Klinefelter syndromes
Familial	6.2%–9.8% of brothers and 4% of fathers

levels, because an elevated LH/FSH ratio with an extremely low testosterone level is indicative of absent testes.

Imaging studies, which include ultrasonography, computed tomography, and magnetic resonance imaging, may assist in locating inguinal or intra-abdominal testes, although the accuracy of ultrasonography and computed tomography is limited.[4] According to one study, the most reliable imaging test is gadolinium-enhanced magnetic resonance angiography.[5] *Surgical exploration*, including laparoscopy or open inguinal exploration/laparotomy, may be needed to confirm the presence of testes. Laparoscopy has mostly replaced imaging studies for localization of a nonpalpable testis and might obviate the need for groin exploration.

Treatment

Pediatric urology specialists should evaluate infants with cryptorchidism in the first 2 to 3 months. Because the testes may continue to descend until 6 to 9 months of age, therapy may be delayed until that time. It is important to remember that the risk of infertility and other complications increase as age advances. In unilateral cryptorchidism, although the risk of infertility is very low irrespective of the age of surgical correction,[6] current information suggests that, even in those cases, placement of the testis in the scrotum should be accomplished by age 1 year.

Hormonal therapy is common in Europe and includes administration of human chorionic gonadotropin (hCG), LH releasing hormone (LHRH), or gonadotropin releasing hormone (GnRH), alone or in combination. The success rate varies from 6% to 30% according to various studies.[2] In one study, hormonal therapy was found to be more effective in bilateral than unilateral cryptorchidism (38% vs 23%, $p = .007$), and monotherapy with hCG or LHRH was equally effective as combination therapy.[7] Some studies have found GnRH to be more effective than hCG (19% vs. 6%).[8] This finding is especially important because GnRH is administered nasally, in contrast to the intramuscular route for hCG. Furthermore, GnRH has fewer side effects, which include increased penile or testicular size, scrotal erythema, and erections.[1]

Surgical placement of one or both testes in the scrotum (orchiopexy) is the treatment of choice. Orchiopexy can be performed by standard surgical techniques or laparoscopically. A hormonal therapy trial can be given before surgical management for the additional benefit of maturation of the testes.

Long-term Prognosis

The incidence of malignancy in a cryptorchid testis case is 1:500, or 20 to 46 times higher than a normally descended testis.[9,10] The risk is higher in cases of abdominal testes compared with undescended inguinal testes.[1] Although orchiopexy makes performance of self-examinations easier, it does not necessarily decrease the risk of testicular cancer.[1]

According to one study, 38% of bilateral cryptorchid males were infertile.[6] In comparison, the infertility rate in a matched control group was 6%, indicating a six times higher risk associated with bilateral cryptorchidism. In the same study, the risk of infertility in unilateral cryptorchid males was 10%, which is closer to infertility rates in other general population studies.[1] Bilateral cryptorchid males are subfertile with a longer period until fertilization is accomplished.[1]

Testicular torsion occurs more frequently in cryptorchidism, particularly in the neonatal/early infancy period. Occasionally it occurs in utero, when the infant may present with unilateral cryptorchidism because of the destruction of an ischemic testis. The diagnosis may be difficult if the testis is located intra-abdominally and torsion occurs postnatally.

Resources for Families and Clinicians

Aetna Intelihealth
www.intelihealth.com
Search for "cryptorchidism" for a short summary for families.

American Academy of Family Physicians
11400 Tomahawk Creek Pathway
Leawood, KS 66211-2672
Phone: (913) 906-6000 or (800) 274-2237
www.familydoctor.org/637.xml

Children's Hospital, Boston
www.childrenshospital.org
Search for "cryptorchidism" for a short summary about cryptorchidism for families.

REFERENCES

1. Kolon TF, Patel RP, Huff DS: Cryptorchidism: diagnosis, treatment, and long-term prognosis. *Urol Clin North Am* 31:469-480, 2004.
2. Dahms WT, Danish RK: Abnormalities of sexual differentiation. In Fanaroff AA, Martin RJ, editors: *Neonatal-perinatal medicine: diseases of the fetus and infant.* St. Louis, 2002, Mosby.
3. Hyun G, Kolon TF: A practical approach to intersex in the newborn period. *Urol Clin North Am* 31:435-443, 2004.
4. Hrebinko RL, Bellinger MF: The limited role of imaging techniques in managing children with undescended testes. *J Urol* 150:458-460, 1993.
5. Yeung CK, Tam YH, Chan YL, et al: A new management algorithm for impalpable undescended testis with gadolinium enhanced magnetic resonance angiography. *J Urol* 162:998-1002, 1999.
6. Lee PA, O'Leary LA, Songer NJ, et al: Paternity after unilateral cryptorchidism: a controlled study. *Pediatrics* 98:676-679, 1996.

7. Esposito C, De Lucia A, Palmieri A, et al: Comparison of five different hormonal treatment protocols for children with cryptorchidism. *Scand J Urol Nephrol* 37:246-249, 2003.
8. Rajfer J, Handelsman DJ, Swerdloff RS, et al: Hormonal therapy of cryptorchidism. A randomized, double-blind study comparing human chorionic gonadotropin and gonadotropin-releasing hormone. *N Engl J Med* 314:466-470, 1986.
9. Zdeb MS: The probability of developing cancer. *Am J Epidemiol* 106:6-16, 1977.
10. Chilvers C, Dudley NE, Gough MH, et al: Undescended testis: the effect of treatment on subsequent risk of subfertility and malignancy. *J Pediatr Surg* 21:691-696, 1986.

Chapter 9B

Inguinal and Umbilical Hernias

Pankaj B. Agrawal, MD, MMSc

Inguinal hernias (IHs) occur in 1% to 5% of full-term infants and 8% to 30% of premature infants.[1] The highest incidence of IH occurs in extremely-low-birth-weight infants, with rates ranging from 17% to 30%.[1,2] IHs are more common in males (7:1) and often are right sided (2:1). On clinical examination, IHs are bilateral in half the cases, although on surgical exploration the number may be as high as 80%.[1]

Evaluation

An IH usually presents as an asymptomatic bulge in the groin. Upon palpation, a smooth, firm, sausage-shaped mass is appreciated. The mass often becomes more prominent during crying or straining. The hernia can extend into the scrotum. If the IH is not reducible, concern for incarceration and/or strangulation arises.

In the differential diagnosis of an IH, the possibility of a hydrocele or testicular torsion must be eliminated. A hydrocele is a fluid-filled sac, an outpocketing of peritoneum that results from incomplete obliteration of the processus vaginalis. Transillumination usually is positive. However, sometimes an ultrasound is needed to confirm the diagnosis. Most hydroceles usually disappear by 1 year of age.

A testicular torsion usually presents in an infant without a history of IH. The infant experiences sudden onset of pain/irritability and tenderness of the testis. Surgery is urgently required because of the high risk for testicular damage within a few hours. Sometimes only surgery can distinguish an incarcerated hernia from a testicular torsion.[3]

Inguinal Hernias in the Premature Infant

Several studies have found a higher incidence of IH in infants with bronchopulmonary dysplasia (BPD).[1,4] Elevated intra-abdominal pressure associated with BPD is a significant risk factor for the increased occurrence.[5] Surgical repair of IH is delayed in infants with BPD to prevent exacerbation of the disease. Unfortunately, this delay is not always ideal, and one study found lower oxygen requirements in the majority of infants following a herniotomy.[6]

Premature infants have a significantly higher risk of developing apnea after IH surgery, particularly if they had a history of apnea before surgery.[7] The risk decreases with advancing postmenstrual age. All general anesthetics, sedatives, hypnotics, and opioids can cause alterations in respiratory mechanics and central respiratory control.[8] The risk of developing apnea can be reduced by using spinal instead of general anesthesia and by delaying the surgery as long as possible (perhaps to a few days before discharge home).[9,10] A caffeine citrate bolus given perioperatively has been shown to reduce the occurrence of apnea in a small number of premature infants less than 44 weeks' postmenstrual age.[11] Although routine perioperative administration of caffeine requires further study, it should be considered in infants with excessive postoperative apnea.

Potential Complications

Inguinal hernias can become incarcerated or herniated. An incarcerated or nonreducible IH is most common in the first year of life. The younger the infant, the greater the risk of incarceration. Potential signs of an incarcerated IH that previously was reducible include an abrupt onset of irritability, refusal to feed, and/or vomiting that may become bilious and sometimes even feculent. Following incarceration, strangulation or impaired perfusion to the bowel may occur. Signs include marked tenderness, bilious or feculent vomiting, fever, tachycardia, erythema/swelling of inguinal region, and abdominal distention.[3] Plain abdominal films can help to determine the diagnosis. A strangulated hernia can lead to perforated bowel, peritonitis, sepsis, and/or death. Thus, a strangulated hernia is a surgical emergency in order to maintain bowel integrity.

Management

An uncomplicated IH is surgically managed by herniotomy. A herniotomy involves ligation and excision of the patent processus vaginalis. Formal repair of the abdominal wall is not required in neonates. In most cases of unilateral IH, the contralateral side also is explored.[1] Surgical complications include recurrent hernias, testicular damage, iatrogenic testicular ascent, spermatic cord injury, hydrocele, and intestinal injury. Postoperative risks include worsening lung disease and/or apnea of prematurity.

If there is concern for an incarcerated or strangulated IH, surgical consultation is urgently required. Reduction can be attempted with the infant placed in the Trendelenburg position, application of local ice packs, and pain medication. Reduction involves moving the knees in a frog-leg position to relax the abdominal wall muscles, then holding the hernia with one hand to fix it in place while the other hand presses the incarcerated mass upward toward the canal.[3] Hernias should be repaired within the next 24 to 48 hours after reduction. An irreducible incarcerated hernia and a strangulated IH require emergent surgical intervention.

Umbilical Hernia

Failure of the umbilical ring to close completely after ligation of the umbilical cord at birth results in an umbilical hernia. The incidence of umbilical hernias is higher in premature infants and darkly pigmented infants. It presents as a swelling of the umbilical region during crying or straining. Because it is mostly benign and typically closes spontaneously by 3 years of age, only observation is needed. In rare cases, an incarceration can occur. Surgical treatment is required only if the umbilical hernia remains open at 4 to 5 years of age.[12]

Resources for Families and Clinicians

American Urological Association
http://www.urologyhealth.org/search/index.cfm?topic=95&search=inguinal%20AND%20hernia&searchtype=and

Cincinnati Children's Hospital Medical Center
3333 Burnet Avenue
Cincinnati, OH 45229-3039
Phone: (513) 636-4200 or (800) 344-2462
http://www.cincinnatichildrens.org
Search for "inguinal hernia."

Children's Hospital, Boston
www.childrenshospital.org
Search for "inguinal hernia" for a short summary for families.

REFERENCES

1. Kumar VH, Clive J, Rosenkrantz TS, et al: Inguinal hernia in preterm infants (< or = 32-week gestation). *Pediatr Surg Int* 18:147-152, 2002.
2. Harper RG, Garcia A, Sia C: Inguinal hernia: a common problem of premature infants weighing 1,000 grams or less at birth. *Pediatrics* 56:112-115, 1975.
3. Puder M, Greene A: Inguinal hernia. In Hansen AR, Puder M, editors: *Manual of neonatal surgical intensive care.* Hamilton, Ontario, Canada, 2003, BC Decker.
4. Yeo CL, Gray PH: Inguinal hernia in extremely preterm infants. *J Paediatr Child Health* 30:412-413, 1994.
5. Powell TG, Hallows JA, Cooke RW, et al: Why do so many small infants develop an inguinal hernia? *Arch Dis Child* 61:991-995, 1986.
6. Emberton M, Patel L, Zideman DA, et al: Early repair of inguinal hernia in preterm infants with oxygen-dependent bronchopulmonary dysplasia. *Acta Paediatr* 85:96-99, 1996.
7. Welborn LG, Greenspun JC: Anesthesia and apnea. Perioperative considerations in the former preterm infant. *Pediatr Clin North Am* 41:181-198, 1994.
8. Maxwell LG: Age-associated issues in preoperative evaluation, testing, and planning: pediatrics. *Anesthesiol Clin North Am* 22:27-43, 2004.
9. Welborn LG, Rice LJ, Hannallah RS, et al: Postoperative apnea in former preterm infants: prospective comparison of spinal and general anesthesia. *Anesthesiology* 72:838-842, 1990.
10. Craven PD, Badawi N, Henderson-Smart DJ, et al: Regional (spinal, epidural, caudal) versus general anaesthesia in preterm infants undergoing inguinal herniorrhaphy in early infancy. *Cochrane Database Syst Rev* CD003669, 2003.
11. Welborn LG, Hannallah RS, Fink R, et al: High-dose caffeine suppresses postoperative apnea in former preterm infants. *Anesthesiology* 71:347-349, 1989.
12. Martin CR, Fishman SJ: Umbilical hernia. In Hansen AR, Puder M, editors: *Manual of neonatal surgical intensive care.* Hamilton, Ontario, Canada, 2003, BC Decker.

Chapter 10

Multiple Gestation

Elizabeth Doherty, MD

Over the past decade, the incidence of multifetal gestation has increased significantly. From 1990 to 2002, the twin birth rate has increased by 50% (from 18:1000 to 32:1000), whereas the triplet birth rate has increased by 400% (from 40:100,000 to 190:100,000).[1] For comparison, the natural occurrence of twins and triplets is 1:80 and 1:8000, respectively. In 2002, multifetal gestations in the United States produced more than 130,000 infants, primarily as a result of the widespread use of fertility therapies.[2] Infertility affects approximately 14% of reproductive-aged couples.[3] Although this rate has remained stable over the past several years, the demand for and successful use of assisted reproductive technologies (ARTs) has increased substantially. Fertility treatments have become widely available to infertile couples and to older women who have delayed potential motherhood until their late 30s and 40s.

ART accounts for 1% to 3% of annual live births in western countries. The risk of multiple gestation associated with these therapies may be as high as 25%.[4] Most multiple births are the result of in vitro fertilization (IVF) with transfer of multiple embryos and of ovulation induction resulting in more than one ovum per cycle. Dizygotic (DZ) twinning accounts for the majority of the overall increase in multifetal gestation.

In order to discern the risks associated with multifetal gestation, it is imperative to understand the differences in types of twinning. Twins can be DZ, resulting from fertilization of two eggs by two sperm, or they can be monozygotic (MZ), resulting from a single fertilized egg that subsequently divides in two. DZ twins have separate placentas and membranes (dichorionic, diamniotic), although rarely they are fused and have vascular connections.[5] The type of MZ twinning is determined by the timing of egg division (Table 10A-1). The resultant placenta–membrane connections of MZ twins can be characterized as follows:

- 70% to 75% share one placenta (monochorionic, diamniotic)
- 25% to 30% have separate placentas and membranes (dichorionic, diamniotic)
- 1% to 2% share one placenta and one membrane (monochorionic, monoamniotic)

There is no simple relationship between zygosity and placenta status. All monochorionic twins are MZ, but some MZ twins are dichorionic.

It is clear that DZ twinning has increased significantly with the use of ART, occurring when there is more than one dominant follicle in a single cycle or there is transfer of more than one embryo. What remains unclear is the etiology of the increase in MZ twinning. One study reviewed 218 ART pregnancies and found the incidence of monochorionic twins to be 3.2% versus a background rate of 0.4%.[6] Fertility treatments that involve manipulation of the zona pellucida or extended embryo culture may provoke MZ twinning.[7-10] Aside from ART, simply being advanced maternal age is associated with a higher incidence of naturally occurring multiple births, presumably as a result of age-associated higher levels of follicle-stimulating hormone. The familial risk for DZ multiple gestation is due to an inherited gene associated with superovulation, potentially linked to chromosome 3.[11]

Twins with monochorionic placentas are at risk for vascular compromise, including twin-to-twin transfusion syndrome (TTTS) in monochorionic, diamniotic twins and cord entanglement in monochorionic, monoamniotic twins. Other conditions associated with monochorionic twins are twin reversed arterial perfusion; unequal sharing of the placenta, leading to growth discordance; and congenital anomalies. In addition, neurologic impairment

Table 10-1 Determining the Type of Monozygotic Twinning

Day of Egg Division Postovulation	Type of Monozygotic Twinning
Ovulation to day 3	Dichorionic/diamniotic
Days 3–8	Monochorionic/diamniotic
Days 8–13	Monochorionic/monoamniotic
Days 13–18	Conjoined twins

to one twin may occur if the co-twin should die during fetal life. This occurs via intertwin agonal transfusion and results in a 38% risk of death and a 46% risk of neurologic injury to the co-twin.[12]

Results of several studies suggest a twofold to threefold increase of congenital anomalies in MZ twins.[5] These congenital anomalies of MZ twins can be separated into malformation, disruptions, and deformations.[13] Malformations include cloacal anomalies, neural tube defects, and congenital heart defects. Disruptions include hemifacial macrosomia, limb reduction defects, and amyoplasia. Deformations associated with intrauterine crowding include clubfeet, dislocated hips, and cranial synostosis.

The most obvious risk of multifetal gestation is preterm delivery, accounting for 17% of all births before 37 weeks' gestation, 23% of births less than 32 weeks' gestation, 24% of low-birth-weight infants (<2500 g), and 26% of very-low-birth-weight infants (<1500 g).[14] Studies estimate average weeks' gestation for the following multiple gestations[2]:

- Twins 35.3 weeks' gestation
- Triplets 32.2 weeks' gestation
- Quadruplets 29.9 weeks' gestation

In general, multifetal gestation poses an increased risk for morbidity and mortality, with higher-order gestations having the least favorable outcomes. The *ACOG Practice Bulletin* in October 2004 summarized the characteristics of multifetal gestations (Table 10-2).[14] Compared with singleton pregnancies, the risk of cerebral palsy (CP) occurs four times more frequently in twin pregnancies and 17 times more frequently in triplet pregnancies.[15,16] The higher risk of CP in multifetal gestations is related to low gestational age and low birth weight, the two most important risk factors for CP.[17] In addition, studies from California and Western Australia show that intrauterine fetal demise of a co-twin is associated with a 13- to 15-fold higher risk for CP than twins born alive.[16,18]

Growth may be compromised in DZ or MZ pregnancies and usually is notable by 30 weeks' gestation. At birth, approximately 75% of twins are less than 15% discordant, 20% are 15% to 25% discordant, and 5% are greater than 25% discordant. Multifetal gestations are at higher risk for suboptimal placental implantation or abnormal umbilical cord insertion leading to utero-placental insufficiency.[14] Almost one third of triplets will have at least one fetus with a velamentous cord insertion leading to growth restriction. Other causes of discordant growth include limited intrauterine space, genetic fetal anomalies, discordant infection, placental abruption, or TTTS.

When reviewing anomalies associated with multifetal gestation, it is important to consider the actual process of ART itself and any effect it may have on the developing fetus. Some preliminary studies have reviewed the molecular characterization of epigenetic abnormalities, including the methylation status of imprinted gene clusters. Genetic imprinting is a mechanism of gene regulation whereby only one of the parental copies of a gene is expressed. Beckwith-Wiedemann syndrome and Angelman syndrome are two such syndromes associated with loss of maternal allele methylation. Registry reports from the United States, England, and France all report a higher incidence of Beckwith-Wiedemann syndrome and Angelman syndrome in children conceived via IVF and intracytoplasmic sperm injection.[19-22] Of note, epidemiologic evidence for imprinting defect is tentative and does not establish a definitive link.[19]

Although technology has made significant positive advances in granting fertility to couples who never thought it possible, it does come with some potential medical, financial, and emotional caveats. Multifetal gestations have a higher risk for preterm delivery and the associated complications, such as respiratory distress syndrome, bronchopulmonary dysplasia, infection, apnea of prematurity, retinopathy of prematurity, intraventricular hemorrhage, and periventricular leukomalacia. In addition, multiples are at higher risk for growth discordance and intrauterine growth restriction, congenital anomalies, and developmental delay.

The financial burden to some families and to our healthcare system can be overwhelming. A review of the economic impact of multifetal gestation was performed at Brigham & Women's Hospital in Boston during the years 1986 through 1991. The study concluded that if all of the ART multiple gestations had been singletons, the predicted savings to the healthcare system in the study hospital alone would have been more than $3 million per year.[23]

The emotional impact of multiple births can be devastating, with greater than 25% of parents demonstrating depression or anxiety in the perinatal period.[24] Neonatologists and pediatricians need to continue to support these families with early intervention, social work, and strategies to connect these families with other parents of multiples via

Table 10-2 Morbidity and Mortality in Multiple Gestation

Characteristic	Twins	Triplets	Quadruplets
Average birth weight[4]	2,347 g	1,687 g	1,309 g
Average gestational age at dellivery[1]	35.3 wk	32.2 wk	29.9 wk
Percentage with growth restriction[2]	14–25	50–60	50–60
Percentage requiring admission to neonatal intensive care unit[3]	25	75	100
Average length of stay in neonatal intensive care unit[3–9]	18 days	30 days	58 days
Percentage with major handicap[9,10]	—	20	50
Risk of cerebral palsy[9,10]	4 times more than singletons	17 times more than singletones	—
Risk of death by age 1 year[11–13]	7 times higher than singletones	20 times higher than singletones	—

From ACOG Practice Bulletin #56: Multiple gestation: complicated twin, triplet, and high-order multifetal pregnancy. *Obstet Gynecol* 104(4):869-883, 2004.

[1]Martin JA, Hamilton BE, Sutton PD, Ventura SJ, Menacker F, Munson MS, Births: final data for 2002. *Natl Vital Stat Rep* 2003;52(10):1–102.

[2]Mauldin JG, Newman RB, Neurologic morbidity associated with gestation. *Female Pat* 1998;23(4);27–8, 30, 35–6, passim.

[3]Ettner SL, Christiansen CL, Callahan TL, Hall JE. How low birthweight and gestational age contribute to increased inpation costs for multiple births. *Inquiry* 1997–98;34:325–39.

[4]McComick MD, Brooks-Gunn J, Workman-Daniels K, Tumer J, Peckham GJ. The health and developmental status of very low-birth-weight children at school age. *JAMA* 1992;267:2204–8.

[5]Luke B, Bigger HR, Leurgans S, Sietsema D. The cost of prematurity: a case-control study of twins vs singletons. *Am J Public Health* 1996;86:809–14.

[6]Albrecht JL, Tomich PG. The maternal and neonatal outcome of triplet gastations. *Am J Obsets Gynecol* 1996;174:1551–6.

[7]Newman RB, Hamer C, Miller MC. Outpatients triplet management: a contemporary review. *Am J Obsets Gynecol* 1989;161:547–53; discussion 553–5.

[8]Seoud MA, Toner JP, Kruithoff C, Muasher SJ. Outcome of twin, triplet, and quadruplet in vitro fertilization pregnancies: the Norfolk experience. *Fertil Steril* 1992;57:825–34.

[9]Elliott JP, Radin TG. Quadruplet pregnancy: contemporary management and outcome. *Obstet Gynecol* 1992;80;421–4.

[10]Grether JK, Nelson KB, Cummins SK. Twinning and cerebral palsy: experience in four northern California counties, births 1983 through 1985. *Pediatrics* 1993;92:854–8.

[11]Luke B, Kleinman J. The contribution of gestational age and birth weight to parinatal viability in singletones versus twins. *J Mat-Fetal Med* 1994;3:263–74.

[12]Kiely JL, Kleinman JC, Kiely M. Triplets and higher order multiple births: time trends and infant mortaility. *Am J Dis Child* 1992;146:862–8.

[13]Luke B, Keith LG. The contribution of singletones, twins, and triplets to low birht weight, infant mortality, and handicap in the Unites States. *J Reprod Med* 1992;37:661–6.

organizations such as the National Organization of Mothers of Twins Clubs, Inc.; the Triplet Connection; and Triplets, Moms, and More (see Resources section). Assisted reproduction provides tremendous benefits to families with infertility, but the increased medical risks and associated costs cannot be overlooked.

Resources for Families and Clinicians

The National Organization of Mothers of Twins Clubs, Inc.

www.Nomotc.org

This is a nonprofit corporation that offers advice, encouragement, and practical knowledge to families with multiples. Information about preparing for multiples, tips for new parents of multiples, and feeding multiples is included.

The Triplet Connection

www.Tripletconnection.org

The Triplet Connection is a nonprofit, tax-exempt organization for multiple-birth families. It provides information to families who are expecting triplets, quadruplets, quintuplets, or more, as well as encouragement, resources, and networking opportunities for families who are parents of larger multiples. In addition, it allows access to their quarterly publication.

Triplets, Moms, and More

www.tripletsmomsandmore.org

This is a Massachusetts-based support group for families and families-to-be of triplets, quadruplets, and more, providing educational information and emotional support.

REFERENCES

1. Allen M: The epidemiology of multiple births. Neonatal Core Conference Lecture Series, Children's Hospital, Boston, Massachusetts, 2004.
2. Martin JA, Hamilton BE, Sutton PD, et al: Births: final data for 2002. *Natl Vital Stat Rep* 52(10):1-113, 2003.
3. Petrozza J: Assisted reproductive technology. emedicine, 2004 *(http://www.emedicine.com/med/topic3288.htm).*
4. Jewell SE, Yip R: Increasing trends in plural births in the United States. *Obstet Gynecol* 85(2):229-232, 1995.
5. Hall JG: Twinning. *Lancet* 362(9385):735-743, 2003.
6. Wenstrom KD, Syrop CH, Hammitt DG, et al: Increased risk of monochorionic twinning associated with assisted reproduction. *Fertil Steril* 60(3):510-514, 1993.
7. Schachter M, Raziel A, Friedler, et al: Monozygotic twinning after assisted reproductive techniques: a phenomenon independent of micromanipulation. *Hum Reprod* 16(6):1264-1269, 2001.
8. Edwards RG, Mettler L, Walters DE: Identical twins and in vitro fertilization. *J In Vitro Fert Embryo Transf* 3(2):114-117, 1986.
9. Bressers WM, Eriksson AW, Kostense PJ, et al: Increasing trend in the monozygotic twinning rate. *Acta Genet Med Gemellol (Roma)* 36(3):397-408, 1987.
10. Milki AA, Jun SH, Hinckley MD, et al: Incidence of monozygotic twinning with blastocyst transfer compared to cleavage-stage transfer. *Fertil Steril* 79(3):503-506, 2003.
11. Busjahn A, Knoblauch H, Faulhaber HD, et al: A region on chromosome 3 is linked to dizygotic twinning. *Nat Genet* 26(4):398-399, 2000.
12. Pasquini L, Wimalasundera RC, Fisk NM: Management of other complications specific to monochorionic twin pregnancies. *Best Pract Res Clin Obstet Gynaecol* 18(4):577-599, 2004.
13. Optiz JM, Czeizel AE, Evans JA, et al: Nosologic grouping in birth defects. In Vogel F, Sperling K, editors: *Human genetics.* Berlin, 1987, Springer Verlag.
14. ACOG Practice Bulletin #56: multiple gestation: complicated twin, triplet, and high-order multifetal pregnancy. *Obstet Gynecol* 104(4):869-883, 2004.
15. Yokoyama Y, Shimizu T, Hayakawa K: Incidence of handicaps in multiple births and associated factors. *Acta Genet Med Gemellol (Roma)* 44(2):81-91, 1995.
16. Petterson B, Nelson KB, Watson L, et al: Twins, triplets, and cerebral palsy in births in Western Australia in the 1980s. *BMJ* 307(6914):1239-1243, 1993.
17. Topp M, Huusom LD, Langhoff-Roos J, et al: Multiple birth and cerebral palsy in Europe: a multicenter study. *Acta Obstet Gynecol Scand* 83(6):548-553, 2004.
18. Grether JK, Nelson KB, Cummins SK: Twinning and cerebral palsy: experience in four northern California counties, births 1983 through 1985. *Pediatrics* 92(6):854-858, 1993.
19. Gosden R, Trasler J, Lucifero D, et al: Rare congenital disorders, imprinted genes, and assisted reproductive technology. *Lancet* 361(9373):1975-1977, 2003.
20. Gicquel C, Gaston V, Mandelbaum J, et al: In vitro fertilization may increase the risk of Beckwith-Wiedemann syndrome related to the abnormal imprinting of the KCN1OT gene. *Am J Hum Genet* 72(5):1338-1341, 2003.
21. Orstavik KH, Eiklid K, van der Hagen CB, et al: Another case of imprinting defect in a girl with Angelman syndrome who was conceived by intracytoplasmic semen injection. *Am J Hum Genet* 72(1):218-219, 2003.
22. Cox GF, Burger J, Lip V, et al: Intracytoplasmic sperm injection may increase the risk of imprinting defects. *Am J Hum Genet* 71(1):162-164, 2002.
23. Callahan TL, Hall JE, Ettner SL, et al: The economic impact of multiple-gestation pregnancies and the contribution of assisted-reproduction techniques to their incidence. *N Engl J Med* 331(4):244-249, 1994.
24. Leonard LG: Depression and anxiety disorders during multiple pregnancy and parenthood. *J Obstet Gynecol Neonatal Nurs* 27(3):329-337, 1998.

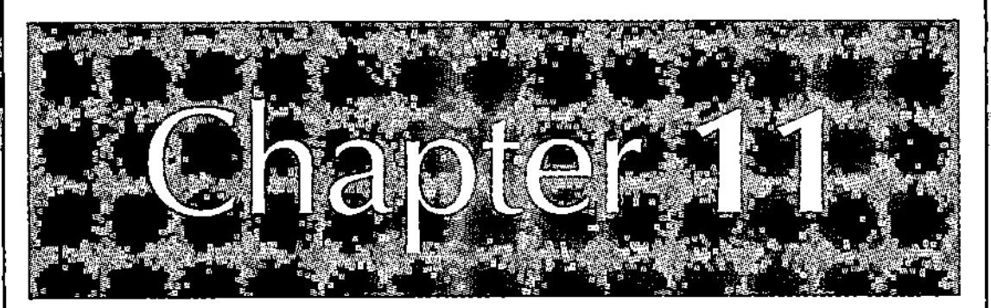

Supporting Parents of Premature Infants: An Infant-Focused, Family-Centered Approach

J. Kevin Nugent, PhD, Yvette Blanchard, ScD, PT, and Jane E. Stewart, MD

The goal of this chapter is to describe the behavioral development of the premature infant during the early months of life and the particular challenges faced by preterm infants as opposed to full-term infants. We present guidelines on how pediatricians and pediatric professionals can help parents respond to the needs of their infants over these early months. We examine the impact of a premature birth on the parents themselves and on the whole family system and show how the pediatric professional can play a supportive role in the health and well-being of the child and family. Finally, we emphasize the importance of relationship building in terms of family support and present a model of family-centered developmental care, based on the Newborn Behavioral Observations (NBO) system,[1] which can be used by pediatric practitioners to support parents in their efforts to meet their premature infant's needs.

Premature birth, followed by the intensity of the experience of the neonatal intensive care unit (NICU), is highly stressful and sometimes traumatic, not only for the baby but also for the parents and the whole family. Health and developmental problems, which are more common in these infants, are also associated with higher rates of psychosocial symptoms in the parents. Mothers of these infants are more likely to have had an illness during the pregnancy, preexisting medical conditions, or a history of fertility treatments, making them more at risk for postpartum illness and depression. In general, they experience higher levels of distress and often are confronted by feelings of disappointment and failure as well as anxieties about their infant's survival and future healthy development, as they mourn the loss of the "imagined" or "wished for baby."[2-5] Moreover, the quality of maternal care for the preterm infant may deteriorate as a result of the stressful events experienced by the mother and by the family, which in turn affects the infant's capacity for recovery and self-regulation.[4,6-9] The stress on parents of meeting a premature infant's daily needs, the associated financial costs, and the strain of preserving marital and family relationships through infancy can place a family at risk of dysfunction, including child abuse and increased rates of family health problems.[10]

However, evidence suggests, that protective factors, such as providing developmental information and strong emotional support to parents, can improve resistance to risk factors and contribute to successful outcomes, adaptation, and child resiliency.[11,12] In a critique of 11 studies on intervention effects for low-birth-weight premature infants, Melnyk et al.[13] concluded that clinical interventions must begin early in the NICU, with an emphasis on providing parents with information on their infant's behavior and development and on how to respond sensitively to the infant's communication cues.

Moreover, it has been found that the long-term outcome of prematurity is influenced to a significant degree by the particular responses of each caregiver to the infant and by the quality of the infant's caregiving environment.[14] We now know that developmentally appropriate interventions, designed to support the parent–child relationship, can enhance the cognitive and social emotional development of the premature infant.[15,16]

A wide range of research studies underscore the need for strengthening parents' knowledge, confidence, and practical skills in caring for their low-birth-weight children after discharge from the hospital, especially during the first months of life. Parents want information, services, and help from doctors on how to get their infants and toddlers off to a good start. Despite evidence for the importance of comprehensive, developmentally appropriate, long-term follow-up for NICU survivors, a meta-analysis of follow-up studies of very-low-birth-weight infants found that many of these children may not receive adequate follow-up and concluded that medically and socially vulnerable children are most likely to be "lost to follow-up."[17] Parents themselves, once they get home, often feel isolated in caring for their at-risk infant.[18,19] Data also suggest that even when parents are included in the decision-making process in the NICU, this collaborative, family-centered care often unravels after discharge because the support is difficult to maintain. Parents want information about their baby's condition, treatment, or prognosis, and they welcome information about early intervention and follow-up services for their babies.[20] The lack of knowledge about expected developmental milestones and parenting techniques may lead to failure to encourage language and other areas of development.[21] The importance of providing parents with information on their child's development and emotional support so that they can respond appropriately to their infant's cues has been well documented as a form of preventative intervention for parents of at-risk infants.[6,11,15,16,22-26]

Despite the challenges that families of premature infants face, support for these families remains an acknowledged concern among healthcare providers, especially after the infants are discharged. Community-based physicians and other caregivers can feel unprepared in dealing with the complex health and developmental issues associated with prematurity. Compounding this problem is the possible lack of a well-established communication system among neonatologists, the primary care clinician, and the family. For that reason, community-based primary care providers may find responding to families' psychosocial needs to be a challenge. Indeed, community support and psychosocial factors often may be left out of discharge planning for preterm infants.

Understanding the Behavior of the Premature Infant

Low birth weight and prematurity place the child at risk for a variety of medical and developmental problems. These infants are much more likely than normal-weight/term infants to experience significant medical complications, chronic illness, developmental delays, and increased use of health services in the first years of life.[27-31] Because the development of the premature infant is affected by a wide range of medical variables, including gestational age, birth weight, time spent on mechanical ventilation in the NICU, incidence and severity of chronic lung disease, need for oxygen, white matter injury, intraventricular hemorrhage status, overall length of time in the NICU, and daily weight gain, the broad range of variability in premature infant behavior prevents consideration of the premature infant from a general typologic viewpoint.

Most preterm infants are discharged from the hospital around the time of their due date; however, until recently, little was known about their specific developmental competencies at that age. The hypersensitivity of the preterm infant to social and environmental stimulation is well documented.[32] For example, research has shown that although infants born as late as 34 and 37 weeks' gestation can visually track, hear, and locate sounds and even seem to have a preference for their mother's voice, they are significantly more reactive and more easily disorganized than their full-term counterparts.[33] Therefore, these infants carry the potential to demonstrate many of the competencies displayed by full-term newborns and are able to demonstrate contingent behavioral responses and preferences to stimulation. However, they may do so at increased cost to their physiologic, motor, and state systems, and for that reason they require a great deal of support and facilitation from the caregiving environment to reach that level of functioning. The task of the pediatrician, then, is to attempt to understand each premature infant as an individual, with his or her own set of strengths and challenges and his or her own unique behavioral repertoire, and the kinds of developmental tasks each infant faces over the first months of life.

Developmental tasks facing the premature infant

The first developmental task to be accomplished by newborns and young infants over the first weeks and months of life is the task of self-regulation, which can be observed through the infant's behavioral adaptations and responses to his or her environment. Self-regulation is achieved through the successful integration of four systems or behavioral dimensions: autonomic, motor, organization of state, and responsivity (Table 11-1). From this developmental perspective, the newborn infant faces a series of hierarchically organized developmental challenges as he or she attempts to adapt to his or her new inanimate and animate extrauterine world.[15,33-35] This includes the infant's capacity first to regulate the physiologic or autonomic system, then the motor and state behavioral dimensions, and finally the affective interactive (responsivity) behavioral dimension, all of which develop in a stagelike progression over the first 2 months of life. These developmental tasks must be successfully negotiated before the infant can develop the capacity for shared mutual engagement that constitutes the major task of the next stage of development.[36-38] Nevertheless, this developmental agenda and the infant's capacity to respond to his or her environment can be achieved only with the support of the caregiver. Under this model, it is assumed that the infant's principal method of communicating is through his or her behavior.[39] Therefore, the behaviors displayed by the infant in each of the four behavioral dimensions form the avenue through which caregivers can understand the current developmental level of self-regulation and maturity of a given infant. It is the recognition of these developmental challenges that will best inform the pediatrician's clinical approach to working with parents and allow them to provide parents with developmentally appropriate information and individualized guidance during this important life transition.[40]

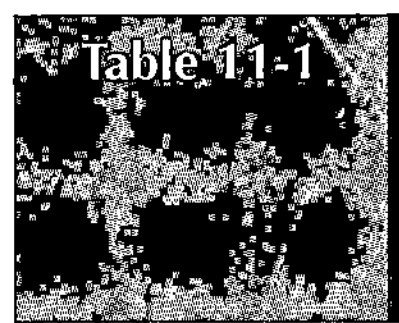

Self-Regulation: Four Behavioral Dimensions Used as Indicators of Self-Regulation and Maturity (AMOR)

Behavioral Dimensions	Specific Behavioral Observations
Autonomic	Breathing patterns: regular, irregular, fast, slow, pause, apnea Changes in skin color: pink, pale, red, mottled, dusky, cyanotic Visceral function: bowel movements, grunting and straining, tremors, twitches and startles
Motor	Tone: normal, low, high or fluctuating Posture: tucked, flexed, extended Motor maturity: reflexes, smoothness of movements, jerkiness, underarm arcs
Organization of state	Clarity and transition patterns in states of consciousness: deep sleep, light sleep, drowsy, alert, active alert and crying Habituation to negative stimuli (light and sound) while asleep Soothability and efforts to self-quiet
Responsivity	Quality and duration of alert state Ability to respond to animate and inanimate visual and auditory stimuli: track human face and voice or toy, locate sounds

The preterm infant's ability to self-regulate appears compromised and limited in duration. Sensory thresholds to stimulation leading to loss of self-regulation are more easily reached as compared with the typical full-term infant. For example, an infant with chronic lung disease may demonstrate the ability to turn to the sound of a voice and may be able to track his mother's face with his eyes, but may be able to do so only with carefully timed stimulation matched to his sensory thresholds. When the parent speaks to the infant, the baby may pause his or her breathing when he or she first hears the parent's voice and after a brief pause, shift his or her eyes toward the parent. These initial behavioral responses (pause in breathing and delayed eye shift toward voice) let the parent know of the infant's initial efforts to respond. The parent, in turn, comes to realize that he or she needs to adapt his or her voice to the infant's level of response before the baby can begin to interact. In this case, if the parent responds by giving the infant a brief "time-out," by not talking for a few seconds, the infant may be able to regulate his or her breathing and orientation responses and turn toward the sound of the parent's voice. On the other hand, if the parent does not read the initial infant behaviors as indicating a need for support or a need for a break in the intensity of the stimulation and continues to ask the infant to respond to his or her voice, the infant may respond by closing his or her eyes and turning away from the parent's voice. The nature and intensity of caregiver facilitation and support required to achieve self-regulation becomes instructive for healthcare professionals and parents and can form the basis for developing individualized developmental goals and strategies for that infant.[41]

An infant is described as organized when his or her self-regulatory abilities are able to support the social and environmental demands placed on him or her, and it is at this time that "approach behaviors" are observed. On the other hand, an infant is described as disorganized when his or her threshold for self-regulation is exceeded, and "avoidance behaviors" are observed.[42] For example, a regular respiratory rate, good color, and stable digestion are noted in physiologically organized infants, whereas infants who are showing signs of disorganization in this behavioral dimension may have irregular breathing, poor color, and signs of unstable digestion. Within the motor subsystem, smooth movements and balanced flexor–extensor tone are considered organized behaviors, whereas jerky movement quality and overuse of extensor movements are considered disorganized behaviors. An infant with a well-organized state system has a broad range of well-defined states available, with smooth transitions from one state to the next. A less well-organized infant may have a narrower range of states, the states may be more diffuse, and the infant may have rapid state changes. Infants with well-organized attention–interaction can achieve and maintain shiny-eyed alertness and well-modulated interactive periods at least briefly. A less well-organized infant may have strained, low-level alertness or conversely may be hyperalert and unable to break away from interaction that may be too intense. It is especially important to share this type of information with parents to help them understand that they are not causing their infant's sensory overload but rather that their preterm infant's ability to self-regulate in varied situations and conditions is still limited in duration and quality. By adjusting their approach on the basis of the behavioral cues of the infant, parents can provide better-matched opportunities for interactions with their child.

Individualized intervention strategies are best accomplished when environmental and social demands support the infant's self-regulatory limits and when they take into account the infant's sensory thresholds. Within this perspective, intervention is aimed at facilitating prolonged periods of organization, thus decreasing the manifestation of disorganized behaviors while reinforcing the infant's individual self-regulatory style. For example, well-organized full-term newborns and infants may be observed bringing themselves into a sleep state by placing one hand against the back of the head or behind the ear with the other hand close to the mouth. Less well-organized preterm infants may attempt to do the same but may not be as successful at maintaining these comfort postures. Building on these observations, the pediatrician or parent can assist the infant by swaddling him or her, by bringing the hand close to the mouth, by offering a finger to hold, or by tucking the legs and allowing the infant to brace his or her feet against one's hand until the infant settles down and is able to maintain a state of organized functioning. Meeting an infant's needs with such individualized and well-timed support leads parents to develop a deeper understanding of their infant's developmental status, strengths, and challenges.

The "Wished for Baby": The Impact on the Parents and Family

In the case of parents of premature infants, the parents themselves can be considered to be "premature parents." Anticipatory grief may set in as parents mourn the loss of their "imagined" or "wished for baby," as they struggle to develop a bond with their "real baby."[2,4] The mother's feelings of anxiety and depression may be rooted in her belief that her inability to bring her baby to term is a personal failure. Moreover, the premature birth is perceived as a violation of the mother's own expectations and the dream of having a perfect "fantasy baby." It is in the immediate postnatal period that parents' perceptions of the infant begin to consolidate, and parents' perceptions of infant behavior play a crucial role in determining the unfolding of the parent–infant relationship.[2,23,38,43-45]

Several investigators have noted interactional difficulties between mothers and their low-birth-weight children.[13] It may be that the difficulty parents of premature infants have in responding to their premature infants is due, in large part, to the fact that these infants not only are less competent than the imagined, "wished for baby" but that they in fact tend to be less responsive, are more fretful, smile less, and give less readable communication signals than full-term infants.[9] Their communication cues are more difficult to decipher, possibly resulting in interactive disturbances—"parental misattunements"—between parent and child. Because the ability to read and attend to their infant's cues both consistently and contingently is important in the development of a secure attachment relationship, the degree to which parents can respond contingently to their preterm infant's cues becomes an important clinical issue. The difficulty that already stressed parents experience in trying to read and understand their infant's behavior may result in feelings of failure, with the result that interactive difficulties begin to emerge, depression deepens, and over time the parent–infant attachment relationship ultimately becomes compromised.[46,47] Helping parents read their baby's cues and providing parents with feedback on how their babies respond to them can help mobilize confidence in their efforts to develop a relationship with their infants.

One of our goals is to help parents develop realistic perceptions of their infants and help them modify their prenatal perceptions in response to their infant's objectively observed behavior patterns. The works of Bruschweiler-Stern,[2] Stern,[38] and Cramer[43,44] clearly indicate that the task of influencing parents' perceptions of their infant is a complex one, because the meanings parents attribute to their infant's behavior may have their origin in the parents' personal history and subconscious. Whereas the resolution of such distorted perceptions may be prolonged and painstaking, we can begin to contribute to the resolution of such perceptions by enabling parents to observe their infant's own unique behavioral makeup and the infant's own interaction capacities, thus helping to prevent the development of maladaptive or noncontingent interaction patterns. The pediatric professional's predominant attitude toward parents is, therefore, both respectful and supportive. The clinician must be able to listen empathically for parents' questions and observations.[48,49] In Cramer's view, paying attention to a mother's verbal reports and what she thinks about her baby is crucial because these attributes play a significant role in determining the unfolding of the mother–infant relationship.[43] We always should provide parents with the opportunity to share their perceptions of their infant and to relate their experience of becoming a parent, in what Zeanah and McDonough[50] refer to as the "family story."

In summary, although prematurity and low birth weight are known risk factors for poor developmental outcome, environmental risk factors that compromise the quality of parenting are more likely to be associated with greater risk.[6,41,51] For that reason, we are proposing that developmentally appropriate interventions, which are designed to enhance parent–child interactions and support the parent–child relationship, can improve outcome and promote the child's cognitive and social emotional development.

Role of the Pediatric Care Provider: Anticipatory Guidance

Pediatricians are in a unique position to address the needs of premature infants and their parents by offering the kind of information and support parents need during the first months of their child's life (Table 11-2).[10,52] Because of the frequency of visits in the first year, primary pediatricians have a great opportunity to develop a supportive relationship with families. The medical home model for family center care, strongly supported by the American Academy of Pediatrics, advocates that the primary pediatrician, "because of his or her unique training, interest and commitment should be a vital member of the early intervention health team" and "offer comprehensive care that is family centered, continuous, compassionate and culturally sensitive."[53,54]

Table 11-2	Role of the Primary Care Provider Caring for a Premature Infant

Ideal to meet with family before infant's discharge home from the NICU
Develop a supportive relationship with family
Screen for developmental problems in infant:
- Use standardized developmental screening tools to measure cognition, language, motor development*
- Use the Newborn Behavioral Observations (NBO) System (Table 11-4) to provide more developmental information to parents, develop a relationship with the parents, and assist with transition from NICU to home
- If developmental delay is identified, refer to early intervention with/without other services, such as neurology, orthopedics, neurodevelopmental specialists, audiology; develop a partnership with the community Early Intervention Services

Screen for behavioral problems in infant
Assess maternal health
- Screen for postpartum depression
- Screen for any domestic concerns

Counsel family about general healthcare issues in premature infants, including:
- Sleep patterns
- Interpretation and management of crying
- Feeding cues
- Infant temperament

NICU, Neonatal intensive care unit.
*Many developmental screening tools are available. Parent report instruments include:
- **Ages and Stages.** Bricker D, Squires J: *Ages & stages questionnaires.* Baltimore, 1995, Paul H Brookes Publishing. Available at: *www.aap.org/healthtopics/stages.cfm.* Available in Spanish and French.
- **Parent's Evaluation of Developmental Status (PEDS).** Glascoe FP: *Collaborating with parents: using parents' evaluation of developmental status to detect and address developmental and behavioral problems.* Nashville, 1998, Ellsworth & Vandermeer Press. Available at: *http://www.pedstest.com* and *www.forepath.org.* Available in Spanish and Vietnamese.
- **Vineland Adaptive Behavior Scales** (VABS) (semistructured interview format).
- **Modified Checklist for Autism in Toddlers** (MCHAT) for older infants. Available at: *www.dbpeds.org/.*

Screening tests that require direct examination by a primary care provider include:
- **Cognitive Adaptive Test/Clinical Linguistic and Auditory Milestone Scale (CAT/CLAMS).** Capute AL: *The Capute scales. CAT/CLAMS. instruction manual.* Baltimore, 1996, Kennedy Fellows Association. Available at: *www.elsevier.com.*
- **Denver Developmental Screening Test (DDST-2).** Frankenburg WK, Dodds J, Archer P, et al: Denver-II screening manual. Denver, 1990, Denver Developmental Materials.

In addition to monitoring the important health issues related to premature birth, the pediatrician is uniquely positioned to screen for infant developmental and behavioral problems as well as for parental medical and mental health issues.[55] Use of standardized developmental screening instruments by the primary care provider and nurse practitioners and referral to a developmental specialist for assessment of early cognitive, language, and motor development not only will identify delays but also will provide ideal opportunities to offer anticipatory guidance to the family about supporting their infant's development. Children identified with developmental delays can be referred promptly to the appropriate community early intervention services. Likewise, a check on maternal health, including screening for postpartum depression or any domestic concerns, should be a routine part of the history obtained by the pediatrician.

Parents of premature infants require special counseling on general healthcare issues, including sleep, crying, feeding, and infant temperament because the parents' level of anxiety often is greatly amplified after a stressful initial NICU stay. Likewise, the transition from the intensive care unit, where there is constant monitoring of the baby's medical status and tremendous social and emotional support from the hospital staff, often is described as extremely isolating and overwhelming. Adding to the complexity of care can be multiple births with twins and triplets, with their unique challenges. Therefore the connection with a "medical home" is of extreme importance and should begin during the NICU hospitalization, with the parents meeting with their pediatrician before their baby's discharge. The NBO system[1] (described in the section on model for supporting parents of premature infants: the NBO system) can be used by practitioners to help parents with the transition from NICU to home. The NBO system can help parents to better understand their baby's behavior and temperament, his or her threshold for responsiveness, sleep patterns, feeding cues, and readiness for interaction, thereby supporting the "goodness of fit" between the baby and his or her new home environment.

Anticipatory Guidance: Specific Caregiving Themes for Care of the Preterm Infant

Sleep issues

Physiologically, premature infants are more likely to have a history of apnea and may have ongoing respiratory issues with chronic lung disease, possibly requiring oxygen therapy or home cardiorespiratory monitoring equipment. Research shows that premature infants have immaturity of their sleep organization when assessed by electroencephalography.[56,57] These infants often are noisy breathers, with snuffling, snoring and grunting, so parents tend to worry about breathing difficulties and are more likely to be awakened by their infant's night waking. In addition, babies who have been in a busy NICU that does not have normal night and day light cycles have been shown to sleep less and do not gain weight as well as those who have been in NICU environments that reduce nighttime light exposure. For these reasons, parents of premature infants are more likely to report that their infants have sleep difficulties and classically complain that their infant has night and day mixed up. This pattern of sleeping can take some time to evolve once a baby has been discharged to home. Premature infants also often require supplemental caloric intake, which requires extra nighttime feedings, or have problems with vomiting related to gastroesophageal reflux that result in frequent parental waking and sleep deprivation.

Maternal posttraumatic reactions have been associated with increased sleep problems in infancy.[58] Parents of a premature infant are more likely to stay with their baby until he or she is asleep and to bring the infant into their own bed when the child does awake.

The pediatrician's role is to identify the presence of sleeping difficulties, try to identify the source of these problems, and advise parents on strategies for possible intervention (Table 11-3). Supportive reassurance regarding the common occurrence of these problems in premature infants and an acknowledgement that these infants' sleeping problems are more complicated and most likely will take longer to resolve than in full-term infants are helpful for anxious parents.

Touch and handling

The importance of positive touch in the NICU is now well recognized, so parents are more likely to be encouraged to hold their premature infants with skin-to-skin contact, practicing "kangaroo care." Research has demonstrated the positive effects of extended skin-to-skin contact or kangaroo care on premature infants and parents alike.[59,60] Meta-analysis on the effects of extended skin-to-skin contact revealed slightly improved Neonatal Behavioral Assessment Scale (NBAS) scores for habituation, motor maturity, and range of state and reduced stress.[61] Likewise, massage therapy has been used in older infants, and results suggest that it may improve weight gain in preterm/low-birth-weight infants and may have an effect of decreasing length of hospital stay.[62,63] Field et al.[64] reported that preterm infants who received regular

Table 11-3 Potential Etiologies and Suggested Interventions for Sleep Difficulties

Sleep Problem	Possible Cause	Suggested Interventions
"Light/dark confusion" (i.e., sleeps in day, awake at night)	Busy NICU exposure	Dark, quiet nighttime nursery Discourage excessive daytime napping
Frequent waking	Neurologic immaturity	Help parents learn to recognize and predict their infant's sleep cycles
	Parental reinforcement of waking	Begin sleep training guidance: Bedtime routine Strategies to encourage self-calming References: Ferber R: *Solve your child's sleep problems.* New York, 2006, Fireside. Mindell J, Owens J: *Take care of your child's sleep.* New York, 2005, Marlowe & Company. Weissbluth M: *Healthy sleep habits, happy child.* New York, 1999, Ballantine Books.
Multiples: twin wakes other twin	Different sleep cycles	Troubleshooting (possibilities include cobedding,* different sleeping locations)

*Co-bedding with parent is contraindicated because of risk for sudden infant death syndrome.

massage (three 15-minute periods per day for 10 days) gained an average of 47% more weight than did control infants. Importantly, no adverse effects from massage have been reported. After discharge to home, massage therapy taught by a trained professional may provide a positive experience for parents and infants. Moreover, the use of infant carriers when the infant reaches the appropriate size may be another way to continue this close contact.

Feeding problems

Feeding problems are common in premature infants during the first year of life.[65-67] The emotional and cultural significance of good weight gain to parents cannot be understated. Pediatricians should review parents' feeding plans, including their desires and priorities (e.g., breastfeeding). NICU parents are very focused on their baby's feedings in terms of volumes, weight gain, and growth. Ideally, parents should be taught from the start about appropriate feeding techniques and how to recognize their baby's cues regarding hunger, feeding tolerance during feedings, and when feedings should stop, as well as how these responses will change developmentally over the first few months of age.

Feeding problems can be categorized as resulting from medical, oral, and behavioral sources.[67] Feeding problems are common, particularly in infants who have undergone prolonged mechanical ventilation and nasogastric tube feedings. In infants with evidence of feeding problems, appropriate oral motor feeding therapy is essential to develop positive feeding experiences and reduce oral sensitivity. Feeding problems are commonly multifactorial, with medical problems such as gastroesophageal reflux resulting in feeding-associated pain that triggers oral sensitivity and oral defensive behavior. Likewise, there is evidence that feeding practices/methods by nursing staff and parents (e.g., forced or prolonged attempts at nipple feedings on a stressed or fatigued infant) may result in the development of oral aversion (see Chapter 4C).

The pediatrician should ask parents appropriate, open-ended questions regarding feeding that will allow for exploration and discovery of the reasons for feeding problems. Detailed feeding histories, including parents' perceived difficulties, mode of feeding, and description of frequency, duration, and environment of feedings, should be obtained. The earlier that feeding difficulties are identified and treated, the less likely it is that long-term oral aversion will develop. In infants with significant chronic respiratory disease and the inability to take appropriate caloric intake, gastrostomy tube (G-tube) placement occasionally is warranted during the NICU hospitalization or after discharge to home if poor weight gain is identified. The importance of prompt referral of these infants to an experienced oral motor therapist who will work with parents to develop a continued plan of positive oral motor stimulation is important and will reduce the duration of G-tube dependency (*www.kidswithtubes.org*).

Crying

Excessive crying is one of the most common problems presented to physicians over the first 3 months of life. Research shows that this is more true of preterm infants than full-term infants. Sobotkova et al.[68] report that at both 6 weeks and at 3 months, mothers of preterm infants, compared with mothers of full-term infants, report that their infants cry more and are more irritable than are full-term infants. Barr et al.[69] compared the crying patterns of healthy full-term infants with those of healthy preterm infants and found that preterm infants still cried significantly more than did the full-term infants after 40 weeks' gestational age, with a peak and evening clustering at 6 weeks' corrected gestational age. This higher threshold for crying may reflect the premature infant's lack of ability to regulate behavioral states. Moreover, many studies have reported that not only do preterm infants cry more but that their cries are rated as more difficult to interpret and more aversive than are the cries of full-term infants. Excessive crying, in turn, has been linked to reduced maternal responsiveness.[24,70]

How then does the pediatrician help parents respond positively to a preterm baby whom they feel cries excessively, has a piercing cry, and is difficult to console? First, it is important to remind parents that over time their baby's cry will become more robust and will sound more like the cry of a full-term infant. For that reason, the clinician can take this opportunity to help parents listen closely to the acoustics and harmonics of the cry in order to "befriend" their baby's cry and to recognize that the strength and robustness of the cry is a reliable index of the baby's well-being and development. Second, we can help parents realize that the cry is their baby's communication system par excellence. When parents take the baby home from the hospital, we can help them to anticipate these crying episodes by suggesting that they attempt the following:

- Set the baby's crib or bassinet somewhere in the house that is not overstimulating in terms of light or sound. This will help the baby protect his or her sleep and thus reduce his or her level of stress.
- Make sure that blanket rolls or supports are available in the crib to provide the baby with the kinds of boundaries he or she may need to sleep longer and conserve energy.[71]
- Throughout the day, try to anticipate the baby's cry by learning his or her early warning signals that indicate overload or overstimulation. Try to learn how the baby reacts to specific situations that are more likely to lead to crying. For example, if the baby usually cries during diaper changing, the caregiver can learn to reduce the level of stimulation or pay attention to the baby's tolerance for different levels of handling.

There is no doubt that caring for a child who cries a lot is extremely stressful for parents. Many parents of premature infants may feel depressed or overwhelmed by the continuous and sometimes inconsolable crying of their infants. Therefore it is especially important to recognize parents' need to talk about their feelings of frustration and inadequacy in the face of their infant's excessive crying. The best form of anticipatory guidance may well be to help parents realize that having a social support network—whether partner, parents, friends, or neighbors—in place is perhaps their most important form of preventative intervention at this time.

Chronological age or corrected age: a dilemma for parents

One of the major sources of variability in premature infant behavior and one that concerns many parents is the question of how to estimate the baby's age, that is, whether to use the concept of "corrected age" or simply the baby's actual "chronological age." Most preterm infants are discharged from the hospital within weeks of their due date. They may match on their corrected age for prematurity, although some may be 4 weeks' chronological age whereas others may be 3 months' chronological age. Parents are unsure which age classification to use as an index of their baby's progress or development. Using the baby's chronological age often results in a comment from the family member or stranger on how small the infant is, whereas using the corrected age requires an explanation from the parents on the infant's prematurity history, a topic of conversation they may prefer to avoid for the moment. Parents also often feel that their infant's development does not fit either age profile and are not sure what to expect in terms of the baby's development.

Once the infant is discharged, the pediatrician becomes one of the main sources of information and support available to parents, to alleviate some of their anxiety over the future outcome of their child and to help them understand their infant's current developmental status. It often is important for the pediatrician to remind the parents of their infant's corrected age and to point out some basic differences between preterm and full-term infants of similar postconceptual ages. Early intervention service providers can be helpful in assisting the pediatrician address these issues with parents. A simple guideline would be to monitor progress in development over time, as seen in the acquisition of early motor skills, and to comment on the quality of the observed skills rather than on the quantity. For example, a premature child may be delayed in sitting, but he or she may display excellent quality of movement in his or her ability to turn, reach, transfer objects, or play with his or her feet. The pediatrician's comments on the quality of movement can reassure the parents that the infant is showing healthy signs of development.

Stimulation and interaction: promoting the "goodness of fit" between parent and infant

The hypersensitivity of the preterm infant to social and environmental stimulation is well documented. Parents and pediatricians need to recognize that preterm infants recently discharged home from the hospital will remain sensitive to stimulation for some months after discharge. Therefore anticipatory guidance given to parents at the hospital or in the pediatrician's office after discharge should include information on the prevention of overstimulation and the support of self-regulation for the sensitive infant.

Preterm infants, even at term age, have limited abilities for multisensory processing.[71] When an infant is showing signs of overstimulation through loss of self-regulation and signs of exhaustion, the simplest advice that pediatricians can give parents is to decrease the amount of stimulation to which the infant is exposed. For example, it often is difficult for a young preterm infant to look at his or her caregiver while being held and talked to at the same time. It is recommended that caregivers take into account the number of modalities they use when interacting with their infants. The pediatrician can suggest that caregivers limit the number of modalities presented all at once by holding (not rocking) and smiling at the infant, but not talking to him or her at the same time. If the infant establishes eye contact and looks relaxed, the caregiver can then greet the infant with a soft voice while watching for his or her behavioral signals of regulation to decide whether voice is appropriate at the moment. To assist the preterm infant's emerging abilities to maintain self-regulation in a variety of settings, taking the baby on outside errands to the grocery store or the shopping mall should be limited for the first few weeks after discharge home from the hospital. Parents often ask about which toys are appropriate for their premature infant. In the first 2 to 3 months of life, the parents themselves are the best "toys" available to their infant. Infants at this age are most interested in faces, especially their parents' faces, and will prefer looking at them rather than at any toy. Parents should avoid battery-powered toys that offer continuous stimulation (light or sound) without pause and should avoid exposing their child to television, in accordance with the guidelines outlined by the American Academy of Pediatrics. Early intervention service providers typically are well versed on what toys are appropriate for very young infants and can assist the pediatrician in making recommendations for activities with developmentally appropriate toys for an infant.

Parents of preterm infants often report that their infant is most alert in the middle of the night. The calm environment in terms of noise and lighting levels typical of the home night setting may be the reason for the increased level of alertness. Changing the intensity of the lighting in the room in which the infant is placed during the day and pulling the shades or dimming the lights may support the infant's efforts at reaching and maintaining an alert state. Swaddling the infant and providing grasping opportunities through finger holding help the infant maintain a relaxed posture for longer periods and can assist the infant in his or her efforts to respond to the parent's voice. In general, a calm daily routine of low-keyed events will appropriately nurture and support the development of the preterm infant's competence.[32] During the day, infants should be in a quiet and calm home environment with opportunities to sleep in a room free of television or conversation noises. Limiting the number of visitors and caregivers will help to establish a predictable routine planned around the infant's developing sleep/wake cycles and feeding schedule.

Caring for the Family of the Preterm Infant: Relationship-Based Care

Research reveals that low birth weight and prematurity place the child at risk for a number of developmental problems and suggests that these infants are much more likely than normal weight/term infants to experience significant medical complications, chronic illness, developmental delays, and increased use of health services in the first years of life. However, compelling evidence suggests that preventive intervention with at-risk infants can positively affect later development. We propose that, especially for the prematurely born infant, an individualized family-centered system of developmentally informed information and support for parents can prevent the compounding of problems that occur when the caregiving environment has difficulty adjusting to the needs of the newborn infant.

For the infant born prematurely, the period from birth to discharge from the NICU through the first months at home after discharge constitutes a major transition stage in the infant's adaptation to his or her new environment and in the development of the parent–infant relationship. This is the time when the earliest patterns of interaction are taking shape, as infant and parent exchange their communication signals in their efforts to achieve a mutually satisfying level of affective mutual regulation. We believe that this period presents the pediatrician with a unique opportunity to intervene preventatively and to support the family, especially under conditions of environmental stress. The transition from hospital to home offers the pediatrician an entry point for supportive intervention in order to counterbalance the risk present within the system itself.[4,38,72] With families that feel anxious or isolated, or that have no support system, this individualized infant-focused, family-centered approach provides reliable developmental information to parents in order to sensitize them to the needs of their infant and thereby enhance their sense of competency as parents. It also can serve as a bridge between the family and the family's healthcare provider and increase the availability of both informal community support for the family and more formal family resource services in the community.[52,73,74]

This kind of pediatric care will be effective only if it is presented in the context of a relationship between the practitioner and the family.[1,40] Inui[75] concludes that a close relationship between a family and the primary care system is helpful in improving the pattern of healthcare utilization by families living in disadvantaged areas. The Pew Health Professions Commission and the Fetzer Task Force for Advancing Psychosocial Health Education have emphasized the centrality of relationship-centered care and the need for pediatric professionals to communicate with patients and include them as partners in the decision-making process (Committee on Practice and Ambulatory Medicine, 2001[76]). The parameters of respect, concern, accommodation, and basic positive regard become crucial as the envelope of the entire "treatment" process. The more concerned or anxious the parent is, the more crucial this reliable emotional context becomes. By valuing the parent's attempts to reach out and understand his or her child, we provide the parent with a more nurturing and supportive relationship. Our hope is that this positive, nurturing, nonjudgmental experience becomes gradually internalized and incorporated into the parent's own internal representation as a parent. For a parent who is feeling alone and vulnerable, "meeting with" a clinician who is supportive and caring can be the first step in enhancing the parent's sense of worth. This, in turn, is an important condition for helping the parent to become more positively invested in his or her child. In order to provide support that is individualized to the baby and to the family, one of our primary tasks as clinicians is to understand each baby's behavior—the baby's language—so that we can provide the kind of individualized developmental information parents need to understand and become attached to their infant.

Model for Supporting Parents of Premature Infants: the NBO System

In our attempts to develop a seamless model of support that will ease the transition of parents from hospital to home, provide them with ongoing information on their baby's development, and help them cope with the challenges they themselves will face as parents, we developed a model of support based on the NBO system.[1] The NBO was developed especially for pediatric professionals as a relationship-building tool with the primary goal of teaching parents about their newborn infants, thus promoting the parent–infant relationship and fostering the development of the practitioner–family relationship. The NBO system consists of 18 neurobehavioral items. It can be described as a brief, structured observation technique that enables pediatric practitioners to make observations of newborn behavior, such as sleep behavior, the baby's interactive capacities and threshold for stimulation, motor capacities, crying and soothability, and state regulation. The practitioner then can offer interpretation in terms of the infant's current level of functioning and provide anticipatory guidance to parents based on these observations (Table 11-4). For example, the interactive items, which record the baby's response to the face or voice, can show the parent how much stimulation the baby can tolerate without being overwhelmed and can provide an example of the kind and level of interaction that is best suited to the baby. The observations on crying and soothability, in the context of the NBO system, can enable the practitioner to offer parents concrete guidelines on how to deal with crying and how best to soothe their baby.

The goal of the NBO system is to help clinicians capture and describe the complexity and uniqueness of the infant's behavioral adaptation over the first months of life, identify the baby's strengths and areas of concern, and then discover how these behaviors are integrated into a coherent set of behaviors that make up the infant's behavioral signature or his or her individuality. In addition, the practitioner can use the NBO system to involve the parents in identifying the kinds of caregiving techniques that are more likely to foster and promote the baby's adaptation to his or her new environment. Because it is conceptualized as an interactive behavioral observation, the NBO system always is administered in the presence of the family so that it can provide a forum for parents and clinician together to observe and interpret the newborn's behavior. In its complete form, the NBO scale takes approximately 5 to 10 minutes to administer and can be conducted from the first day of life up to 3 months' corrected gestational age. It is designed to be used flexibly so that it can be integrated into routine pediatric examinations performed in the hospital, clinic, or home setting in such a way that it is compatible with the demands of a clinical practice. Research suggests that the NBO system may be an effective tool in helping pediatric professionals support parents in their

Table 11-4 Newborn Behavioral Observations (NBO) System*†

Name ______ **Baby's Gender** ______ **Date of Birth** ______ **Date** ______
Gestational Age ______ **Weight** ______ **Apgar** ______ **Parity** ______
Type of Feeding ______ **Setting** ______ **Practitioner's Name** ______

BEHAVIOR	OBSERVATION RECORD 3	2	1	ANTICIPATORY GUIDANCE
1. Habituation to light	with ease	*Habituates* some difficulty	great difficulty	___ Sleep regulation
2. Habituation to sound	with ease	*Habituates* some difficulty	great difficulty	___ Sleep regulation
	3	2	1	
3. Tone: arms and legs	strong	fairly strong	weak	___ Tone
4. Rooting	strong	fairly strong	weak	___ Feeding
5. Sucking	strong	fairly strong	weak	___ Feeding
6. Hand grasp	strong	fairly strong	weak	___ Strength/Contact
7. Shoulder and neck tone	strong	fairly strong	weak	___ Robustness
8. Crawl	strong	fairly strong	weak	___ Sleep positioning safety
	3	2	1	
9. Response to face and voice	very responsive	moderate	not responsive	___ Social interaction
10. Visual response (to face)	very responsive	moderate	not responsive	___ Social readiness
11. Orientation to voice	very responsive	moderate	not responsive	___ Voice recognition
12. Orientation to sound	very responsive	moderate	not responsive	___ Hearing & attention
13. Visual tracking	very responsive	moderate	not responsive	___ Vision/stimulation
	3	2	1	
14. Crying	very little	moderate amount	a lot	___ Crying
15. Soothability	easily consoled	moderate	with difficulty	___ Soothability
	3	2	1	
16. State regulation	well-organized	moderate	not organized	___ Temperament
17. Response to stress: color, tremors, startles	well-organized	moderate	very stressed	___ Stress threshold
18. Activity level	well modulated	mixed	very high/very low	___ Need for support

Behavioral Profile *(Strengths and Challenges)*

Anticipatory Guidance *(Key Points)*

*Nugent JK, Keefer CH, Minear S, et al: *Understanding newborn behavior and early relationship: The newborn behavioral observations (NBO) system handbook.* Baltimore, in press, Paul H. Brookes Publishing.
†Additional information on training for the NBO is available at: *www.brazelton-institute.com.*

efforts to get to know and understand their infant's development and can be effective in promoting a positive relationship between the clinician and the parents.

Conclusion

Although strong evidence suggests that, for parents of premature infants, the stress of meeting the child's daily needs, the associated financial costs, and the strain of preserving family relationships can place a family at risk of dysfunction, we have presented a model of family-centered care that is designed to reduce the level of stress and the risk of family dysfunction and to promote a positive relationship between parents and their infant. We have proposed an infant-focused, family-centered model of pediatric care that can serve to enhance the child's cognitive, social, and emotional development. We pointed out that this infant-focused approach, which is based on describing the baby's strengths and identifying the kinds of challenges their child is likely to face, can help parents to better understand their infant's individuality and temperament and thus can play a powerful role in strengthening the parent–infant relationship. In addition, we have presented the NBO system as an instrument that pediatricians, nurses, or allied healthcare professionals can use to help parents better understand their infant's development and provide the kind of anticipatory guidance parents require to meet their baby's needs.

We believe that establishing a relationship of trust between clinician and family is the cornerstone for the development of family-centered care. In this chapter, we emphasized the importance of developing a partnership with the parents, and we argued that an infant-focused approach may be best suited to addressing the needs of parents who often are under a lot of stress during the early months after their baby's discharge from the NICU. We believe that the infant-focused nature of this approach—because it is based on individualization of the infant, provision of individualized developmental information, and anticipatory caregiving guidance to parents—can lay the foundation for an enduring, supportive relationship between the pediatric professional and the family that will continue to grow as the neonate moves into infancy and early childhood.

Resources for Families and Clinicians

American Academy of Pediatrics
www.medicalhomeinfo.org

Scroll to "Screening Initiatives," then "Developmental Screening," and then "For Providers" or "To Families."

http://www.aap.org/healthtopics/stages.cfm
http://aappolicy.aappublications.org/cgi/content/full/pediatrics;110/1/184?eaf

Provides extensive information about developmental stages and screening.

Brazelton Institute
Brazelton Institute, Children's Hospital, 1295 Boylston Street, Boston, MA 02215
www.brazelton-institute.com

This website provides information about the Newborn Behavioral Observations (NBO) system and NBO training workshops.

Center for Disease Control
http://www.cdc.gov/ncbddd/child/screen_provider.htm

This website discusses the role of the primary care provider in a child's developmental health.

Developmental Screening Tools
www.dbpeds.org/

This website provides information about the specific use of developmental and behavioral screening tools.

Early Intervention Programs for Infants and Toddlers with Disabilities
http://www.nectac.org/partc/partc.asp#overview

This website describes the Individuals with Disabilities Education Improvement Act of 2004 and provides contacts for Early Intervention Programs that are available in the United States.

REFERENCES

1. Nugent JK, Keefer CH, Minear S, et al: *Understanding newborn behavior and early relationships: the newborn behavioral observations (NBO) system handbook.* Baltimore, in press, Paul H. Brookes Publishing.
2. Bruschweiler-Stern N: Mere a terme et mere premature. In Dugnat M, editor: *Le monde relationnel du bebe.* Ramonville Saint-Agne, 1997, ERES.
3. Fleming AS, Flett GL, Wagner VV: Adjustment in first-time mothers: changes in mood and mood content during the early post-partum months. *Dev Psych* 26:137-143, 1990.
4. Klaus MH, Kennell JH, Klaus PH: *Bonding.* Reading, Mass, 1996, Addison-Wesley.
5. Eisengart SP, Singer LT, Fulton S, et al: Coping and psychological distress in mothers of very low birthweight young children. *Parenting Sci Pract* 3:49-72, 2003.
6. Als H, Lawhon G, Duffy FH, et al: Individualized developmental care for the very-low-birth-weight preterm infant. *JAMA* 272(11):853-8585, 1994.
7. Minde K: The assessment of infants and toddlers with medical conditions and their families. In Osofsky J, Fitzgerald H, editors: *Handbook of infant mental health,* vol 2. New York, 2000, Wiley and Sons.
8. Singer LT, Salvator A, Guo S, et al: Maternal psychological distress and parenting stress after the birth of a very low-birth-weight infant. *JAMA* 281:799-805, 1999.
9. Spiker D, Ferguson J, Brookes-Gunn J: Enhancing maternal interactive behavior and child social competence in low birthweight, premature infants. *Child Dev* 64:754-768, 1993.
10. Gray JE, Safran C, Davis RB, et al: Baby CareLink: using the internet and telemedicine to improve care for high-risk infants. *Pediatrics* 106:1318-1324, 2000.
11. Rutter M: Psychosocial resilience and protective mechanisms. In Rolf J, editor: *Risk and protective factors in the development of psychopathology.* New York, 1990, Cambridge University Press.
12. Werner E: Resilience in development. *Curr Dir Psychol Sci* 4(3):503-515, 1995.
13. Melnyk BM., Feinstein NF, Fairbanks E: Effectiveness of informational/behavioral interventions with parents of low birth weight (LBW) premature infants: an evidence base to guide clinical practice. *Pediatr Nurs* 28:511-516, 2002.
14. Sameroff AJ: Models of development and developmental risk. In Zeanah CH, editor: *Handbook of infant mental health.* New York, 1997, Guilford.
15. Nugent JK, Brazelton TB: Preventive mental health: uses of the Brazelton Scale. In Osofsky J, Fitzgerald H, editors: *WAIMH handbook of infant mental health.* New York, 2000, Wiley.
16. Greenspan S, Wieder S, Nover R, et al: *Infants in multirisk families.* Madison, CT, 1987, International Universities Press.
17. Escobar GL, Littenberg B, Petitti DB: Outcome among surviving very low birthweight infants: a meta-analysis. *Arch Dis Child* 66:204-211, 1993.
18. Affleck G, Tennen H, Rowe J, et al: Mothers, fathers and the crisis of neonatal intensive care. *Infant Ment Health J* 11:1, 1990.
19. Madden SL: *The premies parents' companion.* Boston, 2000, The Harvard Common Press.
20. Harrison H: The principles of family-centered neonatal care. *Pediatrics* 92(5):643-650, 1993.
21. Crockenberg S, Litman C: Autonomy as competence in 2 year olds: maternal correlates of child defiance, compliance and self-assertion. *Dev Psych* 26(6):961-971, 1990.
22. Beeghly M, Brazelton TB, Flannery KA, et al: Specificity of preventative pediatric intervention effects in early infancy. *J Dev Behav Pediatr* 16(3):158-166, 1995.
23. Brazelton TB: *Touchpoints: your child's emotional and behavioral development: birth to 3.* Boston, 1992, Perseus Press.
24. Boukydis CFZ, Lester BML: Infant crying, risk status and social support in families of preterm and term infants. *Early Dev Parent* 7:31-39, 1998.
25. Kleberg A, Westrup B, Stjernqvist K: Developmental outcome, child behaviour and mother-child interaction at 3 years of age following Newborn Individualized Developmental Care and Intervention Program (NIDCAP) intervention. *Early Hum Dev* 60:123-135, 2000.
26. Sajaniemi N, Salokorpi T, von Wendt L: Temperament profiles and their role in neurodevelopmental assessed preterm children at two years of age. *Eur Child Adolesc Psychiatry* 7:145-152, 1998.
27. Hack M, Horbar JD, Malloy MH, et al: Very low birthweight outcomes in the NICHD neonatal network. *Pediatrics* 87:587-597, 1991.
28. Hack M, Taylor HG, Klein N, et al: School outcomes in children with birth weights under 750g. *N Engl J Med* 331:753-759, 1994.

29. Hack M, Klein NK, Taylor HG: Long-term developmental outcomes of low birthweight infants. *Future Child* 5: 176-196, 1995.
30. McCormick MC: Has the prevalence of handicapped infants increased with the improved survival rate of the very low birthweight infant? *Clin Perinatol* 20:263-277, 1993.
31. Thompson RA, Nelson CA: Developmental science and the media: early brain development. *Am Psycholt* 56(1):5-15, 2001.
32. Mouradian LE, Als H, Coster WJ: Neurobehavioral functioning of healthy preterm infants of varying gestational ages. *J Dev Behav Pediatr* 21(6):408-414, 2000.
33. Als H: Toward a synactive theory of development: promise for the assessment and support of infant individuality. *Infant Ment Health J* 3(4):229-234, 1982.
34. Brazelton TB: *Neonatal behavioral assessment scale clinics in developmental medicine, no. 50.* London, 1973, Wm. Heinemann Medical Books.
35. Brazelton TB, Nugent JK: *The newborn behavioral assessment scale.* London, 1995, McKeith Press.
36. Adamson, LB: *Communication development during infancy.* Madison, WI, 1993, Brown and Benchmark.
37. Brazelton TB, Koslowski B, Main M: The origins of reciprocity: the early mother-infant interaction. In Lewis M, Rosenblum L, editors: *The effect of the infant on its caregivers.* New York, 1974, Wiley Interscience.
38. Stern DN: *The motherhood constellation.* New York, 1995, Basic Books.
39. Peters KL: Association between autonomic and motoric systems in the preterm infant. *Clin Nurs Res* 10(1):82-90, 2001.
40. Nugent JK, Blanchard Y: Newborn behavior and development: implications for health care professionals. In Theis KM, Travers JF, editors: *Handbook of human development for health care professionals.* Sudbury, MA, 2006, Jones and Bartlett Publishers.
41. Blanchard Y, Mouradian L: Integrating neurobehavioral concepts into early intervention eligibility evaluation. *Infants Young Child* 13(2):41-50, 2000.
42. D'Apolito K: What is an organized infant? *Neonatal Netw* 10(1):23-29, 1991.
43. Cramer B: Objective and subjective aspects of parent-infant relations. In Osofsky J, editor: *The handbook of infant development.* New York, 1987, Wiley.
44. Stern DN: *The interpersonal world of the infant.* New York, 1985, Basic Books.
45. Zeanah CH, Boris NW, Larrieu JA: Infant development and developmental risk: a review of the past 10 years. *J Am Acad Child Adolesc Psychiatry* 36:165-178, 1997.
46. Field T. Affective and interactive disturbances in infants. In Osofsky J, editor: *The handbook of infant development,* ed 2. New York, 1987, Wiley.
47. Murray L, Cooper PJ: The role of infant and maternal factors in postpartum depression, mother-infant interactions, and infant outcomes. In Murray L, Cooper, editors: *Postpartum depression and child development.* New York/London, 1997, Guilford Press.
48. Hirshberg LM: Clinical interviews with infants and their families. In Zeanah CH, editor: *Handbook of infant mental health.* London/New York, 1993, The Guilford Press.
49. MacDonough SC: Interaction guidance: understanding and treating early infant-caregiver disturbances. In Zeanah C, editor: *Handbook of infant mental health.* New York/London, 1993, The Guilford Press.
50. Zeanah CH, McDonough SC: Clinical approaches to families in early intervention. *Semin Perinatol* 13:513-522, 1989.
51. Sameroff AJ: Models of development and developmental risk. In Zeanah CH, editor: *Handbook of infant mental health.* New York/London, 1993, The Guilford Press.
52. Green M, Palfrey J, editors: *Bright futures: guidelines for health supervision of infants, children and adolescents,* ed 2. Arlington, VA, 2000, National Center for Education in Maternal and Child Health.
53. Committee on Children with Disabilities, American Academy of Pediatrics: Role of the pediatrician in family-centered early intervention services. *Pediatrics* 107(5): 1155-1157, 2001.
54. The American Academy of Pediatrics Statement: medical home. *Pediatrics* 110(1):184-186, 2002.
55. Committee on Children with Disabilities, American Academy of Pediatrics: Developmental surveillance and screening of infants and young children. *Pediatrics* 108: 192-195, 2001.
56. Ferri R, Chiaramonti R, Elia M, et al: Nonlinear EEG analysis during sleep in premature and full-term newborns. *Clin Neurophysiol* 114(7):1176-1180, 2003.
57. Sher MS, Steppe DA, Banks DL: Prediction of lower developmental performances of healthy neonates by neonatal EEG-sleep measures *Pediatr Neurol* 14:137-144, 1996.
58. Pierrehumbert B, Nicole A, Muller-Nix C, et al: Parental post-traumatic reactions after premature birth: implications for sleeping and eating problems in the infant. *Arch Dis Child Fetal Neonatal Ed* 88(5): F400-F404, 2003.
59. Anderson GC: Current knowledge about skin-to-skin (kangaroo) care for preterm infants. *J Perinatol* 11(3):216-226, 1991.
60. Ohgi S, Fukada M, Moriuchi H, et al: Comparison of kangaroo care: behavioral organization, development, and temperament in healthy low-birth weight infants through 1 year. *J Perinatol* 22:374-379, 2002.
61. Vickers A, Ohlsson A, Lacy JB, et al: Massage for promoting growth and development of preterm and/or low birth-weight infants. *Cochrane Database Syst Rev* (2):CD00030, 2004.
62. Dieter JN, Field T, Hernandez-Reif M, et al: Stable preterm infants gain more weight and sleep less after five days of massage therapy. *J Pediatr Psychol* 28(6):403-411, 2003.
63. Ferber SG, Kuint J, Weller A, et al: Massage therapy by mothers and trained professionals enhances weight gain in preterm infants. *Early Hum Dev* 67(1-2):37-45, 2002.
64. Field TM, Schanberg SM, Scafidi F, et al: Tactile/kinesthetic stimulation effects on preterm neonates. *Pediatrics* 77: 654-658, 1986.
65. Thoyre SM: Developmental transition from gavage to oral feeding in the preterm infant. *Annu Rev Nurs Res* 21:61-92, 2003.
66. Dodrill P, McMahon S, Ward E, et al: Long-term oral sensitivity and feeding skills of low-risk pre-term infants. *Early Hum Dev* 76(1):23-37, 2004.
67. Rommel N, De Meyer AM, Feenstra L, et al: Complexity of feeding problems in 700 infants and young children presenting to a tertiary care institution. *J Pediatr Gastroenterol Nutr* 37(1):75-84, 2003.
68. Sobotkova D, Dittrichova J, Mandys F: Comparison of maternal perceptions of preterm and fullterm infants. *Early Dev Parent* 5(2):73-79, 1996.
69. Barr RG, Rotman A, Yaremko J, et al: The crying of infants with colic: a controlled empirical description. *Pediatrics* 90(1):14-21, 1992.
70. Worchel FF, Allen M: Mothers' ability to discriminate cry types in low-birthweight premature and full-term infants. *Child Health Care* 26(3):183-195, 1997.
71. Vergara ER, Bigsby R: *Developmental & therapeutic interventions in the NICU.* Baltimore, 2004, Paul H. Brookes Publishing.
72. Garbarino J: *Children and families in the social environment.* New York, 1992, Aldine de Gruyter.
73. Weissbourd B, Kagan S: Family support programs: catalysts for change. *Am J Orthopsych* 59:20-31, 1989.
74. Wolke D, Gray P, Meyer R: Excessive infant crying: a controlled study of mothers helping mothers. *Pediatrics* 94:322, 1994.
75. Inui TS: What are the sciences of relationship-centered primary care? *J Fam Pract* 42(2):171-177, 1996.
76. Tresolini CP, and the Pew-Fetzer Task Force. *Health professions education and relationship-centered care.* San Francisco, 1994 (reprinted 2000), Pew-Health Professions Commission.

Chapter 12A

Newborn Screening in the Premature Infant

Dara Brodsky, MD

Every state in the United States routinely screens all infants for specific genetic, metabolic, infectious, and/or hormonal disorders. In the majority of cases, early detection and treatment can improve outcomes. At present, each state determines the content of its own newborn screening program. There is wide variation by state in both the number and types of conditions that are tested. The National Newborn Screening and Genetics Resource Center's website (see Resources section) provides a list of the specific tests performed in each state. This chapter focuses on newborn screening in the premature infant, emphasizing the timing of the screening test, specific tests that might be altered by the gestational age of an infant, and general responsibilities of the primary care provider.

Timing of Newborn Screening in the Premature Infant

The initial newborn screening for a premature infant, regardless of the infant's gestational age, is sent at the same time as for a full-term infant, which is usually by 72 hours of age. Each state has slightly different recommendations for follow-up testing of premature infants. In Massachusetts, the newborn screening program recommends that premature infants in the neonatal intensive care unit (NICU) should have a second specimen sent at approximately 2 weeks of age or at discharge, whichever is sooner. This state program recommends that additional specimens be sent for infants born weighing less than 1500 g at 2, 4, 6, and 10 weeks of age or until the infant reaches a weight of 1500 g. After the infant's discharge from the hospital, primary care providers may need to repeat the test if the infant had received a blood transfusion (see section on effects of blood transfusion on newborn screening results) or has any abnormal result as per the recommendations of their state program. Sometimes an abnormal result will prompt more specific testing for a disorder, whereas other abnormal tests require repeat screening because they may represent a false-positive result. Thus, it is important that primary care providers be aware of the effect of prematurity on specific newborn screening tests (see next section).

Specific Test Results Potentially Affected by Prematurity

Congenital adrenal hyperplasia

Congenital adrenal hyperplasia as a result of 21-hydroxylase deficiency is screened by measuring 17-hydroxyprogesterone (17-OHP) levels by an enzyme immunoassay or radioimmunoassay.[1] Prematurity is associated with physiologic elevation of 17-OHP. Some newborn screening programs use higher levels of normal values that are adjusted by weight for infants born prematurely. These programs will report an appropriate *normal, borderline*, or *presumptive positive* value for specific weights. For example, some states use a positive value of greater than 90 ng/ml if the infant weighs more than 2250 g, but if an infant weighs less than 1250 g, a positive value of greater than 160 ng/ml is used for the presumptive diagnosis of congenital adrenal hyperplasia. These higher normal values usually are detected while the infant is still in the hospital.

If a premature infant has an elevated 17-OHP level, the clinician should examine the infant for ambiguous genitalia (virilization in females). If there is a high clinical suspicion for congenital adrenal hyperplasia or if the value is presumptive positive, the neonatologist will measure a serum 17-OHP level, evaluate the infant for a salt-losing crisis by measuring electrolyte levels, and obtain an endocrine consultation. If the infant has a normal examination and a borderline high 17-OHP level, a repeat screen is sent as soon as possible. If the repeat 17-OHP value remains elevated, an endocrine consultation usually is obtained.

In addition to the false-positive screen results associated with premature infants, sick infants may have false-positive 17-OHP levels. Infants exposed to maternal steroids or postnatal steroids can have altered results as well.

Congenital hypothyroidism

This section briefly highlights newborn screening for hypothyroidism in the premature infant (See Chapter 7A for a more extensive explanation).

Congenital hypothyroidism is tested in all 50 states by using a radioimmunoassay or fluoroimmunoassay for thyroxine, thyroid-stimulating hormone, or both.[1] Thyroid function varies with the age of sample collection; therefore, age-appropriate reference ranges must be used for proper interpretation of test results. Premature infants may have an abnormal screening result because of physiologic immaturity, transient thyroid dysfunction, or permanent hypothyroidism.

Because a false-negative newborn screen may occur, primary care providers should monitor all infants for signs and symptoms of hypothyroidism, which include prolonged jaundice, a large posterior fontanelle, dry and mottled skin, hypothermia, bradycardia, poor weight gain, constipation, and goiter. If the infant has some of these signs and/or symptoms, the primary care provider should verify that appropriate newborn screening has occurred and consider further evaluation.

Cystic fibrosis

The immunoreactive trypsin (IRT) test, which uses an immunoassay, is the screening test for cystic fibrosis used in the neonatal period.[1] Normal values vary, depending on the test kit and antibody used.[1] Pancreatitis and other conditions, such as prolonged labor, diaphragmatic hernia, and perinatal stress, can affect the IRT. DNA testing followed by a sweat test is the most reliable method for diagnosing cystic fibrosis.

Homocystinuria

Infants with homocystinuria will have elevated methionine levels (>2 mg/dl), usually detected by tandem mass spectrometry. Premature infants may have a false-positive result because of high intake of protein or liver immaturity with transiently decreased activity of enzymes involved in the metabolism of methionine and homocysteine.[1]

Effects of Intake on Newborn Screening Results

Infants with inadequate oral intake or inadequate amino acid intake may have inaccurate testing for maple syrup urine disease, phenylketonuria, and other amino acid disorders.[2] Infants receiving total parenteral nutrition also may have altered newborn screening results for maple syrup urine disease, homocystinuria, and other amino acid disorders.[2] The test for galactosemia is not as reliable if the infant is on a nonlactose diet or is receiving intravenous fluids.[2]

Effects of Blood Transfusion on Newborn Screening Results

The results of the newborn screening test may be unreliable if the infant has received a blood transfusion. A transfusion will alter the results of the hemoglobinopathy by testing donor hemoglobins. Some screens for galactosemia may be altered by blood transfusions. Blood transfusions may give false-negative 17-OHP results in low-birth-weight infants because of hemodilution.

If possible, *before* transfusing an infant, the clinician should obtain a newborn screening test, independent of the age of the infant. If testing has not been completed before blood transfusion, the clinician should repeat a newborn screening test at approximately 2 to 3 days after the last transfusion. In our NICU, an additional specimen also is sent 2 months after the infant's final transfusion.

Primary Care Provider Responsibilities

The primary care provider should be aware of the specific tests that are performed in his or her own state program. If the primary care provider has not officially received the infant's screening result, he or she must not assume that the results are normal. A few reasons why the provider may not have received an abnormal newborn screening result include the following: difficulty finding and notifying the provider, the test may not have been sent, a mistake was made in sending out the results, or the results were sent to a different provider. Sometimes the physician of record during the infant's stay in the NICU may not be the infant's primary care provider. Thus, the provider should obtain an official report of each infant's most recent newborn screening result.

Primary care providers must be aware of the potential false-positive and false-negative results after testing a premature infant and follow the recommendations outlined in this chapter and by their state program. Infants who are born prematurely or who have received blood transfusions may have a normal newborn screening result but still require follow-up testing.

If previous values have been abnormal or if the infant has received a blood transfusion before the most recent newborn screen, the screening test should be repeated. Once an infant is identified as having an abnormal test result, more specific and sensitive testing is warranted. If these tests confirm the abnormal result, the primary care provider should arrange for appropriate follow-up. Because certain tests may identify the carrier state or an asymptomatic carrier state, primary care providers should provide appropriate counseling or referral, because these results can have an impact on the female infant's future pregnancies and on other family members.

Resources for Families and Clinicians

American Academy of Pediatrics (AAP)
www.aap.org/healthtopics/newbornscreening.cfm

This website provides AAP policies about genetic testing resources on Newborn Screening Policy and System Development for the primary care provider.

Action Sheets
www.acmg.net/resources/policies/ACT/condition-analyte-links.htm

This resource is from the American College of Medical Genetics and the Maternal and Child Health Bureau/Health Resources and Services Administration. It provides primary care providers with additional details on many of the conditions detected by expanded newborn screening. The first page of the ACT sheet provides basic and clinical information with follow-up recommendations if an abnormal report is obtained. The second page provides a list of websites to help identify specialists for consultations.

Centers for Disease Control and Prevention, Division of Laboratory Sciences
www.cdc.gov/nceh/dls/newborn_screening.htm

This website contains PowerPoint presentations about quality assurance of newborn screening.

March of Dimes
www.marchofdimes.com/pnhec/298_834.asp

This website provides families with a description of the common disorders tested in newborn screening programs.

National Center of Medical Home Initiatives
www.medicalhomeinfo.org/screening/newborn.html

This website provides a list of state-specific screening tests, national data, and numerous resources available to clinicians.

The National Newborn Screening and Genetics Resource Center
http://genes-r-us.uthscsa.edu/

This organization is a cooperative agreement between the Maternal and Child Health Bureau, Genetic Services Branch, and the University of Texas Health Science Center at San Antonio. This group provides information and resources about newborn screening and genetics to benefit health-care professionals and families, as well as government officials.

Acknowledgments

The author thanks Marvin L. Mitchell, MD, and Inderneel Sahai, MD, for critical review of this chapter.

REFERENCES

1. Committee on Genetics: Newborn screening fact sheets. *Pediatrics* 98(3):473-501, 1996.
2. Metabolic/Genetic Newborn Screening Program in Tennessee: Guide for practitioners. State of Tennessee Department of Health. Available at: *http://www2.state.tn.us/health/Downloads/education.pdf.*

Chapter 12B

Car Seat Safety for the Premature Infant

Michele DeGrazia, RNC, PhD, NNP

When the premature infant is ready to go home from the hospital, the discharging physician must make an important decision: Can the infant safely travel in a car seat? Unlike most full-term infants, premature infants are at risk for oxygen desaturation events while positioned in their car seat. These events encompass a constellation of signs, including apnea or frequent periodic breathing, bradycardia, and/or oxygen desaturations. Maintaining oxygen saturation of premature infants >93% reduces sudden infant death and promotes growth.[1] Recurrent episodes of oxygen desaturation events may lead to hypoxemia and hypoxia and may be associated with adverse behavioral, cognitive, and motor outcomes if these events are not detected.[2-4] Parents may not be able to perceive desaturations because of varying skin tones and hematocrit levels.[5,6]

The American Academy of Pediatrics (AAP) recommends that every infant born less than 37 weeks' gestation be observed in his or her car seat for a period of time before hospital discharge.[7-9] This observation period is called the *infant car seat challenge* (ICSC) and has become standard practice in approximately 75% of hospitals in the United States.[10] Following the lead of the United States, other countries have instituted the practice of predischarge ICSC testing.[11-13]

Although many healthcare institutions in the United States have complied with the AAP's recommendations to perform a car seat test in premature infants, there are no standardized guidelines about how to perform the test. Having acknowledged the lack of standardization, neonatal healthcare providers and institutions have independently addressed this issue and have developed their own set of criteria and procedures for testing.[10,12] Unfortunately, this has led to inconsistencies in infant selection criteria, pass and fail limits, and test duration.[10] The algorithm that we recommend for discharge of a premature infant to a car seat or bed is outlined in Figure 12B-1. In brief, the infant born less than 37 weeks' gestation should be positioned in his or her car seat and monitored for 90 minutes. If the infant has apnea for more than 20 seconds; an irregular respiratory effort, a desaturation <93% for more than 20 seconds, or a heart rate <80 beats/min for more than 10 seconds, the infant has failed the ICSC and should not be discharged home in a car seat.

Collectively, the 10 studies that have examined the results of the ICSC found that 15% to 20% of premature infants experience oxygen desaturation events when positioned in their car seat.[12-21] As outlined in Table 12B-1, these studies have identified several risk factors for oxygen desaturation events. Specifically, the infant's gestational age, posture, tone, and length of time in the car seat are important determinants of car seat tolerance. Primary care providers should be particularly attentive to infants with more than one risk factor.

If the premature infant fails the ICSC, the AAP recommends a crash-tested *car bed* for travel. In addition, because stability testing for the ICSC is not yet complete, risk factors for oxygen desaturation events should be considered when evaluating the need for a car bed. If the infant has several risk factors, especially poor tone, the practitioner may choose to forego the ICSC test and recommend a car bed. Federally approved infant car beds can be purchased in the United States from Mercury Distributing or Cosco. Products designed to stabilize the infant's head, such as inserts and head bands, have not been completely successful at eliminating oxygen desaturation events.[22,23]

ALGORITHM FOR DISCHARGE OF A PREMATURE INFANT TO CAR SEAT OR CAR BED

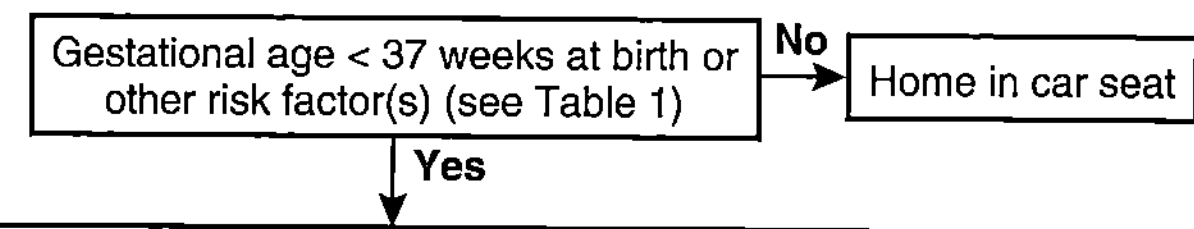

Yes

Infant Car Seat Selection

- The AAP recommends that premature infant car seats should have a distance of 10 inches from lower harness slot to seat and <5 1/2 inches in from the crotch strap to the seat back.
- Infant-only car seat with a 5-point or 3-point restraint system.
- Car seats >5 years old are considered outdated and are not recommended for use.

Infant Car Seat Challenge (ICSC):

- Position infant in (his or her own) car seat according to current AAP infant child safety seat recommendations.
- Monitor breathing, heart rate, and oxygen saturation for 90 minutes.* Note: if the ride home will last longer than 90 minutes, consider testing for that length of time.

Apnea (>20 seconds)*
Oxygen desaturation (<93% for >20 seconds)
Bradycardia (<80 for >10 seconds)*
Irregular breathing pattern = intermittent tachypnea or periodic breathing (frequent pauses lasting <3 seconds), especially if there are brief drops in oxygen saturation below 93%

No → **PASS** → Discharge home in **car seat**

Educate parent(s) that:

- There is no guarantee that the infant will not have a problem in the future.
- They must limit the time the infant spends in car seat to less than 1 hour.
- The infant should be observed by an adult during travel in a car seat.
- The car seat registration card should be mailed in so that they can be contacted about car seat recalls.
- Extra layers of clothing to keep the premature infant warm should be placed <u>over</u> the infant <u>after</u> the buckle is secure to ensure that the straps are not too loose.

Yes → **FAIL** → Discharge home in **car bed**

Retesting:

- Consider retesting while in the car bed if the infant has not been monitored in the supine position prior to the ICSC and/or has known or suspected gastroesophageal reflux.
- If the infant fails the test in the car bed, the infant either needs to be monitored in the hospital for an additional 5–7 days and then retested or needs to be discharged home with a monitor.

Educate parent(s) that:

- The infant should be observed by an adult during travel in a car bed.
- They should not place their infant in other types of seating devices (swings, infant seats) until infant demonstrates good head control in a sitting position.
- The car bed registration card should be mailed in so that they can be contacted about car bed recalls.
- Extra layers of clothing to keep the premature infant warm should be placed <u>over</u> the infant <u>after</u> the buckle is secure to ensure that the straps are not too loose.

Transition to car seat when:

- Passes repeat ICSC 1–2 months after discharge
- If this is impractical, we suggest that the infant remain in the car bed until he/she demonstrates complete head control in a sitting position.

FIGURE 12B-1 *Obtained from: Children's Hospital of Boston (2004) Policy and Procedure References; *AAP* = American Academy of Pediatrics; *ICSC* = The Infant Car Seat Challenge. Please note that this is a recommended algorithm that does not represent a professional standard of care; care should be revised to meet individual patient needs.

Table 12B-1 Risk Factors for Oxygen Desaturation Events in Car Seats

Prematurity	Premature infants have more serious oxygen desaturation events, and these events occur more frequently.[15,17,19,20]
Position of a car seat	The more upright the car seat is positioned (>45 degree angle), the greater chance of oxygen desaturation events.[12,18,20]
Tone	Infants with diminished tone are at greater risk for impaired oxygenation in the car seat.[14,18]
Posture	Flexion of the head on the body leads to narrowing of the upper airway and greater chance of oxygen desaturation.[23]
Time	The longer the premature or term infant remains in the car seat, the greater likelihood he or she will experience a problem.[14,17,18]
Sleep	Sleeping infants in car seats are more likely to spend time in active sleep, which increases the risk of periodic breathing.[16] In addition, relaxation during sleep can result in poor posture.[13]
Genetic disorders	Infants who have genetic disorders that affect their tone and breathing have been described to be at risk for oxygen desaturation events when positioned in their car seat.[14]
Gender	Some studies have not detected any difference between genders,[12,13,17,19] whereas others demonstrated a weak association between oxygen desaturation events and male infants positioned in car seats.[20,21]

Although there are no current AAP recommendations for testing an infant in a car bed, the discharging physician should consider such a test if the infant has not had cardiorespiratory monitoring in the supine position before the ICSC. This is especially important if the infant has known or suspected gastroesophageal reflux. If the infant fails the test in the car bed, the infant either needs to be monitored in the hospital for an additional 5 to 7 days and then retested or needs to be discharged home with a monitor.

Transitioning the infant from the car bed to the traditional car seat has become the responsibility of the primary care provider. Unfortunately, no studies have determined *when* this should occur. Repeating the ICSC test 1 to 2 months after discharge is one way to determine whether an infant is ready for a traditional car seat. If this option is impractical, we suggest that the infant remain in the car bed until he or she demonstrates complete head control while sitting, provided the infant has not outgrown the bed.

Even when an infant passes a car seat test, adult supervision remains essential. Whenever possible, an adult should ride in the back seat to observe the infant. In addition, car travel should be limited for the first 2 months after discharge, and travel time should be limited to less than 1 hour. If travel for longer periods of time is necessary, then ideally parents should briefly stop the motor vehicle at 1-hour intervals and remove their infant from the car seat. Premature infants should not be allowed to sleep in their car seat for long periods of time.

Providers seeking more information about car seat testing should refer to the AAP website for the most current recommendations. In addition, many communities have child passenger safety (CPS) technicians (typically a designated nurse, local police officer, or firefighter), who have been trained in the safe positioning of the car seat in the car. Furthermore, the website of the National Highway Traffic Safety Administration (NHTSA; *www.nhtsa.dot.gov*) provides a wealth of information on car seat safety issues and a listing of CPS technicians by state.

Resources for Families and Clinicians

The Automotive Safety Program
www.preventinjury.org 317-274-2977

The program offers information and a training course on transporting children with special needs.

Available Car Safety Seats
www.aap.org/family/carseatguide.htm

This website describes the different car safety seat options. For a description of car safety seats that are available for children with special needs, refer to the AAP brochure, "Safe Transportation of Children with Special Needs: A Guide for Families and Car Safety Seats: A Guide for Families."

Child Passenger Safety Contact Locator
www.nhtsa.dot.gov/people/injury/childps/Contacts/index.cfm

This website offered by the National Highway Traffic Safety Administration allows one to contact a local car safety seat technician.

REFERENCES

1. Poets CF: When do infants need additional inspired oxygen? A review of the current literature. *Pediatr Pulmonol* 26: 424-428, 1998.
2. Bass JL, Corwin M, Gozal, et al: The effect of chronic or intermittent hypoxia on cognition in childhood: a review of the evidence. *Pediatrics* 114(3):805-816, 2004.
3. Newburger JW, Silbert AR, Buckley LP, et al: Cognitive function and age at repair of transposition of the great arteries in children. *N Engl J Med* 310(23):1495-1499, 1984.
4. Perlman JM, Volpe JJ: Episodes of apnea and bradycardia in the preterm newborn: impact on cerebral circulation. *Pediatrics* 76(3):333-338, 1985.

5. Lees MH: Cyanosis of the newborn infant. *J Pediatr* 77(3):484-498, 1970.
6. Miller MJ, Martin RJ: Apnea in infancy, progress in diagnosis and implications for management. *Neonat Respir Dis* 8(1),1998.
7. American Academy of Pediatrics. Committee on Injury and Poison Prevention and Committee on Fetus and Newborn: Safe transportation of premature infants. *Pediatrics* 87(1):120-122, 1991.
8. American Academy of Pediatrics. Committee on Injury and Poison Prevention and Committee on Fetus and Newborn: Safe transportation of premature and low birth weight infants. *Pediatrics* 97(5):758-60, 1996.
9. American Academy of Pediatrics. Committee on Injury and Poison Prevention: Safe transportation of newborns at hospital discharge. *Pediatrics* 104(4):986-987, 1999.
10. Williams LE, Martin JE: Car seat challenges: where are we in implementation of these programs? *J Perinat Neonatal Nurs* 17(2):158-163, 2003.
11. Fetus and Newborn Committee, CPS: Assessment of babies for car seat safety before hospital discharge. *Paediatr Child Health* 5(1):53-56, 2000.
12. Mullen D, Coutts J: Monitoring premature babies in car seats: the car seat challenge. *J Neonat Nutr* 8(4):129-131, 2002.
13. Nagase H, Yonetani M, Uetani Y, et al: Effects of child seats on the cardiorespiratory function of newborns. *Pediatr Int* 44(1):63, 2002.
14. Bass JL, Mehta KA: Oxygen desaturation of selected term infants in car seats. *Pediatrics* 96(2 pt 1):288-290, 1995.
15. Bass JL, Mehta KA, Camara J: Monitoring premature infants in car seats: implementing the American Academy of Pediatrics policy in a community hospital. *Pediatrics* 91(6):1137-1141, 1993.
16. Hertz G, Aggarwal R, Rosenfeld WN, et al: Premature infants in car seats: effect of sleep state on breathing. *J Sleep Res* 3(3):186-190, 1994.
17. Merchant JR, Worwa C, Porter S, et al: Respiratory instability of term and near-term healthy newborn infants in car safety seats. *Pediatrics* 108(3):647-652, 2001.
18. Smith PS, Turner BS: The physiologic effects of positioning premature infants in car seats. *Neonatal Netw* 9(4):11-15, 1990.
19. Willett LD, Leuschen MP, Nelson LS, et al: Risk of hypoventilation in premature infants in car seats. *J Pediatr* 109(2):245-248, 1986.
20. Willett LD, Leuschen MP, Nelson LS, et al: Ventilatory changes in convalescent infants positioned in car seats. *J Pediatr* 115(3):451-455, 1989.
21. Young B, Shapira S, Finer NN: Predischarge car seat safety study for premature infants. *Paediatr Child Health* 1(3): 202-205, 1996.
22. Dollberg S, Yacov G, Mimouni F, et al: Effect of head support on oxygen saturation in preterm infants restrained in a car seat. *Am J of Perinatol* 19(3):115-118, 2002.
23. Tonkin SL, McIntosh CG, Hadden W, et al: Simple car seat insert to prevent upper airway narrowing in preterm infants: a pilot study. *Pediatrics* 112(4):907-913, 2003.

Chapter 12C

Immunizations

Rosanne K. Buck, RNC, MS, NNP

One of the most important goals of pediatric healthcare maintenance is the prevention of communicable diseases. Immunity of many diseases can be acquired actively and/or passively. Vaccination plays a key role in the acquisition of active immunity. Obtaining active immunity from vaccinations is beneficial because the recipient does not experience the actual disease or its complications. Passive immunity can be conferred by placental transfer of maternal antibodies during the second half of the last trimester.

Because premature infants do not receive the passive immunity and thus lack adequate immune defenses, they are more likely to experience complications of vaccine-preventable diseases. Thus, it is absolutely essential that premature infants receive appropriate active immunity by ensuring the complete schedule of immunizations at the appropriate age. This chapter focuses on specific recommendations for vaccinating the premature infant, including individual vaccines, timing, dosing, method of administration, and potential complications.

Epidemiology

Despite their increased risk for acquiring infections, premature infants are less likely to receive immunizations on time.[1] In one Centers for Disease Control and Prevention (CDC) study assessing immunization rates among premature and low-birth-weight (LBW) infants compared with full-term infants, 52% to 65% of infants weighing less than 1500 g at birth were up to date at age 6 months compared with 65% to 76% of term infants. At age 24 months, 78% to 86% infants weighing less than 1500 g were up to date, significantly less than heavier infants who had rates of 84% to 89%.[2] Although the American Academy of Pediatrics (AAP) Committee on Infectious Diseases recommends that prematurely born infants should receive immunizations at the same chronological age as infants born at term,[3] primary care providers remain hesitant to immunize prematurely born infants who have complicated medical histories. Some primary care providers and parents of prematurely born infants mistakenly believe that other factors, such as birthweight, current weight, or degree of prematurity, should influence the timing of immunizations for children born prematurely.[4] However, gestational age at birth does not appear to alter a person's antibody response. Indeed, prematurely born children immunized at the recommended chronological ages displayed antibody responses similar to those of children born at term for most immunizing antigens in one 3-year follow-up study, displaying less robust antibody levels in only one *Haemophilus* polyribosylribotol phosphate antibody and poliovirus serotype 3.[5] However, even though prematurely born children can mount adequate responses when immunized at the recommended chronological age, they often receive immunizations on a delayed schedule.

Vaccine-Specific Recommendations

Hepatitis B vaccine

Previous recommendations to delay initial administration of hepatitis B (Hep B) vaccine until a body weight of 2000 g have now been revoked. Multiple international studies confirm that preterm infants seroconvert in response to Hep B vaccine by 30 days of age, regardless of gestational age and birth weight.[1] At present, the AAP, the Advisory Committee on Immunizations Practices (ACIP), and the American Academy of Family Physicians (AAFP) recommend that all children be immunized against Hep B virus with a three-dose series. In infants born to hepatitis B surface antigen (HBsAg)-negative mothers, the first dose should be given at hospital discharge, at 1 month of age, or weight of 2000 g, whichever occurs first. If the mother is HBsAg positive *or* the maternal Hep B status is unknown and the infant's weight is less than 2000 g, Hep B vaccine and Hep B immune globulin should be administered within 12 hours of birth. This vaccine dose should *not* be included in the three-dose series; another dose at 1 month of age should be considered the first dose, followed by the routinely recommended schedule. Thus, infants with a birthweight less than 2000 g born to mothers with unknown Hep B status and term or preterm infants born to positive HBsAg mothers should receive a total of four doses of Hep B vaccine. The last dose should never be given before 6 months' chronologic age.[1,6] Table 12C-1 provides a summary of Hep B immunoprophylaxis.

Diphtheria, tetanus, and acellular pertussis vaccine, *Haemophilus influenzae* type B conjugate vaccine, and inactivated poliovirus vaccine

All medically stable preterm and/or LBW infants should begin routine childhood immunization with full doses of diphtheria, tetanus, and acellular pertussis (DTaP) vaccine, *Haemophilus influenzae* type B (Hib) conjugate vaccine, and inactivated poliovirus vaccine licensed by the Food and Drug Administration (FDA) at 2 months' chronologic age, regardless of gestational age or birthweight.[1] Vaccine doses should not be reduced or divided when administered to preterm and/or LBW infants. Although studies have shown decreased immune responses to some vaccines given to very LBW, extremely LBW, and very early gestational age (<29 weeks) neonates, most of these infants produce sufficient vaccine-induced immunity to prevent disease. The severity of vaccine-preventable

Table 12C-1 Hepatitis B Immunoprophylaxis for Premature and Low-Birth-Weight Infants*

Maternal Status	Infant ≥2000 g	Infant <2000 g
HBsAg positive	Hepatitis B vaccine + HBIG (within 12 hours of birth)	Hepatitis B vaccine + HBIG (within 12 hours of birth)
	Immunize with three vaccine doses at 0, 1, and 6 months' chronological age	Immunize with four vaccine doses at 0, 1, 2–3, and 6–7 months' chronological age
	Check anti-HBs and HBsAg at 9–15 months of age[†]	Check anti-HBs and HBsAg at 9–15 months of age[†]
	If infant is HBsAg and anti-HBs negative, reimmunize with three doses at 2-month intervals and retest	If infant is HBsAg and anti-HBs negative, reimmunize with three doses at 2-month intervals and retest
HBsAg status unknown	Hepatitis B vaccine (by 12 hours of age) + HBIG (within 7 days of life) if mother tests HBsAg positive	Hepatitis B vaccine + HBIG (by 12 hours of age)
	Test mother for HBsAg immediately	Test mother for HBsAg immediately and if results are unavailable within 12 hours, give infant HBIG
	Once mother's status is known, follow that protocol for future immunizations	Once mother's status is known, follow that protocol for future immunizations
HBsAg negative	Hepatitis B vaccine at birth preferred	Hepatitis B vaccine dose 1 at 30 days' chronological age if medically stable, or at hospital discharge if before 30 days' chronological age
	Immunize with three doses at 0–2, 1–4, 6–18 months' chronological age	Immunize with three doses at 1–2, 2–4, and 6–18 months' chronological age
	May give hepatitis B-containing combination vaccine beginning at 6–8 weeks' chronological age	May give hepatitis B-containing combination vaccine beginning at 6–9 weeks' chronological age
	Follow-up anti-HBs and HBsAg testing is not needed	Follow-up anti-HBs and HBsAg testing is not needed

Note: This table is modified from the original.
From: Saari TN, American Academy of Pediatrics Committee on Infectious Diseases: Immunization of preterm and low birth weight infants. *Pediatrics* 112(1):196, 2003.
HBs, antibody to HBsAg; *HBIG*, Hepatitis B immune globulin; *HBsAg*, hepatitis B surface antigen.
*Extremes of gestational age and birth weight are no longer a consideration for timing of hepatitis B vaccine doses.
†Some experts prefer to perform serologic testing 1–3 months after completion of the primary series.

diseases in preterm infants precludes any delay in initiating the administration of these vaccines.

Pneumococcal conjugate vaccine

All preterm and LBW infants are considered at increased risk for invasive pneumococcal disease, and medically stable preterm infants should receive full doses of pneumococcal conjugate vaccine (PCV) beginning at 2 months' chronologic age.

Influenza vaccine

All preterm infants are considered at high risk for complications of influenza virus infection and should be offered influenza vaccine beginning at 6 months of age and as soon as possible before the beginning and during the influenza season. Preterm and LBW infants receiving influenza vaccine for the first time will require two doses of the vaccine administered 1 month apart.[1] FluMist, a live attenuated virus intranasal vaccine, is FDA approved for healthy individuals 5 to 49 years old. Because no data are available regarding transmission of attenuated influenza virus to immunocompromised patients from vaccine recipients, it is recommended that persons in contact with such individuals be vaccinated with an inactivated vaccine product.[7] In a severe outbreak of influenza, it could be feasible to administer the attenuated nasal spray to household contacts if the injectible inactivated vaccine were in limited supply.

Hepatitis A vaccine

Administration of hepatitis A vaccine (HAV) is now universally recommended for all children at age 1 year (12–23 months).[3] The two doses in the series should be administered at least 6 months apart. States or communities with preexisting HAV programs for children 2 to 18 years of age are encouraged to continue these programs. Two forms of HAV are available: Havrix and Vaqta. The Havrix vaccine contains a preservative, whereas the Vaqta vaccine does not. Although the vaccines are similar, the AAP recommends that patients should always receive the same product type.[3,7]

Timing

Medically stable preterm and LBW infants should receive all routinely recommended childhood vaccines at the same chronologic age as recommended for full-term infants. Under most circumstances, gestational age at birth and birthweight should not affect the immunization timing of preterm or LBW infants. If an immunization series was initiated while the infant was in the neonatal intensive care unit, documentation and verbal communication should be a priority provision to the accepting primary care provider. Many states provide an immunization record book that is given to the parent or caretaker upon discharge. The parent or caregiver should be instructed to bring the record to the first appointment with the primary care provider. Catch-up immunizations should be considered for infants whose immunizations have been delayed. Figure 12C-1 shows the current recommended immunization schedule in the United States.

Dosing

The dose of a vaccine should not be reduced or divided when it is administered to a preterm or LBW infant. Many practitioners have avoided giving more than three to four injections at one visit, thereby delaying certain immunizations. The CDC recommends giving all scheduled vaccines during each office visit, regardless of the number of injections required. Combination products (Table 12C-2) could ensure that the ACIP/AAP/AFP schedule is followed by reducing the number of injections and appointments.[7,8] Combination vaccines benefit the general public through decreased cost of administration, increased compliance, ease of storage, and improved record keeping and tracking. However, a drawback to the currently available combination products is the overlap in components of the different products.

Administration

The anterolateral thigh is the site of choice when administering vaccines intramuscularly to preterm infants. The choice of needle length used for intramuscularly administered vaccine is made on the basis of available muscle mass of the infant and may be less than the standard ⅞-inch to 1-inch length used for full-term infants.[9]

The Childhood Immunizations Schedule is continually changing and is updated and reviewed annually. Continued monitoring of updated information and review of the recommendations should be a yearly routine of the primary care provider. Current updated information regarding vaccines can be found at the AAP website (*www.cispimmunize.org*) or the CDC pink book online (*http://www.cdc.gov*).

Potential Complications

Primary care providers should be aware of the complications associated with the administration of immunizations. In general, children born prematurely have similar reactions to vaccines as those born at term. Elevated levels of C-reactive protein and interleukin-6, which are associated with bacterial sepsis, have been observed following

DEPARTMENT OF HEALTH AND HUMAN SERVICES • CENTERS FOR DISEASE CONTROL AND PREVENTION

Recommended Immunization Schedule for Ages 0–6 Years UNITED STATES • 2007

Vaccine ▼ Age ▶	Birth	1 month	2 months	4 months	6 months	12 months	15 months	18 months	19–23 months	2–3 years	4–6 years
Hepatitis B[1]	HepB	HepB		see footnote 1		HepB				HepB Series	
Rotavirus[2]			Rota	Rota	Rota						
Diphtheria, Tetanus, Pertussis[3]			DTaP	DTaP	DTaP		DTaP				DTaP
Haemophilus influenzae type b[4]			Hib	Hib	*Hib*[4]	Hib			Hib		
Pneumococcal[5]			PCV	PCV	PCV	PCV				PCV PPV	
Inactivated Poliovirus			IPV	IPV		IPV					IPV
Influenza[6]							Influenza (Yearly)				
Measles, Mumps, Rubella[7]						MMR					MMR
Varicella[8]						Varicella					Varicella
Hepatitis A[9]							HepA (2 doses)			HepA Series	
Meningococcal[10]										MPSV4	

Range of recommended ages

Catch-up immunization

Certain high-risk groups

This schedule indicates the recommended ages for routine administration of currently licensed childhood vaccines, as of December 1, 2006, for children through age 6 years. For additional information see www.cdc.gov/nip/recs/child-schedule.htm. Any dose not administered at the recommended age should be administered at any subsequent visit when indicated and feasible. Additional vaccines may be licensed and recommended during the year. Licensed combination vaccines may be used whenever any components of the combination are indicated and other components of the vaccine are not contraindicated and if approved by the Food and Drug Administration for that dose of the series. Providers should consult the respective ACIP statement for detailed recommendations. Clinically significant adverse events that follow immunization should be reported to the Vaccine Adverse Event Reporting System (VAERS). Guidance about how to obtain and complete a VAERS form is available at www.vaers.hhs.gov or by telephone, 800-822-7967.

1. **Hepatitis B vaccine (HepB).** *(Minimum age: birth)*
   At birth:
   - Administer monovalent HepB to all newborns prior to hospital discharge.
   - If mother is HBsAg-positive, administer HepB and 0.5 mL of hepatitis B immune globulin (HBIG) within 12 hours of birth.
   - If mother's HBsAg status is unknown, administer HepB within 12 hours of birth. Determine the HBsAg status as soon as possible and if HBsAg-positive, administer HBIG (no later than age 1 week).
   - If mother is HBsAg-negative, the birth dose can only be delayed with physician's order and mothers' negative HBsAg laboratory report documented in the infant's medical record.

   Following the birth dose:
   - The HepB series should be completed with either monovalent HepB or a combination vaccine containing HepB. The second dose should be administered at age 1–2 months. The final dose should be administered at age ≥24 weeks. Infants born to HBsAg-positive mothers should be tested for HBsAg and antibody to HBsAg after completion of 3 or more doses in a licensed HepB series, at age 9–18 months (generally at the next well-child visit).

   4-month dose of HepB:
   - It is permissible to administer 4 doses of HepB when combination vaccines are given after the birth dose. If monovalent HepB is used for doses after the birth dose, a dose at age 4 months is not needed.
2. **Rotavirus vaccine (Rota).** *(Minimum age: 6 weeks)*
   - Administer the first dose between 6 and 12 weeks of age. Do not start the series later than age 12 weeks.
   - Administer the final dose in the series by 32 weeks of age. Do not administer a dose later than age 32 weeks.
   - There are insufficient data on safety and efficacy outside of these age ranges.
3. **Diphtheria and tetanus toxoids and acellular pertussis vaccine (DTaP).** *(Minimum age: 6 weeks)*
   - The fourth dose of DTaP may be administered as early as age 12 months, provided 6 months have elapsed since the third dose.
   - Administer the final dose in the series at age 4–6 years.
4. ***Haemophilus influenzae* type b conjugate vaccine (Hib).** *(Minimum age: 6 weeks)*
   - If PRP-OMP (PedvaxHIB® or ComVax® [Merck]) is administered at ages 2 and 4 months, a dose at age 6 months is not required.
   - TriHiBit® (DTaP/Hib) combination products should not be used for primary immunization but can be used as boosters following any Hib vaccine in ≥12 months olds.
5. **Pneumococcal vaccine.** *(Minimum age: 6 weeks for Pneumococcal Conjugate Vaccine (PCV); 2 years for Pneumococcal Polysaccharide Vaccine (PPV))*
   - Administer PCV at ages 24-59 months in certain high-risk groups. Administer PPV to certain high-risk groups aged ≥2 years. See *MMWR* 2000; 49(RR-9):1-35.
6. **Influenza vaccine.** *(Minimum age: 6 months for trivalent inactivated influenza vaccine (TIV); 5 years for live, attenuated influenza vaccine (LAIV)*
   - All children aged 6–59 months and close contacts of all children aged 0–59 months are recommended to receive influenza vaccine.
   - Influenza vaccine is recommended annually for children aged ≥59 months with certain risk factors, healthcare workers, and other persons (including household members) in close contact with persons in groups at high risk. See *MMWR* 2006; 55(RR-10);1-41.
   - For healthy persons aged 5–49 years, LAIV may be used as an alternative to TIV.
   - Children receiving TIV should receive 0.25 mL if aged 6–35 months or 0.5 mL if aged ≥3 years.
   - Children aged <9 years who are receiving influenza vaccine for the first time should receive 2 doses (separated by ≥4 weeks for TIV and ≥6 weeks for LAIV).
7. **Measles, mumps, and rubella vaccine (MMR).** *(Minimum age: 12 months)*
   - Administer the second dose of MMR at age 4–6 years. MMR may be administered prior to age 4–6 years, provided ≥4 weeks have elapsed since the first dose and both doses are administered at age ≥12 months.
8. **Varicella vaccine.** *(Minimum age: 12 months)*
   - Administer the second dose of varicella vaccine at age 4–6 years. Varicella vaccine may be administered prior to age 4–6 years, provided that ≥3 months have elapsed since the first dose and both doses are administered at age ≥12 months. If second dose was administered ≥28 days following the first dose, the second dose does not need to be repeated.
9. **Hepatitis A vaccine (HepA).** *(Minimum age: 12 months)*
   - HepA is recommended for all children at 1 year of age (i.e., 12–23 months). The 2 doses in the series should be administered at least 6 months apart.
   - Children not fully vaccinated by age 2 years can be vaccinated at subsequent visits.
   - HepA is recommended for certain other groups of children including in areas where vaccination programs target older children. See *MMWR* 2006; 55(RR-7):1-23.
10. **Meningococcal polysaccharide vaccine (MPSV4).** *(Minimum age: 2 years)*
    - Administer MPSV4 to children aged 2–10 years with terminal complement deficiencies or anatomic or functional asplenia and certain other high risk groups. See *MMWR* 2005;54 (RR-7):1-21.

The Childhood and Adolescent Immunization Schedule is approved by:
Advisory Committee on Immunization Practices www.cdc.gov/nip/acip • **American Academy of Pediatrics** www.aap.org • **American Academy of Family Physicians** www.aafp.org

SAFER • HEALTHIER • PEOPLE™

FIGURE 12C-1 Recommended childhood and adolescent immunization schedule in the United States 2007. Available at: *http://www.cdc.gov/nip/recs/child-schedule.htm#printable*

Recommended Immunization Schedule for Children and Adolescents Who Start Late or Who Are More Than 1 Month Behind

UNITED STATES • 2007

The tables below give catch-up schedules and minimum intervals between doses for children who have delayed immunizations. There is no need to restart a vaccine series regardless of the time that has elapsed between doses. Use the table appropriate for the child's age.

CATCH-UP SCHEDULE FOR AGES 4 MONTHS THROUGH 6 YEARS

Vaccine	Minimum Age for Dose 1	Minimum Interval Between Doses			
		Dose 1 to Dose 2	Dose 2 to Dose 3	Dose 3 to Dose 4	Dose 4 to Dose 5
Hepatitis B[1]	Birth	4 weeks	8 weeks (and 16 weeks after first dose)		
Rotavirus[2]	6 wks	4 weeks	4 weeks		
Diphtheria, Tetanus, Pertussis[3]	6 wks	4 weeks	4 weeks	6 months	6 months[3]
Haemophilus influenzae type b[4]	6 wks	**4 weeks** if first dose given at age <12 months **8 weeks (as final dose)** if first dose given at age 12-14 months **No further doses needed** if first dose given at age ≥15 months	**4 weeks**[4] if current age <12 months **8 weeks (as final dose)**[4] if current age ≥12 months and second dose given at age <15 months **No further doses needed** if previous dose given at age ≥15 months	**8 weeks (as final dose)** This dose only necessary for children aged 12 months–5 years who received 3 doses before age 12 months	
Pneumococcal[5]	6 wks	**4 weeks** if first dose given at age <12 months and current age <24 months **8 weeks (as final dose)** if first dose given at age ≥12 months or current age 24–59 months **No further doses needed** for healthy children if first dose given at age ≥24 months	**4 weeks** if current age <12 months **8 weeks (as final dose)** if current age ≥12 months **No further doses needed** for healthy children if previous dose given at age ≥24 months	**8 weeks (as final dose)** This dose only necessary for children aged 12 months–5 years who received 3 doses before age 12 months	
Inactivated Poliovirus[6]	6 wks	4 weeks	4 weeks	4 weeks[6]	
Measles, Mumps, Rubella[7]	12 mos	4 weeks			
Varicella[8]	12 mos	3 months			
Hepatitis A[9]	12 mos	6 months			

CATCH-UP SCHEDULE FOR AGES 7–18 YEARS

Vaccine	Minimum Age for Dose 1	Minimum Interval Between Doses			
		Dose 1 to Dose 2	Dose 2 to Dose 3	Dose 3 to Dose 4	Dose 4 to Dose 5
Tetanus, Diphtheria/ Tetanus, Diphtheria, Pertussis[10]	7 yrs[10]	4 weeks	**8 weeks** if first dose given at age <12 months **6 months** if first dose given at age ≥12 months	**6 months** if first dose given at age <12 months	
Human Papillomavirus[11]	9 yrs	4 weeks	12 weeks		
Hepatitis A[9]	12 mos	6 months			
Hepatitis B[1]	Birth	4 weeks	8 weeks (and 16 weeks after first dose)		
Inactivated Poliovirus[6]	6 wks	4 weeks	4 weeks	4 weeks[6]	
Measles, Mumps, Rubella[7]	12 mos	4 weeks			
Varicella[8]	12 mos	**4 weeks** if first dose given at age ≥13 years **3 months** if first dose given at age <13 years			

1. **Hepatitis B vaccine (HepB).** *(Minimum age: birth)*
   - Administer the 3-dose series to those who were not previously vaccinated.
   - A 2-dose series of Recombivax HB® is licensed for 11–15 year olds.
2. **Rotavirus vaccine (Rota).** *(Minimum age: 6 weeks)*
   - Do not start the series later than age 12 weeks.
   - Administer the final dose in the series by 32 weeks of age. Do not administer a dose later than age 32 weeks.
   - There are insufficient data on safety and efficacy outside of these age ranges.
3. **Diphtheria and tetanus toxoids and acellular pertussis vaccine (DTaP).** *(Minimum age: 6 weeks)*
   - The fifth dose is not necessary if the fourth dose was administered at age ≥4 years.
   - DTaP is not indicated for persons aged ≥7 years.
4. ***Haemophilus influenzae* type b conjugate vaccine (Hib).** *(Minimum age: 6 weeks)*
   - Vaccine is not generally recommended for children aged ≥5 years.
   - If current age <12 months and the first 2 doses were PRP-OMP (PedvaxHIB® or ComVax® [Merck]), the third (and final) dose should be administered at age 12–15 months and at least 8 weeks after the second dose.
   - If first dose given at age 7–11 months, give 2 doses separated by 4 weeks plus a booster at age 12–15 months.
5. **Pneumococcal conjugate vaccine (PCV).** *(Minimum age: 6 weeks)*
   - Vaccine is not generally recommended for children aged ≥5 years.
6. **Inactivated poliovirus vaccine (IPV).** *(Minimum age: 6 weeks)*
   - For children who received an all-IPV or all-oral poliovirus (OPV) series, a fourth dose is not necessary if third dose was administered at age ≥4 years.
   - If both OPV and IPV were administered as part of a series, a total of 4 doses should be given, regardless of the child's current age.
7. **Measles, mumps, and rubella vaccine (MMR).** *(Minimum age: 12 months)*
   - The second dose of MMR is recommended routinely at age 4–6 years but may be administered earlier if desired.
   - If not previously vaccinated, administer 2 doses of MMR during any visit with ≥4 weeks between the doses.
8. **Varicella vaccine.** *(Minimum age: 12 months)*
   - The second dose of varicella vaccine is recommended routinely at age 4–6 years but may be administered earlier if desired.
   - Do not repeat the second dose in persons aged <13 years, if administered ≥28 days following the first dose.
9. **Hepatitis A vaccine (HepA).** *(Minimum age: 12 months)*
   - HepA is recommended for certain groups of children including in areas where vaccination programs target older children. See *MMWR* 2006; SS (RR-7) 1-23.
10. **Tetanus and diphtheria toxoids vaccine (Td) and tetanus and diphtheria toxoids and acellular pertussis vaccine (Tdap).** *(Minimum ages: 7 years for Td, 10 years for BOOSTRIX®, and 11 years for ADACEL™)*
    - Tdap should be substituted for a single dose of Td in the primary catch-up series or as a booster if age-appropriate; use Td for other doses.
    - A five-year interval from the last Td dose is encouraged when Tdap is used as a booster dose. A booster (4th) dose is needed if any of the previous doses were administered at age <12 months. Refer to ACIP recommendations for further information. See *MMWR* 2006; SS (RR-3) L34.
11. **Human papillomavirus vaccine (HPV).** *(Minimum age: 9 years)*
    - Administer the HPV vaccine series to females at age 13–18 years if not previously vaccinated.

For information on reporting reactions following immunization, visit www.vaers.hhs.gov or call the 24-hour national toll-free information line 800-822-7967. Report suspected cases of vaccine-preventable diseases to your state or local health department. For additional information including precautions and contraindications for immunization, visit the National Center for Immunization and Respiratory Diseases at www.cdc.gov/ncird or contact 800-CDC-INFO (800-232-4636).

DEPARTMENT OF HEALTH AND HUMAN SERVICES • CENTERS FOR DISEASE CONTROL AND PREVENTION • SAFER • HEALTHIER • PEOPLE

FIGURE 12C-1, cont'd

Table 12C-2 Combination Vaccines

Name	Components	Manufacturer
TriHIBit	DaTP-Hib	Aventis Pasteur
Pediatrix	DaTP-HepB-IPV	GlaxoSmithKline
Comvax	Hib-HepB	Merck Vaccine Corporation

DTaP, Diphtheria, tetanus, and acellular pertussis; *HepB*, hepatitis B; *Hib*, *Haemophilus influenzae* type B; *IPV*, inactivated poliovirus.

immunization of preterm infants. These levels are not as elevated after administration of acellular pertussis vaccine.[10] Although apnea had been reported in extremely LBW infants at less than 31 weeks' gestation after diphtheria, tetanus, and pertussis (DTP) vaccine, apnea has not been observed in these infants after administration of acellular pertussis-containing vaccines (i.e., DTaP vaccine).[3,11] Preterm infants given PCV concomitantly with DTP and Hib vaccine were reported to have benign febrile seizures more frequently than did full-term infants who received the same vaccines.[3] For infants already discharged, families should be made aware of the possibility of adverse reactions and advised to contact the primary care provider immediately if symptoms occur.

Conclusion

Primary care providers are responsible for ensuring that children born prematurely receive the appropriate vaccinations on time. Because recommendations may change, providers must continue to remain aware of any modifications in the vaccination schedule. In addition, they must educate families to prioritize vaccination administration. Because a greater number of premature infants born at lower gestational ages are surviving, correct vaccination of premature infants is more of a priority than ever.

Resources for Families and Clinicians

AAP Immunization Initiative
http://www.cispimmunize.org
This AAP-affiliated website provides immunization information to parents and clinicians. Revised AAP Policy Statements are posted.

Centers for Disease Control and Prevention
www.immunize.org/vis
Provides information packets for families. Available in multiple languages.

National Immunization Program
http://www.cdc.gov/nip/
This CDC-affiliated website provides information for healthcare professionals and families about vaccinations. Information also is provided in Spanish. Recent updates are provided.
http://www.cdc.gov/nip/recs/child-schedule.htm#printable
This CDC-affiliated address provides the immunization schedule.

National Network for Immunization Information
www.immunizationinfo.org
This organization provides the public, health professionals, policy makers, and the media with up-to-date information about immunizations to help them understand the issues and to make informed decisions.

REFERENCES

1. Saari TN: Immunization of preterm and low birth weight infants. *Pediatrics* 112 (1):193-198, 2003.
2. Davis RL, Ruanowice D, Shinefield HR, et al: Immunization levels among premature and low-birth-weight infants and risk factors for delayed up-to-date immunization status. *JAMA* 282 (6):547-553, 1999.
3. American Academy of Pediatrics, Committee on Infectious Diseases: Immunization in special circumstances. Preterm and low birth weight infants. In Pickering LK, editor: *Red book: 2006 report of the Committee on Infectious Diseases,* ed 27. Elk Grove Village, Ill, 2006, American Academy of Pediatrics.
4. Langkamp DL, Hoshaw-Woodard S, Boye M, et al: Delays in receipt of immunizations in low-birth weight children. *Arch Pediatr Adolesc Med* 155:167-172, 2001.
5. Khalak R, Pichichero ME, D'Angio CT: Three-year follow-up of vaccine response in extremely preterm infants. *Pediatrics* 101(4):597-603, 1998.
6. Raucci J, Whitehill J, Sandritter T: Childhood immunizations (part one). *J Pediatr Health Care* 18 (2):95-101, 2004.
7. Whitehill J, Raucci J, Sandritter T: Childhood immunizations (part 2). *J Pediatr Health Care* 18(4):192-199, 2004.
8. Glode MP: Combination vaccines: practical considerations for public health and private practice. *Pediatr Infect Dis J* 20:S19-S22, 2001.
9. Centers for Disease Control: *Pink book: epidemiology and prevention of vaccine-preventable disease,* ed 7. Washington, DC, 2001, US Department of Health and Human Services.
10. Pourcyrous M, Korones SB, Crouse D, et al: Interleukin-6, C-reactive protein, and abnormal cardiorespiratory responses to immunization in premature infants. *Pediatrics* 101(3):E3, 1998.
11. Schloesser RL, Fischer D, Otto W, et al: Safety and immunogenicity of an acellular pertussis vaccine in premature infants. *Pediatrics* 103(5):E60, 1999.

Chapter 12D

Dental Care for the Preterm Infant

Mary Ann Ouellette, MS, APRN, IBCLC

Dental care is frequently an overlooked aspect of anticipatory guidance in the primary care setting for both preterm and term infants. The American Academy of Pediatrics (AAP) policy statement on dental care recommends that all infants should receive an oral health assessment from their primary care provider by the time they are 6 months of age.[1] The AAP and the American Academy of Pediatric Dentistry (supported by the American Dental Association and the Academy of General Dentistry) recommend that infants born prematurely should be referred to a dental provider, on the basis of risk assessment, as early as 6 months of age, 6 months after the first tooth erupts, and no later than 12 months of age. However, these recommendations are not widely practiced. The literature suggests that access to care, family socioeconomic status, cultural issues, and a primary care provider's poor dental education all are contributing factors.

Prematurity affects all areas of an infant's development. The literature suggests that the technology required in the hospital for these infants has an effect on oral development. Eastman[2] describes dental issues associated with prematurity, which includes enamel defects, delayed eruption, decreased tooth crown size, and oral cavity defects as a result of oral endotracheal intubation. Enamel defects can predispose the preterm or low-birth-weight infant to caries.

The development of primary teeth begins to form approximately 4 to 6 weeks in utero and continues through adolescence.[3] Because primary tooth development begins during gestation with permanent teeth starting to form several months before birth, premature delivery may affect the infant's tooth formation.[2] The etiologic factors associated with developmental dentition defects are poorly understood. However, oral and systemic health appear to be related. The nutrients necessary for dental development include calcium, phosphorous, fluoride, and vitamins A, C, and D.[2] The premature infant is at high risk for poor nutrition, mineral deficiency, and metabolic stressors, all of which are contributing factors to development of nutritional deficiencies and therefore enamel defects and hypoplasia.[4]

Tooth decay remains the single most common chronic disease in children. Because preterm infants are at high risk for dental problems, the role of the pediatric provider is to promote good health and to minimize potential problems.[5] Pediatric providers usually are the first healthcare providers to examine the oral cavity. The provider needs to assess family history, feeding practices, nutrition, vitamin and fluoride supplementation, and medications. It is important that the provider perform a thorough oral assessment at each well visit and educate the family about good oral hygiene (Tables 12D-1 and 12D-2). An oral examination should include checking for abnormalities of tooth eruption and soft tissues, checking for plaque on the teeth, and checking for white spots or cavities.[6] It is important that preterm infants be referred to pediatric dentists no later than 1 year of age.

Resources for Families and Clinicians

American Academy of Pediatric Dentistry
www.aapd.org

This organization represents the specialty of pediatric dentistry whose members serve as the primary contributors to professional educational programs concerning dental care for children.

Table 12D-1 Anticipatory Guidance for the Parent or Caregiver*

ORAL HYGIENE

Brush with fluorinated toothpaste twice per day
Floss at least once per day
Rinse every night with an alcohol-free mouth rinse with 0.05% sodium fluoride

DIET

Drink juice only with meals
Avoid carbonated beverages for the first 30 months of the child's life

FLUORIDE

Use fluoride toothpaste approved by the American Dental Association

CARIES PREVENTION

Receive regular dental care
Avoid sharing utensils and cleaning a dropped pacifier with saliva
Maternal use of xylitol gum can prevent dental caries in their children by limiting the transmission of mutans streptococci colonization from mother to child

*Data obtained from: American Academy of Pediatrics, Section on Pediatric Dentistry: Oral health risk assessment timing and establishment of the dental home. *Pediatrics* 111(5):1113-1116, 2003. Available at: *http://aappolicy.aappublications.org/cgi/content/full/pediatrics;111/5/1113#R16.*

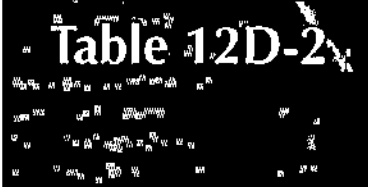

Table 12D-2 Anticipatory Guidance for the Young Patient (Age 0–3 Years)*

ORAL HYGIENE

Cleanse mouth of infant with a damp cloth after feedings
Cleanse teeth after administering medications containing sucrose
Brush the child's teeth twice per day as soon as the teeth erupt
Floss once per day once teeth contact one another

DIET

Provide fruit juice (limited to once per day) only at meals
Avoid carbonated beverages
Do not put the child to bed with a bottle containing anything but water
Do not dip pacifiers in honey or sugar

FLUORIDE

Supplement at 6 months as necessary (for both term and preterm infants)
Use nonfluorinated toothpaste in children younger than 2 years

*Data obtained from: American Academy of Pediatrics, Section on Pediatric Dentistry: Oral health risk assessment timing and establishment of the dental home. *Pediatrics* 111(5):1113-1116, 2003. Available at: *http://aappolicy.aappublications.org/cgi/content/full/pediatrics;111/5/1113#R16.*

American Academy of Pediatrics (AAP)
www.aap.org
http://aappolicy.aappublications.org/cgi/content/full/pediatrics;111/5/1113#R16

The second website provides the AAP's recommendation on dental care.

American Dental Association
www.ada.org

This professional association of dentists is committed to the public's oral health, ethics, science, and professional advancement.

Academy of General Dentistry
www.agd.org

This professional association of dentists is committed to excellence in oral healthcare and continuous, lifelong learning.

Bright Futures
www.brightfutures.org

Bright Futures is a national health promotion initiative dedicated to the principle that every child deserves to be healthy and that optimal health involves a trusting relationship among the health professional, child, family, and community. This organization provides a book about anticipatory guidance titled *Bright Futures: Guidelines for Health Supervision of Infants, Children, and Adolescents.*

REFERENCES

1. American Academy of Pediatrics, Section on Pediatric Dentistry: Oral health risk assessment timing and establishment of the dental home. *Pediatrics* 111(5):1113-1116, 2003. Available at: *http://aappolicy.aappublications.org/cgi/content/full/pediatrics;111/5/1113#R16.*
2. Eastman DL: Dental outcomes of preterm infants. *Newborn Infant Nurs Rev* 3(3):93-98, 2003.
3. Wright JT: Normal formation and development defects of the human dentition. *Pediatr Clin North Am* 47(5):975-1000, 2000.
4. Pimlott JF, Howley TP, Nikiforuk G, et al: Enamel defects in prematurely born, low birth-weight infants. *Pediatr Dent* 7(3):218-223, 1985.
5. Edelstein BL: Public and clinical policy considerations in maximizing children's oral health. *Pediatr Clin North Am* 47(5):1177-1189, 2000.
6. Casamassimo PS: Relationships between oral and systemic health. *Pediatr Clin North Am* 47(5):1149-1157, 2000.

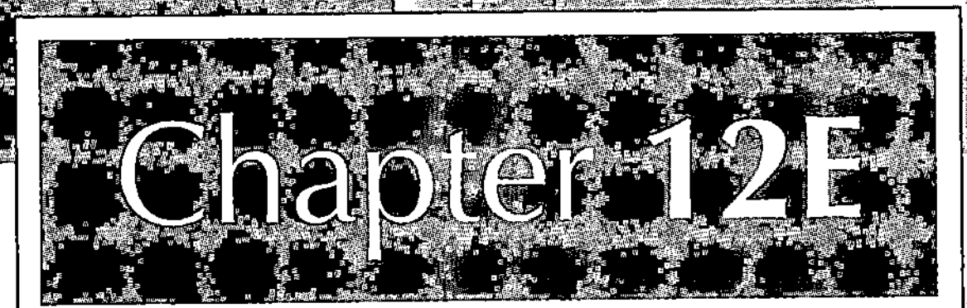

Early Intervention and Follow-Up Programs for the Premature Infant

Jane E. Stewart, MD

Early Intervention

Infants who are born prematurely often are eligible for early intervention (EI) services. The federal Individuals with Disabilities Education Act (IDEA) of 2004 mandates that states provide EI services to infants and toddlers with special developmental and educational needs. Each state has its own policies and laws to enforce the IDEA requirements.

Eligibility criteria

The IDEA states that EI services must be provided to any child younger than 3 years who is (1) experiencing developmental delays or (2) has a physical or mental condition that has a high probability of resulting in developmental delay.[1] States also may choose to provide services to children who are at risk for experiencing a substantial developmental delay if EI services are not provided.[1] Because the instruments for quantitatively measuring the degree of developmental delays in children younger than 2 years may be unreliable, the IDEA regulations require that "informed clinical opinion" also should determine the need for EI services.[1] This "informed clinical opinion" usually is derived from the consensus of a multidisciplinary team, which includes the parents, and information from multiple sources.[1]

Although the IDEA provides these general guidelines, each state uses different criteria to define developmental delay and the degree of developmental delay that leads to eligibility. Thus, there is wide variability for EI eligibility among states. Primary care providers can refer to the State Resource Sheets, which are provided by the National Dissemination Center for Children with Disabilities (NICHCY; available at *http://www.nichcy.org/states.htm*) to determine EI eligibility parameters for their own state.

States frequently use risk factors for adverse developmental outcomes that are categorized by an established risk, a biologic/medical risk, and/or an environmental risk.[1] Some of the conditions associated with each risk factor are listed in Table 12E-1. Although the IDEA requires states to provide EI services to children with conditions of established risk, states are not required to provide EI services to children with conditions associated with biologic/medical risks.[1] Because of recent changes in the IDEA guidelines, children with some environmental risk factors are required to receive EI services (Table 12E-1). Children who are not immediately eligible for EI services (i.e., children with biologic/medical conditions and some environmental risk conditions) should have a comprehensive evaluation by a multidisciplinary team to establish an informed clinical opinion to determine whether EI services are needed. Some states provide services to potentially eligible children if they have multiple (range 3–5) risk factors.

Infants born prematurely do not automatically receive EI services. Some states list specific criteria that apply to premature infants and lead to automatic services. For example, in Massachusetts, infants who are born weighing less than 1200 g at less than 32 weeks' gestation with a neonatal intensive care unit (NICU) admission stay more than 5 days and a total hospital stay of more than 25 days in a 6-month period should receive EI services.

Table 12E-1 Specific Risk Factors for Developmental Delay Recommended by the IDEA

Category	Possible Conditions (Not All-Inclusive)	IDEA Guidelines
Established risk	Chromosomal abnormalities Genetic or congenital disorders Severe sensory (including hearing and vision) impairments Inborn errors of metabolism Disorders reflecting disturbance of nervous system development Congenital infections Disorders secondary to exposure to toxic substances, including fetal alcohol syndrome Severe attachment disorders	The IDEA requires states to provide services to these children, regardless of the presence or absence of a developmental delay.
Biologic/medical risk	Low birth weight (<2500 g) Intraventricular hemorrhage Chronic lung disease Failure to thrive	The IDEA does not require states to provide EI to these children. Often, a comprehensive child and family evaluation by a multidisciplinary team to establish an informed clinical opinion is needed to determine if the child can receive EI services.
Environmental risk	Substantiated child abuse or neglect Withdrawal symptoms because of prenatal drug exposure Other effects of illegal substance abuse	The IDEA recently has required states to provide services to these children, regardless of the presence or absence of a developmental delay.
	Parental substance abuse Family social disorganization Parental age Parental educational attainment Possible child abuse or neglect	The IDEA does not require states to provide EI to these children. Often, a comprehensive child and family evaluation by a multidisciplinary team to establish an informed clinical opinion is needed to determine if the child can receive EI services.

Content gathered from: Shackelford J: State and jurisdictional eligibility definitions for infants and toddlers with disabilities under the IDEA. *National Early Childhood TA Center Notes.* 20, 2006. Available at: *http://www.nectac.org/%7Epdfs/pubs/nnotes21.pdf*
IDEA, Individuals with Disabilities Education Act; *EI,* early intervention.

Thus, primary care providers must know their individual state's requirements for access to EI. When in doubt, primary care providers should err on the side of referral.

Early Intervention services

Once a child is referred to EI, the child is evaluated by a multidisciplinary team and assessed. If the child is determined to be eligible for EI services, the program will develop an individualized family service plan (IFSP), which outlines the services that will be provided in the upcoming year. Services are provided either through individual home visits, clinics, daycare settings, and the hospital, or at Department of Public Health-approved centers individually or through groups. Parent groups sometimes are offered to provide families with information, support, and training.

EI service providers include developmental specialists, nurses, physical therapists, occupational therapists, social workers, psychologists, and speech and language specialists. Services focus on the following five areas of development:

1. Physical development,
2. Cognitive development,
3. Communication,
4. Social or emotional development,
5. Adaptive development.

If an infant has not been referred by the discharging hospital and the infant meets eligibility criteria, the primary care provider should make a referral as early as possible after discharge.

Benefits of Early Intervention

The benefits of an enriched home environment to improve developmental outcome are clear. The simple everyday exposure to words in early life is associated with an increased and more developed vocabulary.[2] Services by EI providers enhance the environment provided by the child's parents and close care providers by emphasizing the importance of reading and recommending developmentally appropriate activities. Data from the Infant Health and Development Program demonstrate that infants who receive intensive EI, including parental education and support at 3 years of age, have developmental scores significantly higher than do infants in the control group who received standard care.[3-5] Early childhood development programs have been associated with reductions in grade retention and placement in special education.[6]

Potential problems with Early Intervention

Occasionally, children are not enrolled in appropriate EI services in a timely manner. Some of the causes for a lack of services are as follows:

- *Initial Referral:* Referral is not made directly from the hospital discharging the infant to home.
- *Parental Reluctance to Participate:* Sometimes parental misperceptions regarding EI exist; parents may think that EI is only for "handicapped" children or that their child will be given a permanent label of needing special education. In addition, some families are reluctant to have strangers come into their home.
- *Inadequate or Inappropriate Services:* Children may receive inappropriate services if a program is short-staffed and does not have the needed specialist. Another potential pitfall occurs when an infant is "graduated" prematurely from EI because he or she no longer strictly qualifies for services despite having a known biologic risk.
- *Lack of Specialized Services for More Rare Diagnoses:* Children with specific diagnoses, such as deafness, blindness, or autism, require very specialized EI services that usually are not provided by the local community EI program. In this case, the child's community EI program should refer the child to another program or subcontract with providers who can provide these services.

Primary care provider's role in Early Intervention

Primary care providers should be familiar with their local, state, and federal programs and requirements for eligibility. If an infant has not been referred from the hospital and the infant meets eligibility criteria, the primary care provider should make a referral as early as possible after discharge. After the infant has received EI services, the primary care provider should obtain detailed information from the families about their visits and the EI services that are being provided. The primary care provider then should determine whether additional services are indicated. A collaboration between the primary care provider's office and the EI program to develop and implement an IFSP is key to optimizing a child's growth and development.[7]

Infant Follow-Up Programs

Infant follow-up programs are sometimes available for developmental and medical consultation for issues related specifically to prematurity. These programs often are affiliated with neonatology academic fellowship training centers. Follow-up programs support optimization of health outcomes for NICU graduates and provide feedback information for improvement of medical care. Activities can include the following:

- Management of sequelae associated with prematurity. As smaller infants survive, the risk for chronic sequelae increases.
- Surveillance for the emergence of a variety of problems that may require referral to and coordination of multiple preventive and rehabilitative services.
- Monitoring outcomes. Information on health problems and use of services by NICU graduates is integral to both the assessment of the effect of services and the counseling of parents regarding an individual child's future. It is extremely important to provide feedback about infant outcomes to the healthcare professionals who provide care in the NICU.

Program structure

The population requiring follow-up care differs with each NICU and with the availability and quality of community resources. Most programs use some combination of birth weight and specific medical complications as criteria. Visits depend on the infant's needs and the community resources. Some programs recommend the first visit within a few weeks of discharge to assess the infant's transition to home. Most programs do not provide primary care for children but work in a consultative mode. In the absence of acute care needs, programs typically assess patients at 6-month intervals from birth until age 3 to 4 years.

Staff team members and consultants may include pediatrician (developmental specialist or neonatologist), neonatology fellows or pediatric residents (for training purposes), pediatric neurology specialist, physical therapist, psychologist, occupational therapist, dietician, speech and language specialist, and social worker.

Program services

Infant follow-up programs provide multiple services, including the following:

1. Complete developmental evaluations using standardized testing to assess cognitive, neuromotor, language, and social developmental progress

2. Physical examination, including a detailed neurologic examination and functional neurosensory developmental assessment
3. Recommendations for optimal EI services
4. Reminders/recommendations for latest guidelines about neurosensory screening, additional hearing and ophthalmologic/visual function assessments
5. Referrals to appropriate medical specialists, such as gastroenterology, pulmonary, neurology, orthopedics, otorhinolaryngology, nutrition, and/or genetics
6. Referral for further developmental therapies that may not be available through EI, such as speech and language, oral motor feeding therapy, sensory integration, augmentative communication, hippotherapy, and/or aquatherapy
7. Most recent recommendations for special immunizations (e.g., respiratory syncytial virus prophylaxis, influenza vaccine) for premature infants

Social work support is an extremely valuable component of infant follow-up programs and may include the following:

- Assistance with transition from the NICU to home
- Assistance with navigating the process of appropriate enrollment in EI programs
- Assistance with transition from EI services to the school system at age 3 years
- Family function assessment/screening for parental depression and possible referrals for supportive therapeutic treatment
- Connect families with a multitude of available community and hospital-based support services that might assist them financially and emotionally (e.g., respite, Women, Infants and Children Program, support groups, bereavement support).

In addition to these services, infant follow-up programs should provide recommendations to the primary care provider and the infant's EI program, as warranted.

Resources for Families and Clinicians

Early Intervention Programs for Infants and Toddlers with Disabilities

http://www.nectac.org/partc/partc.asp#overview

This website describes the Individuals with Disabilities Education Improvement Act of 2004 and provides contacts for early intervention programs that are available in the United States.

National Dissemination Center for Children with Disabilities (NICHCY)

www.nichcy.org

State Resource Sheets are available for each state and can be found at:

http://www.nichcy.org/states.htm

Common questions and answers about early intervention are provided for families at:

http://www.nichcy.org/pubs/parent/pa2txt.htm

National Early Childhood Technical Assistance System

www.nectac.org

This website provides contact information about intervention programs for every state and usually every region for children 0–3 or 3–5 years of age.

Acknowledgment

The author thanks Camilia Martin, MD, MS, for critical review of this chapter.

REFERENCES

1. Shackelford J: State and jurisdictional eligibility definitions for infants and toddlers with disabilities under IDEA. National Early Childhood TA Center Notes. 20, 2006. Available at: *http://www.nectac.org/%7Epdfs/pubs/nnotes21.pdf*
2. Hart B, Risley TR: Meaningful differences in the everyday experience of young American children. Baltimore, 1995, Brookes.
3. McCormick MC, McCarton C, Tonascia J, et al: Early educational intervention for very low birth weight infants. *J Pediatr* 123(4):527-533, 1993.
4. The Infant Health and Development Program: Enhancing the outcomes of low-birth-weight infant, premature infants. A multisite, randomized trial. *JAMA* 263(22):3035-3042, 1990.
5. Ramey CT, Bryant DM, Wasik BH, et al: Infant Health and Development Program for low birth weight, premature infants: program elements, family participation, and child intelligence. *Pediatrics* 89(3):454-465, 1992.
6. Anderson LM, Shinn C, Fullilove MT, et al: The effectiveness of early childhood development programs: a systematic review. *Am J Prev Med* 24(3S):32-46, 2003.
7. American Academy of Pediatrics Committee on Children with Disabilities: The pediatrician's role in development and implementation of an Individual Education Plan (IEP) and/or an Individual Family Service Plan (IFSP). *Pediatrics* 104:124-127, 1999.

GENERAL REFERENCE

Vohr BR: Neonatal follow-up programs in the new millennium. *NeoReviews* 2:e241-e248, 2001.

Chapter 13

Resources for Clinicians and Families

Mary Quinn, NNP, IBCLC, and Deborah S. Kerr, MSW, LICSW

The discharge of a premature infant from the neonatal intensive care unit (NICU) often is bittersweet for parents. Although parents have eagerly anticipated the day when their entire family is at home, they may be overwhelmed by the complexities of emotions and logistic concerns associated with the infant's discharge. Parents leave behind the reassuring technology and constant presence of professionals to negotiate a frightening maze of financial concerns, the healthcare system, and the reorganization of their home lives.

Resources are essential to helping parents cope with the addition of their graduated preemie to their home. The best resource may be another parent who has experienced similar circumstances. The primary care provider usually is the first professional on whom parents rely for guidance and support. Ideally, providers should direct families to organizations and support groups that will benefit them.

Before providing families with a list of resources and referrals, it may be helpful to assess the child(ren) and parent(s). You will be able to choose resources and respond appropriately to their individual needs more successfully after determining the parental concerns and developmental stages of the child. Tables 13-1 through 13-4 highlight the role of the primary care provider in caring for premature children, suggestions for assessing parental perceptions of their child and selves, and recommendations to assist families with resources and referrals.

Federal and state financial and legal supports are available, primarily through federal Social Security programs and state public health departments (Table 13-5). Premature children weighing <1200 g at birth or with specific disabilities, such as trisomy 21, may be eligible for Social Security Insurance (SSI; Table 13-5). State public health departments may have relief funds for "catastrophic illnesses" in children, reimbursing families for ramps, air conditioning, therapeutic horseback riding, and other expensive items that qualify. Most states provide handicapped parking placards for families with children who require supplemental oxygen. Medicaid may cover some over-the-counter generic drugs if the pediatrician provides a prescription to the parent. Utility companies (electric, water, phone, gas, oil) are required by law to maintain services to families of individuals with special healthcare needs regardless of financial limitations, just as hospitals are required to provide free care for uninsured, eligible individuals.

Tax deductions are available for medical expenses, including mileage to and from medical appointments, as well as parking, lodging, and meals that are incurred because of medical need. Medical expenses must meet a certain percentage of the family's annual income in order to be deducted. Tax accountants can assist families with specific details.

All states offer legal services available at no cost or with sliding scale fees. Specific state providers can

Table 13-1 Role of the Primary Care Provider in Assisting Families of Premature Children

- Assess the needs of the parent(s)
- Assess the needs of the child
- Support the parent in being the *care* coordinator for the child
- Refer family members to resources for financial, social, and medical assistance, as well as for emotional and psychological well-being
- Provide written information for referrals and resources
- Remember that there may be a protracted, gradual period of acceptance by parents during which services are needed

Table 13-2 Suggestions for Assessing Parental Perceptions of Their Child

Ideally, begin by explaining that you are "going to ask questions about you and your child so that I may gain a better understanding of your situation and help you as needed."

- Tell me about your child.
- What is he or she doing now? Prompt with questions about feeding, sleeping, playing, communication, cognition, and motor skills as needed.
- How is that different from the last time you were here?
- Does he or she have friends? How does he or she interact with siblings? Peers? Does he or she prefer to play with older children? Younger children? Why do you think that is?
- How well do you think he or she is developing on a scale of 1 to 4, with 1 being poor and 4 being very well?
- What does your child do that makes you proud?
- What concerns do you have about your child?

be identified using the Internet. Some states offer "Lawyer for a Day" programs, enabling families to have one-time free advice from a lawyer. The family should contact its local state or county bar association to determine whether this service is available. The primary care provider should encourage families who seem financially strong to investigate special needs trusts to maintain care for their disabled child in the event of disaster or death of a parent.

The number of available agencies and websites can be overwhelming. In this chapter, we list longstanding resources for primary care providers (Tables 13-6 and 13-7). Issue-specific organizations are listed separately (Table 13-8). Table 13-9 outlines resources for families of premature infants. Although we made every effort to highlight the most longstanding resources, websites may become outdated. Please contact the organization directly if website accessibility is denied.

Table 13-3 Suggestions for Assessing General Parental Perceptions

- What supports and resources do you have in place socially, medically, financially, and emotionally? Which have been helpful?
- Are you involved with any assistance from state or federal agencies, such as:
  - Early Intervention
  - Food Stamps
  - WIC (Women, Infants, and Children) Program
  - Department of Social Services
  - Housing
  - Fuel Assistance
- As the parent of your child, how would you assess your parenting on a scale of 1 to 4, with 1 being poor and 4 being very good?
- What are your coping strategies when you feel challenged as a parent? What or who helps you?

Table 13-4 Recommendations for Assisting Families with Resources and Referrals

- Maintain a list of federal, state, and local agencies in the office, with contact information and eligibility criteria. Be sure to include local school departments and early intervention programs.
- Provide a list of regional counseling agencies and clinicians. Include specifics about which insurances are accepted, as well as provider's interests (grief, blended families, behavioral disorders) and expertise (cognitive behavioral treatment, couples therapy).
- Direct families to *specific* websites and contacts listed in this chapter. If families do not have Internet access in their home, encourage them to go to the public library.
- For financially limited families, provide letters of need to the utility companies so that families can receive lower rates and possibly prevent discontinuance of service for lack of payment. Advocate patient needs to insurance companies.
- Listen to your families. They will tell you what they want and need if you provide them the opportunity to do so.
- Consider hiring a part-time employee to maintain and update your resources.
- Remember that you do not have to have *all* of the answers and resources at your fingertips. Sometimes you will be unable to provide specifics to a parent, but it is hoped that you can refer them to someone or to a website that can help.

Table 13-5 Financial and Legal Resources

Alliance of Special Needs
www.specialneedsalliance.com
Provides information on attorneys in the United States who specialize in legal and financial planning, as well as trusts that will assist in caring for children with special needs.

American with Disabilities Act (ADA)
www.ada.gov
Provides information on technical assistance, regulations, telephone relay services, and publications on the Americans with Disabilities Act.

Center for Medicare and Medicaid Services (formerly the Health Care Financing Administration)
7500 Security Boulevard
Baltimore, MD 21244-1850
Toll-free: (877) 267-2323
Toll-free TTY (866) 226-1819
www.cms.gov
Federal agency that administers Medicare, Medicaid, and Child Health Insurance Programs. The Katie Beckett Waiver is a federally funded, state-regulated program with a long waiting list. Medicaid administers this program for children with disabilities who are not eligible for other Medicaid programs because the income or assets of their parents are too high. The Katie Beckett Waiver for Medically Fragile Children provides Medicaid to parents who make >$24,000 per year. Eligibility criteria include the following:

- The child must be 18 years of age or younger;
- The child must be determined disabled by the SSI* standards of disability;
- The child must require institutional level of care, according to state standards;
- The state must determine that it is appropriate to provide care for the child at home rather than institutional care; and
- The cost to provide care outside the institution must not be greater than it would have been in the appropriate institution.

Children's Health Insurance Program (State Children's Health Insurance Program [SCHIP], Medicaid)
www.cms.hhs.gov/schip/

Center for Health Care Strategies, Inc.
www.chcs.org/
Organization that works to improve health services for people with disabilities and for low-income families. Website offers a wide range of publications, including the following:

- *The Faces of Medicaid*
- *The Complexities of Caring for People with Chronic Illnesses and Disabilities*
- *All About Medicaid: What Is It? Who Qualifies? What Does It Cost? What Services Are Available? What Is Managed Care? What Is Medicaid Managed Care?*
- *Medicaid Managed Care: The Challenges for People with Special Health Care Needs*

Families USA
1334 G Street NW
Washington, DC 20005
Phone: (202) 628-3030
Fax: (202) 347-2417
www.familiesusa.org
National nonprofit organization that advocates high-quality, affordable, and long-term care for all Americans. Includes publications and advocacy information on Medicaid, Medicare, children's healthcare reform, and managed care.

Handicapped Parking Placard
Most states provide handicapped parking placards to families with children who require *oxygen* supplementation. The form is obtained through the state registry of motor vehicles. A physician's signature is required on the form.

Legal Services Corporation (LSC)
3333 K Street NW, Third Floor
Washington, DC 20007-3522
Phone: (202) 295-1500
http://www.lsc.gov/
Organization funded by Congress to provide equal access to the court system for those who are unable to afford legal counsel. The website provides links to states' legal services supported by LSC.

National Dissemination Center for Children with Disabilities
P.O. Box 1492
Washington, DC 20013
Phone: (800) 695-0285
Fax: (202) 884-8441
www.nichcy.org

Continued

Table 13-5 Financial and Legal Resources—cont'd

Center is funded by the U.S. Department of Education, Office of Special Education Programs (OSEP) and serves as a central resource for the Individuals with Disabilities Education Act (IDEA), the nation's special education law, No Child Left Behind (as it relates to children with disabilities), and research-based information on effective educational practices. Patients may qualify for assistance from Part H section of the IDEA, which provides support and services for children younger than 3 years old. Many neonatal intensive unit graduates may qualify.

Needymeds
www.needymeds.com
Good resource for finding information on drug programs for the poor, offered by pharmaceutical manufacturers.

Shriners Hospitals
www.shrinershq.org
Provide medical care free of charge to children younger than 18 years old.

Social Security Administration
Office of Public Inquiries
Windsor Park Building
6401 Security Boulevard
Baltimore, MD 21235
Phone: (800) 772-1213
TTY (800) 325-0778
www.ssa.gov
Administers Social Security programs (SSI, SSDI*), which arrange public health insurance for people with disabilities and their dependents. Search "disability" for information on benefits, application procedures, and childhood listings of impairments (the "Blue Book"). Eligibility for premature infants is based on birth weight, gestational age, and impairment.

WIC (Women, Infants, and Children) Program
www.fns.usda.gov/wic/aboutwic/
Federally funded program that assists financially eligible pregnant and postpartum mothers and children younger than 5 years old with food, nutritional education, and access to healthcare services.

*SSDI, Social Security Disability Insurance; SSI, Social Security Insurance.

Table 13-6 General Resources for Clinicians

American Academy of Pediatrics (AAP)
141 Northeast Point Boulevard
Elk Grove Village, IL 60007
Phone: (847) 434-4000
Fax: (847) 434-8000
www.aap.org
National organization of pediatricians with parent resources, bulletins, and referrals.

Council on Children with Disabilities (The Collaborative)
www.aap.org/visit/cmte10.htm
The AAP is merging the Committee on Children with Disabilities (COCWD) and the AAP Section on Children with Disabilities (SOCWD). A list server for The Collaborative is available. E-mail Stephanie Mucha at *smucha@aap.org* with e-mail address and contact information. For Fellows of the Academy interested in joining the Collaborative, access the "Eligibility and Application" page.

National Center of Medical Home Initiatives for Children with Special Needs
141 Northwest Point Boulevard
Elk Grove Village, IL 60007
Phone: (847) 434-4000
Fax: (847)-228-7035
www.medicalhomeinfo.org
Provides a variety of resources to assist in providing for medical homes, including fact sheets, policy statements, reports/documents, Internet links, and individual state resources. Provides support to physicians, families, and other medical and nonmedical providers who care for children with special needs.

National Perinatal Association
3500 E. Fletcher Avenue, Suite 205
Tampa, FL 33613
Phone: (888) 971-3295 or (813) 971-1008
www.nationalperinatal.org
Professional organization whose mission is to promote the health and well-being of mothers and infants. Publishes the *Journal of Perinatology*.

Society for Developmental and Behavioral Pediatrics
631 6th Avenue South
St. Petersburg, FL 33701
Phone: (727) 502-8035
www.sdbp.org/
National list server whereby professionals can submit questions regarding developmental and behavioral pediatric issues. Articles and links also are available.

Table 13-7 Multiservice Resources

Publications

Exceptional Parent Magazine
65 East Route 4
River Edge, NJ 07661
Phone: (877)-372-7368
www.eparent.com
Provides information, support, ideas, encouragement, and outreach to families and service providers of children with disabilities.

Book
Naseef RA: *Special children, challenged parents: the struggles and rewards of raising a child with a disability.* Baltimore, 2001, Brookes Publishing Company.

Preemie Magazine
LLC, 6412 Brandon Avenue, #274
Springfield, VA 22150
www.preemiemagazine.com
Provides the free and informative publication *Preemie Magazine,* as well as an online community that empowers the preemie parent and educates the preemie professional.

Organizations and Websites

American Academy of Child and Adolescent Psychiatry (AACAP)
3615 Wisconsin Avenue NW
Washington, DC 20016-3007
Phone: (202) 966-7300
Fax: (202) 966-2891
www.aacap.org
Assists families to understand the developmental, behavioral, emotional, and mental disorders affecting children and adolescents. Serves AACAP members. Fact sheets available in English and Spanish.

The Arc link
www.thearclink.org
Provides customized information on the various sources of assistance available to individuals with disabilities and their families on a state-by-state basis, as well as information on almost 30,000 providers.

The Arc of the United States
1010 Wayne Avenue, Suite 650
Silver Spring, MD 20910
Phone: (301) 565-3842
www.thearc.org
National organization of and for people with mental retardation and related developmental disabilities and their families. Services include early intervention, healthcare, public education, and support for families. Publications available in Spanish.

Birth Defects Research for Children, Inc. (BDRC)
930 Woodcock Road, Suite 225
Orlando, FL 32803
Phone: (407) 895-0802
www.birthdefects.org
501(c)(3) nonprofit organization that provides parents and expectant parents with information on birth defects and support services for their children. The organization provides free fact sheets about many birth defects and networking services for families and assists families to research specific birth defects. They maintain a national registry of birth defects.

Children's Disabilities Information
www.childrensdisabilities.info
Comprehensive volunteer family support site providing:

Parenting
Special needs article
Special needs resources
Advocacy
Feeding
Prematurity

Autism, Asperger syndrome
Cerebral palsy

Sensory integration
Speech
Vision
Attention deficit disorder
Link to special needs book list
Links to "list of disabilities" (directory of mailing lists and forums for special needs families

Circle of Inclusion
www.circleofinclusion.org
For families of young children and early childhood service providers. Provides demonstrations and information on the practices of inclusive educational programs for children from birth through age 8 years. Offered in several languages.

Council for Exceptional Children (CEC)
North Glebe Road, Suite 300
Arlington, VA 22201
Phone: (703)-620-3660
TTY: (866)-915-5000
Fax: (703)-264-9494
www.cec.sped.org
Largest international professional organization dedicated to improving outcomes for individuals with exceptionalities, students with disabilities, and/or the gifted.

Easter Seals
230 West Monroe Street, Suite 1800
Chicago, IL 60606
Toll-free: (800) 221-6827
Phone: (312) 726-6200
TTY: (312) 726-4258
Fax: (312) 726-1494
www.easter-seals.org
National agency that offers a variety of services to help individuals with disabilities and their families lead better lives.

The Family Village
www.familyvillage.wisc.edu/
Global community that integrates information, resources, and communication opportunities on the Internet for persons with cognitive and other disabilities, their families, and service providers. The community includes:
- Informational resources on specific diagnoses
- Education
- Communication connections
- Worship
- Adaptive products and technology
- Health issues
- Adaptive recreational activities
- Disability-related media and literature

Family Voices
2340 Alamo SE, Suite 102
Albuquerque, NM 87106
Phone: (505) 872-4774
Toll free: (888) 835-5669
Fax: (505) 872-4780
www.familyvoices.org
Website of a national grassroots network of families that advocates for healthcare that is family-centered, community based, comprehensive, coordinated, and culturally competent for children with disabilities. Offers individual information, links, current events, and Medicaid/Medicare information.

The Father's Network
Washington State Father's Network
Kindering Center
16120 NE Eighth Street
Bellevue, WA, 98008-3937
Phone: (425) 747-4004, extension 4286
www.fathersnetwork.org
Advocates and provides resources and support for all men who have children with special healthcare needs or developmental disabilities. Available in Spanish.

Federation for Children with Special Needs
95 Berkley Street, Suite 104
Boston, MA 02116
www.fcsn.org
The mission of this organization is to provide information, support, and assistance to parents of children with disabilities, the professionals serving them, and their communities. The website provides services primarily to residents of Massachusetts but has a link to the Family Resource database, a national database of agencies across the country, which provides information/services to families of children with special needs.

Federation of Families for Children's Mental Health
1101 King Street, Suite 420
Alexandria, VA 22314

Continued

Table 13-7 Multiservice Resources—cont'd

Phone: (703) 684-7710
Fax: (703) 836-1040
www.ffcmh.org
National parent-managed organization that focuses on the needs of children and youth with emotional, behavioral, or mental disorders and their families.

Government Services
www.firstgov.org
Portal to all government online services.

March of Dimes
1275 Mamaroneck Avenue
White Plains, NY 10605
Phone: 914-997-4488
www.marchofdimes.com/
Supports research, community services, and education about birth defects, premature birth, and infant mortality.

National Center for Latinos with Disabilities
http://clas.uiuc.edu/special/progdesc/cl00480il/cl00480.html
Phone/TTY: (800) 532-3353
Fax: (312)-666-0707
Serves individuals with disabilities and their families, as well as professionals who work with them. Provides linguistically and culturally appropriate advocacy, training, information, and referral programs.

National Clearinghouse on Family Support and Children's Mental Health
Regional Research Institute
Portland State University
P.O. Box 751 Portland, OR 97207-0751
Phone: (503) 725-4040
Fax: (503) 725-4180
www.rtc.pdx.edu

National Dissemination Center for Children with Disabilities
P.O. Box 1492
Washington, DC 20013
Phone: (800) 695-0285
Fax: (202) 884-8441
www.nichcy.org
The Center is funded by the U.S. Department of Education, Office of Special Education Programs (OSEP), and serves as a central source of information for the Individuals with Disabilities Education Act (IDEA), the nation's special education law, No Child Left Behind (as it relates to children with disabilities), and research-based information on effective educational practices. On the website, click on each state to view a myriad of children's services with addresses, phone numbers, e-mail addresses, and website addresses that include:

- State agencies and organizations
- Protection and advocacy
- Programs for infants and toddlers
- Services for the visually, speech, and hearing impaired
- Programs for children
- Disease-specific organizations
- Transition services
- Organizations especially for parents
- Vocational training
- Independent living
- Mental health agencies

Patients may qualify for assistance from Part H section of the IDEA, which provides supports and services for children younger than 3 years old. Many neonatal intensive unit graduates may qualify.

National Early Childhood Technical Assistance Center (NECTAC)
Campus Box 8040 UNC-CH
Chapel Hill, NC 27599-8040
Phone: (919) 962-2001
TDD: (919) 843-3269
Fax: (919) 966-7463
www.nectac.org
Supports the implementation of the early childhood provisions of IDEA. Their mission is to strengthen service systems that ensure that children with disabilities (birth through 5 years of age) and their families receive and benefit from high-quality, culturally appropriate, family-centered supports and services. Center of the Clearinghouse on Early Intervention and Early Childhood Special Education. Available in Spanish.

Table 13-7 Multiservice Resources—cont'd

National Education for Assistance Dog Services (NEADS)
P.O. Box 213
West Boylston, MA 01538
Phone/TDD: (978) 422-9064
Fax: (978) 422-3255
www.neads.org
Provides information on hearing dogs, service dogs (for people who use wheelchairs, canes, walkers, or crutches), service dogs for the classroom, and special dogs for those with two or more disabilities, such as a deaf person who uses a wheelchair.

National Rehabilitation Information Center (NARIC)
8455 Colesville Road, Suite 935
Silver Spring, MD 20910
Phone/TTY: (800) 346-2742
Toll free: (800) 227-0216
www.naric.com
Provides information about disabilities and rehabilitation.

Office of Special Education and Rehabilitative Services (OSERS)
Information Resource Center
Phone: (800) USA-LEARN
Toll free: (800) 872-5327
Available in Spanish
TYY: (800) 437-0833
www.ed.gov/about/offices/list/osers
Provides a wide array of support for parents and individuals, school districts, and states in the areas of special education, vocational rehabilitation, and research.

PACER Center (Parent Advocacy Coalition for Educational Rights)
8161 Normandale Boulevard
Minneapolis, MN 55437
Phone: (952) 838-9000
TTY (952) 838-0190
Toll-free in greater MN: (800) 537-2237
Fax: (952) 838-0197
www.pacer.org
The mission of PACER is to expand opportunities and enhance the quality of life of children and young adults with disabilities and their families. It is based on the concept of parents helping parents. Parents of children with disabilities work collaboratively with 18 disability organizations. This organization can identify resources and services for children with special needs at all stages of childhood and all disabilities.

Office of Families and Advocates for Partnership in Education (FAPE)
www.fape.org
An organization that advocates for families to become informed about the IDEA with the goal of improving educational outcomes for individuals with disabilities.

The National Technical Assistance Center
www.taalliance.org
A project to support technical assistance for individuals with disabilities.

Parent Pals
www.parentpals.com
Internet service for parents and professionals to share information and support.

PRO-ED
8700 Shoal Creek Boulevard
Austin, TX 78757
Phone: (512) 451-3346
(800) 897-3203
www.proedinc.com
Publishes and sells resource and reference texts, professional journals, curricula, and therapy materials in the fields of psychology and special education, including developmental disabilities; rehabilitation; early childhood intervention; occupational and physical therapy; and speech, language, and hearing for professionals and parents.

Special Education Resources on the Internet
www.seriweb.com
Collection of Internet resources for those involved in special education. The goal of this website is to make special education Internet resources more easily and readily available in one location.

Continued

Table 13-7 Multiservice Resources—cont'd

Special Families Guide
www.specialfamilies.com/
The author and psychologist Robert Naseef, PhD, provides information on family life for parents, siblings, and children with special needs. Specifically, he addresses the following issues: autism, developmental disabilities, cerebral palsy, learning disorders, special healthcare needs, and other conditions with an emphasis on the role of fathers. Provides links about parenting, resources, and specific disability organizations.

VORT (Values, Objectives, Resources, Time) Corporation
P.O. Box 60132
Palo Alto, CA 94306
Phone: (650) 322-8282
Fax: (650) 327-0747
www.vort.com
Publishes and sells books and materials for professionals and parents of premature infants about early intervention programs, special education, developmental assessment, and early childhood education.

White House Initiative on Educational Excellence for Hispanic Americans
400 Maryland Avenue SW
Washington, DC 20202-1411
Phone: (202) 401-1411
Fax: (202) 401-8377
www.yosipuedo.gov
www.yesican.gov
Bilingual website with links to "What you need to know if your child has special needs," a list of services, resources, and approaches designed to assist parents of children with mental and/or physical disabilities.

Table 13-8 Issue-Specific Organizations

Assistive Technology

"Assistive Technology (AT) is any item, piece of equipment, or product system, whether acquired commercially off the shelf, modified, or customized, that is used to increase, maintain, or improve the functional capabilities of individuals with disabilities." 29 U.S.c. sec 2202(2).
www.medicalhomeinfo.org/weblinks/asst_tech.html
Site from the AAP page at The National Center of Medical Home Initiatives for Children with Special Needs. Website lists numerous resources for all areas of assistive technology.

Breastfeeding

Academy of Breastfeeding Medicine
www.bfmed.org
International professional organization of physicians that has developed many clinical protocols.

American Academy of Pediatrics
www.aap.org/healthtopics/breastfeeding.cfm
Provides many resources available from the AAP and external organizations to help families initiate and successfully continue breastfeeding.

La Leche League International
www.lalecheleague.org/
Worldwide organization that offers mother-to-mother support, education, information, and encouragement to women who want to breastfeed their babies. It aims to promote a better understanding of breastfeeding.

Lactation Consultants
www.ilca.org
To identify a local consultant, contact International Board of Lactation Consultant Examiners *(www.iblce.org)* or the International Lactation Consultant Association

National Women's Health Information Center
www.womenshealth.gov/breastfeeding
Provides information on breastfeeding to families. Provides a toll-free phone number (800-994-9662) to answer basic breastfeeding questions.

Cardiac Issues

Children's Heart Information Network
1561 Clark Drive
Yardley, PA 19067
Phone: (215) 493-3068
International organization that provides information, support services, and resources to families of children with congenital heart disease.

Car Safety Seats

The Automotive Safety Program
www.preventinjury.org
Phone: (317) 274-2977
Program that offers information and a training course on transporting children with special needs.

Available Car Safety Seats
www.aap.org/family/carseatguide.htm
Describes the different car safety seat options. For a description of car safety seats available for children with special needs, refer to the AAP brochures, *Safe Transportation of Children with Special Needs: A Guide for Families* and *Car Safety Seats: A Guide for Families.*

Child Passenger Safety Contact Locator
www.nhtsa.dot.gov/people/injury/childps/Contacts/index.cfm
Offered by the National Highway Traffic Safety Administration to provide information on contacting a local car safety seat source.

Cerebral Palsy

American Academy for Cerebral Palsy and Developmental Medicine (AACPDM)
http://www.aacpdm.org/index?service=page/Home
6300 North River Road, Suite 727
Rosemont, IL 60018-4226
Phone: (847) 698-1635

Continued

Table 13-8 Issue-Specific Organizations—cont'd

Multidisciplinary scientific society devoted to the study of cerebral palsy and other childhood-onset disabilities; promoting professional education on the treatment and management of these conditions; and improving the quality of life for people with these disabilities.

Kids Health.Org
http://kidshealth.org/kid/health_problems/brain/cerebral_palsy.html
Developed by The Nemours Foundation's Center for Children's Health Media with separate sections for kids, teens, and parents. Contains explanations of medical conditions in language that people at each level can understand. Physicians working in the field review each article for accuracy. The link is for the article on cerebral palsy.

March of Dimes
http://www.marchofdimes.com/professionals/14332_1208.asp
Provides a brief overview of cerebral palsy to families.

National Institutes of Neurological Disorders and Stroke
http://www.ninds.nih.gov/disorders/cerebral_palsy/detail_cerebral_palsy.htm
U.S. government's leading supporter of biomedical research on brain and nervous system disorders, including cerebral palsy. Provides a lengthy overview of cerebral palsy to families.

NICHCY
http://www.nichcy.org/pubs/factshe/fs2txt.htm
NICHCY is the National Dissemination Center for Children with Disabilities. Serves as a centralized source of information on a wide variety of disabilities, special education law, and other information on related laws, such as No Child Left Behind and other information on educational research. The handouts (e.g., the one on cerebral palsy) provided through the website are copyright free so that families may copy and distribute them.

United Cerebral Palsy Foundation (UCP)
http://www.ucp.org
1660 L Street, NW Suite 700
Washington, DC 20036-5602
Phone: (800) 872-5827
The mission of this organization is to advance the independence, productivity, and full citizenship of people with cerebral palsy and other disabilities. They are a leading source about cerebral palsy and a strong advocate for the rights of persons with any disability. Their services include the following:

- Therapy
- Community living
- Assistive technology training
- State and local referrals
- Early intervention programs
- Employment assistance
- Individual and family support
- Advocacy
- Social and recreation programs

Cholestasis

NASPGHAN: North American Society for Pediatric Gastroenterology, Hepatology and Nutrition
http://www.naspghan.org
Provides information to families about specific gastrointestinal disorders. For handouts about biliary atresia in English, Spanish, or French, click on "Public Information" then "Disease Information" and then "Biliary Atresia."

http://www.naspghan.org/PDF/PositionPapers/CholestaticJaundiceInInfants.pdf
Provides the NASPGHAN guidelines for management of cholestasis.

Chronic Lung Disease/Bronchopulmonary Dysplasia

National Heart, Lung and Blood Institute

www.nhlbi.nih.gov/health/dci/Diseases/Bpd/Bpd_WhatIs.html
Provides information on bronchopulmonary dysplasia to families.

Colic and Constipation

NASPGHAN: North American Society for Pediatric Gastroenterology, Hepatology and Nutrition

http://www.naspghan.org
Provides information to families about specific gastrointestinal disorders, including colic. For handouts about colic or constipation in English, Spanish, or French, click on "Public Information" then "Disease Information" and then "Colic" or "Constipation."

Table 13-8 Issue-Specific Organizations—cont'd

Cryptorchidism

Aetna Intelihealth
www.intelihealth.com
Search for "cryptorchidism" for short summary for families.

American Academy of Family Physicians
www.familydoctor.org/637.xml
11400 Tomahawk Creek Pathway
Leawood, KS 66211-2672
Phone: (913) 906-6000; (800) 274-2237

Children's Hospital, Boston
www.childrenshospital.org
Search for "cryptorchidism" for short summary about cryptorchidism for families.

Dental Care

American Academy of Pediatric Dentistry
www.aapd.org and
Organization that represents the specialty of pediatric dentistry. Members serve as the primary contributors to professional educational programs concerning dental care for children.

American Academy of Pediatrics (AAP)
www.aap.org
http://aappolicy.aappublications.org/cgi/content/full/pediatrics;111/5/1113#R16
The second website provides the AAP's recommendation on dental care.

American Dental Association
www.ada.org
Professional association of dentists that is committed to the public's oral health, ethics, science, and professional advancement.

Academy of General Dentistry
www.agd.org
Professional association of dentists that is committed to excellence in oral healthcare and continuous, life-long learning.

Bright Futures
www.brightfutures.org
National health promotion initiative dedicated to the principle that every child deserves to be healthy and that optimal health involves a trusting relationship among the health professional, child, family, and community. Provides a book about anticipatory guidance, *Bright Futures: Guidelines for Health Supervision of Infants, Children, and Adolescents.*

Early Intervention

Early Intervention Programs for Infants and Toddlers with Disabilities
http://www.nectac.org/partc/partc.asp#overview
Describes the Individuals with Disabilities Education Improvement Act of 2004 and provides contacts for early intervention programs available in the United States.

National Dissemination Center for Children with Disabilities (NICHCY)
www.nichcy.org
State Resource Sheets are available for each state and can be found at:
http://www.nichcy.org/states.htm
Common questions and answers about early intervention are provided to families at: *http://www.nichcy.org/pubs/parent/pa2txt.htm*

National Early Childhood Technical Assistance System
www.nectac.org
Provides contact information on intervention programs for every state and usually every region for children 0–3 or 3–5 years of age.

Enteral Tubes

Kids with Tubes
http://www.kidswithtubes.org/
Organization managed by parents offering a variety of support services for parents and caregivers of tube-fed children. Its mission is to provide forums for the sharing of information and mutual support. The organization aims to bring together families whose children have feeding tubes (NG, G, GJ, J, and/or NJ-tubes), without regard to the children's underlying diagnoses.

Continued

Table 13-8 Issue-Specific Organizations—cont'd

Mealtime Notions LLC
http://www.mealtimenotions.com/
Created to provide mealtime support for parents and professionals who feed infants and young children with special feeding challenges. The children served have difficulties coordinating the process of sucking, swallowing, and breathing; handling the sensory aspects of mealtimes; and consuming sufficient calories for growth. Many of these children require supplemental tube feeding to help with nutrition. The organization provides educational opportunities with workshops, therapy consultation and shared information, as well as favorite mealtime resources and materials.

New Visions
http://www.new-vis.com/
Provides continuing education and therapy services to professionals and parents working with infants and children who have feeding, swallowing, oral–motor, and prespeech problems.

The Oley Foundation
http://www.oley.org
National, independent, nonprofit organization that provides up-to-date information, outreach services, conference activities, and emotional support for home parenteral or enteral nutrition support consumers, their families, caregivers, and professionals.

Epilepsy

Epilepsy Foundation (formerly the Epilepsy Foundation of America)
www.efa.org
4351 Garden City Drive
Landover, MD 20785-7223
Phone: (800) 332-1000
501(c)(3) organization that assists people affected by seizures through research, education, advocacy, and service. Provides a forum to respond to online requests for information.

Gastroesophageal Reflux

Children's Digestive Health and Nutrition Foundation
www.CDHNF.org
Provides educational information (including videos) on gastroesophageal reflux disease to families and clinicians.

www.KIDSACIDREFLUX.org
Cartoon sponsored by the Children's Digestive Health and Nutrition Foundation that explains reflux to children.

National Digestive Disease Information Clearinghouse (NDDIC)
http://digestive.niddk.nih.gov/ddiseases/pubs/gerdinfant/
Review of physiologic and pathologic reflux for families.

The North American Society for Pediatric Gastroenterology, Hepatology and Nutrition
www.NASPGHAN.org

Pediatric/Adolescent Gastroesophageal Reflux Association (PAGER)
www.reflux.org
This website of a national parent support group provides information regarding reflux/medication/testing. Available in Spanish.

Genetics

Genetic Alliance, Inc.
www.geneticalliance.org
4301 Connecticut Avenue NW, Suite 404
Washington, DC 20008-2369
Phone: (202) 966-5557
Fax: (202) 966-8552
Nation's leading support, education, and advocacy organization for all those living with genetic conditions. Represents the interests of more than 600 advocacy, research, and healthcare organizations. Website offers links to resources and support groups.

Hearing Impairments

American Academy of Audiology
http://www.audiology.org

American Academy of Pediatrics
www.aap.org/policy/re9846.html and
www.medicalhomeinfo.org/screening/hearing.html
These websites provide the recent AAP policy statement on screening for hearing loss.

Table 13-8 Issue-Specific Organizations—cont'd

American Society for Deaf Children
www.deafchildren.org
P.O. Box 3355
Gettysburg, PA 17325
Phone/TTY: (717) 334-7922
Fax: (717) 334-8808
Parent Hotline: (800) 942-ASDC
National organization for families and professionals, the mission of which is to educate, empower, and support parents and families of the deaf and hard of hearing.

American Speech-Language-Hearing Association (ASHA)
www.asha.org
10801 Rockville Pike
Rockville, MD 20852
Phone/TTY: (800) 638-8255 (public)
(800) 498-2071 (professionals)
The mission of this organization is to ensure that all people with speech, language, and hearing disorders have access to quality services to help them communicate more effectively.

Better Hearing Institute (BHI)
http://www.betterhearing.org/
Not-for-profit corporation that educates the public about the neglected problem of hearing loss and what can be done about it.

Boys Town National Research Center
http://www.babyhearing.org
Team from Boys Town National Research Hospital that provides parents with information on newborn screening and hearing loss. The team consists of audiologists, speech language pathology specialists, teachers of the deaf, geneticists, and parents of deaf and hard of hearing children.

Centers for Disease Control and Prevention (CDC)
http://www.cdc.gov/ncbddd/ehdi/default.htm
Provides information on the Early Hearing Detection and Intervention Program.

Hands & Voices
http://www.handsandvoices.org/
Nonprofit, parent-driven national organization dedicated to supporting families of children who are deaf or hard of hearing.

Harvard Medical School Center for Hereditary Deafness
http://hearing.harvard.edu
Excellent booklets for families are available from this website.

Marion Downs National Center for Infant Hearing
http://www.colorado.edu/slhs/mdnc/
Provides information from the Marion Downs National Center for Infant Hearing that coordinates statewide systems for screening, diagnosis, and intervention for newborns and infants with hearing loss.

Massachusetts Universal Newborn Hearing Screening
http://www.mass.gov/dph/fch/unhsp/index.htm
Organization that oversees statewide implementation of universal hearing screening initiative; ensures access to follow-up services; provides information on newborn hearing screening; provides parent-to-parent support; and helps families pay for audiologic diagnostic tests in Massachusetts.

National Association for the Deaf
www.nad.org
814 Thayer Avenue
Silver Spring, MD 20910-4500
Phone/TTY: (301) 587-1788
Organization established in 1880 that is the oldest and largest constituency organization safeguarding the accessibility and civil rights of deaf and hard of hearing Americans in education, employment, healthcare, and telecommunications.

National Center for Hearing Assessment and Management (NCHAM)
http://www.infanthearing.org/
The goal of NCHAM is to ensure that all infants and toddlers with hearing loss are identified as early as possible and provided with timely and appropriate audiologic, educational, and medical intervention.

National Cued Speech Association
www.cuedspeech.org

Continued

Table 13-8 Issue-Specific Organizations—cont'd

National Deaf Education Center
Gallaudet University
http://clerccenter.gallaudet.edu
800 Florida Ave. NE
Washington, DC 20002
Phone: (202) 651-5051
TTY (202) 651-5052
Provides a centralized source of information on topics dealing with deafness and hearing loss in children and young people younger than 21 years.

National Institute on Deafness and Other Communication Disorders (NIDCD)
www.nidcd.nih.gov
One Communication Avenue
Bethesda, MD 20892
Phone: (800) 241-1044
TTY (800) 241-1055
The NIDCD is part of the National Institutes of Health and is mandated to conduct and support biomedical and behavioral research and research training in the normal and disordered processes of hearing, balance, smell, taste, voice, speech, and language. It addresses special biomedical and behavioral problems associated with people who have communication impairments and supports efforts to create devices that substitute for lost and impaired communication function.

Oberkotter Foundation
www.oraldeafed.org
Phone: (877) 672-5442
TTY: (877) 672-5889
Comprehensive website for parents and professionals providing numerous links. Offers many materials for parents and professionals, including the following:
- Parent Information Kit: A Resource Guide for Parents of Newly-Diagnosed Deaf and Hard of Hearing Children
- The ABCs of Early Intervention.

Hydrocephalus

Hydrocephalus Association (HA)
www.hydroassoc.org
870 Market Street, Suite 705
San Francisco, CA 94102
Phone: (415) 732-7040
Phone: (888) 598-3789 (for personal one-on-one support)

Hydrocephalus Foundation, Inc (HyFI)
www.hydrocephalus.org
910 Rear Broadway
Saugus, MA 01906
Phone: (781) 942-1161
Provides support, educational resources, and networking opportunities to patients and families affected by hydrocephalus.

Hyperbilirubinemia

American Academy of Pediatrics
http://www.aap.org/family/jaundicefeature.htm
Provides clinical practice guidelines for managing hyperbilirubinemia in infants at 35 weeks' gestation and older.

March of Dimes
http://www.marchofdimes.com/professionals/14332_9268.asp
Provides information on jaundice to families.

Mayo Clinic
http://www.mayoclinic.com/invoke.cfm?objectid=EDFE58D5-87F3-4231-91E36178255A37D9&dsection=1
Provides information on jaundice to families.

Tool for Bilirubin Management
http://www.bilitool.org/
The clinical provider can enter the infant's age and bilirubin level and, by use of the Bhutani normogram, the website will determine the level of risk for the infant.

Table 13-8 Issue-Specific Organizations—cont'd

Hypothyroidism

The MAGIC Foundation
http://www.magicfoundation.org/www
National nonprofit organization created to provide support services to families of children with specific diseases that affect a child's growth. Provides detailed information on congenital hypothyroidism to families.

National Newborn Screening & Genetic Resource Center (NNSGRC)
http://genes-r-us.uthscsa.edu/
Provides information and resources about newborn screening to healthcare professionals and families.

Immunizations

AAP Immunization Initiative
http://www.cispimmunize.org
AAP-affiliated website that provides immunization information to parents and clinicians. Revised AAP Policy Statements are posted.

Centers for Disease Control
http://www.cdc.gov/nip/recs/child-schedule.htm#printable
Provides childhood immunization schedule in different formats and in Spanish.

National Immunization Program
http://www.cdc.gov/nip/
CDC-affiliated website provides information on vaccinations for healthcare professionals and families. Information is available in Spanish. Recent updates are provided.

National Network for Immunization Information
www.immunizationinfo.org
Provides the public, health professionals, policy makers, and the media with up-to-date information on immunizations to help them understand the issues and to make informed decisions.

Inguinal Hernias

Cincinnati Children's Hospital Medical Center
http://www.cincinnatichildrens.org
3333 Burnet Avenue
Cincinnati, OH 45229-3039
Phone: (513) 636-4200 or (800) 344-2462
Search for "inguinal hernia."

Children's Hospital, Boston
www.childrenshospital.org
Search for "inguinal hernia" for short summary for families.

Multiple Gestation

The National Organization of Mother's of Twins Clubs, Inc.
www.Nomotc.org
Nonprofit corporation that offers advice, encouragement, and practical knowledge to families with multiples. Information on preparing for multiples, tips for new parents of multiples and for feeding multiples are included.

The Triplet Connection
www.Tripletconnection.org
Nonprofit organization for multiple-birth families. Provides information to families who are expecting triplets, quadruplets, quintuplets, or more, as well as encouragement, resources, and networking opportunities for families who are parents of larger multiples. Allows access to their quarterly publication.

Triplets, Moms, and More
www.tripletsmomsandmore.org
Massachusetts-based support group for families and families-to-be of triplets, quads, and more, providing educational information and emotional support.

Necrotizing Enterocolitis

Parent Resources:
Insurance Considerations
http://www.aetna.com/cpb/data/CPBA0605.html
Insurance payment guidelines for intestinal failure.

Continued

Table 13-8 Issue-Specific Organizations—cont'd

The Oley Foundation
http://c4isr.com/oley/
Phone: (800) 776-OLEY
Founded in 1983, the Oley Foundation is a national organization that provides information and psychosocial support to individuals requiring long-term parenteral nutrition and tube-fed enteral nutrition. All services are free of charge. Many members include children with short bowel syndrome due to necrotizing enterocolitis.

Physician Resources:
American Gastrointestinal Association
http://www.guideline.gov/summary/summary.aspx?ss=15&doc_id=3795&nbr=3021
Provides technical review on short bowel syndrome and intestinal transplantation.

North American Society for Pediatric Gastroenterology, Hepatology and Nutrition
http://www.naspghan.org/
Includes parent information handouts of short bowel syndrome in several languages, including English, Spanish, and French.

Review of Short Bowel Syndrome
http://www.emedicine.com/med/topic2746.htm

Neonatal Diseases and Abnormalities

www.mic.ki.se/Diseases/c16.html
Extensive list of links to medical information on congenital, hereditary, and neonatal diseases and abnormalities.

Neurodevelopmental Issues

American Academy of Pediatrics
www.medicalhomeinfo.org
Scroll to "Screening Initiatives" to "Developmental Screening" to "For Providers" or "To Families"

http://www.aap.org/healthtopics/stages.cfm
http://aappolicy.aappublications.org/cgi/content/full/pediatrics;110/1/184?eaf
Provides extensive information on developmental stages and screening.

http://pediatrics.aappublications.org/cgi/content/full/118/1/405
Provides an AAP policy statement about identifying infants and young children with developmental disorders in the medical home: an algorithm for developmental surveillance and screening. Included within this statement is an easy-to-use algorithm that serves as a decision-making tool for conducting developmental surveillance and screening.

Brazelton Institute
www.brazelton-institute.com
The Brazelton Institute, Children's Hospital
1295 Boylston Street
Boston, MA 02215
Provides information on the Newborn Behavioral Observations (NBO) system.

Centers for Disease Control and Prevention
http://www.cdc.gov/ncbddd/child/screen_provider.htm
This website discusses the role of the primary care provider in a child's developmental health.

Developmental Screening Tools
www.dbpeds.org/ and *http://www.dbpeds.org/articles/detail.cfm?TextID=539*
Provides information on the specific use of developmental and behavioral screening tools.

Early Intervention Programs for Infants and Toddlers with Disabilities
http://www.nectac.org/partc/partc.asp#overview
Describes the Individuals with Disabilities Education Improvement Act of 2004 and provides contacts for early intervention programs that are available in the United States.

Exceptional Parent Magazine
www.eparent.com
Provides information, support, ideas, encouragement, and outreach to families and service providers of children with disabilities.

Table 13-8 Issue-Specific Organizations—cont'd

Federation for Children with Special Needs
www.fcsn.org
95 Berkley Street, Suite 104
Boston MA 02116
The mission of this organization is to provide information, support, and assistance to parents of children with disabilities, the professionals serving them, as well as their communities. Website primarily services Massachusetts but has a link to the Family Resource database, a national database of agencies across the country, which provides information/services to families of children with special needs.

Internet Resources for Special Children
www.irsc.org
Dedicated to children with disabilities and other health-related disorders. Provides a directory for links for families, educators, and medical professionals caring for these children.

National Early Childhood Technical Assistance System
www.nectac.org
Provides contact information on intervention programs for every state and usually every region for children 0–3 or 3–5 years of age.

Other Websites:
www.brightfutures.org
Information on this website is based on published guidelines for health supervision of infants, children, and adolescents. Funded by the U.S. Department of Health and Human Services, under the direction of the Maternal and Child Health Bureau.

www.generalpediatrics.com
Clearinghouse of information, handouts, and problem-based information for clinicians and parents.

Newborn Screening

ACTion Sheets
www.acmg.net/resources/policies/ACT/condition-analyte-links.htm
This resource is from the American College of Medical Genetics and the Maternal and Child Health Bureau/Health Resources and Services Administration. It provides primary care providers with additional details on many of the conditions detected by expanded newborn screening. The first page of the ACT sheet provides basic and clinical information with follow-up recommendations if an abnormal report is obtained. The second page provides a list of websites to help identify specialists for consultations.

American Academy of Pediatrics (AAP)
www.aap.org/healthtopics/newbornscreening.cfm
Provides AAP policies about genetic testing resources on Newborn Screening Policy and System Development for the primary care provider.

Centers for Disease Control and Prevention's Division of Laboratory Sciences
www.cdc.gov/nceh/dls/newborn_screening.htm
Contains PowerPoint presentations about quality assurance of newborn screening.

March of Dimes
www.marchofdimes.com/pnhec/298_834.asp
Provides families with a description of the common disorders tested in newborn screening programs.

National Center of Medical Home Initiatives
www.medicalhomeinfo.org/screening/newborn.html
Provides a list of state-specific screening, national data, and numerous resources available to clinicians.

The National Newborn Screening and Genetics Resource Center
http://genes-r-us.uthscsa.edu/
This organization is a cooperative agreement between the Maternal and Child Health Bureau, Genetic Services Branch and the University of Texas Health Science Center at San Antonio. Provides information and resources on newborn screening and genetics to benefit healthcare professionals and families, as well as government officials.

Nutrition

American Dietetic Association
www.eatright.org
Provides many resources for clinicians as well as a method to identify local dietitians at: http://www.eatright.org/cps/rde/xchg/ada/hs.xsl/home_fanp_business_ENU_HTML.htm

Continued

Table 13-8 Issue-Specific Organizations—cont'd

Growth Charts
http://www.cdc.gov/growthcharts/
The CDC provides growth charts along with frequently asked questions, an interactive web-based training module, and a link to WIC-specific growth charts.

NASPGHAN: North American Society for Pediatric Gastroenterology, Hepatology and Nutrition
http://www.naspghan.org
Provides information to families regarding specific gastrointestinal disorders, including lactose intolerance.

WIC (Women, Infants, and Children) Program
www.fns.usda.gov/wic/aboutwic/
Federally funded program that assists financially eligible pregnant and postpartum mothers and children younger than 5 years old with food, nutritional education, and access to healthcare services.

Oral Aversion

Kids with Tubes
www.kidswithtubes.org
Organization managed by parents that offers a variety of support services for caregivers of tube-fed (nasogastric, gastric, or jejunal) children.

New Visions
www.new-vis.com/
Resources for working with infants and children with feeding, swallowing, oral-motor, and pre-speech problems.

Pediatric/Adolescent Gastroesophageal Reflux Association (GERD)
www.reflux.org
Provides information regarding reflux/medication/testing. Available in Spanish.

Small Wonders Preemie Place
Members.aol.com/_ht_a/Lmwill262/index.html
Resource page, list server, and bulletin board for feeding issues in babies and young children.

Orthopedic Issues

Amputee Coalition of America
www.amputee-coalition.org
900 East Hill Avenue, Suite 285
Knoxville, TN 37915-2568
Phone: (888) 267-5669
Fax: (888) 525-7917
Nonprofit consumer and educational organization for people with limb differences or with amputations.

Helping Hands
www.helpinghandsgroup.org
P.O. Box 332
Medfield, MA 02052
Not-for-profit support group of parents who have children with upper limb differences and who are concerned with the challenges facing the child and the entire family. Emphasizes abilities, not disabilities. Newsletter and links available.

Orthotics and Prosthetics

www.oandp.com
Comprehensive website owned by an Internet software company sponsored by makers of orthotics and prosthetics. Available in Spanish.

Shriners Hospitals for Children
www.shrinershq.org
Provides free prosthetics and corrective surgery to children from low-to-moderate income families with conditions such as spina bifida, cleft lip and palate, and orthopedic anomalies. Contact (800) 237-5055 to determine whether a child qualifies.

World Association of People with Disabilities
www.wapd.org
Many links available. Teen chat room.

Rare Diseases

National Organization for Rare Diseases (NORD)
www.rarediseases.org

Table 13-8 Issue-Specific Organizations—cont'd

55 Kenosia Avenue
P.O. Box 1968
Danbury, CT 06813-1968
Phone: (203) 744-0100 or (800) 999-6673
TDD: (203) 797-9590
Fax: (203) 798-2291
Federation of volunteer health organizations dedicated to helping people with rare diseases and the organizations that serve them. NORD is committed to the identification, treatment, and cure of rare disorders through programs of education, advocacy, research, and service. NORD publishes a comprehensive resource guide and assistance for travel.

Respiratory Syncytial Virus (RSV)

For recent updates about RSV:
http://www.cdc.gov/
http://www.aap.org/

Retinopathy of Prematurity and Visual Impairments

American Academy of Pediatrics
http://www.aap.org/policy/060023.html
Provides a policy statement for screening examinations of premature infants for retinopathy of prematurity.

American Council of the Blind
www.acb.org
1155 15th Street NW, Suite 1004
Washington DC, 2005
Phone: (800) 467-5081
Fax: (202) 467-5085
Strives to improve the well-being of all blind and visually impaired people by improving educational and rehabilitation facilities and opportunities; assisting and encouraging institutions and organizations servicing this population; and educating the public. Provides an extensive list of links to resources and an online store.

American Foundation for the Blind
www.afb.org
Headquarters: 11 Penn Plaza Suite 300
New York, NY 10001
Phone: (800) AFB-LINE (232-5463)
Addresses issues of literacy, independent living, employment, and access through technology for the blind and visually impaired.

Association for Retinopathy of Prematurity and Related Diseases
http://ropard.org/
P.O. Box 250425
Franklin, MI 48025
The purpose of this organization is to fund clinically relevant basic science and clinical research to eliminate retinopathy of prematurity and associated retinal diseases. The organization funds innovative work leading directly to the development of new low-vision devices and teaching techniques and services for children who are visually impaired and their families.

National Association for Parents of Children with Visual Impairment (NAPVI)
http://www.spedex.com/napvi/
APVI is a national organization that enables parents to find information and resources for their children who are blind or visually impaired.

National Federation of the Blind (NFB)
http://www.nfb.org
The purpose of the National Federation of the Blind is twofold: to help blind persons achieve self-confidence and self-respect and to act as a vehicle for collective self-expression by the blind. By providing public education about blindness; information and referral services; scholarships; literature and publications about blindness; aids and appliances and other adaptive equipment for the blind; advocacy services and protection of civil rights; development and evaluation of technology; and support for blind persons and their families, members of the NFB strive to educate the public that the blind are normal individuals who can compete on terms of equality.

National Information Clearinghouse on Children Who Are Deaf-Blind
www.dblink.org
Western Oregon State College
35 North Monmouth Avenue
Monmouth, OR 97361
Phone: (800) 438-9376

Continued

Table 13-8 Issue-Specific Organizations—cont'd

TTY: (800) 854-7013
The goal of this organization is to help parents, teachers, and others by providing them with information to foster the skills, strategies, and confidence necessary to nurture and empower deaf-blind children. DB-LINK is a federally funded service that identifies, coordinates, and disseminates, at no cost, information related to children and youth from birth through 21 years of age.

Tracheostomy Care

Aaron's Tracheostomy Page
www.tracheostomy.com
A comprehensive website covering all aspects of the care of the child with a tracheostomy tube. Provides links and a message board with educational materials. Excellent resource for parents and professionals.

www.nelcor.com
Provides a free guide, Parent Guide to Pediatric Homecare.

www.trachcare.org
A non-profit organization created to provide support and information to parents, caregivers, and healthcare providers of children who have a tracheostomy.

http://ajrccm.atsjournals.org/cgi/content/full/161/1/297
Provides statements adopted by the American Thoracic Society on all aspects of care of the child with a tracheostomy tube. Excellent resource for pediatricians.

www.omronhealthcare.com
Omron Healthcare manufactures a portable, battery-operated, handheld nebulizer system.

Also:
- Companies that design tracheostomy tubes frequently have free educational materials.
- Families can purchase a tracheostomy tube guide, *Just Like You*; contact (260) 351-3555 for information.

Table 13-9 General Resources Related to Prematurity for Parents

Publications

Linden DW, Paroli ET, Doron MW: *Preemies: the essential guide for parents of premature babies.* New York, 2000, Pocket Books.

Madden SL: *The preemie parents' companion: the essential guide to caring for your premature baby in the hospital, at home and through the first years.* Boston, 2000, The Harvard Common Press.

Tracy AE, Maroney DI, Bernbaum JC, et al: *Your premature baby and child: helpful answers and advice for parents.* New York, 1999, Berkley Publishing Group.

Davis DL, Stein MT: *Parenting you premature baby and child: the emotional journey.* Golden, Colorado, 2004, Fulcrum Publishing.

Garcia-Prats JA, Hornfischer SS: *What to do when your baby is premature: A parent's handbook for coping with high-risk pregnancy and caring for the premature infant.* New York, 2000, Three Rivers Press.

Woodwell WA: *Coming to term: A father's story of birth, loss, and survival.* Jackson, Mississippi, 2001, University Press of Mississippi.

Products

Children's Medical Ventures, Inc.
www.childmed.com
275 Longwater Drive
Norwell, MA 02061
Phone: (888) 766-8443 (parents)
Phone: (800) 345-6443 (hospitals)
Develops and sells developmentally appropriate products for premature infants, healthy newborns, and older hospitalized infants. Offers appropriately sized items, safety equipment, positioning aids, car beds, specialty feeding supplies, and educational products and programs.

Organizations and Websites

The Alexis Foundation for Premature Infants and Children
P.O. Box 1126
Birmingham, MI 48012-1126
Phone: (248) 543-4169
www.pages.prodigy.net/thealexisfoundation /THEALEXIS1/html
Organization that provides advocacy and education. The mission is to support parents and professionals in providing the best possible care for premature infants and children. Offers a resource booklet free of charge.

American Association of Premature Infants (AAPI)
P.O. Box 46371
Cincinnati, OH 45246-0371
Phone: (513) 887-2888
www.aapi-online.org
Provides a search link to a comprehensive list of topics related to prematurity.

AAP Department of Community Pediatrics
www.aap.org/commpeds/
Offers extensive links for those in public health and clinical practice to assist in providing optimal care through community services, early detections screenings, training, and education.

Maternal and Child Health Bureau, Division of Services for Children with Special Health Needs
www.mchb.hrsa.gov/programs/default.htm
State resources on children with special healthcare needs.

Parents as Teachers
National Center
Public Information Specialist
2228 Ball Drive
St. Louis, MO 63146
Phone: (314) 432-4330
Toll free: (866) PAT-4YOU (728-4968)
Fax: (314) 432-8963
www.patnc.org
National model for local programs, providing parent education and family support from pregnancy to age 5 years. Trained and certified parent educators work through local programs and provide parenting support and information to families on their developing child through personal visits, parent group meetings, screenings, and resource networking.

www.preemie-l.org/
Registered nonprofit organization that provides support to families and caregivers of premature babies by providing a discussion forum; publishing online information and support resources for parents and professionals; encouraging developmentally supportive care; and listing the availability of outcome statistics and research. Provides a mentor program for parents and sponsor conferences. Provides numerous links to other useful websites. Available in Spanish.

Continued

Table 13-9 General Resources Related to Prematurity for Parents—cont'd

Excellent papers from conferences are available at this website and include the following:
- When life begins in the NICU: understanding the effects of prematurity on the child and family. Estes Park, Colorado, August 24–26 2001.
- Directions for the 21st century: bridging the gap between parents and professional. Chicago, Illinois, July 29–31, 1999.
- Empowering parents of premature babies: a conference for parents and professionals. Detroit, Michigan, July 25, 1998.

www.pediatrics.wisc.edu/patientcare/preemies/resources.html
Website of links to an extensive array of resources and support groups.

www.prematurity.org
Discussion board for preemie parents sharing ideas and support. Website offers links to publications, research, and advocacy for children with special needs or those born prematurely.

www.prematurity.org/preemie-child/index.html
Designed specifically for parents with children 4 years and older who were born prematurely. Addresses special needs that have medical, physical, and psychological impact.

www.emory.edu/PEDS/NEONATOLOGY/DCP/
Information on preemies and developmental issues provided by Emory University Pediatrics.

http://www.neonatology.org
Neonatology on the Internet.

www.mipediatra.com
Mi Pediatra: children's health information in Spanish.

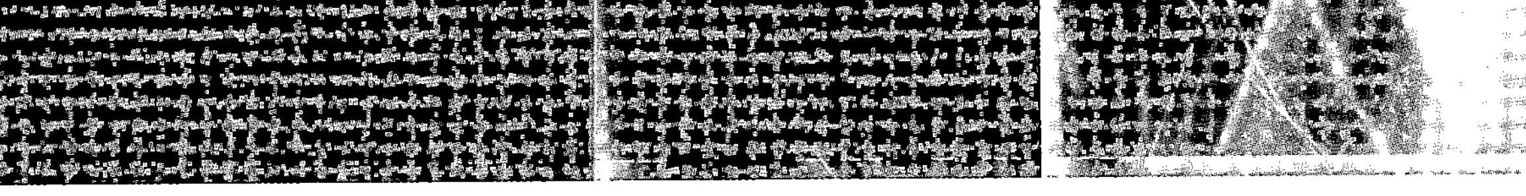

Index

Page numbers followed by f refer to figures; t refer to tables

D